TENTH EDITION

HURST'S
THE HEART.

MANUAL OF CARDIOLOGY

Editors

ROBERT A. O'ROURKE, M.D.

VALENTIN FUSTER, M.D., Ph.D.

R. WAYNE ALEXANDER, M.D., Ph.D.

ROBERT ROBERTS, M.D.

SPENCER B. KING III, M.D.

M.D.

McGraw-Hill
MEDICAL PUBLISHING DIVISION

New York   Chicago   San Francisco   Lisbon
London   Madrid   Mexico City   Milan   New Delhi
San Juan   Seoul   Singapore   Sydney   Toronto

McGraw-Hill

A Division of The McGraw·Hill Companies

HURST'S THE HEART, Tenth Edition
MANUAL OF CARDIOLOGY

1234567890 DOC/DOC 0987654321

ISBN 0-07-135415-8

The book was set in Times Roman by TechBooks.
The editors were Darlene Barela Cooke, Susan R. Noujaim, and
Lester A. Sheinis.
The production manager was Clara B. Stanley.
The production supervisor was Lisa Mendez.
The text designer was Marsha Cohen/Parallelogram Graphics.
The cover designer was Aimee Nordin.
The indexer was Alexandra Nickerson.
R. R. Donnelley & Sons Company was printer and binder.

This book is printed on acid-free paper.

**Library of Congress Cataloging-in-Publication Data are on file for this
title at the Library of Congress.**

INTERNATIONAL EDITION ISBN 0-07-112450-0
Copyright © 2001. Exclusive rights by The McGraw-Hill Companies, Inc.,
for manufacture and export. This book cannot be reexported from the country
to which it is consigned by McGraw-Hill. The International Edition is not
available in North America.

This manual of cardiology is dedicated to the numerous medical students, cardiology trainees, clinical faculty, and cardiovascular researchers who have made major contributions in improving the management of patients with cardiovascular disease and in defining the mechanism responsible for the pathophysiology of many cardiovascular disorders. Much of the information contained in this handbook has resulted from the transition of basic science research findings to the bedside diagnosis and treatment of patients with cardiac disease.

We also wish to acknowledge, as in the tenth edition of *Hurst's The Heart*, the members of our families and the staff of McGraw-Hill's Medical Publishing Division who supported our time and efforts in developing a manual of cardiology describing the improved diagnosis and treatment for cardiovascular disease.

NOTICE

CONTENTS

Contributors   xiii
Preface   xxv

1 THE HISTORY, PHYSICAL
EXAMINATION, AND CARDIAC
AUSCULTATION   1

Nilesh J. Goswami / Robert A. O'Rourke /
James A. Shaver / Mark E. Siverman

2 THE RESTING
ELECTROCARDIOGRAM   21

Agustin Castellanos / Alberto Interian, Jr. /
Robert J. Myerburg

3 CARDIOVASCULAR AGING IN
HEALTH AND THERAPEUTIC
CONSIDERATIONS WITH RESPECT
TO CARDIOVASCULAR DISEASES IN
OLDER PATIENTS   39

Steven P. Schulman

4 DIAGNOSIS AND MANAGEMENT
OF HEART FAILURE   49

Thierry H. LeJemtel / Edmund H. Sonnenblick /
William H. Frishman

5 ARRHYTHMIAS AND CONDUCTION
DISTURBANCES   61

Jeffrey D. Simmons / Simon Chakko /
Robert J. Myerburg

6 ANTIARRHYTHMIC DRUGS   93

Michael J. Kilborn / Raymond L. Woosley

7 THE IMPLANTABLE CARDIOVERTER
   DEFIBRILLATOR   113

Peter A. O'Callaghan / Jeremy N. Ruskin

8 CARDIAC PACEMAKERS   135

Raul D. Mitrani / Robert J. Myerburg /
Agustin Castellanos

9 DIAGNOSIS AND MANAGEMENT
   OF SYNCOPE   151

Harisios Boudoulas / Steven D. Nelson / Stephen
F. Schaal / Richard P. Lewis

10 SUDDEN CARDIAC DEATH   165

Duane S. Pinto / Mark E. Josephson

11 CARDIOPULMONARY
   RESUSCITATION AND THE
   SUBSEQUENT MANAGEMENT
   OF THE PATIENT   207

Nisha Chandra-Strobos / Myron L. Weisfeldt

12 DYSLIPIDEMIA AND RISK FACTORS
   IN THE PREVENTION OF CORONARY
   HEART DISEASE   221

Thomas A. Pearson / David J. Maron /
Paul M. Ridker / Scott M. Grundy

13 DIAGNOSIS AND MANAGEMENT OF
   PATIENTS WITH CHRONIC ISCHEMIC
   HEART DISEASE   237

Raja Naidu / Robert A. O'Rourke /
Robert C. Schlant / John S. Douglas, Jr.

14 DIAGNOSIS AND MANAGEMENT OF PATIENTS WITH UNSTABLE ANGINA 257

Jacob M. Mishell / David D. Waters

15 DIAGNOSIS AND MANAGEMENT OF PATIENTS WITH ACUTE MYOCARDIAL INFARCTION 277

R. Wayne Alexander / Craig M. Pratt / Thomas J. Ryan / Robert Roberts

16 PERCUTANEOUS CORONARY INTERVENTION 327

John S. Douglas, Jr. / Spencer B. King III

17 MECHANICAL INTERVENTIONS IN ACUTE MYOCARDIAL INFARCTION 339

William O'Neill / Bruce R. Brodie

18 HYPERTENSION: DIAGNOSIS, EVALUATION, AND TREATMENT 351

Henry R. Black / William J. Elliott / George L. Bakris

19 PULMONARY HYPERTENSION 373

Lewis J. Rubin

20 PULMONARY EMBOLISM 385

Victor F. Tapson

21 CHRONIC COR PULMONALE 403

John H. Newman / James E. Loyd

22 AORTIC VALVE DISEASE 413

Aly Rahimtoola / Shahbudin H. Rahimtoola

23 MITRAL VALVE DISEASE   431

Shahbudin H. Rahimtoola / Maurice Enriquez-Sarano /
Hartzell V. Schaff / Robert L. Frye

**24 MITRAL VALVE PROLAPSE
     SYNDROME**   451

Raja Naidu / Robert A. O'Rourke

**25 TRICUSPID VALVE AND PULMONIC
     VALVE DISEASE**   463

Nilesh J. Goswami / Robert A. O'Rourke

**26 CLINICAL PERFORMANCE OF
     PROSTHETIC HEART VALVES**   475

Gary L. Grunkemeier / Albert Starr / Shahbudin
H. Rahimtoola

**27 ANTITHROMBOTIC THERAPY FOR
     VALVULAR HEART DISEASE**   483

John H. McAnulty / Shahbudin H. Rahimtoola

**28 CARDIOVASCULAR DISEASES DUE
     TO GENETIC ABNORMALITIES**   493

Jeffrey A. Towbin / Robert Roberts

**29 CONGENITAL HEART DISEASE
     IN ADULTS**   515

Carole A. Warnes / Luc M. Beauchesne

30 DILATED CARDIOMYOPATHIES   527

Michael R. Bristow / Luisa Mestroni /
Teresa J. Bohlmeyer / Edward M. Gilbert

31 HYPERTROPHIC CARDIOMYOPATHY   541

Barry J. Maron

32   RESTRICTIVE, OBLITERATIVE, AND
INFILTRATIVE CARDIOMYOPATHIES   549

Joseph M. Restivo / Brian D. Hoit

33   INFLAMMATORY
CARDIOMYOPATHIES—ENDOCRINE
DISEASE AND ALCOHOL   559

Donna M. Mancini / Ainat Beniaminovitz

34   THE HEART AND NONCARDIAC
DRUGS, ELECTRICITY, POISONS,
AND RADIATION   575

Andrew L. Smith

35   DISEASES OF THE PERICARDIUM   583

Joseph M. Restivo / Brian D. Hoit

36   INFECTIVE ENDOCARDITIS   593

Raja Naidu / Robert A. O'Rourke

37   PERIOPERATIVE EVALUATION AND
MANAGEMENT OF PATIENTS WITH
KNOWN OR SUSPECTED
CARDIOVASCULAR DISEASE
WHO UNDERGO NONCARDIAC
SURGERY   617

Michael J. Lim / Kim A. Eagle

38   DIABETES AND CARDIOVASCULAR
DISEASE   627

Michael E. Farkouh / Elliot J. Rayfield /
Valentin Fuster

39   ADVERSE CARDIOVASCULAR
DRUG INTERACTIONS AND
COMPLICATIONS   647

Lionel H. Opie / William H. Frishman

40   HEART DISEASE AND PREGNANCY   667
      John H. McAnulty / James Metcalfe / Kent Ueland

41   WOMEN AND CORONARY ARTERY
      DISEASE   689
      Pamela Charney

42   DIAGNOSIS AND TREATMENT OF
      DISEASES OF THE AORTA   701
      Joseph Lindsay, Jr.

43   CEREBROVASCULAR DISEASE AND
      NEUROLOGIC MANIFESTATIONS
      OF HEART DISEASE   709
      Louis R. Caplan

44   DIAGNOSIS AND MANAGEMENT
      OF DISEASES OF THE PERIPHERAL
      ARTERIES AND VEINS   721
      Paul W. Wennberg / Thom W. Rooke

45   THE HEART AND OBESITY   733
      Paul Poirier / Robert H. Eckel

      INDEX   751

CONTRIBUTORS

R. WAYNE ALEXANDER, M.D.

R. Bruce Logue Professor and Chair, Department of Medicine, Emory University School of Medicine, Atlanta, Georgia
Chapter 15

GEORGE L. BAKRIS, M.D.

Professor of Preventive and Internal Medicine, Vice-Chairman, Department of Preventive Medicine; Director, Hypertension Clinical Research Center; Rush–Presbyterian–St. Luke's Medical Center, Chicago, Illinois
Chapter 18

LUC M. BEAUCHESNE, M.D.

Fellow, Division of Cardiovascular Diseases and Internal Medicine, Mayo Clinic, Rochester, Minnesota
Chapter 29

AINAT BENIAMINOVITZ, M.D.

Assistant Professor of Medicine; Attending Physician; Columbia Presbyteian Medical Center, New York, New York
Chapter 33

HENRY R. BLACK, M.D.

Charles J. and Margaret Roberts Professor, Associate Dean for Research, Rush Medical College; Chair, Department of Preventive Medicine, Rush–Presbyterian–St. Luke's Medical Center, Chicago, Illinois
Chapter 18

TERESA J. BOHLMEYER, M.D.

Assistant Professor of Medicine, University of Colorado Health Sciences Center, Division of Cardiology, University of Colorado Health Sciences Center, Denver, Colorado
Chapter 30

WENDY M. BOOK, M.D.

Assistant Professor, Division of Cardiology, Emory University School of Medicine, Atlanta, Georgia
Chapter 34

HARISIOS BOUDOULAS, M.D., Ph.D.

Professor of Medicine and Pharmacy, Division of Cardiology, Ohio State University Medical Center, Columbus, Ohio
Chapter 9

MICHAEL R. BRISTOW, M.D., Ph.D.

Professor of Medicine; Head, Division of Cardiology; Director, Temple Hoyne Buell Laboratories; Director, Heart Failure Program; Associate Director, Heart Transplant Program, University of Colorado Health Sciences Center, Denver, Colorado
Chapter 30

BRUCE R. BRODIE, M.D.

Clinical Professor of Medicine; Director, LeBauer, Cardiovascular Research Foundation, University of North Carolina Teaching Service, The Moses H. Cone Memorial Hospital, Greensboro, North Carolina
Chapter 17

LOUIS R. CAPLAN, M.D.

Professor of Neurology, Harvard Medical School, Chief, Cerebrovascular Disease; Director, Stroke Services, Beth Israel Deaconess Medical Center, Boston, Massachusetts
Chapter 43

AGUSTIN CASTELLANOS, M.D.

Director, Clinical Electrophysiology, Professor of Medicine, University of Miami, School of Medicine, Jackson Memorial Hospital, Miami, Florida
Chapters 2, 8

SIMON CHAKKO, M.D.

Professor of Medicine, University of Miami School of Medicine, Chief, Cardiology Section, VA Medical Center, Miami, Florida
Chapter 5

NISHA CHANDRA-STROBOS, M.D.

Professor of Cardiovascular Medicine, Director of Coronary Intensive Care Unit, Division of Cardiology, Johns Hopkins Bayview Medical Center, Baltimore, Maryland
Chapter 11

PAMELA CHARNEY, M.D.

Clinical Professor of Medicine; Clinical Associate Professor of Obstetrics and Gynecology and Women's Health, Albert Einstein College of Medicine, Bronx, New York; Program Director, Internal Medicine Residency, Norwalk Hospital, Norwalk, Connecticut
Chapter 41

JOHN S. DOUGLAS, Jr., M.D.

Professor of Medicine (Cardiology), Emory University School of Medicine, Director, Interventional Cardiology and Cardiac Catheterization Laboratories, Emory University Hospital, Atlanta, Georgia
Chapters 13, 16

KIM A. EAGLE, M.D.

Albion Walter Henleh Professor of Internal Medicine; Chief, Division of Cardiology and Clinical Cardiology, University of Michigan Medical Center, Ann Arbor, Michigan
Chapter 37

ROBERT H. ECKEL, M.D.

Professor of Medicine, Physiology, and Biophysics, Department of Medicine, University of Colorado Health Sciences Center, Denver, Colorado
Chapter 45

WILLIAM J. ELLIOTT, M.D., Ph.D.

Professor of Preventive Medicine, Internal Medicine, and Pharmacology; Attending Physician, Rush University School of Medicine, Rush–Presbyterian–St. Luke's Medical Center, Chicago, Illinois
Chapter 18

MAURICE ENRIQUEZ-SARANO, M.D., F.A.C.C.

Associate Professor of Medicine; Consultant, Cardiovascular Diseases and Internal Medicine, Division of Cardiology, Mayo Clinic, Rochester, Minnesota
Chapter 23

MICHAEL E. FARKOUH, M.D., F.R.C.P., M.Sc.

Assistant Professor of Medicine, Mount Sinai School of Medicine; Director, Telemetry Unit; Consultant, Mount Sinai Diabetes, Mount Sinai Medical Center, New York, New York
Chapter 38

WILLIAM H. FRISHMAN, M.D.

Professor of Medicine and Pharmacology; Director of Medicine, Westchester Medical Center, New York Medical College, Valhalla, New York; Chairman, Department of Medicine, New York Medical College, Valhalla, New York
Chapters 4, 39

ROBERT L. FRYE, M.D.

Rose M. and Morris Eisenberg Professor of Medicine, Mayo Clinic, Rochester, Minnesota
Chapter 23

VALENTIN FUSTER, M.D., Ph.D.

Director, The Zena and Michael A. Wiener Cardiovascular Institute; Richard Gorlin, M.D./Heart Research Foundation; Professor of Cardiology, Vice Chairman, Department of Medicine, The Mount Sinai School of Medicine, New York, New York
Chapter 38

EDWARD M. GILBERT, M.D.

Associate Professor of Medicine, Director, Heart Failure Treatment Program, Division of Cardiology, University of Utah Health Sciences Center, Salt Lake City, Utah
Chapter 30

NILESH J. GOSWAMI, M.D.

Department of Cardiology, University of Texas Health Science Center, San Antonio, Texas
Chapters 1, 25

SCOTT M. GRUNDY, M.D.

Professor, Department of Internal Medicine; Director, Center for Human Nutrition, University of Texas, Southwestern Medical Center, Dallas, Texas
Chapter 12

GARY L. GRUNKENMEIER, M.D.

Director, Medical Data Research Center, Providence Health System, Portland, Oregon
Chapter 26

BRIAN D. HOIT, M.D.

Professor of Medicine, Case Western Reserve University; Co-Director of Echocardiography, Attending Physician, Department of Cardiology, University Hospitals of Cleveland, Cleveland, Ohio
Chapters 32, 35

ALBERTO INTERIAN, Jr., M.D.

Professor of Medicine, Director, Electropathophysiology Laboratory, University of Miami School of Medicine, Division of Cardiology, Miami, Florida
Chapter 2

MARK E. JOSEPHSON, M.D.

Professor of Medicine, Harvard Medical School; Director, Harvard-Thorndike Electrophy, Beth Israel Deaconess Medical Center, Boston, Massachusetts
Chapter 10

MICHAEL J. KILBORN, B.M.B.Ch., D.Phil., F.R.A.C.P.

Assistant Professor of Medicine, Georgetown University School of Medicine, Washington, DC
Chapter 6

SPENCER B. KING III, M.D.

Fuqua Chair of Interventional Cardiology, The Fuqua Heart Center at Piedmont Hospital; Co-Director, Atlanta Cardiovascular Research Institute; Clinical Professor of Medicine, Emory University School of Medicine, Atlanta, Georgia
Chapter 16

THIERRY H. LeJEMTEL, M.D.

Division of Cardiology, Albert Einstein College of Medicine, Bronx, New York
Chapter 4

RICHARD P. LEWIS, M.D.

Professor of Internal Medicine, Ohio State University, Columbus, Ohio
Chapter 9

MICHAEL J. LIM, M.D.

Fellow, Division of Cardiology, University of Michigan Health System, Ann Arbor, Michigan
Chapter 37

JOSEPH LINDSAY, Jr., M.D.

Director, Section of Cardiology, Washington Hospital Center, Professor of Medicine, The George Washington University School of Health Care Sciences, Washington Hospital Center, Washington, DC
Chapter 42

JAMES E. LOYD, M.D.

Professor of Medicine, Division of Allergy, Pulmonary, and Critical Care Medicine, Vanderbilt University School of Medicine, Nashville, Tennessee
Chapter 21

DONNA M. MANCINI, M.D.

Associate Professor of Medicine, Columbia University College of Physicians and Surgeons; Medical Director, Cardiac Transplant, New York Presbyterian Hospital, New York, New York
Chapter 33

BARRY J. MARON, M.D.

Director, Cardiovascular Research Division, Minneapolis Heart Institute Foundation, Minneapolis, Minnesota
Chapter 31

DAVID J. MARON, M.D.

Assistant Professor of Medicine, Director, Preventive Cardiology, Vanderbilt University Medical Center, Division of Cardiovascular Medicine, Nashville, Tennessee
Chapter 12

JOHN H. McANULTY, M.D.

Professor and Head of Cardiology, Oregon Health Sciences University, Portland, Oregon
Chapters 27, 40

LUISA MESTRONI, M.D.

Associate Professor of Medicine, Director, Molecular Genetics, University of Colorado Cardiovascular Institute, Fitzsimons Hospital, Aurora, Colorado
Chapter 30

JAMES METCALFE, M.D.

Professor of Medicine (Emeritus), Oregon Health Sciences University, School of Medicine, Portland, Oregon
Chapter 40

JACOB M. MISHELL, M.D.

Cardiology Fellow, University of California, San Francisco, California
Chapter 14

RAUL D. MITRANI, M.D.

Division of Cardiology, University of Miami Medical Center—Jackson Memorial Hospital, Miami, Florida
Chapter 8

ROBERT J. MYERBURG, M.D.

Director, Division of Cardiology; Professor of Medicine and Physiology, University of Miami School of Medicine, Division of Cardiology, Miami, Florida
Chapters 2, 5, 8

RAJA NAIDU, M.D.

Department of Cardiology, University of Texas Health Science Center, San Antonio, Texas
Chapters 13, 24, 36

STEVEN D. NELSON, M.D.

Associate Professor of Medicine, Director, Cardiac Electrophysiology, Ohio State University Hospitals, Columbus, Ohio
Chapter 9

JOHN H. NEWMAN, M.D.

Chief of Medical Services; Elsa S. Hanigan Professor of Pulmonary Medicine, Vanderbilt University School of Medicine, VAMC Nashville, Nashville, Tennessee
Chapter 21

PETER A. O'CALLAGHAN, M.D.

Research Fellow and Honorary Clinical Registrar, Department of Cardiological Science, St. George's Hospital Medical School, London, England
Chapter 7

WILLIAM O'NEILL, M.D.

Director, Division of Cardiology, William Beaumont Hospital, Royal Oak, Michigan
Chapter 17

LIONEL H. OPIE, M.D., F.R.C.P., D.Phil.

Professor of Medicine; Co-Director, Cape Heart Center, University of Cape Town Medical School, Cape Town, South Africa
Chapter 39

ROBERT A. O'ROURKE, M.D.

Charles Conrad Brown Distinguished Professor in Cardiovascular Disease, University of Texas Health Science Center, San Antonio, Texas
Chapters 1, 13, 24, 25, 36

THOMAS A. PEARSON, M.D., M.P.H., Ph.D.

Albert D. Kaser Professor and Chair, Community and Preventive Medicine, Professor of Medicine, Attending Physician, Department of Medicine; Director, Preventive Cardiology Clinic; Co-Director, Stony Heart Program, University of Rochester Medical Center, Rochester, Minnesota
Chapter 12

DUANE S. PINTO, M.D.

Cardiology Fellow, Clinical Instructor in Medicine, Beth Israel Deaconess Medical Center, Division of Cardiology, Boston, Massachusetts
Chapter 10

PAUL POIRIER, M.D.

Associate Professor of Medicine, Laval University School of Medicine, Quebec Heart Institute, Laval Hospital, Sainte-Foy, Quebec, Canada
Chapter 45

CRAIG M. PRATT, M.D.

Director, Coronary Care Unit, Professor of Medicine, Baylor College of Medicine, The Methodist Hospital, Houston, Texas
Chapter 15

ALY RAHIMTOOLA, M.D.

Fellow in Cardiology, University of Virginia Health Sciences Center, Charlottesville, Virginia
Chapter 22

SHAHBUDIN H. RAHIMTOOLA, M.D., F.R.C.P., M.A.C.P., F.A.C.C.

George C. Griffith Professor of Cardiology, Division of Cardiology, LAC + USC Medical Center, Los Angeles, California
Chapters 22, 23, 26, 27

ELLIOT J. RAYFIELD, M.D.

Clinical Professor of Medicine, Mount Sinai School of Medicine, Attending Physician, Mount Sinai Hospital, New York, New York
Chapter 38

JOSEPH M. RESTIVO, M.D.

Division of Cardiology, University Hospitals of Cleveland and Case Western Reserve University, Cleveland, Ohio
Chapters 32, 35

PAUL M. RIDKER, M.D.

Associate Professor of Medicine, Divisions of Cardiovascular Disease and Preventive Medicine, Harvard Medical School, Brigham and Women's Hospital, Boston, Massachusetts
Chapter 12

ROBERT ROBERTS, M.D.

Don W. Chapman Professor of Medicine and Chief of Cardiology; Professor of Cell Biology, Molecular Physiology and Biophysics; Director, Bugher Foundation Center for Molecular Biology in the Cardiovascular System; Baylor College of Medicine, Director, Specialized Center for Research in Heart Failure, Houston, Texas
Chapters 15, 28

THOM W. ROOKE, M.D.

Professor of Medicine, Gonda Vascular Center, Mayo Clinic, Rochester, Minnesota
Chapter 44

LEWIS J. RUBIN, M.D.

Professor of Medicine, Director, Division of Pulmonary/Critical Care Medicine, University of California, San Diego, California
Chapter 19

JEREMY N. RUSKIN, M.D.

Director, Cardiac Arrhythmia Service, Cardiac Unit, Massachusetts General Hospital, Boston, Massachusetts
Chapter 7

THOMAS J. RYAN, M.D.

Professor of Medicine, Chief of Cardiology, Emeritus Senior Consultant in Cardiology, Boston University School of Medicine, Boston, Massachusetts
Chapter 15

STEPHEN F. SCHAAL, M.D.

Professor of Medicine, The Ohio State University Heart and Lung Research Institute, Ohio State University Hospitals, Columbus, Ohio
Chapter 9

HARTZELL V. SCHAFF, M.D.

Stuart W. Harrington, Professor of Surgery, Division of Cardiology, Mayo Clinic, Rochester, Minnesota
Chapter 23

ROBERT C. SCHLANT, M.D.

Professor of Medicine (Cardiology), Emory University School of Medicine, Atlanta, Georgia
Chapter 13

STEVEN P. SCHULMAN, M.D.

Associate Professor of Medicine, Director of CCU, The Johns Hopkins University School of Medicine, Baltimore, Maryland
Chapter 3

JAMES A. SHAVER, M.D.

University of Pittsburgh Physicians, Cardiovascular Institute, University of Pittsburgh Medical Center Presbyterian, Pittsburgh, Pennsylvania
Chapter 1

MARK E. SILVERMAN, M.D., M.A.C.P., F.A.C.C.

Professor of Medicine (Cardiology), Emory University School of Medicine, Chief of Cardiology, Fuqua Heart Center of Atlanta, Piedmont Hospital, Atlanta, Georgia
Chapter 1

JEFFREY D. SIMMONS, M.D.

Assistant Professor of Medicine, University of Miami School of Medicine, Chief, Electrophysiology Laboratory, VA Medical Center, Miami, Florida
Chapter 5

ANDREW L. SMITH, M.D.

Center for Heart Failure Therapy, Emory University Hospital, Atlanta, Georgia
Chapter 34

EDMUND H. SONNENBLICK, M.D.

Professor of Medicine, Albert Einstein College of Medicine, Department of Medicine, Bronx, New York
Chapter 4

ALBERT STARR, M.D.

Professor of Surgery, Oregon Health Sciences University; Director, Heart Institute, Providence St. Vincent Medical Center, Starr Wood Cardiac Group, Medical Data Research Center, Portland, Oregon
Chapter 26

VICTOR F. TAPSON, M.D.

Associate Professor, Division of Pulmonary and Critical Care; Director, Lung Transplant Program, Duke University Medical Center, Durham, North Carolina
Chapter 20

JEFFREY A. TOWBIN, M.D.

Professor of Pediatrics (Cardiology) and Molecular and Human Genetics; Associate Chief, Pediatrics Director, Heart Failure and Transplant Program, Texas Children's Hospital Foundation; Chair, Pediatric Molecular Cardiac Research, Molecular and Human Genetics, Baylor College of Medicine, Houston, Texas
Chapter 28

KENT UELAND, M.D.

Professor Emeritus, Department of OB/GYN, Stanford University School of Medicine, Stanford, California
Chapter 40

CAROLE A. WARNES, M.D., M.R.C.P., F.A.C.C.

Professor of Medicine, Mayo Medical School; Consultant, Division of Cardiovascular Diseases, Internal Medicine, Pediatric Cardiology, and Adult Congenital Heart Disease Clinic, Cardiovascular Diseases and Internal Medicine, Mayo Clinic, Rochester, Minnesota
Chapter 29

DAVID D. WATERS, M.D.

Division of Cardiology, San Francisco General Hospital, San Francisco, California
Chapter 14

MYRON L. WEISFELDT, M.D.

Chair, Department of Medicine, Samuel Bard Professor of Medicine, Columbia Presbyterian Medical Center, College of Physicians and Surgeons, New York, New York
Chapter 11

PAUL WENNBERG, M.D.

Instructor of Medicine, Senior Associate Consultant, Cardiovascular Division, Mayo Clinic, Rochester, Minnesota
Chapter 44

RAYMOND L. WOOSLEY, M.D., Ph.D.

Professor and Chairman, Department of Pharmacology, Georgetown University Medical Center, Washington, DC
Chapter 6

PREFACE

This manual of cardiology, like its predecessors, was prepared to meet the needs of physicians and students for a concise, portable handbook that they could carry with them and use in the middle of the night or in circumstances when they did not have access to a larger reference textbook of cardiology such as the tenth edition of *Hurst's The Heart*. While it is written by many of the same authors who contributed to the larger textbook, it can be used as a stand-alone source for quick information concerning the presentation, natural history, and treatment of various cardiovascular disorders. It actually contains some tables and algorithms not present in the larger text in order to provide the reader with appropriate, easily accessible indications for specific therapy. Useful information from the ACC/AHA Clinical Guidelines are included in many chapters of this pocket manual.

We express our gratitude to the authors of the individual chapters of this succinct but accurate handbook, many of whom are the authors of corresponding chapters in the tenth edition of *Hurst's The Heart*.

HURST'S
THE HEART
MANUAL OF CARDIOLOGY

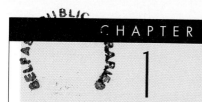

CHAPTER 1

THE HISTORY, PHYSICAL EXAMINATION, AND CARDIAC AUSCULTATION

Nilesh J. Goswami
Robert A. O'Rourke
James A. Shaver
Mark E. Siverman

In the assessment of patients with definite or suspected heart disease, the history and physical examination, along with various noninvasive studies, can provide relevant information. Integration of these data can provide accurate diagnoses and guidance in making appropriate decisions regarding further diagnostic studies and/or therapeutic options. The history and physical examination should be the cornerstone in the evaluation of any patient with known or suspected heart disease.

This chapter is composed of three sections, including salient features of the history, physical examination, and cardiac auscultation.

HISTORY

As in any medical evaluation, the history is the initial step in the assessment of the patient. The most common complaint among patients with heart disease is chest pain; however, particular attention should be paid to the chief complaint with clarification of all relevant symptoms. These may include exercise tolerance, shortness of breath (especially with exertion), orthopnea, and paroxysmal nocturnal dyspnea. Symptoms of edema, ascites, cough, hemoptysis, palpitation, fatigue, and peripheral embolization can be consistent with heart disease. Chest pain is the foremost manifestation of myocardial ischemia and the most commonly encountered symptom. The differential diagnosis of chest pain is extensive and listed in Table 1-1. Extensive effort should be made to evaluate and determine the origin of any chest pains.

1

TABLE 1-1

DIFFERENTIAL DIAGNOSIS OF CHEST PAIN

1. Angina pectoris/myocardial infarction
2. Other cardiovascular causes
   a. Likely ischemic in origin
      (1) Aortic stenosis
      (2) Hypertrophic cardiomyopathy
      (3) Severe systemic hypertension
      (4) Severe right ventricular hypertension
      (5) Aortic regurgitation
      (6) Severe anemia/hypoxia
   b. Nonischemic in origin
      (1) Aortic dissection
      (2) Pericarditis
      (3) Mitral valve prolapse
3. Gastrointestinal
   a. Esophageal spasm
   b. Esophageal reflux
   c. Esophageal rupture
   d. Peptic ulcer disease
4. Psychogenic
   a. Anxiety
   b. Depression
   c. Cardiac psychosis
   d. Self-gain
5. Neuromusculoskeletal
   a. Thoracic outlet syndrome
   b. Degenerative joint disease of cervical/thoracic spine
   c. Costochondritis (Tietze's syndrome)
   d. Herpes zoster
   e. Chest wall pain and tenderness
6. Pulmonary
   a. Pulmonary embolus with or without pulmonary infarction
   b. Pneumothorax
   c. Pneumonia with pleural involvement
7. Pleurisy

Angina pectoris is defined as chest pain or discomfort of cardiac origin that usually results from a temporary imbalance between myocardial oxygen supply and demand. The important characteristics of angina include the quality of the pain, precipitating factors, mode of onset, duration, location, and pattern of disappearance.

The quality of the pain is typically described as "tightness," "pressure," "burning," "heaviness," "aching," "strangling," or "compression." The description of the quality may be influenced by the patient's intelligence, social background, and education; thus other descriptors may also be used, depending upon the patient.

The most common precipitating factor is physical exertion. Angina can be provoked by emotional distress, cold weather, or eating. Angina typically has a crescendo pattern but can occur acutely, as with the acute coronary syndromes. An episode may last up to 20 min. Most patients have relief of symptoms within 5 min after cessation of physical activity or by nitroglycerin lingual spray or sublingual tablets. Failure of rest or nitroglycerin to relieve symptoms suggests another cause of the pain or impending myocardial infarction. Localizing the site of chest discomfort is also helpful in determining the cause. Angina pectoris is usually retrosternal or slightly to the left of midline. Pain tends to radiate into the arms, neck, and jaw. In the arms, the pain radiates down the ulnar aspect and the volar surface to the wrist and the ulnar fingers. Patients with angina pectoris are classified functionally from classes I to IV (Table 1-2).

Other cardiovascular diseases can also precipitate chest pain in the absence of coronary atherosclerosis. Increased oxygen demand resulting in chest pain can be seen with aortic stenosis, hypertrophic cardiomyopathy, and systemic arterial hypertension. In addition, chest discomfort as a result of myocardial ischemia can result from aortic valve regurgitation. Chest pain not related to myocardial ischemia can be caused by pericarditis, aortic dissection, and mitral valve prolapse.

A separate New York Heart Association Functional Classification exists for assessing cardiac disability for patients with heart failure (Table 1-3). Patients should be asked sufficient questions to allow proper assessment in this classification. The classification according to symptoms is used frequently in medical literature multicenter research trials and clinical practice.

PHYSICAL EXAMINATION

Important information concerning the patient with definite or suspected heart disease is often obtained by a careful and deliberate physical examination, which includes a general inspection of the

TABLE 1-2

CANADIAN CARDIOVASCULAR SOCIETY FUNCTIONAL CLASSIFICATION OF ANGINA PECTORIS

I. Ordinary physical activity, such as walking and climbing stairs, does not cause angina. Angina results from strenuous or rapid or prolonged exertion at work or recreation.

II. Slight limitation of ordinary activity. Walking or climbing stairs rapidly, walking uphill, walking or stair climbing after meals, in cold, in wind, or when under emotional stress, or only during the few hours after awakening. Walking more than two blocks on the level and climbing more than one flight or ordinary stairs at a normal pace and under normal conditions.

III. Marked limitations of ordinary physical activity. Walking one to two blocks on the level and climbing more than one flight under normal conditions.

IV. Inability to carry on any physical activity without discomfort—anginal syndrome may be present at rest.

SOURCE: Modified from Campeau L. Letter to the editor. *Circulation* 19, 54:522. Reproduced with permission from the American Heart Association, Inc., and the author.

TABLE 1-3

THE OLD NEW YORK HEART ASSOCIATION FUNCTIONAL CLASSIFICATION

Class 1	No symptoms with ordinary physical activity.
Class 2	Symptoms with ordinary activity. Slight limitation of activity.
Class 3	Symptoms with less than ordinary activity. Marked limitation of activity.
Class 4	Symptoms with any physical activity or even at rest.

SOURCE: The Criteria Committee of the New York Heart Association: *Diseases of the Heart and Blood Vessels: Nomenclature and Criteria for Diagnosis of the Heart and Great Vessels.* 6th ed. New York: New York Heart Association/Little Brown; 1964. Reproduced with permission from the New York Heart Association, Inc., and the publisher.

patient, an indirect measurement of the arterial blood pressure in both arms and one or both lower extremities, an examination of central and peripheral arterial pulses, an evaluation of the jugular venous pressure and pulsations, palpation of the precordium, and cardiac auscultation. Based on this rather inexpensive evaluation, a definite diagnosis is often made and noninvasive and invasive testing is unnecessary.

ARTERIAL PRESSURE PULSE

The arterial pulse wave begins with aortic valve opening and the onset of left ventricular ejection (Fig. 1-1). The rapid-rising portion of the arterial pressure curve is often termed the *anacrotic limb* (from the Greek, meaning "upbeat"). During isovolumic relaxation, a transient reversal of flow from the central arteries toward the ventricle just prior to aortic valve closure is associated with an incisura on the descending limb of the aortic pressure pulse.

A small weak pulse, *pulsus parvus*, is common in conditions with a diminished left ventricular stroke volume, a narrow pulse pressure, and increased peripheral vascular resistance. A hypokinetic pulse may be due to hypovolemia, left ventricular failure, restrictive pericardial disease, or mitral stenosis. In aortic valve stenosis, the delayed systolic peak, *pulsus tardus*, results from obstruction to left ventricular ejection. In contrast, a large, bounding (hyperkinetic) pulse is usually associated with an increased left ventricular stroke

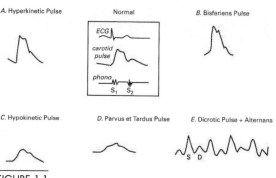

FIGURE 1-1

Schematic representation of the normal carotid arterial pulse, five types of abnormal pulses, and pulsus alternans. ECG, electrocardiogram; phono, phonocardiogram; S_1, S_2, first and second heart sounds; S, systole; D, diastole.

volume, a wide pulse pressure, and a decrease in peripheral vascular resistance. This pattern occurs characteristically in patients with an elevated stroke volume, with hyperkinetic circulation, or with a rapid runoff of blood from the arterial system—i.e., such as with an atrioventricular (AV) fistula. Patients with mitral regurgitation or a ventricular septal defect also may have a bounding pulse. In aortic regurgitation, the rapidly rising, bounding arterial pulse results from an increased left ventricular volume and an increased rate of ventricular ejection. The *bisferiens* pulse, which has two systolic peaks, is characteristic of aortic regurgitation (with or without accompanying stenosis) and of hypertrophic cardiomyopathy. The *dicrotic* pulse has two palpable waves, the second in diastolic, and occurs most frequently in patients with a very low stroke volume, including in those with dilated cardiomyopathy.

Pulsus alternans is a pattern in which there is regular alteration of the pressure pulse amplitude, despite a regular rhythm. It denotes severe impairment of left ventricular function and commonly occurs in patients who also have a loud third heart sound. In *pulsus paradoxus*, the decrease in systolic arterial pressure that normally accompanies the reduction in arterial pulse amplitude during inspiration is accentuated. In patients with pericardial tamponade, airway obstruction (asthma), or superior vena cava obstruction, the decrease in systolic arterial pressure frequently exceeds the normal decrease of 10 mmHg, and the peripheral pulse may disappear completely during inspiration.

JUGULAR VENOUS PULSE

The two main objectives of the examination of the neck veins are inspection of their waveforms and estimation of the central venous pressure (CVP). In most patients, the right internal jugular vein is best for both purposes. Usually, the pulsation of the internal jugular vien is optimal when the trunk is inclined less than 30 degrees. In patients with elevated venous pressure, it may be necessary to elevate the trunk further, sometimes to as much as 90 degrees. Simultaneous palpation of the left carotid artery aids the examiner in determining which pulsations are venous and in relating the venous pulsations to their timing in the cardiac cycle.

The normal jugular venous pulse (JVP) consists of two to three positive waves and two negative troughs (Fig. 1-2). The positive, presystolic *a wave* is produced by venous distention due to right atrial contraction and is the dominant wave in the JVP. Large *a waves* indicate that the right atrium is contracting against increased resistance, as occurs with tricuspid stenosis or more commonly with

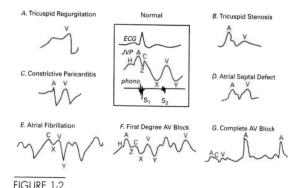

FIGURE 1-2

Schematic representation of the normal JVP, four types of abnormal JVPs, and the JVPs in three arrhythmias. See text under "Jugular Venous Pulse" for definition of H, A, Z, C, X, V, and Y.

increased resistance to right ventricular filling. Large *a waves* ("cannon" *a waves*) also occur during arrhythmias whenever the right atrium contracts while the tricuspid valve is still closed. The *a wave* is absent in patients with atrial fibrillation and there is an increased delay between the *a wave* and the carotid arterial pulse in patients with first-degree atrioventricular block.

The *c wave* is a positive wave produced by the bulging of the tricuspid valve into the right atrium during right ventricular isovolumetric systole and by the distention of the carotid artery located adjacent to the jugular vein. The *x descent* is due both to atrial relaxation and to the downward displacement of the tricuspid valve during ventricular systole. The *x descent* is reversed in tricuspid reguitation. The positive late systolic *v wave* results from right atrial filling during ventricular systole, when the tricuspid valve is closed. Tricuspid regurgitation causes the *v wave* to become more prominent; when tricuspid regurgitation becomes severe, the combination of a prominent *v wave* and obliteration of the *x descent* results in a single large, positive systolic wave (i.e., "ventricularization"—a pattern similar to the right ventricular pressure tracing). The negative descending limb, the *y descent* of the JVP, is produced by the opening of the tricuspid valve and the rapid inflow of blood into the right ventricle. A venous pulse characterized by a sharp *y descent*, a deep *y* trough, and a rapid ascent to the baseline is seen in patients with constrictive pericarditis or with severe right-sided heart failure and a high venous pressure.

The right internal jugular vein is the best vein to use for accurate estimation of the CVP. The sternal angle is used as the reference point, because the center of the right atrium lies approximately 5 cm below the sternal angle. The patient is best examined at the optimal degree of trunk elevation for visualization of the jugular venous pulsations. The vertical distance between the top of the oscillating venous column and the level of the sternal angle is determined; generally, it is less than 3 cm (3 cm + 5 cm = 8 cm blood or water; multiply by 0.8 to convert to millimeters of mercury). In patients suspected of having right ventricular failure who have a normal CVP at rest, the abdominojugular reflux test may be helpful. The palm of the examiner's hand is placed over the abdomen and firm pressure is applied for 10 s or more. When right heart function is impaired, the upper level of venous pulsations usually increases. A positive abdominojugular reflux test is best defined as an increase in the JVP during 10 s of firm midabdominal compression followed by a rapid drop in pressure by 4 cm blood on release of the compression. *Kussmaul's sign*—an increase rather than the normal decrease in the CVP during inspiration—is most often caused by severe right-sided heart failure; it is a frequent finding in patients with constrictive pericarditis or right ventricular infarction.

PRECORDIAL PALPATION

The location, amplitude, duration, and direction of the cardiac impulse usually can be best appreciated with the fingertips. Left ventricular hypertrophy results in exaggeration of the amplitude, duration, and often size (normal is <3 cm) of the normal left ventricular thrust. The impulse may be displaced laterally and downward into the sixth or seventh interspace, particularly in patients with a left ventricular volume load, as in the case of aortic regurgitation or dilated cardiomyopathy (Fig. 1-3).

Additional abnormal features detectable at the left ventricular apex include marked presystolic distention of the left ventricle, which is often accompanied by a fourth heart sound (S_4) in patients with an

$\longrightarrow$

FIGURE 1-3

Graphic representation of apical movements in health and disease. Heavy line indicates palpable features. P_2, pulmonary component of second heart sound; A, atrial wave, corresponding to a fourth heart sound (S_4) or atrial gallop; F, filling wave, corresponding to third heart sound (S_3) or ventricular gallop. (From Willis P IV: Inspection and palpation of the precordium. In: Hurst JW, ed: *The Heart*, 7th ed. New York: McGraw-Hill; 1990:164. Reproduced with permission from the publisher and author.)

Graphic Representation
(palpable features in heavy line)

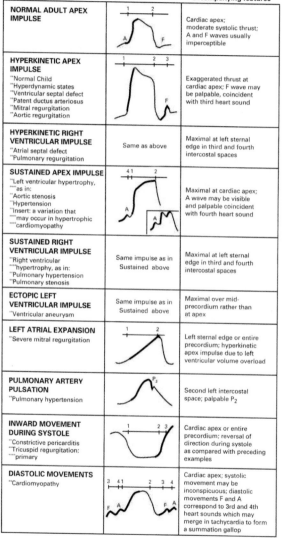

Type of movement and associated clinical condition	Location and accompanying features
NORMAL ADULT APEX IMPULSE	Cardiac apex; moderate systolic thrust; A and F waves usually imperceptible
HYPERKINETIC APEX IMPULSE *Normal Child *Hyperdynamic states *Ventricular septal defect *Patent ductus arteriosus *Mitral regurgitation *Aortic regurgitation	Exaggerated thrust at cardiac apex; F wave may be palpable, coincident with third heart sound
HYPERKINETIC RIGHT VENTRICULAR IMPULSE *Atrial septal defect *Pulmonary regurgitation	Same as above	Maximal at left sternal edge in third and fourth intercostal spaces
SUSTAINED APEX IMPULSE *Left ventricular hypertrophy, as in: *Aortic stenosis *Hypertension *Insert: a variation that *may occur in hypertrophic *cardiomyopathy	Maximal at cardiac apex; A wave may be visible and palpable coincident with fourth heart sound
SUSTAINED RIGHT VENTRICULAR IMPULSE *Right ventricular *hypertrophy, as in: *Pulmonary hypertension: *Pulmonary stenosis	Same impulse as in Sustained above	Maximal at left sternal edge in third and fourth intercostal spaces
ECTOPIC LEFT VENTRICULAR IMPULSE *Ventricular aneurysm	Same impulse as in Sustained above	Maximal over mid-precordium rather than at apex
LEFT ATRIAL EXPANSION *Severe mitral regurgitation	Left sternal edge or entire precordium; hyperkinetic apex impulse due to left ventricular volume overload
PULMONARY ARTERY PULSATION *Pulmonary hypertension	Second left intercostal space; palpable P_2
INWARD MOVEMENT DURING SYSTOLE *Constrictive pericarditis *Tricuspid regurgitation: *primary	Cardiac apex or entire precordium: reversal of direction during systole as compared with preceding examples
DIASTOLIC MOVEMENTS *Cardiomyopathy	Cardiac apex; systolic movement may be inconspicuous; diastolic movements F and A correspond to 3rd and 4th heart sounds which may merge in tachycardia to form a summation gallop

excessive left ventricular pressure load or myocardial ischemia/infarction, and a prominent early diastolic rapid-filling wave, which is often accompanied by a third heart sound (S_3) in patients with left ventricular failure or mitral valve regurgitation.

Right ventricular hypertrophy often results in a sustained systolic lift at the lower left parasternal area, which starts in early systole and is synchronous with the left ventricular apical impulse.

A left parasternal lift is present frequently in patients with severe mitral regurgitation. This pulsation occurs distinctly later than the left ventricular apical impulse, is synchronous with the *v wave* in the left atrial pressure curve, and is due to anterior displacement of the right ventricle by an enlarged, expanding left atrium. Pulmonary artery pulsation is often visible and palpable in the second left intercostal space. While it may be normal in children or thin young adults, in others, this pulsation usually denotes pulmonary hypertension, increased pulmonary blood flow, or poststenotic pulmonary artery dilation.

CARDIAC AUSCULTATION

To obtain the most information from cardiac auscultation, the observer should keep several principles in mind: (1) Auscultation should be performed in a quiet room. (2) Attention must be focused on the phase of the cardiac cycle during which the auscultory event is expected to occur. (3) The timing of a heart sound or murmur can be determined accurately from its relation to other observable events in the cardiac cycle. (4) It is often necessary to observe alterations in its timing or intensity during various physiologic and/or pharmacologic interventions.

HEART SOUNDS

The intensity of the first heart sound (S_1) is influenced by (1) the position of the mitral valve leaflets at the onset of ventricular systole, (2) the rate of rise of the left ventricular pressure pulse, (3) the presence or absence of structural disease of the mitral valve, and (4) the amount of tissue, air, or fluid between the heart and the stethoscope. The S_1 sound is louder if diastole is shortened (tachycardia) or if atrial contraction precedes ventricular contraction by an unusually short interval, reflected in a short PR interval. The loud S_1 in mitral stenosis usually signifies that the valve is pliable (Fig. 1-4).

A reduction in the intensity of S_1 may be due to poor conduction of sound through the chest wall, a long PR interval, or imperfect closure, as in mitral regurgitation.

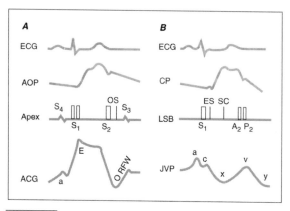

FIGURE 1-4

A. schematic representation of electrocardiogram, aortic pressure pulse (AOP), phonocardiogram recorded at the apex, and apex cardiogram (ACG). On the phonocardiogram, S_1, S_2, S_3, and S_4 represent the first through fourth heart sounds; OS represents the opening snap of the mitral valve, which occurs coincident with the O point of the apex cardiogram. S_3 occurs coincident with the termination of the rapid-filling wave (RFW) of the ACG, while S_4 occurs coincident with the *a* wave of the ACG. *B*. Simultaneous recording of electrocardiogram, indirect carotid pulse (CP), phonocardiogram along the left sternal border (LSB), and indirect jugular venous pulse (JVP). ES = ejection sound; SC = systolic click.

Splitting of the two high-pitched components of S_1 is a normal phenomenon. The first component of S_1 is attributed to mitral valve closure and the second to tricuspid valve closure. Widening of S_1 is due most often to complete right bundle-branch block.

Splitting of S_2 into aortic (A_2) and pulmonic (P_2) components occurs normally during inspiration. Physiologic splitting of S_2 is accentuated in conditions associated with right ventricular volume overload and a distensible pulmonary vascular bed. However, in patients with an increase in pulmonary vascular resistance, narrow splitting of S_2 is present. Splitting that persists with expiration (heard best at the pulmonic or left sternal border) is usually abnormal when the patient is in the upright position. Such splitting may be due to delayed activation of the right ventricle (right bundle branch block), left ventricular ectopic beats, a left ventricular pacemaker, pulmonary embolism or pulmonic stenosis, or atrial septal defect.

In pulmonary hypertension, P_2 is increased in intensity, and splitting of the second heart sound may be diminished, normal, or accentuated. Early aortic valve closure, occurring with mitral regurgitation or a ventricular septal defect, also may produce splitting that persists during expiration. In patients with an atrial septal defect, the volume and duration of right ventricular ejection are not significantly increased by inspiration, and there is little inspiratory exaggeration of the splitting of S_2. This phenomenon, termed *fixed splitting* of the second heart sound, is of considerable diagnostic value.

A delay in aortic valve closure causing P_2 to precede A_2 results in reversed (*paradoxic*) splitting of S_2. Splitting is then maximal in expiration and decreases during inspiration. The most common causes of reversed splitting of S_2 are left bundle branch block and delayed excitation of the left ventricle from a right ventricular ectopic beat. Mechanical prolongation of left ventricular systole, resulting in reversed splitting of S_2, also may be caused by severe aortic outflow obstruction, a large aorta-to-pulmonary artery shunt, systolic hypertension, and ischemic heart disease or cardiomyopathy with left ventricular failure. A P_2 that is greater than A_2 suggests pulmonary hypertension, except in patients with atrial septal defect.

The third heart sound (S_3) is low-pitched sound produced in the ventricle after A_2. In patients over 40 years old, an S_3 usually indicates impairment of ventricular function, AV valve regurgitation, or other conditions that increase the rate or volume of ventricular filling. The left-sided S_3 is best heard with the bell of the stethoscope at the left ventricular apex during expiration and with the patient in the left lateral position. The right-sided S_3 is best heard at left sternal border or just beneath the xiphoid and usually is louder with inspiration.

Third heart sounds often disappear with the treatment of heart failure. The *opening snap* (OS) is a brief, high-pitched, early diastolic sound that is usually due to stenosis of an AV valve, most often the mitral valve. It is generally heard best at the lower left sternal border and radiates well to the base of the heart. The A_2–OS interval is inversely related to the mean left atrial pressure. The OS of tricuspid stenosis occurs later in diastole than the mitral OS and is often overlooked in patients with more prominent mitral valve disease.

The fourth heart sound (S_4) is a low-pitched, presystolic sound produced in the ventricle during ventricular filling; it is associated with an effective atrial contraction (thus is absent in atrial fibrillation) and is best heard with the bell of the stethoscope. The S_4 is present frequently in patients with systemic hypertension, aortic stenosis, hypertrophic cardiomyopathy, ischemic heart disease, and acute mitral regurgitation. Most patients with an acute myocardial infarction and sinus rhythm have an audible S_4. It peaks in intensity at the left ventricular apex when the patient is in the left lateral position and is accentuated by mild isotonic or isometric exercise in the supine position. In patients with chronic obstructive pulmonary disease (COPD) and increased anteroposterior (AP) diameter of the chest, the fourth heart sound may be heard best at the base of neck or in the infra- or supraclavicular areas.

The *ejection sound* is a sharp, high-pitched event occurring in early systole and closely following the first heart sound. Ejection sounds occur in the presence of semilunar valve stenosis and in conditions associated with dilatation of the aorta or pulmonary artery. The aortic ejection sound is usually best heard at the left ventricular apex and the second right intercostals space; the pulmonary ejection sound is strongest at the upper left sternal border. The latter, unlike most other right-sided acoustical events, is heard better during expiration. *Nonejection* or *midsystolic clicks*, occurring with or without a late systolic murmur, often denote prolapse of one or both leaflets of the mitral valve.

HEART MURMURS

The intensity of murmurs may be graded from I to VI. A grade I murmur is so faint that it can be heard only with special effort; a grade VI murmur is audible with the stethoscope removed from contact with the chest. The configuration of a murmur may be crescendo, decrescendo, crescendo-decrescendo (diamond-shaped), or plateau. The precise time of onset and time of cessation of a murmur depend on the instant in the cardiac cycle at which an adequate pressure difference between two chambers arises and disappears (Fig. 1-5).

The location on the chest wall where the murmur is best heard and the areas to which it radiates can be helpful in identifying the cardiac structure from which the murmur originates.

In addition, by noting changes in the characteristics of the murmur during maneuvers that alter cardiac hemodynamics, the auscultator often can identify its correct origin and significance.

Accentuation of murmur during inspiration implies that it originates on the right side of the circulation. The Valsalva maneuver reduces the intensity of most murmurs by diminishing both right and left ventricular filling. The systolic murmur associated with hypertrophic cardiomyopathy and the late systolic murmur due to mitral valve prolapse are exceptions and may be paradoxically accentuated during the Valsalva maneuver. Murmurs due to flow across a normal or obstructed semilunar valve increase in intensity in the cycle following a premature ventricular beat or a long RR interval in atrial fibrillation. In contrast, murmurs due to AV valve regurgitation or a ventricular septal defect do not change appreciably during the beat following a prolonged diastole. Standing accentuates the murmur of hypertrophic cardiomyopathy and occasionally the murmur due

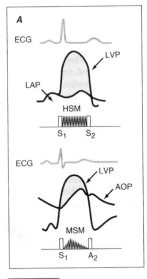

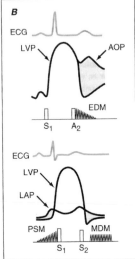

FIGURE 1-5

A. Schematic representation of ECG, aortic pressure (AOP), left ventricular pressure (LVP), and left atrial pressure (LAP). The shaded areas indicated a transvalvular pressure difference during systole. HSM = holosystolic murmur; MSM = midsystolic murmur. *B.* Graphic representation of ECG, aortic pressure (AOP), left ventricular pressure (LVP), and left atrial pressure (LAP), with shaded areas indicating transvalvular diastolic pressure difference. EDM = early diastolic murmur; PSM = presystolic murmur; MDM = middiastolic murmur.

to mitral valve prolapse. Squatting increases most murmurs except those caused by hypertrophic cardiomyopathy and mitral regurgitation due to a prolapsed mitral valve. Sustained hand-grip exercise often accentuates the murmurs of mitral regurgitation, aortic regurgitation, and mitral stenosis but usually diminishes those due to aortic stenosis or hypertrophic cardiomyopathy. Pharmacologic interventions include inhalation of amyl nitrate, which increases the intensity of murmurs due to valvular stenosis while diminishing those due to aortic and mitral regurgitation. Transient arterial occlusion by the inflation of bilateral arm cuffs to 20 mmHg above the systolic pressure for 5 s usually intensifies murmurs due to left-sided regurgitant lesions.

SYSTOLIC MURMURS

Holosystolic (pansystolic) murmurs are generated when there is flow between two chambers that have high pressure gradients throughout systole. Therefore, holosystolic murmurs accompany mitral or tricuspid regurgitation and ventricular septal defect. Although the typical high-pitched murmur of mitral regurgitation usually continues throughout systole (Fig. 1-6), the shape of the murmur may vary considerably. The holosystolic murmurs of mitral regurgitation and ventricular septal defect are augmented by transient exercise and are diminished by inhalation of amyl nitrate. The murmur of tricuspid regurgitation associated with pulmonary hypertension is holosystolic and frequently increases during inspiration. Midsystolic murmurs, also called *systolic ejection murmurs*, which are often crescendo-decrescendo in shape, occur when blood is ejected across the aortic or pulmonic outflow tracts (Fig. 1–6). When the semilunar valves are normal, an increased flow rate, ejection into a dilated vessel beyond the valve, or increased transmission of sound through a thin chest wall may be responsible for this murmur. Most benign functional murmurs are midsystolic and originate from the pulmonary outflow tract. Valvular or subvalvular obstruction of either ventricle also may cause such a midsystolic murmur.

The murmur of aortic stenosis is the prototype of the left-sided midsystolic murmur. In valvular aortic stenosis, the murmur is usually maximal in the second right intercostal space, with radiation into the neck. In supravalvular aortic stenosis, the murmur is occasionally loudest above the second intercostal space, with disproportionate radiation into the right carotid artery. In hypertrophic cardiomyopathy, the midsystolic murmur originates in the left ventricular cavity and is usually maximal at the lower left sternal edge and apex, with relatively little radiation to the carotids. When the aortic valve is immobile (calcified), the aortic closure sound (A_2) may be soft and inaudible, so that the length and configuration of the murmur are difficult to determine. Midsystolic murmurs also occur in patients with mitral regurgitation resulting from papillary muscle dysfunction.

Midsystolic aortic and pulmonic murmurs are intensified after amyl nitrate inhalation and during the cardiac cycle following a premature ventricular beat, while those due to mitral regurgitation are unchanged or softer. Aortic systolic murmurs are diminished by interventions that increase aortic impedance, such as intravenous phenylephrine administration.

Early systolic murmurs begin with the first heart sound and end in midsystole. An early systolic murmur is a feature of tricuspid regurgitation occurring in the absence of pulmonary hypertension. Patients with acute mitral regurgitation into a noncompliant left atrium and a

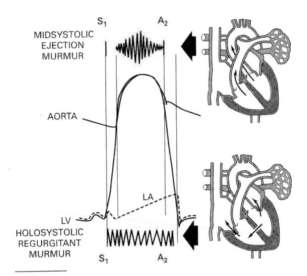

S₁ ... A₂ labels shown in figure

MIDSYSTOLIC
EJECTION
MURMUR

AORTA

LA

LV
HOLOSYSTOLIC
REGURGITANT
MURMUR

FIGURE 1-6

Midsystolic ejection murmurs are caused by forward flow across the LV or RV outflow tract, whereas pansystolic regurgitant murmurs are caused by retrograde flow from a high-pressure cardiac chamber to a low-pressure one. (*Left*) Diagrammatic representation of the midsystolic ejection murmur and the pansystolic regurgitant murmur, as related to LV, aortic, and left atrial (LA) pressures. The systolic ejection murmur occurs during the period of LV ejection; the onset of the murmur is separated from S_1 by the period of isovolumic contraction and the crescendo-decrescendo murmur terminates before A_2. The pansystolic regurgitant murmur begins with, or may replace, S_1, and the murmur continues up to and through A_2 as LV pressure exceeds left atrial pressure during the period of isovolumic relaxation. The murmur has a plateau configuration and varies little with respiration. (*Right*) Flow diagram. (Left panel reproduced from Reddy PS, Shaver JA, Leonard JJ: Cardiac systolic murmurs: Pathophysiology and differential diagnosis. *Prog Cardiovasc Dis* 1971; 14:19. Entire figure reproduced with permission from Shaver JA: Systolic murmurs. *Heart Dis Stroke* 1993; 2:10.)

large v wave often have a loud early systolic murmur that diminishes as the pressure gradient between the left ventricle and the left atrium decreases in late systole.

Late systolic murmurs are faint or moderately loud, high-pitched apical murmurs that start well after ejection and do not mask either heart sound. They are probably related to papillary muscle dysfunction and may appear only during angina, but they are common in patients with myocardial infarction of diffuse myocardial disease. Late systolic murmurs following midsystolic clicks are due to late systolic mitral regurgitation caused by prolapse of the mitral valve into the left atrium.

DIASTOLIC MURMURS

Early diastolic murmurs begin with or shortly after S_2 (Fig. 1-7). The high-pitched murmurs of aortic regurgitation or of pulmonic regurgitation due to pulmonary hypertension are generally decrescendo.

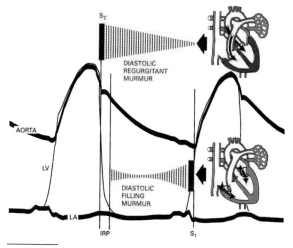

FIGURE 1-7

Diastolic filling murmurs or rumbles are caused by forward flow across the AV valves, whereas diastolic regurgitant murmurs are caused by retrograde flow across incompetent semilunar valves. (*Left*) Diagrammatic representation of the diastolic filling murmur and the diastolic regurgitant murmur as related to LV, aortic, and left atrial (LA) pressures. The diastolic filling murmur occurs during the diastolic filling period and is separated from S_2 by the isovolumic relaxation period. The rumbling murmur is most prominent during rapid, early ventricular filling and presystole, terminating with S_1. The diastolic regurgitant murmur begins immediately after S_2 and continues in a decrescendo fashion up to S_1, closely paralleling the aortic LV diastolic pressure gradient. (*Right*) Flow diagram. (From Shaver JA: Diastolic murmurs. *Heart Dis Stroke* 1993; 1:98–103. Reproduced with permission from the American Heart Association.)

Faint, high-pitched murmurs of aortic regurgitation are difficult to hear unless they are specifically sought by applying firm pressure with the diaphragm over the left midsternal border while the patient sits, leaning forward, and holds a breath in full expiration. The diastolic murmur of aortic regurgitation is enhanced by hand-grip exercise; it diminishes with amyl nitrate inhalation.

Middiastolic murmurs, usually arising from the AV valves, occur during early ventricular filling. Such murmurs may be quite loud (grade III) despite only slight AV valve stenosis. Conversely, the murmurs may be soft or even absent despite severe obstruction if the cardiac output is markedly reduced. When the stenosis is marked, the diastolic murmur is prolonged, and the duration of the murmur is more reliable than its intensity as an index of the severity of valve obstruction.

The low-pitched, middiastolic murmur of mitral stenosis characteristically follows the OS. It should be specifically sought by placing the bell of the stethoscope at the site of the left ventricular impulse, which is best localized with the patient in the left lateral position. Frequently, the murmur of mitral stenosis is present only at the left ventricular apex, and it may be increased in intensity by mild supine exercise or by inhalation of amyl nitrate. In tricuspid stenosis, the middiastolic murmur is localized to a relatively limited area along the left sternal border and may be stronger during inspiration.

A soft, middiastolic murmur may sometimes be heard in patients with acute rheumatic fever (Carey-Coombs murmur). In acute, severe aortic regurgitation, the left ventricular diastolic pressure may exceed the left atrial pressure, resulting in middiastolic murmur due to "diastolic mitral regurgitation." In severe, chronic aortic regurgitation, a murmur is frequently present that may be either middiastolic or presystolic (Austin-Flint murmur).

Presystolic murmurs begin during the period of ventricular filling that follows atrial contraction and therefore occur in sinus rhythm. They are usually due to stenosis of the AV valve and have the same quality as the middiastolic filling rumble, but they are usually crescendo, reaching peak intensity at the time of a loud S_1. It is the presystolic murmur that is most characteristic of tricuspid stenosis and sinus rhythm.

CONTINUOUS MURMURS

These begin in systole, peak near S_2, and continue into all or part of diastole. A patent ductus arteriosus causes a continuous murmur as long as the pressure in the pulmonary artery is much below that in the aorta. The murmur is intensified by elevation of the systemic arterial pressure and reduced by amyl nitrate inhalation. When pulmonary hypertension is present, the diastolic portion may disappear, leaving the murmur confined to systole.

Continuous murmurs may result from congenital or acquired systemic arteriovenous fistulas, coronary arteriovenous fistula, anomalous origin of the left coronary artery from the pulmonary artery, and communications between the sinus of Valsalva and the right side of the heart.

In nonconstricted arteries, continuous murmurs may be due to rapid flow through a tortuous bed. Such murmurs typically occur within the bronchial arterial collateral circulation in cyanotic patients with severe pulmonary outflow obstruction.

PERICARDIAL FRICTION RUB

These adventitious sounds may have presystolic, systolic, and early diastolic scratchy components; they may be confused with a murmur or extracardiac sound when heard only in systole. A pericardial friction rub is best appreciated with the patient upright and leaning forward and may be accentuated during inspiration.

SUGGESTED READING

Ewy GA: Venous and arterial pulsations: Bedside insights into hemodynamics. In: Chizner M (ed): *Classic Teachings in Clinical Cardiology: A Tribute to W. Proctor Harvey*. Cedar Grove, NJ: Laennec; 1996.

Leon DF, Shaver JA (eds): *Physiologic Principles of Heart Sounds and Murmurs*. Monograph 46. New York: American Heart Association; 1975.

O'Rourke RA: The history, physical examination, and cardiac auscultation. In: Fuster V, Alexander RW, O'Rourke RA, et al (eds): *Hurst's The Heart*, 10th ed. New York: McGraw-Hill; 2001: 193–280.

O'Rourke RA: Approach to the patient with a murmur. In: Goldman L, Braunwald E (eds): *Primary Cardiology*. Philadelphia: Saunders; 1998:155–173.

O'Rourke RA, Braunwald E: Physical examination of the cardiovascular system. In: Fauci AS, Braunwald E, Isselbacher KJ, et al (eds): *Harrison's Principles of Internal Medicine*, 14th ed. New York: McGraw-Hill; 1998.

2

THE RESTING
ELECTROCARDIOGRAM

Agustin Castellanos
Alberto Interian, Jr.
Robert J. Myerburg

INTRODUCTION

The electrocardiogram (ECG) has many uses: it may serve as an independent marker of myocardial disease; it may reflect anatomic, hemodynamic, molecular, ionic, and drug-induced abnormalities of the heart; and it may provide information that is essential for the proper diagnosis and therapy of many cardiac problems. In fact, it is the most commonly used laboratory procedure for the diagnosis of heart disease. All physicians who interpret ECGs as well as those learning electrocardiographic interpretation should read the *Guidelines for Electrocardiography of the American College of Cardiology, American Heart Association Task Force.*

VENTRICULAR DEPOLARIZATION
AND REPOLARIZATION

In the resting or polarized state, the charges are at rest. A unipolar electrode facing the epicardial side of a left ventricular strip, such as V_6, registers an isoelectric line. When depolarization occurs, it does so with an endocardium-to-epicardium *sequence*. Depolarization has been described as a moving wave *with the positive charges in front of* the negative charges. The unipolar lead will record a positivity because it consistently faces positive charges throughout the entire depolarization sequence. On the other hand, the *sequence* of ventricular repolarization is from epicardium to endocardium but with the negative charges in front. Thus, V_6 will record a positive deflection because it constantly faces positive charges. The earlier epicardial end of repolarization has been attributed to the shorter duration of repolarization that epicardial cells have in comparison to endocardial cells. Therefore, repolarization finishes at the epicardium while it still has not been completed at the endocardium. This simplistic view is of didactic value only since it fails to take into consideration the role played by the M cells described by Antzelevitch and coworkers. According to these authors M cells play a determining role in the inscription of the T wave, since currents flowing down voltage gradients on either side of the usual (but not necessarily) mid-myocardial cells determine both the height and width of the T wave as well as the degree to which the ascending or descending limbs of the T wave are interrupted.

ELECTROCARDIOGRAPHIC LEADS

Standard and Extremity Leads

An ECG lead can be defined as a pair of terminals with designated polarity, each of which is connected either directly or via a passive-active network to recording electrodes. Einthoven et al first developed a method of studying the electrical activity of the heart by representing it graphically in a *two-dimensional* geometric figure—namely, an equilateral triangle. Although there are three bipolar leads and three unipolar extremity leads, the information contained in limb leads is redundant. If any two of the six are recorded, the other four can be derived according to Einthoven's equation (III = II − I) and to the relationship between bipolar and unipolar limb leads (I = V_L−V_R, II = V_F−V_R, and III = V_F−V_L). When the electrodes are placed proximally to the roots of the extremities, they lose their relatively "far" distance from the heart. Hence, Einthoven's equilateral theory does not hold. This explains why leads placed proximally to the roots of the extremities such as those used for exercise testing, monitoring in the coronary care unit, and ambulatory ECG recordings, by being only "equivalent" to the corresponding bipolar leads, are in some cases markedly different than the "true" standard bipolar leads.

Unipolar Precordial Leads

Unipolar precordial leads should be viewed in a slightly different context. Precordial (V) leads yield a positive deflection when facing positive charges and negative deflections when facing negative charges. They do this according to what Wilson called the *solid angle*, which is merely an imaginary cone extending from the site in the chest throughout the heart. The precordial electrode is at its apex, and its base is at the opposite epicardial surface. According to Wilson's scalar concept of electrocardiography, this occurs because the solid angle subtended by the corresponding lead records the electrical activity from the regions of the heart over which it is placed as well as from distant regions. Thus, if V_2 is placed over (thereby facing) the right ventricle, part of the initial positive ventricular deflection reflects right ventricular activation, with the corresponding electrical forces moving toward the electrode. Most portions of the terminal S wave represent activation of muscle other than the right ventricle (septum and free left ventricular wall), reflecting electrical forces moving away from the electrode. Acceptance that the amount of muscle activity recorded by various unipolar leads is not the same implies different "real" duration of depolarization and repolarization, irrespective of the one supposedly resulting from the projections of a vector on an idealized horizontal plane of a "corrected" spatial vectorcardiographic (such as the Frank) system.

NORMAL ACTIVATION OF THE HEART: VENTRICULAR DEPOLARIZATION

After emerging from the sinus node, the cardiac impulse propagates throughout the atria in its journey toward the atrioventricular (AV) node. The sequence of atrial depolarization occurs in an inferior, leftward, and somewhat posterior direction. The PR interval (used to estimate AV conduction time) includes conduction through the "true" AV structures (AV node, His bundle, bundle branches, and main divisions of the left bundle branch) as well as through those parts of the atria located between sinus and AV nodes. The onset of ventricular depolarization (given by the beginning of the normal q wave) reflects activation of the left side of the interventricular septum. Hence, the normal initial depolarization is oriented from left to right, therefore explaining the small q wave in lead V_6 and the small r wave in V_1. Thereafter the interventricular septum is activated in both directions. Septal activation is encompassed within or neutralized by subsequent free-wall activation. The greater mass of the left ventricular (LV) free wall explains why LV free-wall events overpower those of the interventricular septum and right ventricular free wall.

ELECTRICAL AXIS

The electrical axis (EA) may be defined as a vector originating in the center of Einthoven's equilateral triangle. When applied to the EA of the QRS complexes, the vector that represents it also gives the direction of the activation process as projected in the plane of the limb leads. The classical school recommends calculating the net *areas* enclosed by the QRS complex in leads I, II, and III. A simpler, though less precise, method of calculating the quadrant (or parts of a quadrant) in which the EA is located consists of using the maximal QRS deflection in leads I and aV_F and, when necessary, lead II.

VENTRICULAR GRADIENT

The relationship between the EA of the QRS complex and the T wave was referred to by Wilson as the *ventricular gradient*. In the human heart, both sequences and pathways of ventricular depolarization and repolarization are not exactly the same. Because of the latter a gradient is said to exist. The ventricular gradient can be calculated by determining the electrical axis of the QRS and T (using *areas*) and then obtaining the resultant by the parallelogram method. The ventricular gradient differentiates between T-wave inversion of various causes (primary changes) and the obligatory secondary T-wave changes resulting from abnormalities in depolarization, such as bundle branch block, ventricular hypertrophy, ventricular pacing, and preexcitation syndromes.

Apparent Challenges to the Concept of the Ventricular Gradient Cardiac Memory

Rosenbaum et al. studied the prolonged depolarization occurring during long periods of ventricular stimulation and found two types of altered ventricular repolarization. One, corresponding to Wilson's classic theory, was primary and proportional in magnitude to the QRS complex but of opposite polarity. The other, concealed by (and during) the former, required a longer time (even days) to reach maximal effect as well as to disappear, becoming apparent *only when* normal activation recurred. The latter type was attributed to modulated electrotonic interactions occurring during cardiac activation in such a way that repolarization was accelerated at ventricular sites where depolarization begins and delayed in areas where depolarization terminates. Abnormal T-wave changes occurring after disappearance of prolonged periods of abnormal repolarization induced by abnormal depolarization showed accumulation and (fading) *long-term* memory for variable time. The occurrence of *short-term* effects memory after periods of altered ventricular depolarization (and repolarization) as short as 1 min in duration has recently been reported. In addition, the term *memory* has also been applied to gradual adjustments of action potential duration (roughly corresponding to QT intervals) after abrupt changes in cycle lengths (events influenced by past history) without necessarily requiring previous abnormal ventricular repolarization.

ABNORMAL ST-SEGMENT CHANGES

In orthodox ECG language, *injury* implies *abnormal* ST-segment changes, *necrosis* or *fibrosis* implies *abnormal* Q waves, and *ischemia* implies *symmetrical* T-wave inversion (or elevation). Various hypotheses have been postulated to explain how the injury-related diastolic hypopolarization is manifest as abnormal ST-segment shifts. One hypothesis is based on the existence of a *diastolic* current of "injury" and the other presupposes a true, active, *systolic* displacement. Most likely, injury reflects both disappearance of diastolic baseline shifts plus active ST elevation. In addition, loss or depression of the action potential dome in epicardium but not endocardium underlies the development of prominent ST elevation. Some authors consider ST changes in ventricular aneurysms as a result of the earlier repolarization of a ring of persistently viable tissue surrounding the aneurysm; however, others believe they reflect functional (echocardiographic) dyskinesia. ST-segment elevation from the epicardial injury due to pericarditis should be differentiated from the benign "early repolarization" pattern, a normal variant. Although the mechanism of early repolarization has not been fully elucidated, it has been related to enhanced activity of the right sympathetic nerves.

SELECTIVE NON-ISCHEMIC ST-SEGMENT ELEVATION IN THE RIGHT PRECORDIAL LEADS

High-take-off ST segments of either the caved or saddle-back type localized to the right chest leads associated with different degrees of right bundle branch block (RBBB) with or without T-wave inversion are seen in the Brugada syndrome. Strong sodium channel blocking drugs can produce ST-segment elevations even in patients without any evidence of syncope or ventricular fibrillation. Slight ST-segment elevation with an incomplete RBBB pattern showing an epsilon wave has been described in some patients with arrhythmogenic right ventricular dysplasia. Hyperkalemic "injury" can produce an anteroseptal myocardial infarction (MI) pattern (dialyzable current of injury).

ABNORMAL Q WAVES

Abnormal Q waves appearing several hours after total occlusion of a coronary artery result from the necrosis secondary to the decreased blood supply. The number of affected cells has to be large enough to produce changes reflected at the body surface. The following changes have been said to be equivalent to Q waves in non-Q-wave myocardial infarctions: R/S ratio changes, acute frontal plane right axis deviation, new left axis deviation or left bundle branch block (LBBB), initial and terminal QRS notching, and some types of "poor r-wave progression." Although the concept of non-Q-wave MI as a discrete clinicopathologic entity that differs from Q-wave MI has gained almost universal acceptance, it was recently challenged by a group of respectable electrocardiographers.

ISCHEMIC T-WAVE CHANGES

Symmetrical T waves, inverted, or upright (as in "hyperacute" T waves) characteristic of ECG "ischemia" have been considered to reflect a type or degree of cellular affection resulting in action potentials of increased and different duration with regional alterations of the duration of the depolarized state. T-wave inversions do not always reflect "physiologic" ischemia (due to decreased blood supply), since they can also be seen in evolving pericarditis, myocardial contusion, increased intracranial pressure, and in the right chest leads of young patients (persistent juvenile pattern).

SECONDARY ST-T-WAVE CHANGES

Alterations in the sequence of (and sometimes delay in) ventricular depolarization (as produced by BBBs, ventricular pacing, ectopic ventricular impulse formation, preexcitation syndromes, and ventricular hypertrophy) result in an obligatory change in the sequence of ventricular repolarization. This causes nonischemic T-wave inversions (secondary T-wave changes) in leads showing predominantly positive QRS deflections. Disappearance of these alterations of ventricular depolarization may be followed by narrow QRS complexes with negative T waves due to cardiac memory, as previously stated.

NONSPECIFIC ST-T-WAVE CHANGES

Non-specific (or rather, nondiagnostic) ST-T-wave changes are the most commonly diagnosed ECG abnormalities. They have not been adequately categorized and represent different findings for various interpreters. When analyzed without clinical information, this diagnosis was made in 40 percent of 410 abnormal ECGs, this number being reduced to 10 percent when clinical data became available. In the absence of structural heart disease, these changes can be due to a variety of physiologic, pharmacologic, and extracardiac factors.

ACUTE MYOCARDIAL INFARCTION

Myocardial infarctions are no longer classified as transmural and subendocardial but as Q wave and non Q wave. In the thrombolytic era, the prevalence of non-Q-wave MI seems to be greater (see Chap.15). The pre-thrombolytic "classic" evolution of acute Q-wave MI has been transformed by pharmacologic therapy and interventional techniques. The succession of events in the course of a classic Q-wave MI is from hyperacute positive T waves (on occasion) to ST-segment elevation to abnormal Q waves to T-wave inversion. Acceleration of these phases can occur with effective reperfusion. The time course of ST-segment elevation is a good predictor of reperfusion. Because pre-thrombolytic 12-lead ECG studies on ST-segment evolutions were based on static recordings obtained at fixed time intervals, it became clear that continuous monitoring in the coronary care unit was essential to adequately record the dynamics of ST-segment trends (Figs. 2-1 and 2-2). Sensitivity increases as frequency of monitoring increases. Continuous monitoring is thus essential to evaluate occurrence of reperfusion. Resolution of ST-segment elevation has been defined as a progressive decrease within 40 to 60 min to less than 50 percent of its maximally elevated value. It has been suggested that in patients treated with thrombolytics, the dichotomization for Q and non-Q-wave MI should be made by the predischarge rather than the 24-h ECG due to possible crossover from one group to another (see also Chap. 14).

EVOLUTION OF ACUTE
CORONARY SYNDROMES

ECG changes indicative of *physiologic* ischemia that may progress to MI (see also Chap. 15):

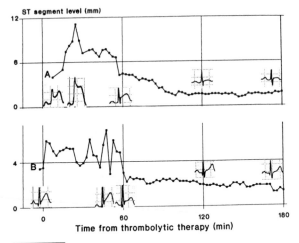

FIGURE 2-1

Plots of ST-segment levels versus time from therapy in two selected patients with patency of the infarct-related vessel at 60 min. Note that a 50 percent decrease in ST-segment levels within 60 min occurred only when measurements were made from the peak ST-segment level (highest ST-segment level measurement within the last 60 min).

1. Patients with ST-segment elevation: new or presumed new ST-segment elevation in two or more contiguous leads with the cut-off points ≥ 0.2 mV in leads V_1, V_2, or V_3 and ≥ 0.1 mV in other leads (contiguity in the frontal plane is defined by the lead sequences aV_L, inverted aV_R, II, aV_F, III. There can be evolution into Q-wave MI or non-Q-wave MI.
2. Non-Q-wave MI may also present with ST-segment elevation as well as with T-wave abnormalities only.

LOCATION OF THE SITE OF Q-WAVE MYOCARDIAL INFARCTION

Table 2-1 shows an acceptable classification for the ECG location of MI according to leads showing abnormal Q waves while also depicting other processes that may result in false patterns of Q-wave MI.

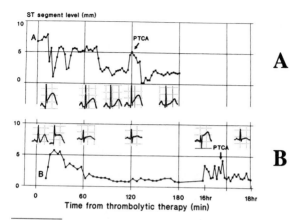

FIGURE 2-2

Assessment of thrombolytic therapy in patients with acute myocardial infarction by ST-segment monitoring. Plots of ST-segment levels versus time from initiation of therapy in two selected patients with angiographic reocclusion. Patient A showed wide ST-segment shifts in the first 40 min, angiographic and electrocardiographic reperfusion at 90 min, and reocclusion at 120 min that required percutaneous transluminal coronary angioplasty (PTCA). Patient B had successful thrombolysis within 60 min of initiation of therapy. At 16 h, ST-segment elevation recurred and PTCA was performed.

PERICARDITIS

In acute pericarditis, ST segments can be elevated in all leads except aV_R and, rarely, in V_1. Symmetrical T-wave inversion (due to epicardial "ischemia") usually develops after the ST segments have returned to the baseline (but it can appear during the injury stage). Neither reciprocal ST-segment changes nor abnormal Q waves are seen. In most cases of acute pericarditis, the PR segment is depressed. Average ECG resolution occurs in close to 2 weeks (see also Chap. 15).

INTRAVENTRICULAR CONDUCTION DEFECTS

The following classification is the most commonly accepted and widely known. Consequently, only important pointers are presented.

TABLE 2-1
ELECTROCARDIOGRAPHIC LOCATION OF INFARCTION SITES BASED ON THE PRESENCE OF ABNORMAL Q WAVES

Site	Leads	False Patterns
Inferior (diaphragmatic)	II, III, aV_F	WPW (PSAP), HCM
Inferolateral	II, III, aV_F, V_F, V_4–V_6	RVH, "atypical" incomplete RBBB, WPW (LFWAP)
"True" posterior (posterobasal)	V_1*	WPW (left PSAP), HCM
Inferoposterior	II, III, aV_F, $V_1{}^a$	ASMI
Inferior–right ventricular	II, III, aV_F plus V_{4R}–V_{6R} or V_1–V_3	
Anteroseptal	V_1, V_2, V_3	LVH, chronic lung disease, LBBB, chest electrode misplacement, right ventricular MI
Extensive anterior	I, aV_L, V_1–V_6	
High lateral	I, aV_L	Extremely vertical hearts with aV_L resembling aV_R
Anterior (apical)	V_3–V_4	
Posterolateral	V_4–V_6, V_1*	WPW (LFWAP)
Right ventricular	V_{4R} with V_{4R}–V_{6R} or V_1–V_3	ASMI

aTall R wave, "reciprocal" to changes in "indicative" back leads.

KEY: ASMI = anteroseptal myocardial infarction; HCM = hypertrophic cardiomyopathy; LBBB = left bundle branch block; LFWAP = left free-wall accessory pathway; PSAP = posteroseptal accessory pathway; WPW = Wolff-Parkinson-White syndrome; RVH = right ventricular hypertrophy.

Left Anterior Fascicular Block

1. Abnormal left superior (rarely right superior) axis with rS complexes in II, III, and aV_F. Peak of R in aV_L occurs before that of aV_R.
2. Left precordial leads may show RS complexes when the electrical axis is markedly superior.
3. Other causes of left axis deviation—such as extensive inferior wall MI, Wolff-Parkinson-White syndrome (posteroseptal accessory pathway), hyperkalemia, ventricular pacing, and pulmonary emphysema—should be excluded.
4. QRS widening (over normal values) does not exceed 0.025 s.
5. Usually there are no interferences with the diagnosis of MI, or RBBB.

Left Posterior Fascicular Block

1. Generally diagnosed only when coexisting with complete RBBB.
2. Right (and inferior) axis deviation should not be due to right ventricular hypertrophy or lateral MI.
3. The QRST pattern resembles that of inferior ischemia or infarction.

Left Middle Septal Blocks

1. There are discrepancies regarding this entity, since several contradictory, diagnostic criteria have been proposed:
   a. Large R waves in V_1 (similar to those seen in true posterior MI or right ventricular hypertrophy)
   b. Small Q waves in V_1, V_2, and V_3
   c. Absence of the expected normal Q waves in V_5 and V_6

Complete Right Bundle Branch Block

1. Does not deviate the electrical axis (determined by maximal deflections) *abnormally* to the left or to the right.
2. Although true posterior MI cannot be diagnosed in its presence, it does not interfere with the diagnosis of MI of other locations.
3. It may masquerade as LBBB when the expected wide S wave is not present in lead I, presumably because the terminal vectors are perpendicular to this lead.
4. An upright T wave in right chest leads may be reciprocal to posterior ischemia or may reflect a primary change in repolarization in anteroseptal leads.

Incomplete Right Bundle Branch Block

1. An r' or R' in V_1 with QRS duration of less than 0.10 s may be referred to as a normal IRBBB "pattern."
2. It need not always reflect a conduction delay in the trunk of a normal right branch since it has been attributed to:
   a. An increased conduction time due to a right ventricular enlargement, stretch-related *delay* in an elongated right branch or in the Purkinje-myocardial junction.
   b. An interruption of a subdivision of the right bundle branch or
   c. A physiologic later-than-usual arrival of excitation at the crista supraventricularis

Complete Left Bundle Branch Block

1. May simulate anteroseptal MI.
2. Interferes with the diagnosis of lateral and inferior MI but not anteroseptal, MI.
3. A normal q wave before an otherwise typical wide R wave indicates anteroseptal, not lateral MI.
4. MI of any location may be present without any change in its basic features.
5. Acute inferior and anterolateral MIs can be diagnosed by characteristic ST-segment changes.
6. A positive T wave always reflects a primary change in repolarization.

NONSPECIFIC INTRAVENTRICULAR CONDUCTION DEFECT

This condition is associated with a wide QRS complex (with repolarization abnormalities) not having a left- or right-BBB pattern. The EA may be normal, left, or right.

Wide QRS Complexes in Patients with Manifest Preexcitation Syndromes

The characteristic pattern of manifest Wolff-Parkinson-White (WPW) syndrome during sinus rhythm is well known. The ventricular complex is a fusion beat resulting from ventricular activation by two wave-fronts. The degree of preexcitation (amount of muscle activated through the accessory pathway) is variable and depends on many factors. Foremost among these are the distance between the sinus node and atrial insertion of the accessory pathway and, more important, the differences in duration of the refractory period and in conduction time through the normal pathway and accessory pathway. If there is total block at the AV node or His-Purkinje system, the impulse will be conducted exclusively via the accessory pathway. Consequently, the QRS complexes are different than fusion beats, though the direction of the delta wave remains the same. Moreover, the QRS complexes are as wide as (and really simulating) those produced by artificial or spontaneous beats arising in the vicinity of the ventricular end of the accessory pathway. Initial noninvasive determination of the anatomic position of the accessory pathway is of great clinical importance because of introduction of surgical and catheter ablative techniques for symptomatic cases of pre-excitation. Many ECG algorithms have been proposed for this task. Although useful as approximations, most are extremely complex for the average electrocardiographer, who finds them difficult to remember. Furthermore, the currently used nomenclature for accessory pathway location was recently discussed and challenged by a group of notable experts in the field of pre-excitation.

Wide QRS Complexes Produced by Ventricular Pacing from Different Sites

In determining the location of the stimulating electrodes, what is relevant is the polarity of the *properly positioned* V_1 and V_2 electrodes and the direction of the EA. For example, endocardial or epicardial stimulation of the *anteriorly* located right ventricle at any site [apical (inferior), or mid/outflow tract (superior)] yields predominantly negative deflections in the right chest leads due to the *posterior* spread of activation. The reverse (positive deflections in V_1 and V_2) occurs when the epicardial stimulation of the superior and lateral portions of the posterior left ventricle by catheter electrodes in the distal coronary sinus or great and middle cardiac veins (or by implanted electrodes in the nearby muscle) results in *anteriorly* oriented forces. Right ventricular apical pacing may rarely produce positive deflections in V_1 specifically if this lead is (mis)placed above its usual level. On the other hand, *superior* deviation of the electrical axis only indicates that a spatial *inferior* ventricular site has been stimulated, regardless of whether this site is the apical portion of the right ventricle or the inferior part of the left ventricle, the latter being paced through the middle cardiac vein. Conversely, an *inferior*, vertical axis is simply a consequence of pacing from a *superior* site, which can be the endocardium of the right ventricular outflow tract or the epicardium of the posterosuperior and lateral portions of the left ventricle. The top of the catheter is determined by the antero-posterior and lateral x-ray views. The method discussed above to locate the site of impulse initiation during pacing is simpler than the more complicated ones used to determine the ventricular sites of exit from accessory pathways (crossing the AV junction), which require the use of right anterior oblique and especially left anterior oblique projections.

LEFT VENTRICULAR HYPERTROPHY

Multiple criteria have been proposed to diagnose left ventricular hypertrophy (LVH) using necropsy or echocardiographic information. Of these, the Sokolow-Lyon criterion ($SV_1 + RV_{5-6} \geq 35$ mm) is the most specific (>95 percent) but is not very sensitive (around 45 percent). The Romhilt-Estes score has a specificity of 90 percent and a sensitivity of 60 percent in studies correlated with echocardiography. The following are some of the other criteria: The Casale (modified Cornell) criterion ($RaV_L + SV_3 > 28$ mm in men and >20 in women) is somewhat more sensitive, but less specific than the Sokolow-Lyon criterion. The Talbot criterion ($R \geq 16$ mm in aV_L) is very specific (>90 percent), even in the presence of myocardial infarction and ventricular block but not very sensitive. The Koito and Spodick criterion ($RV_6 > RV_5$) claims a specificity of 100 percent and a sensitivity of more than 50 percent. According to Hernandez Padial, a total 12-lead QRS voltage > 120 mm is a good ECG criterion of LVH in systemic hypertension and is better than those most frequently used. With echocardiography as the "gold standard," several authors postulated ECG criteria for diagnosis of LVH in the presence of complete LBBB and left anterior fascicular block (LAFB), which are not widely used.

PROCESSES PRODUCING OR LEADING TO RIGHT VENTRICULAR HYPERTROPHY AND ENLARGEMENT

The ECG manifestations of right ventricular hypertrophy (RVH) or enlargement can be subdivided into the following main types: (1) the posterior and rightward displacement of the QRS forces associated with low voltage, as seen in patients with pulmonary emphysema; (2) the incomplete RBBB pattern *with right axis deviation* occurring in patients with chronic lung disease and some congenital cardiac malformation resulting in volume overloading of the right ventricle; (3) the true posterior wall myocardial infarction pattern with normal-to-low voltage of the R wave in V_1 of mitral stenosis with abnormal P wave or big f waves (which can be as large as the QRS complexes); (4) and the classic RVH and strain pattern seen in young patients with congenital heart disease (producing pressure overloading) or in adult patients with high right ventricular pressures, such as "primary" pulmonary hypertension. (See also Chap. 19.)

QT Interval: Normal, Prolonged, and Dispersed

The QT interval (considered as some to be a surrogate of action potential duration) is manually measured from the beginning of the Q wave to the point at which the T-wave downslope crosses the baseline. However, there has been considerable debate and speculation regarding the accurate measurement of the QT interval. For example, according to Coumel et al., the human interobserver variability was 30.6 ms. Similarly, the machine interautomatic comparison of 19 systems yielded standard deviations as great as 30 ms. At present there seems to be a trend toward the acceptance of the (automatic) values obtained with the QT Guard package (Marquette). With this system the end of the T wave is determined using the intersection of the isoelectric line with the tangent to the *inflection point* of the descending part of the T. The QT interval is affected by autonomic tone and catecholamines and has day-night differences. It varies with heart rate and sex. Several formulas have been proposed to take these variables into account and provide a corrected measurement (QTc interval), of which that proposed by Bazett is the most used. In general, the unadjusted (noncorrected), usually resting QT interval decreases linearly from ±0.42 s at rates of 50/min to ±0.32 s at 100/min to ±0.26 s at 150/min. On the contrary, during exercise, when the rate becomes faster, the QTc first increases until reaching a maximum at approximately a rate of 120/min, thereafter again decreasing. Although the value of the normal QTc is open to question, it is still used in routine computer interpretations.

Because the 12-lead ECG shows a normal degree of QT and QTc dispersion, indexes have been used to quantify the extent of what has been called "the heterogeneity in ventricular repolarization." The difference between the longest and shortest QT interval is referred to as *QT dispersion*. Since 1990 it has been used as a prognostic marker not only in patients with congenitally prolonged QT intervals but also in those with acute MI and those taking drugs with proarrhythmic properties; it has also been used to predict mortality in general epidemiologic studies. However, recent reports have challenged the values of QT dispersion. The upper limits of normal vary with different investigators; a value of 60 to 65 ms may be an acceptable compromise. Some may disagree with this range.

Coumel emphasized that QT dispersion could be an illusion or a reality. Inferred from the oncoming section on spatial vectorcardiography, the fact is that a truly spatial (Frank system) QRS-T loop cannot yield abnormal QT dispersion. For in planar projections of this spatial loop (as well as in the plane of the standard and unipolar extremity leads of the ECG), the shortest interval occurs because the terminal forces are perpendicular to the plane or derived lead. On the other hand, if precordial leads are considered scalar leads capable of recording local potentials with different durations, then QT dispersion is a reality. The same can be said regarding measurements performed from vectorcardiographic systems using precordial leads (electrovectorcardiographic methods).

The M-cell studies of Antzelevitch allow for the differentiation of this global "dispersion" (derived from *multiple* leads, if it exists at all) from "local" transmural dispersion in *single* precordial leads (reflecting the electrical activity of the region explored by it) by measuring time elapsing between the peak of the T wave (given by the end of the composite epicardial action potentials) and the end of the T wave (given by the end of the composite M-cell action potentials).

SPATIAL VECTORCARDIOGRAPHY

Space: The Final Frontier

The theory of the truly spatial vectorcardiography (VCG)is theoretically attractive. Because the heart is a tridimensional structure (located in space), its electrical activity should best be recorded by a spatial method. This is also true for the purposes of anatomic description, as previously stated for the location of accessory pathways and pacing electrodes. In this sense, space, as conceived by physicists through objects and their motion, has three dimensions, and positions are characterized by three numbers. The instant of an event is the fourth number. Four definite numbers correspond to every event; a definite event corresponds to any four numbers. Therefore, the world of events really forms a four-dimensional continuum. Unfortunately, judging by what is being published in the literature, the quest for an optimal method of visualizing the truly spatial loop apparently has been abandoned. A truly spatial method requires three *corrected* orthogonal leads with the following features. (1) Mutual perpendicularity, with each lead being parallel to one of the rectilinear coordinate axes of the human body. Such axes are the horizontal, X (left-to-right and right-to-left) axis; the vertical, Y (inferosuperior or superoinferior) axis; and sagittal, Z (anteroposterior or posteroanterior) axis. (2) Equal amplitude from the vectorial viewpoint. (3) The lead vectors of the three leads would not only be of equal amplitude and mutually perpendicular for a single point within the heart but would also retain the same magnitude and direction for all points where cardiac electromotive forces are generated. The most widely used, corrected spatial VCG method probably is the one introduced by Frank. Since the spatial loop cannot be analyzed tridimensionally, it is customary to study its planar projections. By proper attachment to the oscilloscope, the X and Y leads are used for the frontal plane, the X and Z leads for the horizontal plane, and the Z and Y leads for the sagittal plane (of which the right side has been the most popular).

Differences between Electrovectorcardiography and Spatial Vectorcardiography

Truly spatial VCG is distinctly different from the various vectorial methods of ECG interpretation, such as those of Sodi-Pallares et al. and Grant. In clinical practice and in teaching, both seem to be considered equal, but this is so only for pragmatic and didactic reasons. Although the spatial VCG and the ECG should each be studied as distinct methods, most electrocardiographers either memorize loop patterns or attempt to derive the leads with which they are familiar from the corresponding QRS loops. Thus bipolar standard and unipolar extremity leads are derived from the frontal plane more or less as when, in clinical ECG, they are derived from the electrical axis. To do this in spatial vector loops, the electrical axis is equated with the maximal QRS vector that extends from the point of the loop to its farthest point. The unipolar precordial leads are derived from the horizontal plane loops. Leads thus derived are different from the usual precordial ECG leads. The latter, as mentioned previously, record electrical forces moving toward or away from them, including local potentials that can be of different duration in different precordial leads. In the 12-lead ECG (especially when the precordial electrodes are misplaced), however, these forces can move spatially not only in a left-to-right and anteroposterior direction but also in an inferosuperior direction, as in leads V_5 and V_6 in patients with a very superior and leftward deviation of the EA. On the other hand, the theory of spatial VCG states that the horizontal plane and unipolar leads derived from them just record left-to-right and anteroposterior forces and that they do not record local potentials, so that any difference in the duration of intervals is merely an illusion. In spatial VCG, electrical forces oriented superiorly or inferiorly cannot be reflected in the horizontal plane but only in the frontal and sagittal planes.

Most of the information contained in the sagittal plane is present in the frontal and horizontal planes.

VCG loops obtained with the Frank system need not resemble those obtained by the methods discussed in the year 2000 by Malik's group, since the latter used a technology based on the ECG, thus being different (in respect to Frank's loops) in their ability to record nondipolar components. Moreover, their main application initially was in evaluation of QT dispersion by studying T-loop characteristics such as "true" dispersion, area, morphology, and angle with maximal QRS vector.

SUGGESTED READING

Antzelevitch C, Shimizu W, Yan GX, et al: The M cell: Its contribution to the ECG and to normal and abnormal electrical function of the heart. *J Cardiovasc Electrophysiol* 1999; 10:1124-1152.

Bayes de Luna A: *Clinical Electrocardiography: A Textbook.* Mt. Kisco, NY: Futura; 1993: 450.

Castellanos A, Interian A Jr, Myerburg RJ: The resting electrocardiogram. In: Fuster V, Alexander RW, O'Rourke RA, et al (eds): *Hurst's The Heart,* 10th ed. New York: McGraw-Hill; 2001: 281–314.

Chou TC, Helm RA, Kaplan S: *Clinical Vectorcardiography,* 2d ed. New York: Grune & Stratton; 1974.

Macfarlane PW, Lawrie TDV (eds): *Comprehensive Electrocardiology: Theory and Practice in Health and Disease.* New York: Pergamon Press; 1989.

Malik M, Acar B, Gang Y, et al: QT dispersion does not represent electrocardiographic interlead heterogeneity of ventricular repolarization. *J Cardiovasc Electrophysiol* 2000; 11:835-843.

Rosenbaum MB, Elizari MV, Lazzari JO: *The Hemiblocks.* Oldsmar, FL: Tampa Tracings; 1970.

Wagner GS: *Marriott's Practical Electrocardiography,* 10th ed. New York: Lippincott Williams & Wilkins; 2000.

CHAPTER

3

CARDIOVASCULAR AGING IN HEALTH AND THERAPEUTIC CONSIDERATIONS WITH RESPECT TO CARDIOVASCULAR DISEASES IN OLDER PATIENTS

Steven P. Schulman

INTRODUCTION

The elderly make up the fastest-growing segment of the world's population. It is estimated that by the year 2035, nearly one in four individuals will be 65 years of age or older. Cardiovascular diseases—such as coronary artery disease, congestive heart failure, and hypertension—are the leading causes of morbidity and mortality in the elderly. The manifestations and severity of cardiovascular disease in the elderly may be modified to a certain extent by the cardiovascular changes that occur with normal aging. This chapter reviews the age-associated changes in the cardiovascular system in healthy humans and how the manifestations and prognosis of cardiovascular disease may be influenced by these age-associated changes.

CARDIOVASCULAR STRUCTURE

The age-associated structural changes in the cardiovascular system of healthy humans are shown in Table 3-1. Echocardiographic left ventricular wall thickness and aortic wall thickness and dimensions increase with increasing age. Autopsy studies confirm that older subjects without apparent cardiovascular disease have cardiac myocyte enlargement with a decrease in myocyte number due to apoptosis (programmed cell death). Myocardial collagen and elastin content

TABLE 3-1
AGE-ASSOCIATED STRUCTURAL CHANGES IN THE CARDIOVASCULAR SYSTEM

Structural	Age-Associated Change	Structural	Age-Associated Change
LV wall thickness	→ Increased	Large arteries	→ Dilate
Myocyte size	→ Increased	Arterial intima	→ Thickened
Myocyte number	→ Decreased	Arterial collagen	→ Increased
Myocardial collagen/elastin	→ Increased	SAN pacemaker cells	→ Decreased

KEY: LV = left ventricle; SAN = sinus node.

also increase with aging; this is notable also in the conduction system, with a resultant decrease in the number of pacemaker cells in the sinus node.

RESTING CARDIOVASCULAR FUNCTION

Resting left ventricular early diastolic filling declines linearly with increasing age (Table 3-2). Decreased left ventricular relaxation and the increase in collagen within the left ventricle likely contribute to this decline. The decline in early left ventricular filling is compensated by an augmented left atrial contraction, such that resting left ventricular end-diastolic volume index does not change with increasing age. Resting end-systolic volume and stroke volume indices are also unchanged with increasing age. Heart rate is also unrelated to age; thus, cardiac index and ejection fraction at rest do not change in older healthy subjects as compared with younger subjects.

The vascular load on the heart has four components, all of which change with aging: conduit artery compliance, reflected waves, inertance, and resistance. The age-associated increase in collagen and fragmentation in elastin in large arteries result in a decrease in conduit artery compliance in healthy elderly subjects. One manifestation of this increased stiffness (the inverse of compliance) is an increase in arterial pulse-wave velocity, resulting in reflected waves reaching the left ventricle in late systole, thus increasing systolic blood pressure. An important blood pressure change in healthy elderly is an increase in systolic blood pressure and a decline in diastolic blood pressure, resulting in large increases in pulse pressure. Systemic vascular resistance also increases with increasing age. Finally, inertance, which is determined by the mass of blood in the large arteries that requires acceleration, also increases with aging due to enlargement of the aorta.

The increase in arterial stiffness is matched by an increase in left ventricular stiffness, such that resting ventricular-vascular coupling remains unchanged in healthy older subjects. A consequence of an increase in ventricular stiffness is that older subjects are more preload-sensitive than younger subjects, with greater increases and decreases of systolic blood pressure for changes in left ventricular end-diastolic volume.

EXERCISE CARDIOVASCULAR FUNCTION

Aerobic capacity declines 50 percent from the second to eight decades due to an age-associated decline in both oxygen utilization and

TABLE 3-2

AGE-ASSOCIATED CHANGES IN RESTING SUPINE CARDIOVASCULAR FUNCTION

Cardiac Function	Age-Associated Change	Vascular Function	Age-Associated Change
Early diastolic filling	→ Decreased	Arterial compliance	→ Decreased
Atrial contraction	→ Increased	Aortic pulse-wave velocity	→ Increased
Cardiac volumes	→ Unchanged	Reflected waves	→ Early
Heart rate	→ Unchanged	Systemic vascular resistance	→ Increased
Cardiac index	→ Unchanged	Systolic blood pressure	→ Increased
Ejection fraction	→ Unchanged	Pulse pressure	→ Increased
Ventricular-vascular coupling	→ Unchanged	Inertance	→ Increased

TABLE 3-3

AGE-ASSOCIATED CHANGES IN MAXIMAL EXERCISE
CARDIOVASCULAR FUNCTION

Cardiac Function	Age-Associated Change	Cardiac Function	Age-Associated Change
EDVI	$\longrightarrow$ Increased	SVI	$\longrightarrow$ Unchanged
ESVI	$\longrightarrow$ Increased	Cardiac index	$\longrightarrow$ Decreased
Heart rate	$\longrightarrow$ Decreased	Ejection fraction	$\longrightarrow$ Decreased

KEY: EDVI = end-diastolic volume index; ESVI = end-systolic volume index; SVI = stroke volume index.

cardiac index. The age-associated changes in cardiovascular function during exercise are listed in Table 3-3. Peak exercise end-diastolic volume and end-systolic volume indices rise linearly with increasing age. In young healthy subjects, the end-systolic volume index progressively declines from rest to increasing levels of exercise. By contrast, older subjects have a much smaller decline in end-systolic volume index from rest to peak exercise but utilize the Frank-Starling mechanism to augment exercise stroke volume. These volume changes cause an age-associated decline in maximal exercise ejection fraction. Maximal exercise heart rate declines by about one-third from the second to eighth decades, resulting in an age-associated decline in peak cardiac index.

These age-associated changes in the cardiovascular response to exercise likely result from a change in the inotropic state, an increase in afterload, and a decrease in the β-adrenergic response. Critical among these is the decrease in the beta-adrenergic response, due to a decline in the efficiency of postsynaptic beta-adrenergic signaling. Supporting this latter view is the fact that acute beta-adrenergic blockade changes the exercise hemodynamic profile of younger persons to resemble that of older ones. Physical deconditioning also contributes to the age-associated decline in aerobic capacity. Moderate aerobic training in sedentary elderly subjects increases peak oxygen consumption, improves peak exercise ejection fraction, and increases arterial compliance.

ISCHEMIC HEART DISEASE IN THE ELDERLY

Sixty percent of myocardial infarctions occur in patients above 65 years of age and one-third of all infarcts occur in those older than 75 years (see also Chaps. 13–15). Eighty percent of all infarct-related mortality occurs in patients over 65 years and 60 percent in those greater than 75 years of age. In unstable angina and non-Q-wave infarction cohorts and in patients suffering a Q-wave myocardial infarction, age is the most important demographic predictor of short- and long-term mortality. Table 3-4 shows some of the common features of ST-segment elevation myocardial infarction in the elderly.

Even in older patients with a first ST-segment elevation myocardial infarction and who are thrombolytic eligible, the in-hospital morbidity and mortality is much greater than in younger patients. This is true despite the fact that indices of infarct size, such as creatinine phosphokinase levels and QRS scores, do not change with age. The incidence of heart failure and cardiogenic shock is three- to four-fold greater among the elderly than among younger infarct patients. Their age-associated decreased left ventricular filling, aortic compliance, and beta-adrenergic responsiveness may contribute to the high incidence of these complications in the elderly.

Thrombolytic therapy reduces mortality in subjects aged 65 to 75 in both randomized and observational trials. There is less agreement about the benefits of thrombolytic therapy given to otherwise eligible patients greater than 75 years of age with ST-segment elevation infarction. In high-volume centers, direct percutaneous coronary interventions (PCI) appear to be a reasonable alternative in this age group.

Like younger patients, older patients have large reductions in morbidity and mortality with appropriate postinfarction therapy, including beta-adrenergic receptor blockers, lipid-lowering agents, angiotensin-converting enzyme (ACE) inhibitors, and aspirin. In spite of randomized, placebo-controlled trials and observational trials supporting the use of these agents in the older postinfarct patient, these drugs are underutilized in this age group.

The use of PCI and coronary artery bypass (CAB) surgery has increased in older patients with chronic coronary artery disease over the last 10 to 20 years. Although short- and long-term mortality is greater among the very elderly than in younger subjects, mortality in this group with revascularization procedures has declined and procedural success improved over the last decade. Increasing age is a significant predictor of mortality and stroke during CAB surgery. Although lipid-lowering therapy benefits older patients with chronic coronary artery disease, hormone replacement therapy does not reduce events in postmenopausal women.

TABLE 3-4

FEATURES AND TREATMENT OF ST-SEGMENT ELEVATION MYOCARDIAL INFARCTION IN THE ELDERLY

Feature	Age-Associated Change	Treatment	Result
Complications	→ Shock, CHF, rupture, death	Thrombolytics	Lifesaving for 65- to 75-yo patients; controversial in those >75 yo
Prior symptoms	→ Angina	Direct angioplasty	Lifesaving in high-volume centers
Symptoms	More often atypical	Beta blockers	Lifesaving
Unrecognized	≈ $\frac{1}{2}$	Aspirin	Lifesaving
Recurrent ischemia	More frequent	ACE inhibitors	Lifesaving
Gender	Female	Lipid lowering	Reduces recurrent events

KEY: MI = myocardial infarction; yo = year(s) old; ACE = angiotensin-converting enzyme inhibitor; CHF = congestive heart failure.

CONGESTIVE HEART FAILURE IN THE ELDERLY

The prevalence of congestive heart failure is dramatically increasing. As older patients live longer with chronic coronary artery disease, hypertension, valvular heart disease, and post–myocardial infarction, congestive heart failure is epidemic in this population. Congestive heart failure is a lethal diagnosis in the elderly as well as a leading cause of recurrent hospital admissions (see also Chap. 4). It is likely that the age-associated decreased left ventricular filling, decreased beta-adrenergic response, and increased vascular load make the burden of left ventricular damage greater in the older patient.

Older patients with newly diagnosed heart failure symptoms need careful evaluation, including a noninvasive study to determine whether the primary problem is systolic dysfunction. Up to 40 percent of older individuals with heart failure have normal systolic function. Patients need careful evaluation for ischemic and hypertensive disease, which frequently leads to congestive heart failure in this age group. In patients with systolic dysfunction, angiotensin converting enzyme inhibitors are the cornerstone of therapy. Diuretics usually improve symptoms, and recent studies suggest that beta-blocker therapy as well as aldosterone inhibitors reduce morbidity and mortality in patients with systolic dysfunction and heart failure despite standard treatment. This observation probably extends to the older population.

HYPERTENSION IN THE ELDERLY

Hypertension is extremely common in the elderly, particularly isolated systolic hypertension (see also Chap. 18). The increased arterial stiffness that occurs with aging likely contributes to the high frequency of isolated systolic hypertension in the elderly. Elevated pulse pressure is a powerful predictor of coronary artery disease, heart failure, and mortality in this age group. Numerous randomized, placebo-controlled trials have shown that therapy with thiazide diuretics and dihydropyridine calcium channel blockers reduce stroke and cardiovascular events in the elderly hypertensive subject. Nonpharmacologic therapies—including restricted sodium intake, weight reduction, and exercise—are efficacious in many older hypertensives. The selection of an individual antihypertensive agent should be based on data from randomized trials while also tailoring therapy to associated comorbidities that are common in the elderly, including coronary artery disease, congestive heart failure, diabetes, and renal insufficiency.

AORTIC STENOSIS IN THE ELDERLY

Calcific aortic stenosis is by far the most frequent clinically significant valvular abnormality afflicting the elderly (see also Chap. 22).
The development of clinically significant aortic stenosis may be
rapid in this age group (months to several years). The predictors
of rapid progression to symptoms or death in the elderly with initially asymptomatic calcific aortic stenosis include a heavily calcified
valve and rapid yearly progression of the echocardiographic Doppler
gradient across the aortic valve. This noninvasive technique is the
most helpful study to detect aortic stenosis. Asymptomatic older patients require careful follow-up for the development of symptoms,
including angina, syncope, and heart failure. Aortic valve replacement often results in marked improvement in symptoms and survival, even in the very elderly. Age itself should not be an exclusion
for valve replacement; and other surgical risk factors—including
low ejection fraction, atrial fibrillation, need for coronary artery
bypass grafting, and a small-sized aortic root—need be taken into
consideration.

For elderly patients requiring valve replacement, the choice of
a mechanical valve with the bleeding risk of lifelong anticoagulation must be balanced against the risk of structural deterioration
and need for repeat surgery with a bioprosthetic valve. Considerations include age of the patient, anticoagulation risk, and valve position, with mitral bioprosthetic valves deteriorating at a higher rate
than bioprosthetic valves in the aortic position (see also Chaps. 26
and 27).

ATRIAL FIBRILLATION IN THE ELDERLY

As a result of an increased frequency of hypertensive and coronary
heart disease plus age-associated loss of pacemaker and conduct-
ing cells with fibrosis, atrial fibrillation and sick sinus syndrome
are common arrhythmias in the elderly. In an older population, approximately 5 to 6 percent of subjects have atrial fibrillation. Older
subjects are more likely to experience symptoms of heart failure with
atrial fibrillation, probably because of the age-associated decrease in
early diastolic filling and increased dependence on atrial contraction. The risk of embolic stroke in atrial fibrillation is also increased
with age; several large randomized studies involving patients with
a mean age of 69 years show that chronic anticoagulation reduces
stroke risk. Careful monitoring is needed to reduce the risk of intracranial hemorrhage with anticoagulation in the elderly (see also
Chap. 5).

SUGGESTED READING

Aviolio AP, Fa-Quan D, Wei-Qiang L, et al: Effects of aging on ar-
    terial distensibility in populations with high and low prevalence
    of hypertension: Comparison between urban and rural commu-
    nities in China. *Circulation* 1985; 71:202–210.

Fleg JL, O'Connor F, Gerstenblith G, et al: Impact of age on the
    cardiovascular response to upright exercise in healthy men and
    women. *J Appl Physiol* 1995; 78:890–900.

Franklin SS, Gustin W IV, Wong ND, et al: Hemodynamic pat-
    terns of age-related changes in blood pressure. *Circulation* 1997;
    96:308–315.

Lakatta EG. Cardiovascular regulatory mechanisms in advanced age.
    Physiol Rev 1993; 73:413–467.

Lakatta EG, Schulman SP, Gerstenblith G: Cardiovascular aging in
    health and therapeutic considerations with respect to cardiovas-
    cular diseases. In: Fuster F, Alexander RW, O'Rourke R, et al
    (eds): *Hurst's The Heart,* 10th ed. New York: McGraw-Hill;
    2001:2329–2355.

White HD, Barbash GI, Califf RM, et al: Age and outcome with
    contemporary thrombolytic therapy. Results from the GUSTO-I
    trial. *Circulation* 1996; 94:1826–1833.

CHAPTER

4

DIAGNOSIS AND MANAGEMENT OF HEART FAILURE

Thierry H. LeJemtel
Edmund H. Sonnenblick
William H. Frishman

Chronic heart failure is a syndrome that evolves from damage to the myocardium resulting in significant reduction in left ventricular (LV) function, whether from a persistent overload, such as hypertension, or loss of myocardium, as may occur from a myocardial infarction or myocarditis.

PATHOPHYSIOLOGY

With mild LV damage, repair and adaptations (remodeling) occur, including hypertrophy, and—if this is inadequate—modest LV dilatation. Hence, LV performance may be adequate to meet metabolic needs and the symptoms associated with limited pump capacity; i.e. exertional fatigue and dyspnea are absent. When extensive LV damage substantially reduces the capacity of the left ventricle to eject blood, heart failure is referred to as systolic. LV filling pressure rises, causing pulmonary congestion, further limiting cardiac output. Thus, systolic heart failure is characterized by an increasing end-diastolic volume (EDV) with initially a sustained stroke volume (SV), resulting in a reduced LV ejection fraction (EF). Increased EDV helps maintain SV by the Frank-Starling effect, but at the cost of elevated LV filling pressure. Further, LV dilatation begets LV dilatation, with stretch-induced myocyte death and an increasing amount of mitral regurgitation.

Pulmonary congestion may also result from elevated LV filling pressure without LV dilatation or reduced LVEF, a clinical entity commonly referred as chronic heart failure with preserved LV systolic function, or diastolic heart failure. Diastolic heart failure occurs when the LV wall is thickened due to systemic hypertension or hypertrophic cardiomyopathy or also becomes fibrotic with an increased amount of collagen. Symptoms of diastolic heart failure are often triggered or exacerbated by tachycardia due to atrial fibrillation, which results in loss of atrial contraction and reduction in the time for diastolic ventricular filling, further impeding LV filling.

The process of ventricular remodeling commonly proceeds over months to years without symptoms, although LV enlargement continues to progress. Recurrent myocardial damage, such as reinfarction or further myocyte loss, may hasten the process. Modest activation of the sympathetic nervous system occurs early, with concomitant decreased parasympathetic tone as the process ensues.

Eventually the marked elevation of LV filling pressure during exertion results in shortness of breath and a limited cardiac output, leading to exercise intolerance and fatigue. At this point, several months to years after initial myocardial damage has occurred, the symptomatic phase of the syndrome, referred to as congestive heart failure (CHF), ensues. Local cytokine and neurohormonal activation accompanies initial myocardial damage and progresses to accelerate the remodeling process by increasing damage to the myocardium. Systemic activation of the sympathetic and renin-angiotensin-aldosterone system (RAAS) occurs at some variable point in time. Systemic activation results in renal vasoconstriction, increased aldosterone secretion, sodium accumulation, and peripheral edema. Loop diuretic therapy leads to further RAAS activation.

DIAGNOSIS

The diagnosis of heart failure at the asymptomatic phase of the syndrome may be suggested by an enlarged heart on chest film; a definitive diagnosis depends on cardiac imaging by echocardiography, nuclear medicine, or left ventriculography during cardiac catheterization. The need to image the heart in patients with vascular and metabolic diseases such as hypertension, peripheral or coronary atherosclerosis, diabetes mellitus, and dyslipidemias cannot be overstated. Further, in view of the difficulty in obtaining an adequate cardiac examination in many patients with chronic lung disease, the diagnosis often relies heavily on cardiac imaging studies and/or therapeutic response to cardiac medications.

At the symptomatic phase of heart failure, physical examination is more fruitful, often detecting the presence of pulmonary rales on inspiration that do not clear after cough, a displaced and weak LV maximal impulse, an S_3 reflecting LV dilatation, and an S_4 reflecting LV hypertrophy (see also Chap. 1). Jugular vein distension, an enlarged liver that is tender at palpation with hepatojugular reflux, a murmur of tricuspid regurgitation, and pitting or peripheral edema suggest the presence of biventricular failure due to elevated pulmonary artery pressure. Overall, the severity of symptoms does not parallel the magnitude of LV systolic dysfunction as reflected by LV ejection fraction (EF). The severity of symptoms reflects the development and progression of vascular and metabolic abnormalities in skeletal muscles that are in part secondary to a deconditioned state. It is difficult to differentiate LV systolic from diastolic dysfunction by physical examination. A markedly elevated systolic blood pressure, a loud S_4, and accentuated A_2 and a sustained non-displaced maximal LV impulse favor diastolic dysfunction. However, these clinical findings are often not evident and, as a rule, a definite diagnosis of systolic versus diastolic heart failure is made by 2D Doppler echocardiography (see also Chap. 1). The primary target of therapy depends on the presence or absence of symptoms.

Treatment of Patients with LV Systolic Dysfunction in the Absence of Symptoms

At the so-called asymptomatic phase of CHF, the major aim is to prevent, attenuate, or even reverse LV dilatation and hypertrophy. The first step for controlling LV remodeling is to vigorously treat the cardiovascular and metabolic conditions that lead initially to CHF. Vigorous control of hypertension, diabetes mellitus, and dyslipidemias, as well as optimal treatment of coronary artery disease, is essential.

Angiotensin-Converting Enzyme Inhibition

The impressive results of the Heart Outcomes Prevention Evaluation (HOPE) trial now mandate long-term angiotensin-converting enzyme (ACE) inhibition in the medical regimens of most patients with high-risk vascular disease or diabetes mellitus. Absolute contraindications to ACE inhibitors are few. They include bilateral renal artery stenosis, pregnancy, and previously documented angioedema. Moderate chronic renal insufficiency as evidenced by serum creatinine <3.5 mg/dL does not preclude the use of ACE inhibitors but points out the need to closely monitor renal function at the initiation of therapy, especially in diabetic patients with class IV renal tubular acidosis. Patients who cannot tolerate ACE inhibition due to cough or angiodema are likely to benefit from angiotensin II type 1 receptor blockade (ARB), although definite evidence is not yet available (Table 4-1). Of note, intolerance to ACE inhibitors due to symptomatic hypotension, hyperkalemia, and worsening renal function is

TABLE 4-1
SOME CLINICAL TRIALS WITH ANGIOTENSIN-RECEPTOR BLOCKADE IN HEART FAILURE

Trial	Number of Patients	Drugs Studied	Primary Endpoints/Results
CHARM[a] ELITE II	6500 3152	Candesartan vs. placebo Losartan vs. captopril	Mortality and morbidity (in progress) Captopril better than losartan in reduction of all-cause mortality; losartan better than captopril in continuation of treatment.
RESOLVD	768	Candesartan alone, candesartan + enalapril, enalapril alone	Combination better for preventing LV remodeling than either drug alone; study terminated prematurely because of possible increase in number of events in patients treated with candesartan
Val-HeFT[a]	5000	Valsartan vs. placebo	Time to death; time to first significant medical event related to chronic heart failure (in progress)

[a]No results are given for CHARM or Val-HeFT; only endpoints are listed.

52

highly dependent on the experience of the physician. Fifty percent of patients referred to specialized heart failure centers for intolerance to ACE inhibition end up being treated with ACE inhibitors. For example, symptomatic hypotension is often caused by intravascular volume depletion that, in turn, is due to excessive diuretic therapy. Temporarily withdrawing loop-diuretics and resuming at lower doses often alleviates symptomatic hypotension. The list of ACE inhibitors approved by the U.S. Food and Drug Administration (FDA) for various indications is detailed in Table 4-2. It is presently unclear whether all ACE inhibitors exert similar therapeutic properties, a phenomenon often referred to as "class effect." ACE inhibitors with high sensitivity for tissue ACE, such as ramipril, quinapril, and perindopril, appear to offer additional vascular benefits over those with low tissue ACE sensitivity. However, a direct comparison of the vascular effects of tissue-specific and tissue-nonspecific ACE inhibitors is not presently available. Independent from the issues related to the selection of a given ACE inhibitor, present wisdom strongly suggests that the dose of the selected ACE inhibitor should be increased to that maximally tolerated or recommended. In any event, the dose should be at least equal to that administered in relevant large trials showing positive outcomes.

Beta-Adrenergic Blockade

Beta-adrenergic blockade must be initiated as soon as LV dilatation is detected by cardiac imaging. Currently beta-adrenergic blockade is approved by the FDA for postmyocardial infarction patients independent of the presence or absence of heart failure and for the treatment of CHF in patients with LV systolic dysfunction and symptoms compatible with functional class II–III of the New York Heart Association (NYHA). In view of the unique effect of beta-adrenergic blockade on LV remodeling, all patients with enlarging LVs should receive this pharmacologic intervention independent of the presence or absence of symptoms of coronary artery disease. Long-term beta-adrenergic blockade improves LVEF while reducing LV end-diastolic and systolic volumes. This is the only pharmacologic intervention that thus far reverses LV dilatation. Not uncommonly, LV volumes and function return toward normal values. Beta-adrenergic blockade with selective beta$_1$ antagonists such as metoprolol and bisoprolol and nonselective beta antagonist such as carvedilol lowers mortality by 35 to 40 percent and reduces morbidity in patients with symptomatic CHF (Table 4-3). Whether selective or nonselective beta-adrenergic blockade is preferable in patients with CHF is presently unknown. This issue may be settled by the results of the ongoing Carvedilol or Metoprolol Evaluation Trial (COMET), which compares the effects

TABLE 4-2
FDA-APPROVED INDICATIONS FOR ACE INHIBITORS

ACE Inhibitor	Hypertension	CHF	Acute MI	LV Dysfunction	Diabetic Nephropathy
Benazepril	+				
Captopril	+	+		+[a]	+
Enalapril	+	+		+[b]	
Fosinopril	+	+			
Lisinopril	+	+	+		
Perindopril	+				
Quinapril	+	+[c]			
Ramipril	+	+[d]			
Trandolapril				+[d]	

[a]Captopril is indicated in clinically stable patients with left ventricular (LV) dysfunction (ejection fraction ≤40%) after myocardial infarction (MI), to improve survival and to reduce the incidence of overt heart failure.

[b]Enalapril is indicated in clinically stable asymptomatic patients with LV dysfunction (ejection fraction ≤35%) to decrease the rate of development of overt heart failure and to decrease the incidence of hospitalization due to congestive heart failure (CHF).

[c]Ramipril is indicated in stable patients who have demonstrated clinical signs of CHF within the first few days after sustaining acute MI, to decrease mortality and progression to severe heart failure.

[d]Trandolapril is indicated for treatment of heart failure after MI and of LV dysfunction after MI.

SOURCE: Reproduced with permission from Cheng A, Frishman WH: Use of angiotensin converting enzyme inhibitors as monotherapy and in combination with diuretics and calcium channel blockers. *J Clin Pharm* 1998; 38:477–491

54

TABLE 4-3

BETA-BLOCKER MORTALITY TRIALS IN PATIENTS WITH CONGESTIVE HEART FAILURE

Trial	Number of Patients	Drug(s)	NYHA Class	EF (%)	Mean Follow-up (months)	Progress
CIBIS II	2647	Bisoprolol	III–IV	≤35	17	Benefit
MERIT-HF	3991	Metoprolol XL	II–IV	≤40	12	Benefit
COPERNICUS	2000	Carvedilol[a]	IIIb–IV	≤25	36	Benefit
COMET	3073	Carvedilol/metoprolol	II–IV	≤35	36	In follow-up

[a]Carvedilol is already approved for use in patients with class II and III heart failure.

KEY: NYHA = New York Heart Association; EF = ejection fraction; CIBIS = Cardiac Insufficiency Bisoprolol Study; MERIT-HF = Metoprolol CR/XL Randomized Intervention Trial in Heart Failure; COPERNICUS = Carvedilol Prospective Randomized Cumulative Survival Trial; COMET = Carvedilol or Metoprolol Evaluation Trial.

SOURCE: Adapted from *Internal Medicine World Report*, ACC Symposium Issue, April 1999; 14:4. Medical World Business Press, Inc.

of carvedilol and metropolol on mortality in patients with CHF. Of note, LVEF is reduced below baseline value during the first 4 weeks that follow initiation of beta-adrenergic blockade, even when this therapy is initiated at a low dose. Tolerability is highly dependent on the level of cardiac reserve and severity of baseline symptoms. The admonition "start low and go slow" is appropriate. Beta-adrenergic blockade is extremely well tolerated by clinically stable patients with moderate to severe reduction in LV systolic function and moderate symptoms. Ease of initiation is somewhat less, but tolerability is still very high in stable patients with severe LV systolic dysfunction and symptoms compatible with true functional class IV (NYHA). Thus, severe but stable CHF does not contraindicate beta-adrenergic blockade. However, initiation of beta-adrenergic blockade in patients with severe CHF always requires close monitoring and occasionally an increase in the dose of diuretics for a few days. Beta-adrenergic blocking agents that have vasodilating properties, such as carvedilol, are preferable in patients with severe LV systolic dysfunction and little cardiac reserve. Beta-adrenergic blockade should not be attempted in unstable, ambulatory patients with CHF and especially not in patients hospitalized for decompensated heart failure.

Treatment of LV Dysfunction Associated with Symptoms

Until the late stages of the syndrome, symptoms related to heart failure are characteristically related to exertion. The time course of symptoms is different in patients with systolic and diastolic heart failure. Symptoms are exacerbated during an episode of decompensation in patients with systolic heart failure, and they persist once the episode of decompensation has resolved, even if more manageable. Thus, constant therapy is needed. In fact, noncompliance to medications and diet is by far the most frequent cause of hospitalization in patients with systolic heart failure. Symptoms are mostly paroxysmal in nature in patients with diastolic heart failure and are often triggered by poorly controlled hypertension, rapid atrial fibrillation, myocardial ischemia, or excessive sodium intake. Aside from paroxysmal episodes, patients with diastolic heart failure may not experience symptoms. Chronic therapy is often not needed or even harmful when the doses of medications are not reduced after the acute episode.

Diuretics

The presence of symptoms—such as ankle edema, exertional dyspnea, and fatigue—mandates treatment with loop diuretics in patients with CHF, either by intravenous or oral administration depending on the severity of symptoms. If patients are already treated with ACE inhibitors, this therapy should be continued. If the patient is not receiving ACE inhibition, this therapy should be rapidly initiated while the patient is still somewhat volume-overloaded. The dose of loop diuretics should be tailored according to renal function and previous diuretic therapy when relevant. Overall, the aim of therapy is to promote a diuresis that amounts to a weight loss of 3 to 5 lb/day. Electrolytes must be closely monitored and potassium supplemented in order to maintain serum potassium above 4 meq/L. Contrary to widespread belief, borderline systolic blood pressure does not contraindicate the use of loop diuretics in patients with clinically overt pulmonary congestion. When patients with overt fluid overload do not respond to oral administration of loop diuretics, intravenous administration, including repeated boluses or continuous intravenous administration, is recommended. The combination of metolazone and loop diuretics is often successful. A poor response to loop diuretic therapy, especially in the absence of overt pulmonary congestion, should always raise the question of the need for this therapy.

Digitalis Glycosides and Aldosterone Receptor Antagonism

Other pharmacologic modalities for the treatment of symptomatic CHF include digitalis glycosides and aldosterone receptor antagonists. Digitalis glycosides are recommended for the treatment of patients with heart failure due to LV systolic dysfunction who have symptoms compatible with functional class III–IV (NYHA). Digitalis glycosides act centrally to reduce sympathetic tone and increase parasympathetic tone. When atrial fibrillation is present, digitalis glycosides are useful in controlling heart rate, especially with the concomitant judicious use of beta-blocking agents. The effect of increasing myocardial contractility tends to be modest. Measurement of serum digoxin levels is helpful for preventing overdose and toxicity, especially in patients treated with amiodarone, verapamil, or quinidine. Serum digoxin levels should be kept around 1 ng/mL to optimize the risk:benefit ratio.

In view of the impressive results of the Randomized Aldactone Evaluation Study (RALES), aldosterone-receptor blockade with aldactone is usually recommended for patients with severely symptomatic CHF. Mortality was reduced by 39 percent in patients randomized to aldactone as compared with that of patients randomized to placebo. Of note, episodes of hyperkalemia occur more frequently than initially reported by the RALES investigators, and serum potassium levels must be monitored.

UNRESOLVED ISSUES

Several issues are unresolved regarding the treatment of severely symptomatic patients with CHF due to LV systolic dysfunction:

1. Whether temporary positive inotropic support with dobutamine or milrinone is beneficial has never been proven in a placebo-controlled randomized trial. Ultimately, the preferred therapy of heart failure is prevention or limitation of primary damage with close attention to patients with risk factors that predispose to heart failure. In view of the symptomatic relief routinely observed with administration of dobutamine or milrinone in patients with severe heart failure, most heart failure experts are convinced of the efficacy of these agents and unwilling to randomize patients to placebo or inotropic support.

2. Whether beta-adrenergic blockade should be discontinued in patients hospitalized for severely decompensated CHF is also unknown. A pragmatic approach is to initiate temporary inotropic support with a specific phosphodiesterase inhibitor such as milrinone. When patients can be returned to their baseline state by temporary inotropic support with milrinone, beta-adrenergic blockade therapy should be continued. When patients do not improve despite inotropic support and intravenous loop diuretic therapy, beta-adrenergic therapy may have to be progressively withdrawn.

3. The treatment of patients with severe CHF with frequent episodes of asymptomatic nonsustained ventricular tachycardia is still not well codified. Present trends favor insertion of an implantable cardioverter/defibrillator (ICD) in patients with ischemic cardiomyopathy, while inducible ventricular tachycardia must be documented before insertion of an ICD in patients with nonischemic cardiomyopathy (see also Chap. 7).

SUGGESTED READING

Bristow MR: β-Adrenergic receptor blockade in chronic heart failure. *Circulation* 2000; 101:558–569.

Consensus Recommendations for the Management of Chronic Heart Failure. *Am J Cardiol* 1999; 83(2A).

Francis GS, Gassler JP, Sonnenblick EH: Pathophysiology and diagnosis of heart failure. In: Fuster V, Alexander RW, O'Rourke RA, et al (eds): *Hurst's The Heart*, 10th ed. New York: McGraw-Hill; 2001:655–685.

Frishman WH: Carvedilol. *N Engl J Med* 1998; 339:1759–1765.

Hunt SA, Frazier OH, with the technical assistance of Myers TJ: Mechanical circulatory support and cardiac transplantation. *Circulation* 1998; 97:2079–2090.

Hunt SA, Schroeder JS, Berry GJ: Cardiac transplantations, mechanical ventricular support, and endomyocardial biopsy; In: Fuster V, Alexander RW, O'Rourke RA, et al (eds): *Hurst The Heart*, 10th ed. New York: McGraw-Hill; 2001:725–747.

Lejemtel TH, Sonnenblick EH, Frishman WH: Diagnosis and management of heart failure, In: Fuster V, Alexander RW, O'Rourke RA, et al (eds): *Hurst's The Heart*, 10th ed. New York: McGraw-Hill; 2001:687–724.

The Heart Outcomes Prevention Evaluation Study Investigators: Effects of an angiotensin-converting-enzyme inhibitor, ramipril, on cardiovascular events in high-risk patients. *N Engl J Med* 2000; 342:145–153.

Vasan RS, Larson MG, Benjamin EJ, et al: Left ventricular dilatation and the risk of congestive heart failure in people without myocardial infarction. *N Engl J Med* 1997; 336:1350–1355.

ARRHYTHMIAS AND CONDUCTION DISTURBANCES

Jeffrey D. Simmons
Simon Chakko
Robert J. Myerburg

Effective management of cardiac arrhythmias and conduction disturbances requires accurate identification of the specific rhythm disturbances, analysis of the clinical settings in which they occur, and identification of a safe and effective endpoint of therapy. Clinical settings may be divided into those that cause acute and transient electrophysiologic abnormalities and those that are chronic and provide the substrate for persistent or recurrent arrhythmias. The former include acute ischemia, the acute phase of myocardial infarction, electrolyte abnormalities, and proarrhythmic drugs; the latter include chronic ischemic heart disease, cardiomyopathies, and the anatomic and physiologic substrate for the various supraventricular tachyarrhythmias. Arrhythmias may be aggravated by hemodynamic, electrolyte, metabolic, and respiratory abnormalities, which mandate correction for effective treatment. The treatment decision depends upon the presence and type of symptoms and the potential for morbidity and mortality. Some arrhythmias may produce bothersome symptoms but may not affect long-term prognosis, whereas other arrhythmias that cause few or no symptoms may portend a poor outcome.

PRINCIPLES OF RHYTHM ANALYSIS

The standard 12-lead electrocardiogram (ECG) and rhythm strips are the most easily accessible tools for the diagnosis of a cardiac rhythm disturbance. Recognition of the P wave and QRS morphology and their relative timing may be the only information needed for correct arrhythmia diagnosis. When the standard ECG does not provide enough information, special lead systems, such as a bipolar esophageal lead (to record left atrial activity) or an intraatrial electrode catheter (to record right atrial activity) may be used simultaneously with the standard ECG to help identify P waves and provide further information.

Continuous monitoring of cardiac rhythm at the bedside or with ambulatory recording devices with simultaneous two-lead recordings (lead II and MCL-1) can improve diagnostic yield. For infrequently occurring arrhythmias, patient- or observer-activated event recorders are used. These allow device activation when an event occurs and subsequent retrieval of the arrhythmia recording for physician review at a later time.

Exercise stress testing is useful for evaluating exercise-induced arrhythmias, particularly premature ventricular contractions (PVCs) and ventricular tachycardia; to diagnose ischemic heart disease; for sinus node or atrioventricular (AV) node dysfunction; and to evaluate for rate-dependent proarrhythmic effects of antiarrhythmic drugs. Stress testing also may be used to estimate the refractory period of the accessory pathway in patients with Wolff-Parkinson-White syndrome. Signal-averaged ECG measures terminal QRS low-amplitude signals using high-amplification techniques. These signals represent inhomogeneous activation of the left ventricular muscle mass. The absence of late potential after healing of myocardial infarction identifies a greater than 97 percent probability of remaining free of ventricular arrhythmias. However, the positive predictive value is poor.

Heart rate variability estimates the sympathetic and parasympathetic balance by measuring the variations in sinus rate from Holter (ambulatory ECG) recordings. Blunted heart rate variability is found in subgroups of myocardial infarction and cardiac arrest survivors who appear to be at increased risk for recurrent events.

Intracardiac electrophysiologic testing is used to diagnose arrhythmias and conduction disturbances when surface ECG is insufficient. Multielectrode catheters positioned in various intracardiac sites allow mapping of the sequence of activation in the atria, AV junction, and ventricle, permitting the localization of sites of anomalous pathways and the mechanism of supraventricular and ventricular tachyarrhythmias. In addition, the level of AV block can be identified during electrophysiologic testing.

Intraoperative mapping of both supraventricular and ventricular tachyarrhythmias may be performed using hand-held probes or specialized multielectrode arrays to identify areas for surgical ablation. Previously, the management of cardiac arrhythmias was limited to pharmacologic or surgical therapy. However, surgical mapping for most supraventricular arrhythmias and some forms of ventricular arrhythmias has largely been replaced by catheter mapping and ablation techniques performed in the electrophysiology laboratory.

Implantable devices are commonly used for long-term management of both tachyarrhythmic episodes and bradyarrhythmic events.

SUPRAVENTRICULAR ARRHYTHMIAS

Sinus Rhythm and Sinus Tachycardia

Normal sinus rhythm is defined as a rate of 60 to 100 beats per minute, originating in the sinus node; the rhythm is regular. *Sinus arrhythmia* is present when the variation between the longest and the shortest cycle on a resting tracing is above 0.12 s. This is a normal variant seen most commonly in children; it decreases with age.

Sinus tachycardia results from automatic discharge of the sino-atrial pacemaker cells at a rate that exceeds 100 beats per minute. It is characterized by normal sinus P waves at a rapid rate that usually does not exceed 130 to 140 beats per minute under resting conditions but can be as high as 180 to 200 beats per minute, particularly during exercise. Sinus tachycardia is a normal physiologic response to exercise or emotional stress or may be pharmacologically induced by such drugs as epinephrine, ephedrine, or atropine. Exposure to alcohol, caffeine, or nicotine can also cause sinus tachycardia. Persistence of sinus tachycardia usually signals an underlying disorder (such as heart failure, pulmonary embolism, hypovolemia, or hypermetabolic states). Vagotonic maneuvers, such as carotid sinus massage or Valsalva maneuver, may help differentiate sinus tachycardia from other supraventricular tachycardias (SVTs). Gradual slowing of the rapid rate followed by gradual return to that rate is typical for sinus tachycardia. In contrast, vagal maneuvers may abruptly terminate other SVTs by blocking conduction in the AV node. Sinus tachycardia usually requires no specific treatment; management should be directed toward the underlying disorder. When pharmacologic slowing of sinus tachycardia is desired, beta-adrenergic blocking agents often are effective. However, it must first be determined that the tachycardia is not a necessary compensatory response, as in heart failure.

Premature Atrial Impulses

Atrial extrasystoles or premature atrial contractions (PACs) are impulses that arise in an ectopic atrial focus and are premature in relation to the prevailing sinus rate. The early P wave has a different vector than the sinus P wave, and the PR interval of the conducted PAC may be normal or minimally prolonged but occasionally may be markedly prolonged. If the coupling interval of the PAC to the previous sinus P wave is short, aberrant intraventricular conduction may occur, making the diagnosis dependent on recognition of the

P wave distorting the previous T wave. The *hallmark* of timing of PACs is the less than fully compensatory pause; however, this may not always occur. The significance of atrial extrasystoles depends on the clinical setting in which they occur. Often they are found in completely normal individuals; however, they may be associated with myocardial ischemia, rheumatic heart disease, myopericarditis, congestive heart failure, and a variety of systemic abnormalities including acid-base/electrolyte disturbances and pulmonary diseases. Caffeine, tobacco, or alcohol use as well as emotional stress may initiate or exacerbate premature atrial contractions. Asymptomatic patients with no underlying heart disease require no treatment other than removal of the underlying or precipitating factors. If patients are symptomatic, beta-adrenergic blocking agents may provide relief. Both digitalis and verapamil have been tried, but their efficacy has not been proven.

Supraventricular Tachyarrhythmias

All tachyarrhythmias that originate above the bifurcation of the bundle of His are classified as supraventricular arrhythmias. The atrial rate must be 100 or more beats per minute for a diagnosis, but the ventricular rate may be less when AV conduction is incomplete. SVTs usually have narrow QRS configurations, but they may be wide because of aberrant conduction through the intraventricular conduction tissue, preexisting bundle branch block, or conduction via an accessory pathway. Atrial activity may be identified by using a long rhythm strip with multiple leads. Recording the rhythm strip at rapid paper speed (e.g., 50 mm/s) may be helpful. Other diagnostic aids include vagal maneuvers to slow the ventricular response rate or an esophageal lead to identify atrial activity. Intraatrial electrograms are occasionally required.

SVTs may be classified as *paroxysmal* (lasting seconds to hours), *persistent* (lasting days to weeks), or *chronic* (lasting weeks to years). Consideration not only of the duration of the tachyarrhythmia but also its electrophysiologic mechanism is essential to the appropriate management.

Paroxysmal SVT (PSVT) may occur in the presence or absence of heart disease and in patients of all ages. It is most often due to reentry involving the AV node or an accessory pathway; infrequently, sinus node reentry or intraatrial reentry is the mechanism.

SUPRAVENTRICULAR TACHYCARDIA DUE TO ATRIOVENTRICULAR NODAL REENTRY

AV nodal reentry is the most common mechanism of SVT and is characterized electrophysiologically by two functionally distinct pathways (slow and fast) within or near the AV node. In the common form of AV nodal reentrant tachycardia, antegrade conduction occurs over the slow pathway and retrograde conduction over the fast pathway, resulting in almost simultaneous activation of the atria and ventricles. Electrocardiographically, retrograde P waves are hidden within the QRS complex or appear immediately after it. In the uncommon form, in which antegrade conduction occurs over the fast pathway, the retrograde P wave occurs well after the end of the QRS complex and is characterized by a long R-P interval and a short PR interval with an inverted P wave in II, III, and AVG. In the absence of structural heart disease, PSVT due to AV nodal reentry is a benign rhythm and may be treated acutely with rest, sedation, and vagotonic maneuvers. If these physiologic interventions are unsuccessful, intravenous adenosine, intravenous calcium antagonists, digoxin, or beta-adrenergic blockers may be used (Table 5-1). Adenosine, 6 mg intravenously, followed by one or two

TABLE 5-1

DRUGS FOR ACUTE MANAGEMENT OF SUPRAVENTRICULAR TACHYCARDIA

Drug	Dosage
Adenosine	IV: 6 mg rapidly; if unsuccessful within 1–2 min, 12 mg rapidly
Diltiazem	IV: 0.25 mg/kg body wt over 2 min; if response inadequate, wait 15 min, then 0.35 mg/kg over 2 min; maintenance of 10–15 mg/h
Digoxin[a]	IV: 0.5 mg over 10 min; if response inadequate 0.25 mg q 4 h to a maximum of 1.5 mg in 24 h
Esmolol	IV: 500 μg/kg per min × 1 min followed by 50 μg/kg per min × 4 min, repeat with 50-μg increments to maintenance dose of 200 μg/kg/min
Procainamide	IV: 10–15 mg/kg at 25 mg/min as loading dose, then 1–4 mg/min
Propranolol	IV: 0.1 mg/kg in divided 1-mg doses
Verapamil	IV: 5 mg ovaer 1 min; if unsuccessful, 1–2 5-mg boluses 10 min apart

[a]Contraindicated in patients with Wolff-Parkinson-White syndrome.

TABLE 5-2
ANTIARRHYTHMIC DRUGS: DOSAGE AND KINETICS

Drug	Usual Dosing Range[a]	Half-Life, h	Therapeutic Range, μg/mL	Plasma Protein Binding, %	Major Route of Excretion
Class IA: Quinidine	Oral sulfate: 200–600 mg q 6 h; Oral long acting: 330–660 mg, q 8 h or q 6 h	5–7	2.3–5	80	H
Procainamide	Oral: 250–750 mg, q 4 h or q 6 h; Oral long acting: 500–1500 mg, q 8 h or q 6 h; IV: 10–15 mg/kg at 25 mg/min, then 1–6 mg/min	3–5	4–10	15	R[b]
Disopyramide	Oral: 100–200 mg q 8 h or q 6 h	8–9	2–5	35–95	H/R
Moricizine[c]	Oral: 150–300 mg q 12 h to q 8 h	6–13	—	95	H
Class IB: Lidocaine	IV: 1–3 mg/kg at 20–50 mg/min, then 1–4 mg/min	1–2	1–5	60	H
Tocainide	Oral: 400–600 mg 8–12 h	15	4–10	10	H
Mexiletine	Oral: 200–400 mg q 8 h	10–12	0.5–2.0	55	H
Class IC: Flecainide	Oral: 100–200 mg q 12 h	20	0.4–1.0	40	H
Encainide	Oral: 25–50 mg q 8 h	3–4+	0.5–1.0[d]	80	H
Propafenone[d]	Oral: 150–300 mg q 8 h	2–10	0.5–1.5[d]	95	H
Class II: Propranolol	Oral: 10–100 mg q 6 h; IV: 0.1 mg/kg in devided 1-mg doses	4–6	0.04–0.10	95	H
Esmolol	IV: 500 μg/kg per min × 1 min followed by 50 μg/kg per min × 4 min, repeat with 50-μg increments to maintenance dose to 200 μg/kg per min	9 min	—	55	H
Acebutolol	Oral: 200–600 mg bid	3–4	—	26	H/R

Class III: Amiodarone	Oral: 600–1600 mg/day × 1–3 weeks, then 200–400 mg/day; IV: 5 mg/min × min, then 1 mg/min × 6 h, then maintenance at 0.5 mg/min	50 days	96	1–2.5	H
Bretylium	IV: 5–10 mg/kg at 1–2 mg/kg, then 0.5–2.0 mg/min	8–14	?	?	R
Sotalol[d]	Oral: 80–320 mg q 12 h	10–15	0	0.5–1.5	R
Ibutilide	IV: (for >60 kg): 1 mg over 10 min, may repeat × 1 10 min after completion of initial dose[c]	2–12	40	—	H
Class IV: Verapamil	Oral: 80–320 mg q 6–8 h; IV: 5–10 mg in 1–2 min	3–8	90	0.1–0.15	H
Diltiazem	IV: 0.25 mg/kg body wt over 2 min; if response inadequate, wait 15 min, then 0.35 mg/kg over 2 min; maintenance 10–15 mg/h	3.5–5.0	70–80	0.1–3.0	H
Other: Digoxin	Oral: 1.25–1.5 mg in divided doses over 24 h followed by 0.125–0.375 mg/day; IV: Approximately 70% of oral dose	36	30	0.8–1.4 ng/mL	R
Adenosine	IV: 6 mg rapidly; if unsuccessful within 1–2 min, 12 mg rapidly	10s	—	—	—

[a] All dosing should follow FDA-approved guidelines as outlined in package insert or Physicians' Desk Reference. See also Chap. 45. Does not include pediatric use in infants and young children.

[b] Parent compound metabolized to active metabolite (NAPA) in liver; both active metabolite and unmetabolized parent compound excreted by kidneys.

[c] Shares classes IB, IC activities.

[d] Active metabolite limits significance of these measurements.

[e] Shares class II activity.

[f] D/C upon arrhythmia conversion or for ventricular or prolongation of QT or QT_c.

KEY: H = hepatic; R = renal.

12-mg boluses if necessary, has an extremely short half-life (10 s), causes no hemodynamic complications, and is the first choice for treatment of PSVT. Intravenous verapamil in a 5-mg bolus, followed by one or two additional 5-mg boluses 10 min apart if the initial bolus does not convert the arrhythmia, has been effective in up to 90 percent of patients. Intravenous diltiazem beginning with a bolus of 0.25 mg/kg over 2 min also is effective. If the response is not satisfactory, a repeat bolus of 0.35 mg/kg may be given after 15 min. Intravenous digoxin, 0.5 mg over 10 min, followed by an additional 0.25 mg every 4 h to a maximum dose of 1.5 mg in 24 h, may be used. Intravenous beta-adrenergic blockers such as propranolol or esmolol may be effective. Class IA antiarrhythmic agents occasionally may be effective if the other drugs fail (Table 5-2). Hemodynamic instability dictates immediate cardioversion; low-energy synchronized shocks (10 to 50 J) are usually sufficient. Rapid atrial pacing is an alternative if other methods fail or cardioversion should be avoided.

Although the QRS complexes usually are narrow in SVT due to AV nodal reentry, occasionally aberrant intraventricular conduction with resultant wide QRS complexes [patterns of either right bundle branch block (RBBB) or left bundle branch block (LBBB)] may occur. However, unless preexisting BBB or aberrant conduction has *clearly* been documented, a wide-QRS complex tachycardia should be assumed to be ventricular tachycardia. The use of verapamil for the treatment of a wide complex tachycardia on the *assumption* that it is a SVT with aberration may lead to severe hemodynamic compromise and even death if the arrhythmia has been incorrectly diagnosed. Low-energy cardioversion or class I antiarrhythmic agents are logical alternatives when the diagnosis of the arrhythmia is uncertain.

Long-term therapy for control of recurrent SVT due to AV nodal reentry is most frequently achieved today with either pharmacologic methods or catheter ablation techniques. No chronic therapy may be necessary in patients who have infrequent, short-lived, well-tolerated attacks and/or who respond to physiologic maneuvers. Patients who have more frequent attacks, who are intolerant to medications, and/or whose SVTs cause hemodynamic compromise are offered radiofrequency catheter ablation for curative therapy. Ablation of the common form of AV nodal reentry is achieved by selective ablation of the slow pathway to abolish the reentrant loop. Less commonly, ablation of the fast pathway will be performed, but the risk of iatrogenic heart block is higher. In either case, experience has demonstrated that this is a safe and effective technique for the management of AV nodal reentry.

Pharmacologic therapy is an alternative for patients who do not desire radiofrequency ablation or who have few, well-tolerated occurrences. Beta-adrenergic blocking agents, verapamil, or digoxin in standard doses may be used. In patients with no structural heart disease, class IC agents may be used (Table 5-2).

SUPRAVENTRICULAR TACHYCARDIA DUE TO WOLFF-PARKINSON-WHITE SYNDROME

This is the second most common form of reentrant SVT. When conduction during an SVT occurs antegrade through the AV node and retrograde via the accessory pathway, it is referred to as an *orthodromic* reciprocating tachycardia. This is the common form of SVT in Wolff-Parkinson-White (WPW) syndrome; the ECG pattern is a narrow QRS tachycardia at rates ranging from 160 to 240 per minute. Vagal maneuvers, adenosine, verapamil, diltiazem, propranolol, and the class IA antiarrhythmic agents may be used acutely to convert the arrhythmia. However, digoxin is contraindicated, since it may shorten the refractory period of the bypass tract and cause extremely rapid conduction across the bypass tract during atrial flutter (>250 beats per minute), leading to hemodynamic collapse or ventricular fibrillation. If the patient has a history of atrial fibrillation or flutter, verapamil should also be avoided, as it may accelerate the ventricular rate. *Antidromic* SVT, referring to retrograde conduction through the normal pathway and antegrade conduction via accessory pathway, is uncommon; the QRS complexes are wide and are similar to fully preexcited impulses during sinus rhythm or premature atrial contractions. Differentiation from ventricular tachycardia may be difficult.

Intracardiac electrophysiologic studies permit characterization of the accessory pathway and its associated tachyarrhythmias. Electrophysiologic testing is recommended for patients who have frequent or poorly tolerated tachyarrhythmias or a history of atrial fibrillation or atrial flutter (particularly with antegrade bypass tract conduction). Radiofrequency catheter ablation of the accessory pathway has revolutionized the treatment of SVT due to WPW syndrome, and today it is the preferred method. Intracardiac mapping utilizing multielectrode catheters allows for localization of the accessory pathway and subsequent application of radiofrequency energy to abolish the reentrant loop, preventing the recurrence of arrhythmias. Medical therapy with class IC agents may be used temporarily in patients without structural heart disease while the patient awaits ablative therapy or in patients who do not desire ablation. Class III agents (Table 5-2) are also effective, but not all are approved for this indication. The threshold for use of amiodarone should be high because of this side-effect profile. Surgical therapy currently is reserved for patients whose arrhythmias have not been amenable to catheter ablation.

Concealed WPW syndrome is an entity in which the accessory pathway is incapable of antegrade conduction. However, the ability to conduct retrograde across the bypass tract permits orthodromic SVT. There is little if any danger of atrial fibrillation degenerating to ventricular fibrillation in this instance. Class IC agents, calcium channel antagonists, and beta-adrenergic blocking agents may be utilized in patients with documented SVTs. Catheter ablation provides definitive, curative therapy.

OTHER REENTRANT SUPRAVENTRICULAR TACHYCARDIAS

Sinus node reentry or intraatrial reentry is distinguished electrocardiographically from SVT due to AV node reentry of WPW syndrome by the presence of P waves preceding the QRS complexes, with normal or short PR intervals. Nodoventricular pathways (Mahaim's tracts) may cause PSVT with wide QRS complexes having a LBBB pattern. There is no standard effective treatment for these SVTs; membrane-active antiarrhythmic agents, beta-adrenergic blockers, and calcium-channel antagonists have all been used. Radiofrequency catheter ablation is helpful in some instances. Intracardiac electrophysiologic studies may be required to optimize therapy in some patients.

ECTOPIC ATRIAL TACHYCARDIAS

These arrhythmias are characterized by an abnormal P-wave vector, a tendency to low P-wave amplitude, and rapid atrial rates (range, 160 to 240 beats per minute), although ectopic atrial rates in excess of 200 beats per minute usually are accompanied by 2:1 AV conduction. An ectopic atrial rhythm associated with a high-grade block and a relatively slow ventricular rate [so-called paroxysmal atrial tachycardia (PAT) with block] suggests digitalis intoxication.

Antiarrhythmic agents may provide effective treatment if no reversible cause can be found. Cardioversion is rarely helpful. Ectopic atrial tachycardias commonly have precipitating factors; therefore removal, reversal, or control of the inciting factors (e.g., digitalis intoxication, decompensated chronic obstructive pulmonary disease, electrolyte imbalance, metabolic abnormalities, hypoxia, thyrotoxicosis) is the primary therapy. In patients in whom no reversible cause can be identified, intracardiac localization of the arrhythmia's focus and subsequent radiofrequency ablation may be attempted.

MULTIFOCAL ATRIAL TACHYCARDIA

This tachycardia is identified electrocardiographically by three of more P-wave morphologies and a chaotic, irregular rhythm. The rate is usually <150 beats per minute. When the average rate is <100 beats per minute, it is not a tachycardia and is referred to as a chaotic or multifocal atrial *rhythm,* but the implications are similar.

It occurs most commonly in chronic lung disease but is also seen in patients with severe metabolic abnormalities or sepsis. Although calcium channel antagonists have been tried with some success, the most effective approach to therapy has been to correct the underlying hypoxia or other metabolic disturbance. There is no role for cardioversion, surgery, or catheter ablation.

ATRIAL FLUTTER

Atrial flutter is characterized electrocardiographically by broad, atrial deflections—"F" or flutter waves—which have a sawtooth configuration in leads II, III, and aV$_F$. There are two types of atrial flutter: type I, or classic, and type II. Type I flutter can be entrained and interrupted with atrial pacing techniques. It has an atrial rate of 280 to 320 per minute. Type II flutter has an atrial rate faster than 340 per minute and cannot be terminated by pacing. The usual atrioventricular conduction ratio is 2:1 or 4:1. However, partial treatment with antiarrhythmic drugs (especially class IC drugs) may slow the flutter rate to as low as 220 beats per minute, facilitating 1:1 conduction. The *paroxysmal* form of atrial flutter may rarely occur in healthy individuals or transiently in acute pulmonary embolism or thyrotoxicosis. Most commonly it is associated with some form of chronic heart disease, such as valvular disease, congenital heart disease, or cardiomyopathy.

Carotid sinus massage may slow the ventricular response, but it tends to increase the flutter rate; occasionally it will convert flutter to fibrillation and very rarely to sinus rhythm. The treatment of choice in hemodynamically compromising atrial flutter is low-energy (10 to 50 W/s) electrical cardioversion (Table 5-3). Otherwise treatment is directed first to controlling the ventricular rate with digoxin, verapamil, or diltiazem and then adding a class IA antiarrhythmic agent to convert the rhythm to sinus. Class IC antiarrhythmic agents are less effective in converting atrial flutter to sinus rhythm. If antiarrhythmic agents are unsuccessful, elective cardioversion is an alternative. Patients receiving digoxin who do not have signs of digoxin toxicity may safely undergo cardioversion with digoxin levels under 1.9 mg/mL.

Although recent studies using transesophageal echocardiography have demonstrated a significant incidence of thrombus in the left atrial appendage, an increased incidence of thromboembolic events after cardioversion has not been documented. Anticoagulation, therefore, is controversial. If cardioversion is contraindicated, rapid atrial pacing may convert the atrial flutter rate. A special pacemaker generator is required for overdrive pacing, and insertion of a right atrial catheter usually requires fluoroscopy. In the patient who has recently undergone open-heart surgery, atrial pacing wires are usually in place, and these may be used. Chronic control of recurrences of

TABLE 5-3

ENERGIES FOR EXTERNAL
CARDIOVERSION/DEFIBRILLATION

Atrial flutter	10–50 W/s (synchronized)
Atrial fibrillation	50–200 W/s (synchronized)
Supraventricular tachycardia	25–50 W/s (synchronized)
Ventricular tachycardia	50–200 W/s (synchronized, except for very rapid VT)
Ventricular fibrillation	200–360 W/s (asynchronized)
Torsades de pointes	Not indicated; use methods to increase HR, e.g., temporary external or transvenous pacing, isoproterenol $1\,\mu$g/min and titrate to increased HR (contraindicated in ischemia)

paroxysmal and persistent atrial flutter includes class IA antiarrhythmics or catheter ablation to prevent the arrhythmia and digitalis AV nodal blocking agents to control the ventricular response rate during recurrences. Class III agents, particularly amiodarone, also are effective. A new class III drug, intravenous ibutilide, has been reported to convert 63 percent of patients with atrial flutter, but it must be used under close monitoring, since it may prolong the QT interval acutely with the risk of short-term torsades de pointes. Radiofrequency catheter ablation should be considered for rhythm control of both paroxysmal and chronic forms of atrial flutter. Intracardiac catheter mapping confirms the location of the arrhythmia circuit, and the catheter ablation success rate approaches 90 percent. If drugs are ineffective or poorly tolerated for controlling ventricular response during recurrences, catheter ablation of the AV node offers a permanent solution. Permanent pacing is required, however, in most patients.

ATRIAL FIBRILLATION

Atrial fibrillation is characterized by disorganized atrial deflections and an irregular AV conduction sequence resulting in a grossly irregular pattern of the QRS complexes. Atrial fibrillatory waves are best seen in standard lead V_I and are usually evident in II, III, and aV_F. They may be large and coarse or fine to imperceptible. In the latter case, the grossly irregular ventricular rhythm suggests atrial fibrillation.

First Episode of Atrial Fibrillation   The first episode of atrial fibrillation requires a thorough clinical investigation to determine whether the arrhythmia is a primary electrical abnormality or secondary to an underlying cause. The incidence of atrial fibrillation increases with age and the presence of structural heart disease. Atrial fibrillation occurring in the absence of structural heart disease is called *lone atrial fibrillation.* Significant mitral or aortic valve disease, hypertension, coronary artery disease, cardiomyopathy, atrial septal defect, and myopericarditis are all disease processes frequently associated with atrial fibrillation. Pulmonary emboli and thyrotoxicosis are well-known causes of atrial fibrillation. Consumption of coffee, tobacco, or alcohol and extreme stress or fatigue also predispose to atrial fibrillation.

In the absence of organic heart disease or WPW syndrome, removal of precipitating factors and observation for recurrences are sufficient. In the presence of significant heart disease, however, therapy should be directed toward treatment of that particular cardiac abnormality; otherwise, recurrence, seen with pharmacologic therapy and/or electrical cardioversion, is high (Table 5-3). Cardioversion is warranted for the first episode of atrial fibrillation if the patient requires the benefit obtained from the hemodynamic contribution of atrial contraction (e.g., aortic stenosis) or slowing of the ventricular rate to prolong the diastolic filling period (e.g., mitral stenosis).

Paroxysmal Atrial Fibrillation   In the absence of underlying heart disease, rest, sedation, and treatment with digitalis is the treatment of choice for short paroxysms. Chronic therapy is based on the need to control the ventricular rate during recurrences and may be accomplished with digitalis, beta blockers, or calcium channel blockers, as described for atrial flutter.

In the presence of heart disease, the development of hemodynamic compromise or congestive heart failure (CHF) requires immediate reversion to sinus rhythm. Immediate cardioversion is mandatory to prevent or reverse the development of pulmonary edema when atrial fibrillation occurs in the presence of hemodynamically significant mitral or aortic stenosis. Direct-current countershock synchronized to the QRS complex using energies ranging from 100 W/s for the initial shock to 200 W/s for the second and subsequent shocks is the preferred method. If the patient is hemodynamically stable, the ventricular rate can be controlled with intravenous digoxin, beta blocker, or calcium channel antagonists. Digoxin is effective at rest but does not provide adequate rate control during exercise. Currently, intravenous verapamil or diltiazem is preferred because of their rapid onset of action and better rate control during exercise. The class IA antiarrhythmics—quinidine, procainamide, and disopyramide—are effective in chemically converting atrial fibrillation to sinus rhythm. Quinidine has been the most frequently used. Conventional dosing schedules (200 to 600 mg orally every 6 to 8 h) are now used—unlike the highly aggressive, potentially toxic quinidine protocols of the past. During attempted chemical cardioversion, careful monitoring of QT intervals for excessive prolongation (i.e., QTc 25 percent greater than QTc prior to initiation of treatment) should be performed in addition to monitoring of serum drug levels. The class IC agents (flecainide and propafenone) may convert atrial fibrillation to sinus rhythm when class IA agents have failed. They have also been useful for maintaining sinus rhythm. Intravenous formulations of these drugs are also effective but are not available in the United States. A new class III drug, intravenous ibutilide, has also been demonstrated to restore sinus rhythm in 31 percent of patients, but it must be used under close monitoring, since it may prolong the QT interval acutely, with the risk of short-term torsades de pointes.

Amiodarone, a class III agent, is effective for preventing recurrences of atrial fibrillation. The major limitation of amiodarone is its adverse side-effect profile and its extraordinarily long half-life, which limits flexibility in changing therapy. However, low doses of amiodarone (Cordarone) (200 to 300 mg daily) have been shown to decrease the adverse side effects significantly. Sotalol (Betapace), another class III agent, also may be useful in preventing recurrence of atrial fibrillation. In patients with atrial fibrillation refractory to all medical therapy and in whom the arrhythmia is accompanied by severe disabling symptoms due to tachycardia, catheter ablation adjacent to the His bundle to produce complete AV block is an alternative. However, because this often results in pacemaker dependency, the procedure should be used as a last resort for the control of ventricular rate during atrial fibrillation.

Persistent Atrial Fibrillation   If recurrent episodes of persistent atrial fibrillation (lasting days to weeks) are well tolerated hemodynamically, most physicians avoid repeated electrical cardioversions. This pattern of atrial fibrillation leads eventually to chronic atrial fibrillation; therefore, the best approach is control of ventricular rate during recurrences. Membrane-active antiarrhythmic agents may be used in an attempt to decrease the frequency of recurrences, but their efficacy is unpredictable and the risk of side effects is high. Prevention of episodes of atrial fibrillation may be achieved with class IA, IC, or III drugs. Efficacy is uneven and proarrhythmic or toxic adverse effects are of concern. In the absence of structural heart disease, class IC drugs may be used. Amiodarone, a class III agent, is also effective and is preferred in patients with cardiomyopathies. If symptoms during recurrences are disturbing enough, catheter ablation of the AV node should be considered.

Chronic Atrial Fibrillation   Pharmacologic or electrical cardioversion of chronic atrial fibrillation is indicated primarily if the patient will gain some hemodynamic benefit. Usually no more than one attempt at electrical cardioversion is warranted in the presence of adequate levels of a membrane-active antiarrhythmic agent, since the chance of long-term maintenance of sinus rhythm is very low if the patient reverts back to chronic atrial fibrillation after cardioversion. Management of the patient is then directed toward control of the ventricular response rate, as outlined above.

Anticoagulation of Patients with Atrial Fibrillation   The purpose of anticoagulation is to limit the morbidity and mortality from systemic and pulmonary embolization. The decision to initiate anticoagulation for atrial fibrillation depends on the balance between the relative risk of an embolic event versus the risk of a major bleeding complication secondary to anticoagulant therapy. Table 5-4 lists indications for anticoagulation in patients with atrial fibrillation. These same indications apply to elective cardioversion of recent-onset persistent atrial fibrillation and to chronic atrial fibrillation. Anticoagulation with warfarin (Coumadin) is begun 3 weeks before elective cardioversion and maintained for 4 weeks after cardioversion because of the higher risk of embolic phenomena in the early days after reversion to sinus rhythm. When anticoagulation is used, warfarin is given in doses sufficient to prolong the prothrombin time to an International Normalized Ratio (INR) of 2.0 to 3.0.

An alternative is earlier cardioversion of the patient with recent onset of atrial fibrillation and no evidence of atrial thrombus or transaesophageal echocardiography. The patient is started on warfarin and heparin, 24 to 48 h before cardioversion and continues on warfarin for 2 to 3 weeks after reversion to sinus rhythm.

ATRIOVENTRICULAR JUNCTIONAL AND ACCELERATED VENTRICULAR RHYTHMS

AV junctional rhythms originate within or just distal to the immediate vicinity of the AV node. This category includes premature AV junctional impulses, accelerated junctional rhythms, and AV junctional tachycardias that may be automatic or reentrant. Various forms of reentrant tachyarrhythmias that incorporate the AV junction as a part of a larger reentrant pathway are discussed in the section on PSVTs, above. In AV junctional rhythm, the impulse travels antegrade and retrograde at the same time from the AV junction and is characterized

TABLE 5-4

RISK OF STROKE AND GENERAL APPROACHES TO ANTICOAGULATION IN ATRIAL FIBRILLATION

Age Group %	Risk Factors[a]	Annual Event Rate if Untreated (95% Confidence Intervals)	Recommendation
<65	Absent	1.0 (0.3–3.1)	Aspirin or no therapy
	Present	4.9 (3.0–8.1)	Warfarin
65–75	Absent	4.3 (2.7–7.1)	Warfarin (aspirin)
	Present	5.7 (3.9–8.3)	Warfarin
>75	Absent	3.5 (1.6–7.7)	Warfarin
	Present	8.1 (4.7–13.9)	Warfarin

[a] Presence of one or more of the following features: previous stroke or transient ischemic attack, hypertension, heart failure (HTN), coronary artery disease (CAD), prosthetic heart valve or hyperthyroidism.

NOTE: Contraindications to warfarin include inability to monitor prothrombin times (target INR 2–3), prior major bleeding event on warfarin, history of major gastrointestinal hemorrhage, history of falls or unstable gait, alcohol abuse or serious liver disease, or uncontrolled hypertension in an elderly patient.

SOURCE: Adapted from American College of Chest Physicians recommendations for anticoagulation for patients with atrial fibrillation. Laupacis A. Albergs G, Dalen J, et al. Antithrombotic therapy in atrial fibrillation, *Chest* 1995; 108:3525–3595; and Atrial Fibrillation Investigators. Risk factors for stroke and efficacy of antithrombotic therapy in atrial fibrillation: Analysis of pooled data from five randomized controlled trials, *Arch Intern Med* 1994; 154:1449–1457. With permission.

by a normal QRS complex (unless coexistent BBB or aberrancy is present) and a retrograde P wave. Depending on the site of origin and the rate of conduction in each direction, the P wave may occur shortly before the QRS complex, follow the QRS, or be lost within it. The rates of AV junctional escape rhythms are usually in the range of 40 to 60 beats per minute; therefore, these rhythms become manifest only when the sinus impulse fails to reach the AV node within physiologic ranges of rate. These rhythms are secondary, occurring as a result of sinus depression or sinoatrial block, and are a normal physiologic phenomenon. Failure of these escape rhythms can result in significant bradycardia. This is discussed in the section on bradyarrhythmias, below.

Another type of secondary rhythm is an *accelerated ventricular rhythm*. This occurs because the sinus rate is slow enough to permit an ectopic ventricular rhythm to escape. The ectopic pacemaker is accelerated above its normal physiologic rate of 20 to 40 beats per minute and overrides the sinus rate, which may be relatively depressed. The rate of an accelerated ventricular rhythm is usually between 50 and 100 beats per minute, and the QRS complexes are wide. The rhythm commonly begins with one or two fusion beats and then is regular; however, it may show progressive acceleration or deceleration until it terminates spontaneously.

Atrioventricular Junctional Premature Beats

An AV junctional premature beat or AV nodal extrasystole arises from the AV nodal or junctional focus; these beats are premature in relation to the prevailing sinus rhythm. They are relatively uncommon and may be difficult to distinguish from atrial or ventricular extrasystoles. They usually require no active treatment. Correction of any hemodynamic abnormalities present may abolish the arrhythmias.

Accelerated Junctional and Ventricular Rhythms

If the AV junctional rate exceeds 60 beats per minute but is less than 100 beats per minute, it is referred to as an *accelerated junctional rhythm*. These rhythms are seen commonly in patients with acute myocardial infarction (MI), particularly when the inferior wall is involved. They have also been associated with digitalis intoxication, electrolyte abnormalities, hypertensive heart disease, cardiomyopathy, and congenital and rheumatic heart disease. In ischemia, ventricular pacemaker acceleration is associated with sinus node depression. Accelerated ventricular rhythms are discussed here with accelerated junctional rhythms because both are due to enhanced automaticity. AV junctional rhythms, however, are supraventricular in origin, whereas accelerated ventricular rhythms originate in the His-Purkinje network of the ventricles. These rhythms usually require no treatment; in fact, the use of antiarrhythmic agents may suppress a subordinate pacemaker required for maintenance of an adequate rate. If a faster ventricular rate is required to maintain adequate hemodynamics, atropine, 0.6 to 1.2 mg intravenously, may be given to increase the sinus rate, or temporary pacing may be used.

Atrioventricular Junctional Tachycardia

Occasionally, the rate of accelerated AV junctional rhythm increases abruptly to the tachycardia range (i.e., ≥ 100 beats per minute). This phenomenon probably represents an autonomic focus firing at the faster rate, with 2:1 exit block that abruptly changes to 1:1 conduction. Usually no treatment is needed except in ischemia, when faster heart rates are unacceptable.

Persistent AV junctional tachycardia (sometimes referred to as *nonparoxysmal* junctional tachycardia) occasionally occurs in patients with chronic heart disease. The response to treatment is unpredictable, and the rhythm may be resistant to conventional antiarrhythmics. Catheter ablation has been utilized in some patients.

VENTRICULAR ARRHYTHMIAS

Effective management of ventricular arrhythmias depends on identification of the risk associated with a particular clinical setting, assessment of the risk-benefit ratio of antiarrhythmic drug treatment, awareness of nonpharmacologic methods of treatment, and an ability to set realistic goals of therapy. The equilibrium between the risk implied by an arrhythmia and the proarrhythmic risk of a drug has been dramatically emphasized by the CAST study. The conventional definition of ventricular tachycardia (VT)—three or more consecutive ventricular ectopic impulses at a rate of ≤ 120 beats per minute—is no longer applicable to current methods of evaluation and treatment. A distinction between short runs or *salvos* of three to five consecutive impulses, bursts of nonsustained VT lasting 30 s or less (not resulting in hemodynamic compromise), and sustained VT lasting more than 30 s is necessary to evaluate patients properly. In addition, the ECG pattern of the VT (monomorphic, polymorphic, torsades de pointes, right ventricular outflow pattern, and bidirectional tachycardia) has clinical implication for risk and treatment. Finally, the presence or absence of heart disease and the left ventricular function (ejection fraction) markedly influence the management approach. Risk increases with the severity of structural heart disease and left ventricular dysfunction.

Premature Ventricular Contractions

A ventricular extrasystole or premature ventricular contraction (PVC) is an impulse that arises in an ectopic ventricular focus and is premature in relation to the prevailing rhythm. PVCs are characterized by a tendency to constant coupling intervals, wide QRS complexes, and secondary ST-segment and T-wave changes.

Occasionally, PVCs will have narrow complexes, and the QRS and/or T vector will change only minimally. The sinus cycle length usually is not interrupted, resulting in a fully compensatory pause.

PREMATURE VENTRICULAR CONTRACTIONS IN THE ABSENCE OF SIGNIFICANT STRUCTURAL DISEASE

Routine treatment of PVCs in this setting is not indicated because there is little or no increased risk of lethal arrhythmias in patients with no underlying cardiac disease. If a patient is bothered by symptoms of palpitations, particularly if frequent, the problem must be addressed to improve the quality of life. First, aggravating factors such as tobacco, caffeine, stress, or other stimulants should be removed. If the symptoms persist, therapy with a mild antianxiety medication or low-dose beta-adrenergic blocking agent, such as 5 to 20 mg propranolol qid or an equivalent dose of another beta blocker, may be helpful. Class I antiarrhythmic agents are rarely indicated because of their potential side effects. In the absence of structural heart disease, even more advanced forms of PVCs, such as salvos, need not be treated because there is no increased risk of sudden death.

Although PVCs are common in mitral valve prolapse (MVP), only a subgroup of patients with MVP appear to be at higher risk for serious ventricular arrhythmias (see also Chap. 24). Patients with nonspecific ST-T wave changes in leads II, III, and aV$_F$ as well as more advanced forms of arrhythmias and a redundant valve by echocardiography may require more aggressive treatment. Management of MVP patients with sustained VT or VF is similar to that used in other clinical settings.

PREMATURE VENTRICULAR CONTRACTIONS IN ACUTE SETTINGS

PVCs are frequently seen in acute MI. Although the classic teaching is that PVCs are a "warning" of more severe arrhythmias and therefore require aggressive treatment, the predictive value of such warning arrhythmias is not substantiated. Intravenous lidocaine, 50- to 200-mg bolus, followed by a 2- to 4-mg/min continuous infusion, is the treatment of choice for PVCs associated with an acute MI. Second, intravenous procainamide, 100 mg every 5 min to a total dose of 10 to 20 mg/kg body weight, followed by a 1- to 4-mg/min continuous infusion, may be used if lidocaine cannot be used or has proved ineffective. Both drugs have significant side effects, particularly with improper dosing. The use of these drugs to suppress PVCs has not been shown to alter hospital mortality in patients for whom prompt medical attention and electrical defibrillation are available.

Other acute syndromes associated with the appearance of PVCs are those characterized by transient myocardial ischemia and coronary reperfusion, such as Prinzmetal's angina, thrombolysis in acute MI, and balloon deflation during percutaneous transluminal coronary angioplasty (PTCA). Reperfusion arrhythmias are usually transient and self-limiting, but they do have the potential to progress to sustained VT or VF. Arrhythmias associated with acute ischemia initially may be treated with intravenous lidocaine or intravenous procainamide, although prevention of recurrences should include control of the ischemia.

Frequent and advanced forms of PVCs are common in severe heart failure and acute pulmonary edema as well as in acute and subacute myocarditis and myopericarditis. Antiarrhythmic therapy is given until the hemodynamic abnormality or acute disease process has resolved. In the case of myocarditis and myopericarditis, antiarrhythmic therapy should be continued for at least 2 months after resolution of clinical symptoms. At that time, after discontinuing antiarrhythmic medications, the patient should be reevaluated by 24-h ECG monitoring. If no advanced forms reappear, antiarrhythmic therapy is not restarted. If complex forms do reappear, drug therapy is reinstituted for 2 to 3 months, after which a drug-free 24-h ECG monitoring is repeated. Usually no antiarrhythmic therapy is required after 6 months.

PREMATURE VENTRICULAR CONTRACTIONS IN CHRONIC CARDIAC DISEASES

The presence of chronic heart disease heightens the clinical significance of PVCs. Sudden and total death rates are increased in patients having frequent or repetitive PVCs in the presence of chronic ischemic heart disease, hypertensive heart disease, and the cardiomyopathies. A reduced ejection fraction (<30 percent) further increases mortality risk. Conversely, patients with ejection fractions >40 percent and single PVCs have a much smaller increase in mortality risk.

In post-MI patients, the management of frequent and repetitive forms of PVCs moved away from the use of membrane-active agents after the CAST study demonstrated that PVC suppression with the class IC agents, flecainide and encainide, demonstrated a significant excess risk of sudden and total cardiac death among the treatment groups. In addition, meta-analyses of data from previous small randomized studies testing the effect of antiarrhythmic drugs on mortality in post-MI patients also suggest an adverse effect of most antiarrhythmic agents. Accordingly, the drugs used in CAST are now contraindicated in post-MI patients with asymptomatic or mildly symptomatic PVCs, and there is a trend away from the use of any membrane-active agent for asymptomatic PVCs in this setting. Beta-adrenergic agents, however, have a beneficial effect on long-term outcome and have evolved as the drugs of choice for post-MI patients with asymptomatic or mildly symptomatic PVCs. Patients with repetitive forms of PVCs, especially when accompanied by low left ventricular ejection fraction, are at a higher risk for sudden death. Regardless of the depressed ejection fraction, beta-adrenergic blocking agents should be tried first. Use of antiarrhythmic therapy guided by programmed electrical stimulation has been reported to be effective. The MADIT trial—comparing conventional antiarrhythmic therapy (80 percent amiodarone) with implantable defibrillators in a population of patients with nonsustained VT, ejection fraction ≤35 percent, and inducible sustained VT resistant to intravenous procainamide—demonstrated a major mortality benefit in favor of automatic implanted defibrillator.

Cardiomyopathies represent the other major category of heart disease associated with PVCs. The risk of sudden cardiac death is high in both dilated and hypertrophic cardiomyopathies; the efficacy of antiarrhythmic medications in the suppression and prevention of ventricular arrhythmias is not certain. In patients with heart failure secondary to idiopathic dilated or ischemic cardiomyopathy, chronic PVCs are very common and nonsustained VT is a marker for sudden death; but in the CHF-STAT study, amiodarone did not improve survival. Subgroup analysis of the CHF-STAT study and the GESICA trial suggest that amiodarone may improve survival in patients with heart failure secondary to idiopathic dilated cardiomyopathy.

The selection of antiarrhythmic medications for suppression of chronic PVCs in higher-risk patients involves several considerations: incidence of proarrhythmia, occurrence of intolerable side effects, and myocardial depression. Hospitalization of patients during initiation of antiarrhythmic therapy is recommended because of the increased risk of proarrhythmia. Class IA agents are all associated with significant risks of proarrhythmia, but most of these responses are not life-threatening. Torsades de pointes is a high-risk proarrhythmic effect. Procainamide may be associated with a lupus-like reaction, gastrointestinal discomfort, or agranulocytosis. Quinidine most commonly causes diarrhea but is also associated with cinchonism, allergic reactions, or thrombocytopenic purpura. Disopyramide has such side effects as urinary retention, dry mouth, and abdominal discomfort attributed to the drug's anticholinergic properties. Importantly, in the patient with reduced ejection fraction, disopyramide may induce CHF.

Although the class IB agents tocainide and mexiletine may be effective, they are associated with a high incidence of gastrointestinal and neurologic side effects. Based on data from CAST, flecainide and encainide, class IC agents, are contraindicated for the treatment of PVCs after MI.

Occasionally, a combination of antiarrhythmic agents such as classes IA and IB may be effective when a single agent is not effective. Class III agents have been approved only for life-threatening arrhythmias, although amiodarone may be useful in patients with severe LV dysfunction and long runs of nonsustained VT. The class II agents, beta-adrenergic blockers, suppress PVCs. The class IV agents, calcium channel blockers, have no role in the treatment of chronic PVCs.

The appropriate endpoint of therapy for chronic PVCs appears to be suppression of advanced forms of PVCs (couplets, salvos, nonsustained VT) if these forms were present on baseline ambulatory monitoring. The goal of therapy includes suppression of 70 to 80 percent of total PVCs in a 24-h period and complete suppression of salvos and nonsustained VT.

Nonsustained Ventricular Tachycardia

Nonsustained runs of VT (salvos of 3 to 5 consecutive ventricular impulses) and nonsustained VT of 6 to 30 s are considered indicators of high risk for potentially lethal arrhythmias (sustained VT or VF) in all patients except those with no underlying or only limited heart disease. Patients with cardiomyopathies or advanced coronary artery disease and low ejection fractions are among those at highest risk. Treatment for these conditions is similar to that for other forms of PVCs, although recent data suggest that patients with prior MI who have a low ejection fraction, nonsustained VT, and are inducible into sustained VT during electrophysiologic testing may benefit from the implantation of a defibrillator (see also Chap. 7).

REPETITIVE MONOMORPHIC VENTRICULAR TACHYCARDIA

This unusual form of ventricular tachycardia is characterized by short paroxysms of VT that last a few beats or a few seconds. The paroxysms may be separated by only one sinus beat and are not aggravated by effort. Occasionally the paroxysms become continuous, and then the arrhythmia becomes a sustained VT. This rhythm disturbance is more common in women and usually is benign. The QRS pattern of the tachycardia on a 12-lead ECG suggests an origin in the right ventricular outflow tract. Treatment usually is not needed unless there is concomitant structural heart disease or the patient is extremely symptomatic. Beta-adrenergic blocking agents or calcium antagonists are effective in some patients. Catheter ablation also may be considered.

Sustained Monomorphic Ventricular Tachycardia

Sustained VT is defined as a succession of ventricular impulses at a rate ≥ 100 per minute and lasting more than 30 s or resulting in severe hemodynamic compromise in less than 30 s. In the absence of hemodynamic compromise, intravenous antiarrhythmia therapy may be used. In addition, a 12-lead ECG should be recorded to characterize VT morphology. On ECG, the distinction between sustained ventricular tachycardia and supraventricular tachyarrhythmias with aberrant intraventricular conduction is based on a complex set of ECG criteria (Table 5-5). Ventricular/atrial dissociation with clearly discernible P waves independent of a regular QRS rhythm is strongly suggestive of VT. In the presence of ventricular/atrial dissociation, a sinus impulse fused with the wide QRS complex due to VT and producing a single cycle having an altered (usually narrowed) QRS complex known as a *fusion beat* helps to distinguish VT from SVT. A QRS duration above 0.14 s favors VT but also can occur in patients with SVT and a preexisting BBB. Concordantly positive or negative QRS complexes across the precordium from V_1, a RBBB pattern that is monophasic or biphasic (qR), suggests VT, while a triphasic pattern (rSR) suggests SVT with aberrant conduction. R-wave amplitude in V_1 during tachycardia that exceeds that during sinus rhythm favors VT. Polymorphic tachyarrhythmias, wide QRS tachycardias with a LBBB configuration in the precordial leads and right axis deviation in the frontal leads, and bidirectional tachycardias are almost always ventricular in origin.

TABLE 5-5

ELECTROCARDIOGRAPHIC SIGNS THAT FAVOR THE DIAGNOSIS OF VENTRICULAR TACHYCARDIA

AV dissociation

Fusion beats

QRS duration >0.14 s

Positive or negative concordance of QRS complexes across precordium

RBBB pattern with monophasic (R) or biphasic (qR)

Polymorphic tachyarrhythmias

Wide QRS tachycardias with LBBB in precordial leads, right axis deviation in frontal leads

Bidirectional tachycardias

MANAGEMENT OF SUSTAINED MONOMORPHIC VENTRICULAR TACHYCARDIA

Management of this form of ventricular tachycardia depends on the clinical characteristics of the VT and the setting in which it occurs. When it appears within the first 24 h of an acute MI, aggressive treatment is mandatory because of the high risk that the VT will degenerate into VF. If the patient is hemodynamically unstable, immediate DC cardioversion is required, followed by an infusion of lidocaine that is maintained for 24 to 48 h. If the patient is hemodynamically stable, intravenous lidocaine, 75 to 100 mg, followed by an infusion of 1 to 4 mg/min, is the first line of therapy (Table 5-6). Cardioversion is necessary if the arrhythmia does not revert immediately or the patient develops hemodynamic compromise (Table 5-3). If VT recurs in spite of lidocaine therapy, procainamide is the next drug of choice. If neither lidocaine nor procainamide is effective in suppressing the arrhythmias, intravenous amiodarone (Cordarone) may be used. Hypotension is the most common adverse effect. Antiarrhythmic therapy may be discontinued 48 to 72 h later, since the risk of recurrence is small at that point.

TABLE 5-6

ANTIARRHYTHMIC AGENTS FOR VENTRICULAR ARRHYTHMIAS IN ACUTE MYOCARDIAL ISCHEMIA/INFARCTION

Drug	Dosage
Lidocaine[a]	IV: 50–200 mg bolus, followed by 2–4 mg/min continuous infusion
Procainamide	IV: 100 mg every 5 min to a total dose of 10–20 mg/kg body weight, followed by 1–4 mg/min continuous infusion
Bretylium	IV: 5 mg/kg body weight over 15 min, repeated if necessary, and followed by 0.5–2.0 mg/min infusion; total dose not to exceed 25 mg/kg per 24 h
Amiodarone	IV: 150 mg over 10 min, followed by a continuous infusion of 1 mg/min for 6 h, then maintenance infusion 0.5 mg/min

[a]Treatment of choice.

VT occurring during the convalescent phase after MI, which is most common in patients with large anterior wall infarctions, has a far more serious long-term implication and higher mortality rate than VT occurring during the acute phase. Patients should undergo both cardiac catheterization and invasive electrophysiologic studies to define the effective therapy. For both convalescent VT (72 h after infarction) and VT appearing later (i.e., chronic phase), electrophysiologic testing is used to demonstrate the characteristics of arrhythmias induced at baseline study and to guide therapy. Left main coronary artery disease or unstable angina are relative contraindications to baseline testing. At least 80 percent of patients with chronic ischemic heart disease and recurrent monomorphic VT can have their clinical VT induced at baseline off all antiarrhythmic drugs. Identification of a drug or combination of drugs that will prevent induction of the same VT is associated with a lower risk of recurrent VT at 1 year compared with the risk of VT if the patient remains inducible on therapy (10 to 15 percent versus 30 to 40 percent). However, in a recent clinical trial including patients with hemodynamically unstable VT randomized to antiarrhythmic therapy or implantable cardioverter/defibrillator (ICD), the ICD offered improved total mortality.

Alternatives to pharmacologic antiarrhythmic therapy include antiarrhythmic surgery, catheter ablation, and defibrillator implantation. Patients with discrete ventricular aneurysms and bypassable coronary artery lesions may undergo coronary bypass, aneurysmectomy, and surgical cryoablation guided by E-P mapping if VT was induced preoperatively. If this approach is unsuccessful, an implantable ICD is indicated (see also Chap. 7). The development of ICDs with antitachycardia pacing and programmed tiered therapy has expanded therapeutic options for patients with inducible ventricular tachycardias that can be pace-terminated. The technique avoids electrical cardioversions in patients with frequent VT. Medication may be used to slow the rate of VT in some patients, thus rendering the VT pace-terminable. ICDs are also indicated for patients who have life-threatening recurrent arrhythmias that cannot be managed surgically and are refractory to medical therapy. The relative proportion of patients managed by these different techniques (i.e., pharmacologic, surgical, catheter ablation, and ICD) is changing, with fewer surgical interventions and broader use of ICD therapy. ICDs with antitachycardia pacing capabilities obviate the need for antiarrhythmic surgery in some cases.

Less Common Causes of Sustained Ventricular Tachycardia

Sustained VT may be mediated by catecholamines or other neurophysiologic influences. Beta-adrenergic blocking agents are useful for those sustained VTs seen in association with emotion and stress, as they probably are catecholamine-related. Another small group of patients with VT may respond to calcium antagonists. This group includes adenosine-sensitive VT and VT with RBBB/left axis deviation originating in the low interventricular septum. Arrhythmogenic right ventricular dysplasia is commonly associated with nonsustained or sustained VT. The VT in this condition has a LBBB morphology, reflecting its origin from the right ventricle. During sinus rhythm anterior precordial T-wave inversions are commonly present.

Sustained VT or VF that may be seen years after repair of complex congenital heart defects—such as tetralogy of Fallot and transposition of the great vessels—are potentially lethal and must be treated. Bidirectional VT is very infrequent and usually associated with digitalis toxicity.

Polymorphic Ventricular Tachycardia

VT with a continuously varying QRS morphology is called *polymorphic VT*. It is often associated with acute ischemia and tends to be more electrically unstable than monomorphic VT. Hemodynamic collapse is common and serial electrophysiologic testing is not informative.

Polymorphic VT includes a specific variant referred to as torsades de pointes—characterized by QRS peaks that "twist" around the baseline—that occurs in the presence of repolarization abnormalities. Most commonly, it occurs as a proarrhythmic response to a class IA or III antiarrhythmic agent, but it may also be seen rarely in association with class IC agent. Other causes of torsades de pointes include chronic bradycardia (complete AV block with a slow ventricular response rate), hypokalemia, hypomagnesemia, phenothiazines, tricyclic antidepressants, and the use of drugs such as terfenadine or cisapride in combination with cytochrome-P450 inhibitors (ketoconazole, miconazole, erythromycin). Treatment is first directed toward the correction of precipitating factors. Cardioversion usually interrupts the torsades de pointes only transiently. Intravenous magnesium sulfate, 2 g over 2 min, is often effective. Acceleration of the heart rate by pacing or isoproterenol will shorten the QT interval, but the latter may precipitate ischemia.

Torsades de pointes may also be caused by congenital long-QT syndromes that are present from childhood and characterized by the presence of long-QT intervals and/or prominent U waves on the 12-lead ECG. Arrhythmias may occur at rest, under emotional stress, or with exercise. Recent progress in molecular genetics has clearly demonstrated that inherited defects in the molecular structure and function of the membrane ion channel underlie the disease.

Congenital QT prolongation with associated symptomatic ventricular arrhythmias may require beta-adrenergic blockade and/or partial sympathectomy. Placement of an ICD should be considered in patients with resistant arrhythmias.

Ventricular Fibrillation

Ventricular fibrillation is a terminal rhythm characterized electrocardiographically by gross disorganization without identifiable repetitive waveforms or intervals. It requires immediate defibrillation with 200 W/s or more. Cardiopulmonary resuscitation (CPR) measures should be performed until defibrillation is successful. Some antiarrhythmic drugs may increase the defibrillation threshold, and thresholds may be decreased by the use of lidocaine or epinephrine. Once the patient's rhythm has returned to normal, prophylactic antiarrhythmic agents (lidocaine or procainamide, or, in resistant recurrent cases, bretylium) should be administered and all metabolic and electrolyte disturbances corrected. Ventricular fibrillation occurs most commonly in acute ischemia warranting the determination of coronary anatomy and LV function, especially if it is noted 48 h after a MI. The published clinical trials in patients after cardiac arrest have supported ICD implantation as opposed to antiarrhythmic therapy for improving cardiac mortality.

BRADYARRHYTHMIAS

Bradyarrhythmias may be secondary to abnormalities of cardiac impulse formation or to AV conduction abnormalities. Although bradyarrhythmias are often asymptomatic, symptoms of hypoperfusion may occur, necessitating immediate treatment. The first step in management is to increase the heart rate. Atropine sulfate, 0.5 to 1.0 mg (0.01 mg/kg), should be administered intravenously and repeated two to three times if necessary. Sympathomimetic amines such as isoproterenol (Isuprel) may be used, but with caution; they should be avoided in patients with ischemic symptoms. Temporary external pacing is a simple, noninvasive way to increase the heart rate and in some instances has supplanted transvenous pacing. It offers a rapid alternative for patients in whom venous access is difficult or is relatively contraindicated (e.g., patients receiving thrombolytic agents). Moreover, it is ideal for patients who have transient bradycardic episodes. Its limitation is the number of patients in whom capture is inconsistent or fails. Temporary transvenous demand pacing provides a stable and reliable increase in ventricular rate when necessary. Dual-chamber pacing is indicated for patients who will benefit from synchronized atrial contraction.

In addition to increasing the heart rate, any medications known to cause bradycardia should be discontinued. Beta-adrenergic blocking agents, calcium channel blockers, digitalis, clonidine, and lithium are common offenders; less frequently, quinidine, procainamide, and lidocaine cause bradyarrhythmias. Patients with persistent symptomatic bradyarrhythmias and no identifiable reversible cause require permanent pacing.

Sinus Bradycardia

Sinus bradycardia is a rhythm in which each cardiac impulse arises normally from the sinoatrial node, but the rate is <60 beats per minute. The P-wave morphology is identical to that observed in normal sinus rhythm; occasionally the P-R interval is prolonged. Sinus bradycardia occurs normally in patients with no underlying heart disease (particularly in well-conditioned individuals), in acute inferior MI, and in association with certain medications, autonomic imbalance, hypothermia, hypothyroidism, or hyperkalemia. The rhythm requires no treatment unless the patient is symptomatic. Removal of aggravating factors is the first step in therapy. If this is not successful, or if the patient requires negative chronotropic agents as part of the medical management, permanent pacing may be necessary.

Sick Sinus Syndrome

Sick sinus syndrome is a condition characterized by abnormal cardiac impulse formation, commonly accompanied by disordered intraatrial electrical activity and atrioventricular conduction. The syndrome is associated with a wide spectrum of brady- and tachyarrhythmias. Some patients exhibit fixed or intermittent sinus bradyarrhythmias; others have sinus bradyarrhythmias alternating with normal sinus rhythm and/or supraventricular tachyarrhythmias (the "tachy/brady syndrome"). Therapy should be reserved for patients with ECG documentation of bradyarrhythmias or tachyarrhythmias and symptoms corresponding to the periods of arrhythmias. Patients with sick sinus syndrome may be particularly susceptible to bradycardias induced by beta-adrenergic blocking agents, calcium channel blockers, and antiarrhythmic drugs. If these medications are needed to treat the tachyarrhythmias associated with sick sinus syndrome, concomitant permanent pacing may be required.

First-Degree Atrioventricular Block

Isolated first-degree AV block is characterized electrocardiographically by a PR interval that exceed 200 ms. It may occur as the result of increased vagal tone, vagotonic drugs, digitalis, beta-adrenergic receptor blockade, hypokalemia, acute carditis, tricuspid stenosis, Chagas' disease, and some forms of congenital heart disease. A prolonged PR interval may occur in normal individuals, reflecting increased vagotonia. Isolated first-degree AV block is never symptomatic and temporary or permanent pacing is not indicated.

Second-Degree Atrioventricular Block

Mobitz type I AV block, or the Wenckebach phenomenon, is characterized electrocardiographically by consecutively conducted impulses with progressively increasing PR intervals until an impulse is blocked and the P wave is not followed by a QRS complex. This is the most common form of second-degree AV block and is usually not symptomatic. It usually does not progress to high-grade AV block; therefore, prophylactic pacing is not necessary unless the patient is symptomatic and vagolytic therapy is ineffective. The presence of Mobitz type I AV block usually does not adversely affect a patient's prognosis.

In contrast, the less common Mobitz type II block implies more significant distal or infrahisian conduction system disease. It is characterized by consecutively conducted impulses with fixed PR intervals and a sudden block of impulse conduction. It is almost always associated with organic heart disease, including disease in the AV conduction system distal to the AV node, and may progress to complete AV block. For this reason permanent pacing may be indicated, primarily to protect the patient from symptomatic events.

Complete Atrioventricular Block

Complete heart block, or third-degree AV block, is characterized by a complete interruption of conduction within the AV junctional tissues; supraventricular impulses are unable to propagate to and activate the ventricles. The ventricles are subsequently activated by a subsidiary idionodal or idioventricular pacemaker at a rate of 20 to 50 beats per minute. Two independent pacemakers then control the rhythm of the heart: one for the atria and one for the ventricles. The two rhythms are asynchronous, since each pacemaker discharges at its own rate.

Acute, symptomatic complete heart block required immediate treatment with either pharmacologic agents (atropine or isoproterenol) or temporary external or transvenous intracardiac pacing. Isoproterenol should be avoided in ischemia. Complete heart block in the setting of an acute inferior MI usually is transient but may take up to 2 weeks to resolve. In contrast, complete AV block in association with acute anterior wall MI may be permanent and require permanent pacing; even if AV block is not permanent, it indicates a high risk for future events. Some have proposed permanent pacemakers for transient high-degree AV block complicating anterior infarction.

Congenital Block

Complete heart block may occur as an isolated congenital anomaly. The QRS complex usually is normal or near normal, since the site of the block is almost always within the AV node or the bundle of His. The resting heart rate usually is in the range of 45 to 65 beats per minute, and the patients frequently are asymptomatic; syncopal attacks are rare. Diagnostic evaluation should include exercise testing to ascertain whether the patient can mount an adequate heart rate in response to stress. If the patient is asymptomatic and the heart rate increases appreciably with exercise, no further therapy may be needed. On the other hand, congenital complete AV block associated with structural congenital cardiac abnormalities implies higher risk.

Atrioventricular Dissociation

Electrocardiographically, the diagnosis of AV dissociation is made when the P waves of sinus rhythm (or other forms of atrial electrical activity) are dissociated from and bear no fixed relationship to the QRS complexes of the ectopic idionodal or idioventricular rhythm. The presence of AV dissociation suggests an abnormality of normal intrinsic pacemaker activity. AV dissociation may occur as a result of slowing of normal pacemaker activity, acceleration of a subordinate focus, or the presence of complete AV block. The diagnosis of AV dissociation, however, is not synonymous with complete AV block.

If a patient with AV dissociation is symptomatic, the underlying rhythm disturbance responsible for the symptoms must be identified and treatment directed toward that rhythm disturbance. For example, a ventricular ectopic focus may become predominant during extreme sinus bradycardia. Suppression of these ventricular escape beats with antiarrhythmic therapy may worsen the underlying bradycardia and the patient's symptoms. Appropriate treatment in this instance would be directed toward the bradycardia; pacing would alleviate the bradycardia, abolish the patient's symptoms, and suppress the ventricular ectopy.

Indications for Pacing

Cardiac pacing is indicated for the treatment of symptomatic brady-arrhythmias that are unresponsive to medical therapy. In the setting of an acute anterior wall MI, temporary pacing is indicated for AV block if it is associated with excessively slow heart rates and/or a reduction in cardiac output. The development of a new LBBB or RBBB particularly in association with a left hemiblock frequently heralds the development of complete heart block and traditionally requires prophylactic pacing.

External pacing techniques in some instances have supplanted the need to insert temporary transvenous pacemakers. This is particularly applicable in acute inferior wall MI, where AV block is usually transient. New LBBB or a preexisting RBBB or LBBB does not require pacing. Permanent pacing is often recommended for patients who have had transient complete heart block during an acute anterior MI. Permanent pacing is the therapy of choice for fixed or intermittent symptomatic bradyarrhythmias that have no identifiable or reversible cause.

SUGGESTED READING

Chakko S, Mitrani R: Recognition and management of cardiac arrhythmias. Part I. General principles and supraventricular tachyarrhythmias. *J Intens Care Med* 1998; 13:68–77.

Crawford MH, Bernstein SJ, Deedwania PC: ACC/AHA guidelines for ambulatory electrocardiography. *J Am Coll Cardiol* 1999; 34:912–948.

Echt DS, Liebson RP, Mitchell B, et al: Mortality and morbidity in patients receiving encainide, flecainide, or placebo: The Cardiac Arrhythmia Suppression Trial. *N Engl J Med* 1991; 324:781–788.

Gregoratos G, Cheitlin MD, Conill A, et al: ACC/AHA guidelines for implantation of cardiac pacemakers and antiarrhythmia devices. *J Am Coll Cardiol* 1998; 31:1175–1209.

Kennedy HL, Whitlock JA, Spague MK, et al: Long-term follow-up of asymptomatic healthy subjects with frequent and complex ventricular ectopy. *N Engl J Med* 1985; 313:193–197.

Laupacis A, Albers GW, Dalen J, et al: Antithrombotic therapy in atrial fibrillation. *Chest* 1998; 114:579S–588S.

Mitrani RD, Simmons JD, Interian A, et al: Cardiac pacemakers: Current and future status. *Curr Probl Cardiol* 1999; 24:341–420.

Moss AM, Hall WJ, Cannom DS, et al: For the Multicenter Automatic Defibrillator Implantation Trial Investigators: Improved survival with an implanted defibrillator in patients with coronary artery disease at high risk for ventricular arrhythmia. *N Engl J Med* 1996; 335:1933–1940.

Myerburg RJ, Kloosterman EM, Castellanos A: Recognition, clinical assessment, and management of arrhythmias and conduction disturbances. In: Fuster V, Alexander RW, O'Rourke RA, et al (eds): *Hurst's The Heart,* 10th ed. New York: McGraw-Hill; 2001:797–873.

Prystowsky EN, Benson W, Fuster V, et al: Management of patients with atrial fibrillation. A statement for health care professionals from the Subcommittee on Electrocardiography and Electrophysiology, American Heart Association. *Circulation* 1996; 93:1262–1277.

Singh SN, Fletcher RD, Fisher SB, et al: For the CHF STAT Investigators: Amiodarone in patients with congestive heart failure and asymptomatic ventricular arrhythmia. *N Engl J Med* 1995; 333:77–82.

Stewart RB, Bardy GH, Greene LH: Wide complex tachycardia: Misdiagnosis and outcome after emergent therapy. *Ann Intern Med* 1986; 104:766–771.

Subcommittee on Advanced Cardiac Life Support: *Advanced Cardiac Life Support*. Dallas: American Heart Association; 1997.

Zipes DP, DiMarco J, Gollette PC, et al: Guidelines for clinical intracardiac electrophysiological and catheter ablation procedures. *J Am Coll Cardiol* 1995; 26:555–573.

CHAPTER

6

ANTIARRHYTHMIC DRUGS

Michael J. Kilborn
Raymond L. Woosley

Antiarrhythmic drugs were developed with the expectation that they would extend and improve life for many patients with heart disease. Their usefulness, however, has been limited by ineffectiveness and/or toxicity. Meanwhile, effective nonpharmacologic treatments for some tachyarrhythmias have emerged. In most mortality trials with antiarrhythmic drugs, benefit has not been clearly demonstrated. Indeed, worsened mortality rates have been observed with a number of drugs in some patient populations. For example, the Cardiac Arrhythmia Suppression Trial (CAST) tested the hypothesis that suppression of asymptomatic ventricular arrhythmias in patients with recent myocardial infarction would reduce mortality rates. Encainide, flecainide, and moricizine were chosen because they were well tolerated and had reasonable ability to suppress ventricular arrhythmias. The trial was terminated prematurely, initially for encainide and flecainide, because of a two- to threefold increase in mortality rates, and then for moricizine, due to a similar trend toward harm, with no reasonable chance of finding a beneficial effect on mortality. Care must be taken, therefore, in deciding on the mode of treatment or, in fact, whether to treat at all. Drug selection is often empiric. The side-effect profiles of the available drugs are very different and are often the determining factors in drug selection. Because of the narrow margin between effective and potentially toxic dosages, physicians must be thoroughly familiar with the clinical pharmacology, dosages, and adverse effects of these agents.

CLASSIFICATION OF ANTIARRHYTHMIC DRUGS

Antiarrhythmic drugs are classified according to their electrophysiologic effects. The scheme most often employed was originally proposed by Vaughan Williams as a classification of drug actions that should be antiarrhythmic, not a classification of drugs. This subtle

DRUG	Vaughan Williams Class	CHANNELS Na Fast	Na Med	Na Slow	Ca	K	α	β	M₂	P	Na/K ATPase	Pro-Arrhy	LV Fx	Heart Rate	Extra Cardiac
Lidocaine	IB														
Mexiletine	IB														
Tocainide	IB														
Moricizine	IC														
Procainamide	IA														
Disopyramide	IA														
Quinidine	IA														
Propafenone	IC														
Flecainide	IC														
Encainide	IC														
Bepridil	IV														
Verapamil	IV														
Diltiazem	IV														
Bretylium	III														
Sotalol	III														
Amiodarone	III														
Ibutilide	III														
Propranolol	II														
Atropine	Misc.														
Adenosine	Misc.														
Digoxin	Misc.														

FIGURE 6-1

Summary of the potentially most important actions of drugs on membrane channels, receptors, and ionic pumps in the heart. Listed are drugs used to modify cardiac rhythm. Most are marketed as antiarrhythmic agents. The drugs (rows) are ordered in a fashion similar to the columns so that generally the darker symbols for their predominant action or actions form a diagonal. Drugs with multiple actions (e.g., amiodarone) depart strikingly from the diagonal trend. The actions of drugs on the sodium, calcium, and potassium channels are indicated. Sodium channel blockade is subdivided into three groups of actions characterized by fast (300 ms), medium (Med; 300–1500 ms), and slow (greater than or equal to 1500 ms) time constants for recovery from block. This parameter is a measure of "use dependence" and predicts the likelihood that a drug will decrease conduction velocity of normal sodium-dependent tissues in the heart and perhaps the propensity of a drug for causing bundle-branch block or proarrhythmia. Drug interactions with receptors alpha, beta, M₂, and P (alpha- and beta-adrenergic, muscarinic subtype, and A, purinergic) and drug distinction is important, because most antiarrhythmic drugs have multiple actions; with such complex pharmacology, a simple drug classification scheme can be misleading. Furthermore, the actions of a given drug differ in different cardiac tissues.

Drugs having class I action slow intracardiac conduction by blocking fast inward sodium channels and have been subclassified into classes IA, IB, and IC. Drugs having class IA actions also produce measurable increases in ventricular refractoriness and prolongation of the QT interval. Drugs with class IB actions generally exert little effect on PR, QRS, or QT intervals. Drugs with class IC actions slow conduction velocity the most (increasing the PR and QRS intervals) while having little effect on repolarization and the QT interval. Class II action refers to beta-adrenergic antagonism. Although the mechanism is unknown, class II agents are the only antiarrhythmic drugs found clearly effective in preventing sudden cardiac death in patients with prior myocardial infarction (discussed in Chap. 5). Drugs whose predominant effect is to prolong the duration of the cardiac action potential and refractoriness have class III action. Class IV action is calcium channel antagonism (discussed in Chap. 5).

Because of the many limitations of the Vaughan Williams classification, a new approach termed the "Sicilian gambit" (see Fig. 6-1) has been proposed. This classification system is based on the differential effects of the drugs on (1) channels, (2) receptors, and (3) transmembrane pumps. The grouping is based primarily on the predominant action of drugs but also considers other ancillary actions that may be clinically relevant. The increased detail of the new system reflects the current state of knowledge at a level necessary for optimal use of these drugs. This chapter reviews the clinical pharmacology and applications of the currently available antiarrhythmic drugs excluding digoxin, beta-receptor antagonists, and calcium channel blockers, which are addressed in other chapters. The pharmacokinetics, usual dosages, and ranges of plasma concentration for the major drugs are listed in Tables 6-1 and 6-2.

---

effects on the sodium-potassium pump (Na/K ATPase) are indicated. Symbols indicate the type of actions at receptors or channels (Antagonist relative potency: O low; ●, moderate; ●, high; △, agonist; ▲, agonist/antagonist). Filled triangles for bretylium indicate its biphasic action to initially stimulate alpha and beta receptors by release of norepinephrine, followed by blocking of norepinephrine release and indirect antagonism of these receptors. (Adapted from the Task Force of the Working Group on Arrhythmias of the European Society of Cardiology,[9] with permission.)

TABLE 6-1

PHARMACOKINETICS OF ANTIARRHYTHMIC DRUGS

Agent	Inactivation or Elimination,[a] %	Protein Binding, %	V_D, L/kg	Elimination Half-life, h	Bioavailability, %	Apparent Oral Clearance, mL/min
Quinidine	Hepatic, 50–90 Renal, 10–30	80–90	2.5	3–19	70	200–400
Procainamide	Hepatic, 40–70[b] Renal, 30–60	15	2	2–4	100	400–700
Disopyramide	Hepatic, 20–30 Renal, 40–50	20–50	0.6	6–8	80–90	90
Lidocaine	Hepatic, 90	40–70	1.1	1.5–4	35[c]	700–1000[c]
Tocainide	Hepatic, 30–40 Renal, 40	10	1.5–3	8–20	90	150–200
Mexiletine	Hepatic, 85–90[b] Renal, 10–15	70	5.5–9.5	8–20	90	400–700
Flecainide	Hepatic, 70[b] Renal, 30	40	7–10	7–26	90–95	200–800
Propafenone	Hepatic, 99[b]	90	3–4	2–24[b]	10–50[b]	800–5000[b]
Sotalol	Renal, 90	low	1.5–2.5	8–12	90–100	100–300
Amiodarone	Hepatic, 99	95	20–200	13–103 days	20–80	6500–11,000
Bretylium	Renal, 90	Low	3–4	4–16	25[c]	1300
Ibutilide	Hepatic, 93	40	11	2–12	—	—
Dofetilide	Renal, 80	60–70	3	10	>90	—

[a] Renal elimination of unchanged drug.
[b] Dependent on metabolic phenotype (see text).
[c] Not recommended for oral administration.

TORSADES DE POINTES

A potential side effect often seen with a number of commonly used antiarrhythmic drugs, in particular those with class III or IA actions, is torsades de pointes, a polymorphic ventricular tachycardia occurring in the context of a long-QT interval. Risk factors (in addition to prolonged QT interval) for this potentially lethal arrhythmia include: female sex, left ventricular dysfunction, bradycardia, and electrolyte disturbances, especially hypokalemia and hypomagnesemia. Prevention, therefore, relies upon careful patient selection, maintenance of potassium levels above 4 meq/L, and monitoring of the electrocardiogram (ECG) for degree of QT prolongation after drug initiation and dosage increases. Recommended immediate treatment for torsades de pointes includes intravenous magnesium sulfate (2 g over 10 to 20 min), and measures to increase heart rate (pacing or isoproterenol infusion). This should be followed by correction of hypokalemia, if necessary, and discontinuation or dose reduction of QT-prolonging drugs. Clinically, it is essential to distinguish torsades de pointes from polymorphic ventricular tachycardia occurring in the setting of a normal QT interval, because the latter should be treated with "local anesthetic" antiarrhythmic drugs such as lidocaine and may be worsened by the treatment outlined above for torsades de pointes.

DRUGS

Lidocaine (Xylocaine)

Lidocaine, introduced as a local anesthetic, is still the most widely used intravenous antiarrhythmic drug. It is effective for the acute suppression of sustained ventricular arrhythmias, especially in the presence of acute myocardial ischemia or infarction. Extensive first-pass metabolism makes it unsatisfactory for oral use. Because of lidocaine's complex pharmacokinetics, measurement of blood level is essential for dosage adjustment, and a monitored environment is desirable to permit evaluation of response and detection of toxicity.

Regimens employing a series of loading doses and a maintenance infusion should be used. Single boluses achieve only transient therapeutic effects because the drug is rapidly redistributed. For a stable patient, a total loading dose of lidocaine should be 3 to 4 mg/kg body weight administered over 20 to 30 min, starting with 1 mg/kg over 2 min. At the time of initiation of loading, a maintenance infusion should also be started.

TABLE 6-2
DOSAGE AND PLASMA CONCENTRATION RANGE FOR ANTIARRHYTHMIC AGENTS[a]

Agent	Usual Initial Dosage[b]	Modification of Dosage in Disease[c]	Dosage Range	Maximum Single Dose	Therapeutic Ranges,[d] μg/mL
Quinidine (sulfate)	200 mg q 6 h	None	800–2400 mg/day	600	0.7–5.5
Procainamide (sustained release)	500 mg q 6 h	$\rightarrow$ CHF $\rightarrow$ RI	2000–6000 mg/day	1500	4–8
Disopyramide	100 mg q 6 h	$\rightarrow$ CHF $\rightarrow$ HI $\rightarrow$ RI	300–1200 mg/day	300	2–5
Lidocaine	See text	$\rightarrow$ CHF $\rightarrow$ HI	1–4 mg/min IV	—	1.5–5
Tocainide	400 mg q 8 h	$\rightarrow$ CHF $\rightarrow$ HI $\rightarrow$ RI	1200–2400 mg/day	800	4–10
Mexiletine	200 mg q 8 h	$\rightarrow$ CHF $\rightarrow$ HI?	600–1200 mg/day	400	0.7–2
Flecainide	50–100 mg q 12 h	$\rightarrow$ CHF $\rightarrow$ HI?	200–400 mg/day	200	0.2–1

98

Propafenone	150 mg q 8 h	See text	300–900 mg/day	300	0.5–3?
Sotalol	40–80 mg q 12 h	→ RI	160–640 mg/day	320 mg	—
Amiodarone	600–1400 mg/day (load)	None	200–600 mg/day	600	1–2
Bretylium	See text	→ RI	1–4 mg/min IV	—	—
Ibutilide	1 mg, repeat after 10 min	—	0.01 mg/kg–1 mg × 2	1 mg	—
Dofetilide	500 mcg bid	→ RI	125–1000 mcg/d	500 mcg	0.001–0.003

[a] These are general guidelines only. Dosage should be determined for each patient based on clinical presentation, disease states, clinical response, and tolerance to the drug.

[b] Dosage usually recommended in absence of significant cardiac, renal, or hepatic failure.

[c] CHF = congestive heart failure; HI = hepatic insufficiency; RI = renal insufficiency. See text for details.

[d] The range of therapeutic plasma concentrations is a statistical range that should be considered only a guideline to therapy.

Desired plasma concentration (about 3 μg/mL)
× expected clearance = initial maintenance infusion rate
(usually in the range of 20 to 60 μg/kg/ min)

There is great variability in peak plasma concentrations. Therefore, during loading and after dose increases, the patient's ECG,
blood pressure, and mental status should be monitored; the process
should be stopped at the first sign of lidocaine excess. The time required to reach steady-state conditions is approximately 8 to 10 h
in normal individuals and up to 20 to 24 h in patients with liver
disease and/or heart failure. If the maintenance infusion has reached
steady state and the arrhythmia reappears while side effects are absent and the plasma level is nontoxic, it is appropriate to administer
a small bolus of lidocaine (25 to 50 mg over 2 min) and increase the
maintenance infusion rate proportionally. The plasma concentration
can be used to estimate the final maintenance infusion—i.e.

Maintenance dosage = clearance × desired plasma concentration

where clearance = infusion rate ÷ steady state plasma concentration. The risk of toxicity increases at plasma concentrations above
5 μg/mL and becomes prohibitive above 9 μg/mL.

When a lidocaine infusion is being terminated, it should not be
tapered off, particularly if oral antiarrythmic therapy has already been
initiated. The half-life of decline of lidocaine levels after termination
of an infusion can be estimated from the equation

$$T_{1/2} = \text{plasma concentration} \times \text{VD} \times 0.693/\text{infusion rate}$$

where VD is the final volume of distribution, usually 1.1 L/kg, but
reduced by 50 percent or more in patients with heart failure. In patients with congestive heart failure, loading doses as well as maintenance and infusion rates should be reduced by about half, with little
change in the time to reach steady state. In patients with liver disease,
initial loading regimens require no adjustment, but maintenance infusions must be decreased, and steady state may not be reached for
20 to 24 h. With mechanical ventilation, a decrease in cardiac output and hepatic blood flow may necessitate a decrease in lidocaine
dosage.

The most frequent side effects of lidocaine involve the central
nervous system. Boluses can induce tinnitus or seizures. With more
gradual attainment of excessive levels, drowsiness, dysarthria, confusion, hallucinations, and dysesthesia may occur. Excessive lidocaine
can also cause coma, which should be a consideration in patients after
cardiac arrest. Lidocaine can depress cardiac function, decreasing its
own clearance, and producing an even greater increase in plasma concentration. Advanced degrees of sinus node dysfunction have been
reported in isolated instances. In patients with known conduction

abnormalities below the AV node, some studies have found slowing of ventricular escape rate or potentiation of infranodal block; therefore, lidocaine should be administered cautiously if at all in such patients unless a temporary pacemaker is readily available. Additive depression of myocardial function or conduction may occur when lidocaine is used in combination with other antiarrhythmic agents. Beta-adrenergic blockers can cause decreased lidocaine clearance. In patients receiving cimetidine, both loading and maintenance dosages may require downward adjustment due to a complex interaction.

Mexiletine (Mexitil)

Mexiletine, an orally active lidocaine congener with class IB sodium channel-blocking activity, is used in the treatment of ventricular arrhythmias. Success rates vary between 6 and 60 percent, and more than half of published studies suggest limited efficacy (less than 20 percent). Mexiletine does not prolong the QT interval and therefore can be useful for patients with a history of drug-induced torsades de pointes or long-QT syndrome. Mexiletine has been combined successfully with quinidine, propranolol, or procainamide for possible additive or synergistic antiarrhythmic response produced by the combination of agents. Lower than usual dosages of both agents can be used. Mexiletine exerts minimal effect on hemodynamics and myocardial contractility, even in patients with severe congestive heart failure.

Mexiletine therapy should be initiated with a low dosage, which is increased at 2- to 3-day intervals until efficacy or intolerable side effects develop. The usual wide variation in clearance, which is seen for most drugs having extensive hepatic metabolism, is especially marked for mexiletine, because the CYP2D6 enzyme responsible for its metabolism is absent in 7 percent of the Caucasian population. Also, consideration of dosage adjustment to compensate for the action of agents that induce (e.g., phenytoin) or inhibit (e.g., quinidine) hepatic mexiletine metabolism is required. Adverse reactions to mexiletine are dose-related and include tremor, visual blurring, dizziness, dysphoria, and nausea. Both thrombocytopenia and a positive antinuclear antibody test result have been reported to occur infrequently. Severe bradycardia has been reported in patients with sick sinus syndrome; at high concentrations, worsening in heart block has been reported.

Procainamide (Pronestyl-SR, Procan-SR)

Procainamide is effective against both supraventricular and ventricular arrhythmias, including atrial fibrillation and flutter associated with Wolff-Parkinson-White syndrome. It can be used intravenously to suppress recurrent nonsustained ventricular arrhythmias or to terminate hemodynamically tolerated sustained ventricular tachycardia. Its main disadvantage compared to lidocaine in this context is its longer loading time (about 20 min). Compared to quinidine, procainamide has very little vagolytic activity. Its active metabolite, N-acetylprocainamide (acecainide, or NAPA) produces antiarrhythmic actions different from those of procainamide. NAPA has predominantly class III antiarrhythmic activity, prolonging the QT interval and refractoriness in both atrial and ventricular myocardium. Slightly more than half of the general population are rapid acetylators of procainamide and quickly convert it to NAPA. When each is given as the sole agent, the usually effective plasma concentration is 4 to 8 μg/mL for procainamide and 7 to 15 μg/mL for NAPA. During oral procainamide therapy, both agents are present in variable amounts, and there is no way to determine readily the contribution of NAPA to arrhythmia suppression. Monitoring plasma concentrations for prevention of toxicity or determination of compliance is recommended.

When administered intravenously, procainamide can be initiated as a loading infusion over 20 to 50 min or by a series of doses (100 mg delivered over 3 min) given every 5 min, up to a total dose of 1g. If the loading dose is well tolerated, with no hypotension and less than 25 percent QRS or QT widening, a maintenance intravenous infusion of 20 to 60 μg/kg per minute can then be given. For *oral* therapy, the initial recommended maintenance dose is 50 mg/kg per day if renal and cardiac function are normal. With its short half-life of elimination and the availability of various sustained-release preparations, the dosing frequency may be every 3, 6, 8, or 12 h, depending on the formulation used. This can create confusion, so care is needed to avoid dangerous mistakes in dosing. The elimination half-life of NAPA is much longer than that of procainamide. Therefore dosage should be initiated at conservative levels, and the patient should be monitored carefully until both procainamide and NAPA have reached steady state. The practice of using the sum of the plasma concentrations of procainamide and NAPA is not recommended.

Intravenous procainamide depresses myocardial contractility and lowers blood pressure, but worsening of heart failure is uncommon during oral therapy at usual doses. Side effects associated with long-term procainamide therapy limit its usefulness. Up to 40 percent of patients discontinue therapy in the first 6 months due to adverse reactions. Procainamide should not be used in patients with a long-QT syndrome or a history of torsades de pointes. Potassium levels should be maintained above 4 meq/L. Heart block and sinus node dysfunction can occur in patients with preexisting conduction system abnormalities. Between 15 and 20 percent of patients receiving chronic oral procainamide therapy develop a lupus-like syndrome, which usually begins insidiously as mild arthralgia but progresses to frank arthritis, fever, malar erythematous rash, and pleural and/or pericardial effusions (potentially fatal), with serum antibodies against nucleoprotein (histone) appearing as antinuclear antibodies with a "smooth" or "diffuse" pattern. These symptoms abate if procainamide is discontinued. Almost all patients treated chronically develop antinuclear antibodies. The patient should be fully informed of the symptoms, so that therapy can be discontinued at the earliest symptoms or signs of the lupus syndrome. It is dangerous to continue procainamide after the development of the early symptoms of the lupus syndrome.

Due to the risk of agranulocytosis, it is recommended that a white blood cell count be obtained every 2 weeks for the first 3 months. There are few reports of interactions with other drugs. Procainamide's clearance is reduced by cimetidine and by NAPA. Ranitidine reduces both its renal clearance and its absorption, the former by 14 to 23 percent and the latter by 10 to 24 percent, depending on dose.

Disopyramide (Norpace)

Disopyramide is useful for supraventricular arrhythmias, including those associated with WPW syndrome; but because of its negative inotropic effect, its utility for ventricular arrhythmias is limited to patients with preserved ventricular function. The drug's anticholinergic actions make it a suitable choice for the subset of patients with paroxysmal atrial fibrillation whose arrhythmia is "vagally mediated" (onset of episodes always occurs during sleep or rest). A sustained-release formulation allows dosing every 12 h.

Plasma concentration monitoring is of little value because of variable and saturable binding to plasma proteins. A doubling of total concentration in blood may actually be associated with a sixfold increase in the *free* drug level, potentially toxic. For this reason, loading doses or rapid increases in dosage are dangerous and not recommended. Dose-related anticholinergic side effects (urinary retention, dry mouth, blurred vision) limit therapy in many patients. There is little organ toxicity associated with chronic therapy, however; if the drug is initially tolerated, chronic therapy is usually without problems. Agents that induce hepatic metabolism (phenytoin, rifampicin, barbiturates) can cause levels to fall.

Quinidine

Quinidine has been used successfully for treating a variety of supraventricular and ventricular arrhythmias. Care must be taken to minimize the risk of ventricular proarrhythmia. A grouped analysis of six small placebo-controlled trials in patients with atrial fibrillation showed a statistically significant increase in mortality for the patients treated with quinidine.

The effective dosage of quinidine varies considerably among individuals. The drug is available commercially in at least three different forms: the sulfate, the gluconate, and the polygalacturonate. Since the quinidine content varies among these at 83, 62, and 60 percent, respectively, dosage adjustment should be considered if one form is substituted for another. Intravenous therapy with quinidine is usually avoided if alternatives are feasible. If quinidine is given intravenously (as the gluconate), the patient should be carefully monitored, the infusion rate should be no greater than 16 mg/min, and the drug should be discontinued if hypotension is observed or the QRS is prolonged by more than 30 percent. For patients with renal or hepatic disease, slower dose titration is advisable; but dosage for these patients is not markedly different. Elderly patients often require lower dosages.

Dose-related increases in PR, QRS, and QTc intervals in the ECG are seen. Patients with congenital long-QT syndrome, hypokalemia, or a history of torsades de pointes should not be given quinidine. For patients with congestive heart failure, problems associated with use of quinidine are proarrhythmia and digoxin toxicity. Torsades de pointes is likely to be the major cause of quinidine syncope—which occurs in as many as 5 to 10 percent of patients within the first days of quinidine treatment—and of quinidine-induced sudden death. Torsades de pointes is preceded by marked prolongation of the QT interval, but most cases occur with low serum concentrations of quinidine.

Hypotension may occur with quinidine therapy, especially in patients concomitantly receiving nitrates or other vasodilators. Other adverse effects include a high incidence of diarrhea and vomiting and the syndrome of *cinchonism* (tinnitus, blurred vision, and headache) at high plasma levels. Rarer adverse effects are thrombocytopenia and AV conduction block in patients with existing conduction system disease. Patients with atrial flutter and normal AV nodal conduction should be receiving an AV nodal blocking agent (beta blocker, non-dihydropyridine calcium channel blocker, or digitalis) before being treated with quinidine; so as to minimize the potential for dangerous sudden increases in ventricular rates up to 200 to 250 beats per minute (which can occur when quinidine causes a slight reduction of the flutter rate and anticholinergic enhancement of AV nodal conduction, permitting 1:1 conduction through the AV node).

Quinidine metabolism is inhibited by cimetidine and induced by phenytoin, phenobarbital, and rifampicin. Prudent use of quinidine in individuals taking digitalis requires the following: (1) that titration begin at a reduced dosage; (2) that dosage of the digitalis be reduced; and (3) that plasma potassium be maintained above 4 meq/L. Quinidine is a potent inhibitor of the metabolism (by the hepatic CYP2D6 enzyme) of many drugs, including propafenone, mexiletine, flecainide, metoprolol, timolol, sparteine, and bufuralol. It also worsens neuromuscular blockade in patients with myasthenia gravis and may prolong the effects of succinylcholine.

Propafenone (Rythmol)

Propafenone has a role in the treatment of many types of arrhythmias, particularly supraventricular arrhythmias. It has class IC antiarrhythmic activity. Having a marked structural similarity to propranolol, it can produce significant beta-adrenergic inhibition at high plasma concentrations. Dosage should not be changed more frequently than every 3 days; there is slow elimination of the parent drug in poor metabolizers and slow accumulation of the metabolite(s) in extensive metabolizers. If propafenone is used in the context of reduced ventricular function, patients should be carefully monitored for heart failure resulting from beta-adrenergic receptor antagonism and/or the drug's direct negative inotropic effect. Dosage recommendations for patients with cardiac, renal, or hepatic dysfunction are not yet available. An interaction has already been documented between propafenone and metoprolol, and it is very likely that there are interactions with other agents that utilize or inhibit cytochrome CYP2D6 for their metabolism (e.g., timolol, many antidepressants, many neuroleptics).

Flecainide (Tambocor)

Flecainide has class IC actions and is effective in suppressing a variety of ventricular and supraventricular tachycardias. The finding of increased mortality when it is given to patients with ischemic heart disease has led to restricted usage; however, there has been no evidence to indicate that this increase in mortality is seen when flecainide is given to treat supraventricular arrhythmias in patients without known coronary artery disease. Its negative inotropic effect further restricts its use to patients having well-preserved ventricular function. Flecainide therapy should start with a low dosage that is maintained for at least 4 days and then gradually titrated to clinical response. With cardiac failure, the usual initial dose is 50 to 100 mg every 12 h. Patients with renal failure should be given very low dosages and that are titrated very carefully. Plasma concentration monitoring is essential in patients with renal, cardiac, or hepatic dysfunction.

Flecainide has the potential to induce proarrhythmic events, even when prescribed as recommended. It produces a measurable decrease in left ventricular function in most patients, though the increased mortality seen in CAST seemed to be confined to patients with structural heart disease. Other side effects of flecainide include exacerbation of sinus node dysfunction and prolongation of QRS and PR intervals on the surface ECG. If they are below 25 percent, these effects do not necessarily indicate excessive dosage. Flecainide increases thresholds for pacing and electrical defibrillation and should therefore be used with caution in patients dependent upon pacemakers or implanted defibrillators. Cimetidine reduces flecainide clearance and prolongs elimination half-life. Amiodarone can elevate plasma flecainide concentration, necessitating reduction of flecainide dosage. Flecainide can cause an increase in the plasma concentrations of digoxin and propranolol.

Bretylium (Bretylol)

Bretylium is effective for acute therapy of ventricular tachycardia and/or ventricular fibrillation, but it is usually employed only after patients have not responded to lidocaine. In addition to the indirect electrophysiologic changes caused by the drug's biphasic action on postganglionic autonomic neurons, the drug has a direct class III action. The usual intravenous dosage is 5 mg/kg given at a rate dependent upon the clinical setting. During cardiac emergencies, it should be given by rapid injection into a central intravenous line. In less acute situations, giving the same dose but over 10 to 20 min will reduce the incidence of nausea and vomiting. A total loading dose of 20 mg/kg may be required, and dosages up to 9 g in 24 h have been given without serious adverse effects. Maintenance infusion rates should be 1 to 4 mg/min, depending upon body size and renal function. In patients with renal insufficiency, the maintenance infusion should be reduced to the lowest effective dosage. When bretylium is given by rapid intravenous injection, increased frequency of ventricular arrhythmias is often seen and can lead to the need for more frequent cardioversion. Hypotension can occur in volume-depleted patients. In stable patients, doses of bretylium can cause a transient increase in heart rate, blood pressure, contractility, peripheral vascular resistance, and arrhythmia frequency, followed by a fall in standing blood pressure. Other than those with tricyclic antidepressants, no drug interactions have been reported. However, competition for renal tubular secretion with procainamide, NAPA, cimetidine, and other organic bases might be expected.

Sotalol (Betapace)

Unlike other beta-adrenergic antagonists, sotalol markedly prolongs refractoriness of atrial and ventricular tissues. This unique combination of properties makes sotalol effective in a variety of supraventricular and ventricular arrhythmias. In patients with relatively normal renal function, steady state is reached in 2 to 3 days. Dosage must be adjusted for altered renal function. The recommended dosing interval is every 12 h for patients with a creatinine clearance greater than 60 mL/min but 24 h if the creatinine clearance (CL CR) is between 30 and 60 mL/min. For patients with CL CR between 10 and 30 mL/min, the interval should be every 36 to 48 h or the usual dose halved and given every 24 h. The dosage for patients with CL CR below 10 mL/min should be individualized. Because of the increased risk of proarrhythmia and congestive heart failure, patients with reduced cardiac output should be given lower doses and monitored carefully.

A major concern with sotalol treatment has been the occurrence of torsades de pointes, with an overall incidence around 2 percent (4 percent of patients with sustained ventricular tachycardia and 1.5 percent of patients with supraventricular arrhythmias). The incidence of torsades de pointes should be minimized by careful screening and consideration of predisposing factors; careful dose escalation beginning at 80 or 160 mg/day; and limiting the maximum QT interval prolongation to less than 550 ms. The incidence of new or worsened congestive heart failure is about 3 percent. Other side effects typical of beta blockers are to be expected, including bronchospasm in asthmatic patients, masking the signs and symptoms of hypoglycemia in diabetic patients, and catecholamine hypersensitivity withdrawal syndrome. No pharmacokinetic interactions have been seen with sotalol and warfarin, digoxin, cholestyramine, or hydrochlorothiazide.

Amiodarone (Cordarone)

The U.S. Food and Drug Administration (FDA) has recommended amiodarone only for life-threatening ventricular arrhythmias refractory to other available forms of therapy, however, there are now numerous trials in the literature describing the efficacy of amiodarone in the treatment of atrial fibrillation and other supraventricular tachycardias. The reasons for amiodarone's limited labeling are (1) the potentially lethal complications of chronic amiodarone therapy, (2) the complications associated with its variable onset of action, and (3) multiple dangerous drug interactions. Meta-analyses of the many trials with amiodarone in patients at risk of ventricular arrhythmias have generally confirmed a modest reduction in mortality. One study concluded that the benefit could be extended to patients with congestive heart failure, but another did not. Three controlled trials demonstrated the value of *intravenous* amiodarone in patients with recurrent life-threatening ventricular tachycardia or fibrillation.

Amiodarone has many diverse pharmacologic actions. It can cause torsades de pointes proarrhythmia but there appears to be a lower incidence of this than that due to other drugs with similar degrees of QT prolongation. It is a highly lipid-soluble compound with extremely variable and complex pharmacokinetics. Bioavailability varies over a fourfold range. Amiodarone is extensively metabolized to desethylamiodarone (DEA), which has antiarrhythmic potency equal to or greater than that of amiodarone in animal models. Without a loading dose regimen, amiodarone requires several weeks to months before it produces its antiarrhythmic action. For intravenous administration, the manufacturer recommends a three-phase infusion over the first 24 h: 150 mg over 10 min, followed by 360 mg over the next 6 h, followed by 0.5 mg/min. The drug can be continued at this rate, but monitoring of plasma concentrations is recommended. An additional 150 mg can be infused over 10 min for those patients who continue to have ventricular tachycardia or fibrillation or whose arrhythmia recurs during downward titration of the infusion. Concentrations of drug greater than 3 mg/mL should be infused through a central catheter to prevent phlebitis. Pumps that count drops will give approximately 30 percent less drug than intended because of the surfactant properties of the drug. Oral loading dosages have varied, but a currently accepted loading regimen is 600 to 800 mg daily for 14 days. The dosage should then be tapered over a period of several weeks. The usual maintenance dose varies from 100 to 600 mg/day, and because of variable bioavailability and the severe nature of adverse reactions, the lowest effective dosage should be prescribed. Once tissues become saturated, the decline in plasma levels is slow and extremely variable, with half-lives ranging from 13 to 103 days at steady state.

Intravenous amiodarone can decrease cardiac contractility and peripheral vascular resistance, producing severe hypotension in some instances. The safety of amiodarone for chronic therapy is controversial. The most serious adverse reaction is interstitial pneumonitis and pulmonary fibrosis. Monitoring (for example, by clinical assessment and chest x-ray every 3 months) is essential, since the pneumonitis can be lethal and is reversible if detected early. Serial pulmonary function tests are of little value for follow-up. Hyper- or hypothyroidism is seen in about 4 percent of patients treated chronically. Accumulation of corneal microdeposits is almost uniform during long-term therapy and can progress to the point of interfering with vision. Photosensitivity and development of a bluish-gray discoloration of sun-exposed areas of the skin in Caucasian patients can be prevented or alleviated with sunscreens, protective garments, and minimization of dosage. Thirty percent or more of patients have abnormally elevated serum hepatic enzyme levels, and progression to jaundice and cirrhosis has been reported.

Serial laboratory tests to screen for amiodarone toxicity can be costly and generally are of limited value; however, it is wise to obtain a reliable assessment of baseline tests, including complete blood count, blood chemistry, tests of thyroid and pulmonary function, a slit-lamp examination, and measurement of blood levels of other drugs. Amiodarone interferes with the clearance of many drugs including warfarin, quinidine, procainamide, disopyramide, mexiletine, propafenone, and digoxin.

Ibutilide (Corvert)

Ibutilide was approved by the FDA in 1995 for the rapid conversion of recent-onset atrial fibrillation or flutter, for which it has a success rate of 45 to 60 percent. When combined with electrical cardioversion within an hour of administration, the chance of acute success approaches 100 percent. Ibutilide is an analog of sotalol and has class III action. It should not be given to patients who have hypokalemia, hypomagnesemia, or QTc prolongation at baseline >440 ms. Dosing is recommended on the basis of body weight for patients under 60 kg (0.01 mg/kg should be given). Ibutilide is given as an infusion over 10 min. For patients whose arrhythmias have not converted by 10 min after completion of the first dose, a second dose of equal size can be administered provided that excessive QT prolongation has not occurred. It is essential that patients receiving ibutilide be treated in a carefully monitored environment during and at least 4 h after treatment. Personnel, facilities, and medication for defibrillation or resuscitation must be readily available. Patients with severe left ventricular dysfunction have a higher risk of developing ventricular arrhythmias, including torsades de pointes. Despite exclusion of patients with a QTc > 440 ms or potassium concentrations <4 meq/L in trials before marketing, the incidence of sustained polymorphic ventricular tachycardia requiring cardioversion was 1.7 percent. Another 7.6 percent developed nonsustained ventricular tachycardia (some polymorphic, some monomorphic), and 1.5 percent had AV block. Bradycardia, multiple episodes of sinus arrest, and a single case of acute renal failure have been reported. No specific drug interaction studies have been performed. The manufacturer's labeling warns against combining ibutilide with other drugs that prolong the QT interval.

Dofetilide (Tikosyn)

Dofetilide was approved and marketed in 2000 for oral therapy of atrial fibrillation and flutter. Its success rate (about 30 percent) for conversion of atrial fibrillation appears to be inferior to that of ibutilide but superior to that of safe dosages of available oral agents. Prevention of recurrence at 5 months has been demonstrated, with a success rate at least comparable to that of sotalol. Extensive screening and monitoring for potential harm, particularly from torsades de pointes, appears necessary for safe use. For this reason, the manufacturer requires physicians to receive special training prior to prescribing dofetilide and, on the labeling, the FDA has required inclusion of a warning that therapy must be initiated in the hospital with continuous ECG monitoring for at least 3 days. Dofetilide does not depress cardiac function at usual dosages even in patients with reduced ejection fraction. Lower dosages are recommended for patients who develop excessive QTc prolongation on 500 μg bid. In the largest clinical trial "excessive" was defined as >550 ms or >20 percent longer than baseline. Dosage should be reduced in patients with renal disease (250 mg bid for a creatinine clearance 60 to 40 mL/min and 250 mg daily for a creatinine clearance 40 to 20 mL/min). Data are not available for adjustment of dosage in patients with liver disease. Concomitant administration of dofetilide with verapamil, ketoconazole, or cimetidine (but not ranitidine) results in increased plasma concentrations of dofetilide, especially in patients with reduced renal function. There may be other important interactions with erythromycin, other macrolides, or antifungals. No interactions have been seen between dofetilide and digoxin or warfarin.

Adenosine (Adenocard)

Adenosine is very effective for the acute conversion of paroxysmal supraventricular tachycardia (PSVT) due to reentry involving the AV node (see also Chap. 5). Sixty percent of patients respond at a dose of 6 mg, and an additional 32 percent respond when given a higher dose of 12 mg. Adenosine potently slows AV nodal conduction, which can result in transient AV block for 5 to 20 s. It usually has no effect on accessory pathway conduction except in pathways that demonstrate decremental conduction. Half-life of elimination has ranged from 1.5 to 10 s. The drug is rapidly metabolized in the plasma and in cells. Adenosine should be injected rapidly into a proximal site on an intravenous line and flushed quickly with saline. Maximal pharmacologic effects are seen within 30 s after injection into a peripheral intravenous line but occur within 10 to 20 s when given into a central line. For adults, the initial dose is 6 mg. If the arrhythmia persists, a 12-mg dose can be injected 1 to 2 min later. Higher doses may be required for patients who have received caffeine or theophylline, because of their antagonistic effects at A1 receptors. Lower doses are recommended if the patients are receiving dipyridamole or carbamazepine. Cardiac transplant patients appear to require one-third to one-fifth of the usual dose because of denervation hypersensitivity.

Adenosine is contraindicated in patients with sick sinus syndrome or second- or third-degree heart block unless the patient has a functioning artificial pacemaker. Patients should be warned beforehand about side effects such as facial flushing, dyspnea, and chest pressure, which last less than 60 s. Bronchospasm in asthmatic patients has not been reported with intravenous administration. Other less frequent side effects include nausea, light-headedness, headache, sweating, palpitations, hypotension, and blurred vision. Intravenous theophylline has been recommended to reverse the effects of adenosine if necessary.

SUGGESTED READING

CAST investigators: Preliminary report: Effect of encainide and flecainide on mortality in a randomized trial of arrhythmia suppression after myocardial infarction. *N Engl J Med* 1989; 321:406–412.

Connolly SJ: Meta-analysis of antiarrhythmic drug trials. *Am J Cardiol* 1999; 84:90R–93R.

Mason JW, ESVEM Investigators: A comparison of seven antiarrhythmic drugs in patients with ventricular tachyarrhythmias. *N Engl J Med* 1993; 329:452–458.

Task Force of the Working Group on Arrhythmias of the European Society for Cardiology: The Sicilian gambit: A new approach to the classification of antiarrhythmic drugs based on their actions on arrhythmogenic mechanisms. *Circulation* 1991; 84(4):1831–1851.

Vaughan Williams EM: A classification of antiarrhythmic actions reassessed after a decade of new drugs. *J Clin Pharmacol* 1984; 24:129–147.

Woosley RL: Antiarrhythmic drugs. In: Fuster V, Alexander RW, O'Rourke RA, et al (eds): *Hurst's The Heart*, 10th ed. New York: McGraw-Hill; 2001:899–924.

7

THE IMPLANTABLE CARDIOVERTER DEFIBRILLATOR

Peter A. O'Callaghan
Jeremy N. Ruskin

BACKGROUND

Sudden and unexpected cardiac death (SCD) is estimated to claim 300,000 lives annually in the United States. In more than 80 percent of cases, sudden death is caused by the abrupt onset of ventricular tachycardia (VT) that progresses to ventricular fibrillation (VF). Since self-termination of VF is exceedingly rare, the single most important factor determining survival is the time between event onset and first defibrillation attempt. The implantable cardioverter/defibrillator (ICD) was designed to circumvent the delay in providing therapy to ambulatory individuals with life-threatening ventricular tachyarrhythmias. The ICD delivers an internal electric shock within 10 to 15 s of arrhythmia onset—a time frame in which the potential for arrhythmia reversal approaches 100 percent.

Mirowski and coworkers implanted the first implantable defibrillator at the Johns Hopkins University Medical Center in 1980. In the original article, the authors state "It is intended to protect patients at particularly high risk of sudden death whenever and wherever they are stricken by these lethal arrhythmias . . . . the only purpose of this device is to achieve defibrillation automatically, before the victim of a lethal arrhythmia can be reached by a cardiac resuscitation team." Since then the indications for ICD implantation have greatly expanded, devices have become small enough for pectoral implantation, and the number implanted annually has markedly increased.

THE EVIDENCE BASE FOR ICD THERAPY

As a therapeutic modality, the ICD is unsurpassed in its ability to prevent sudden cardiac death. Nevertheless, despite a marked reduction

TABLE 7-1
SECONDARY PREVENTION ICD TRIALS

Trial	Study Population	Treatment Groups	Number of Patients	Primary Endpoint	Study Period	Outcome
AVID (Antiarrhythmics Versus Implantable Defibrillators)	(i) Cardiac arrest survivors or (ii) VT with either syncope or hypotension+EF<40%	ICD vs. amiodarone or guided sotalol therapy	1016	Total mortality	1993 to 1997	31% reduction in total mortality at 3 years with the ICD (25 vs. 36%, $p < 0.02$)
CIDS (Canadian Implantable Defibrillator Study)	(i) Cardiac arrest survivors or (ii) syncopal VT or (iii) symptomatic VT+ EF <35% or (iv) SUO + documented spontaneous or induced VT	ICD vs. amiodarone	~600	Total mortality	1990 to 1997	20% reduction in total mortality at 3 years with the ICD (25 vs. 30%, $p < 0.07$, NS)
CASH (Cardiac Arrest Study Hamburg)	Cardiac arrest survivors and inducible VT or VF	ICD vs. amiodarone vs. metoprolol vs. propafanone[a]	346	Total mortality	1987 to 1995	37% reduction in total mortality with the ICD compared with amiodarone or metoprolol (12 vs. 20%, one-sided $p = 0.047$)

KEY: SUO = syncope of undetermined origin.
[a] Propafanone limb terminated 1993 due to excess mortality.

in sudden death rates, overall mortality in ICD recipients remains high, with nearly 20 percent 2 year mortality in most series. The degree of survival benefit is usually dependent on the sudden cardiac death rate relative to the progressive pump failure death rate, a ratio that is largely unknown. In the past, it was argued that ICDs may have little effect on overall survival in patients with heart failure. First, as New York Heart Association (NYHA) functional class deteriorates, the proportion of deaths which are sudden decreases. Second, successfully terminating an episode of VF will have little effect on overall survival if the patient dies shortly thereafter of progressive pump failure. Therefore, prospective randomized trials were conducted to test the hypothesis that implantable defibrillators significantly improve total survival.

Secondary Prevention of Sudden Cardiac Death

The results of three large prospective ICD trials (AVID, CIDS, and CASH) comparing implantable defibrillators versus antiarrhythmic drug therapy (mainly amiodarone) in patients with life-threatening ventricular tachyarrhythmias have consistently shown that the implantable defibrillator improves overall survival (Table 7-1, Fig. 7-1).

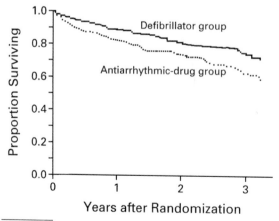

FIGURE 7-1

The Antiarrhythmic Versus Implantable Defibrillator (AVID) trial. Overall survival in the defibrillator group and the antiarrhythmic drug group up to 3 years after randomization in the AVID trial. Survival was better among patients treated with the implantable defibrillator ($p < 0.02$).

TABLE 7-2
PRIMARY PREVENTION ICD TRIALS

Trial	Study Population	Treatment Groups	Number of Patients	Primary Endpoint	Study Period	Outcome
MADIT (Multicenter Automatic Defibrillator Implantation Trial)	Prior MI with EF <35%, NSVT and inducible, nonsuppressible VT or VF	ICD vs. conventional medical therapy	196	Total mortality	1990 to 1996	Total mortality in ICD group significantly less than that in conventional group (16 vs. 39%, $p < 0.01$)
MUSTT (Multicenter Unsustained Tachycardia Trial)	CAD with EF <40%, NSVT and inducible VT or VF	Antiarrhythmic therapy (ICD or EP-guided antiarrhythmic drug) vs. no antiarrhythmic therapy	704	Cardiac arrest or death from arrhythmia	1990 to 1998	5-year incidence of cardiac arrest or death from arrhythmia significantly less among 'antiarrhythmic therapy' compared to 'no antiarrhythmic therapy' patients (25 vs. 32%, $p = 0.04$)

Trial	Population	Comparison	N	Endpoint	Years	Results
CABG Patch (Coronary Artery Bypass Graft Patch Trial)	CABG with EF <36% and positive SAECG	ICD + CABG vs. CABG only	900	Total mortality	1990 to 1997	At 4-year follow-up total actuarial mortality in ICD group no different from control group (27 vs. 24%, $p = 0.7$)
SCD-HeFT (Sudden Cardiac Death in Heart Failure Trial)	Ischemic or dilated cardiomyopathy with CHF(NYHA II–III) and EF <35%	ICD vs. amiodarone vs. conventional group	~2500	Total mortality	1996 to present	Ongoing
MADIT II (Second Multicenter Automatic Defibrillator Implantation Trial)	Prior myocardial infarction with EF <30%	ICD vs. conventional group	~1200	Total mortality	1998 to present	Ongoing

KEY: VT = ventricular tachycardia; VF = ventricular fibrillation; EF = ejection fraction; MI = myocardial infarction; NSVT = nonsustained ventricular tachycardia; CAD = coronary artery disease; EP = electrophysiologic; CABG = coronary artery bypass graft; SAECG = signal-averaged electrocardiogram; ICD = implantable cardioverter defibrillator; vs. = versus; NYHA = New York Heart Association functional classification.

Although each of these three studies found lower total mortality rates in ICD recipients, only the AVID trial reached clear statistical significance. A meta-analysis of these trials was presented at the North American Society of Pacing and Electrophysiology Annual Scientific Sessions, 1999. In total there were 200 deaths among patients treated with implantable defibrillators and 255 deaths among patients treated with amiodarone. Compared to amiodarone, the ICD reduced total mortality by 27 percent ($p < 0.05$). As a result of these clinical trials, the implantable defibrillator is now accepted as the therapy of first choice in survivors of symptomatic sustained ventricular tachyarrhythmias.

Primary Prevention of Sudden Cardiac Death

The majority of patients at risk of sudden cardiac death have not previously experienced a sustained ventricular tachyarrhythmia. Primary (prophylactic) ICD implantation involves placing the device in a patient who is at high risk but has never had a spontaneous episode of sustained VT or VF, with the aim of effectively treating the first episode. Defining populations of patients who are at high enough risk to justify primary ICD implantation is the focus of several clinical trials (Table 7-2). Included are select patients with left ventricular dysfunction and nonsustained VT (MADIT and MUSTT trials), high-risk coronary artery disease patients who have undergone surgical revascularization (CABG-Patch trial), and patients with either ischemic or nonischemic dilated, cardiomyopathy (SCD-HeFT, and MADIT II trials).

Nonsustained VT (NSVT) in the setting of a previous myocardial infarction and left ventricular dysfunction is associated with a 2-year mortality rate of 20 to 30 percent. In the Multicenter Automatic Defibrillator Implantation Trial (MADIT), ICD implantation in such patients with inducible, nonsuppressible VT or VF improved survival compared to conventional medical therapy. In the Multicenter UnSustained Tachycardia Trial (MUSTT), patients randomized to antiarrhythmic therapy (ICD or electrophysiological-guided drug therapy) had a significantly reduced arrhythmic mortality. Of note, the improvement in outcome was due to ICD patients; electrophysiologically guided drug therapy (mostly class I agents) did not improve and may have worsened outcome (Fig. 7-2). Therefore MADIT and MUSTT trials confirm that, in patients with coronary artery disease, left ventricular dysfunction, spontaneous nonsustained VT, and inducible sustained ventricular tachyarrhythmias, the ICD is effective in significantly reducing the risk of sudden cardiac death and in prolonging overall survival.

The CABG-Patch trial randomized patients with left ventricular dysfunction and a positive signal averaged electrocardiogram (ECG)

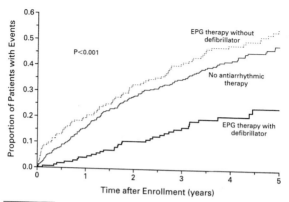

FIGURE 7-2

The Multicenter UnSustained Tachycardia Trial (MUSTT). Kaplan-Meier estimates of overall mortality according to whether the patients received treatment with electrophysiologically guided (EPG) therapy without defibrillator (i.e., antiarrhythmic drug therapy), no antiarrhythmic therapy, or electrophysiologically guided therapy with a defibrillator. Mortality rates were significantly less in the ICD-treated patients than in the other two groups.

who were undergoing coronary artery bypass surgery to an ICD or no specific antiarrhythmic therapy. There was no survival benefit from ICD implantation. These patients were at relatively low risk of arrhythmic death compared with the MADIT or MUSST populations, and the outcome also underscores the survival benefit of coronary artery revascularization. The results of negative ICD trials such as CABG-Patch emphasize the fact that ICDs prolong survival only in a population that has a sufficiently high incidence of life-threatening ventricular tachyarrhythmias.

Despite conventional medical therapy, the mortality rate associated with heart failure and left ventricular dysfunction remains unacceptably high, and sudden cardiac death is responsible for approximately half of all cardiac deaths. The Sudden Cardiac Death in Heart Failure Trial (SCD-HeFT) and the second Multicenter Automatic Defibrillator Implantation Trial (MADIT-II) were designed to address the issue of whether the ICD improves survival in a population of cardiomyopathy patients regardless of the presence or absence of arrhythmia markers (inducibility, NSVT, etc.). The real challenge over the next few years will be to develop means of accurately identifying patients in whom ICD therapy is both efficacious and cost-effective.

TABLE 7-3

ACC/AHA GUIDELINES FOR ICD IMPLANTATION

Class I: ICD indicated
1. Cardiac arrest due to VT or VF not due to a transient or reversible cause.
2. Spontaneous sustained VT.
3. Syncope of undetermined origin with clinically relevant, hemodynamically significant sustained VT or VF induced at electrophysiologic study when drug therapy is ineffective, not tolerated, or not preferred.
4. Nonsustained VT with coronary artery disease, prior myocardial infarction, left ventricular dysfunction, and inducible VF or sustained VT at electrophysiology study that is not suppressible by a class I antiarrhythmic drug.

Class II: ICD may be indicated
1. Cardiac arrest presumed to be due to VF when electrophysiologic testing is precluded by other medical conditions.
2. Severe symptoms attributable to ventricular tachyarrhythmias while awaiting cardiac transplantation.
3. Familial or inherited conditions with a high risk for life-threatening ventricular tachyarrhythmias such as long-QT syndrome or hypertrophic cardiomyopathy.
4. Nonsustained VT with coronary artery disease, prior myocardial infarction, LV dysfunction, and inducible sustained VT or VF at electrophysiologic study.
5. Recurrent syncope of undetermined etiology in the presence of ventricular dysfunction and inducible ventricular arrhythmias at electrophysiological study when other causes of syncope have been excluded.

Class III: ICD contraindicated

1. Syncope of undetermined cause in a patient without inducible ventricular tachyarrhythmias.
2. Incessant VT or VF.
3. VF or VT resulting from arrhythmias amenable to surgical or catheter ablation; for example, atrial arrhythmias associated with Wolff-Parkinson-White syndrome, right ventricular outflow tract VT; idiopathic left ventricular tachycardia, or fascicular VT.
4. Ventricular tachyarrhythmias due to a transient or reversible disorder; for example, acute myocardial infarction, electrolyte imbalance, drugs, trauma.
5. Significant psychiatric illnesses that may be aggravated by device implantation or preclude systematic follow-up.
6. Terminal illness with projected life expectancy ≤ 6 months.
7. Patients with coronary artery disease, left ventricular dysfunction, and prolonged QRS duration in the absence of spontaneous or inducible sustained or nonsustained VT who are undergoing coronary bypass surgery.
8. NYHA class IV drug-refractory CHF in patients who are not candidates for cardiac transplantation.

ICD THERAPY IN SPECIFIC CLINICAL SETTINGS

The American College of Cardiology/American Heart Association advise ICD therapy in cardiac arrest survivors, in patients with spontaneous sustained VT, in select patients with syncope of undetermined origin, and in select patients with coronary artery disease, left ventricular dysfunction, and nonsustained VT (Table 7-3). In these clinical circumstances, the implantable defibrillator is now the treatment of first choice. Antiarrhythmic therapy is mainly limited to adjunctive therapy in ICD recipients who have other tachyarrhythmias (e.g., atrial fibrillation) or who are receiving frequent shocks and require suppressive drug therapy.

Cardiac Arrest Survivors

Aborted sudden cardiac death is, in the majority of cases, caused by life-threatening ventricular tachyarrhythmias (VF and hypotensive VT). Structural heart disease is almost invariably present; in adult populations, the cause is most frequently coronary artery disease. Survivors of cardiac arrest are at high risk of future recurrence, and ICD therapy is usually indicated. Cardiac catheterization identifies survivors who have critical obstructive coronary artery disease. It is our practice to also revascularize these patients whenever feasible. Cardiac arrest occurring in the setting of acute clinical ischemia or within 48 h of an acute myocardial infarction is, with rare exception, treated in the conventional manner without electrophysiologic workup or ICD implantation.

Sustained Monomorphic Ventricular Tachycardia

In patients with sustained monomorphic VT (SMVT) that has resulted in a cardiac arrest or syncope, the ICD is usually employed as first-line therapy. In patients with SMVT that is tolerated hemodynamically, other potential therapeutic options include amiodarone therapy, catheter ablation, and arrhythmia surgery. Amiodarone therapy is associated with high rates of drug discontinuation due to adverse side effects. Catheter ablation is usually employed only as adjunctive therapy in patients with underlying structural heart disease, typically in patients with implanted devices. Arrhythmia surgery is the only therapy with long-term sudden death rates similar to those associated with ICD therapy, but it carries a higher perioperative mortality. Combined aneurysmectomy and arrhythmia surgery yields a low rate of arrhythmia recurrence and may be indicated in highly selected patients who have a discrete left ventricular aneurysm. In summary, compared to the other available treatments, ICD therapy is widely applicable, well tolerated, and associated with good short- and long-term results. Today it is the preferred mode of therapy in the majority of SMVT patients with structural heart disease. In individual patients, more than one therapy may be indicated.

Syncope of Undetermined Origin

When it is associated with structural heart disease and inducible VT, syncope carries a high risk of sudden cardiac death, similar to that of patients presenting with documented spontaneous VT or VF. ICD therapy is recommended in these patients. Patients with idiopathic dilated cardiomyopathy who present with syncope have high mortality, and in them, unlike coronary artery disease patients, the role of electrophysiologic study is ill defined. Prospective studies are needed to identify which patients with dilated cardiomyopathy and undetermined syncope may benefit from ICD implantation. Meanwhile, these patients need careful clinical assessment, and select patients may benefit from implantable event loop-recording devices.

Symptomatic Patients with Severe Left Ventricular Dysfunction

Patients with poor left ventricular function who have experienced a spontaneous episode of life-threatening ventricular tachyarrhythmia are a high risk of both sudden cardiac death and death due to progressive pump failure. Somewhat surprisingly, subgroup analysis of both the AVID and CIDS trials has found that patients with a left ventricular ejection fraction (LVEF) ≤ 35 percent derive the greatest survival benefit from defibrillator therapy. Patients with an LVEF $>$ 35 percent had similar survival benefit up to 3 years after randomization with either amiodarone or device therapy, probably due to a lower arrhythmia recurrence rate.

Patients awaiting heart transplantation are not only at risk of sudden tachyarrhythmic death, they are also at high risk of sudden death due to bradyarrhythmias or electromechanical dissociation and of death due to progressive pump failure. Nevertheless, it has been reported that cardiac transplant candidates who have experienced a spontaneous episode of life-threatening ventricular tachyarrhythmia can be effectively protected against sudden arrhythmic death. It is argued that ICDs should be implanted in all NYHA class III patients as a "bridge" to transplantation. To date, no prospective randomized trial has been conducted to assess the benefit of such a strategy.

Asymptomatic High-Risk Patients

As the prognosis associated with a first cardiac arrest is very poor, an effective primary prevention strategy is required to identify and effectively treat patients at high risk of sudden death. The results of the MADIT and MUSST trials confirm that, in a clearly defined high-risk group of patients with coronary artery disease, the ICD is effective in significantly reducing the risk of SCD and prolonging overall survival. *In practice we do not recommend routine screening of coronary artery disease patients with left ventricular dysfunction to detect the presence of nonsustained VT.* However, in select patients with severe left ventricular dysfunction who are brought to our attention because of recurrent nonsustained VT, we recommend electrophysiologic testing and, if MADIT or MUSST criteria are met, ICD implantation.

FUNCTIONAL CHARACTERISTICS

The ICD system consists of two basic components: a pulse generator and lead electrode(s) for arrhythmia detection and for therapy delivery. In addition to internal defibrillation, ICDs also provide pacing (antitachycardia and bradycardia), synchronized cardioversion, telemetry, and diagnostics (event electrograms and history logs).

Detection of Tachyarrhythmia

Reliable sensing of ventricular depolarizations is essential for proper functioning of the ICD. Sensing electrodes transmit unfiltered electrograms to the sense amplifier of the ICD. The sense amplifier amplifies, filters, and rectifies the incoming signals. It then compares them to a sensing threshold and produces a set of RR intervals for the detection algorithm to use (Fig. 7-3A). Intracardiac electrogram amplitude can vary markedly between rhythms such as sinus rhythm, VT, and VF. Therefore all ICDs utilize some form of automatically adjusting signal amplifier. Sensed events are then analyzed using a detection algorithm. The range of all possible ventricular cycle lengths is divided into rate zones that do not overlap. These include a VF zone, VT zone(s), normal rate zone, and bradycardia zone.

Devices employ rate criteria as the sole method of detecting VF. Any tachycardia with a programmable proportion of cycle lengths less than the tachycardia detection interval will be detected as VF and therapy will be initiated. At the end of capacitor charging and prior to the delivery of therapy, a reconfirmation algorithm must be fulfilled. This prevents inappropriate shock therapy for self-terminating events such as nonsustained VT.

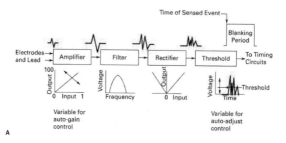

A

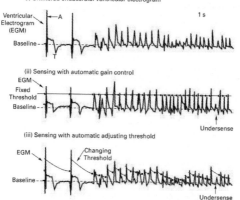

B

FIGURE 7-3

Sensing of electrogram signals by implantable cardioverter defibrillators. *A.* Functional block diagram for an ICD sense amplifier consists of an amplifier that may be fixed or have automatic gain control, a bandpass filter to reject low-frequency T waves and high-frequency noise, a rectifier to eliminate polarity dependency, and a threshold detector that may be fixed or autoadjusting. The net result is a single pulse for each ventricular depolarization that is used by timing circuits to determine a series of cycle lengths. The effects of each block on a biphasic electrogram are shown above the blocks and each functional operation is shown below each block. *B.* Sinus rhythm and ventricular fibrillation signals are shown for the raw electrogram in panel i, for automatic gain control in panel ii, and for automatic adjusting threshold in panel iii. With automatic gain control, the small electrograms are amplified compared to panel i and sensing is shown by the dots where the signal crosses the fixed threshold. With automatic adjusting threshold, the electrograms are the same as in panel i and the threshold varies according to the amplitude of the electrogram. Sensing is again shown by the dots where the signal crosses the variable threshold.

Although rate is the principal detection criterion, the VT detection algorithm is different from that in the VF zone. Most VT detection algorithms require a programmable number of consecutive intervals shorter than the VT detection interval. Any interval longer than the detection interval (e.g., due to RR variability in atrial fibrillation) resets the counters. Both ventricular and supraventricular tachycardias (e.g., sinus tachycardia, atrial fibrillation) may result in ventricular rates within the VT zone. Up to 25 percent of ICD discharges are inappropriate when rate is employed as the sole criterion for VT therapy. These inappropriate discharges are poorly tolerated by patients and constitute a major clinical problem. To increase specificity, optional VT detection enhancements are programmable (Table 7-4). This approach should be limited to tachycardias that are hemodynamically tolerated. Although programming of these options improves specificity, it does so at the risk of prolonging detection times and of failure to detect an episode of VT. As a safety feature "sustained rate duration" is a programmable maximum period of time (e.g., 30 to 120 s) during which therapy is inhibited if the enhancement criteria are not met. If the tachycardia persists at the end of this period, therapy is be delivered.

Dual-chamber ICDs, requiring an additional atrial lead, provide the benefits of dual-chamber pacing and also dual-chamber detection algorithms. These algorithms reduce the number of inappropriate shocks, but it is unknown whether dual-chamber ICDs will perform better than optimally programmed single-chamber devices.

Ventricular Fibrillation Therapy

ICDs employ electrical defibrillation as the sole therapy option for the treatment of VF. Successful defibrillation may require voltages up to 100 times greater than the voltage of the ICD battery ($\sim$6.4 V). A capacitor is used to store charge immediately prior to therapy delivery. This energy is then delivered between the high-voltage electrodes and depolarizes the intervening myocardium, thereby restoring baseline rhythm. Reversing electrode polarity during capacitor discharge (biphasic waveform) lowers defibrillation energy requirements and is one of the main factors that facilitated the introduction of smaller, lower-energy pectoral devices. The time interval between VF onset and delivery of defibrillation energy is usually 10 to 15 s, with capacitor charge time accounting for most of the delay. During this time the subject may experience syncope, with restoration of consciousness after successful defibrillation and restoration of cardiac output. One study of ICD recipients found that 16 percent of patients experienced syncope during follow-up, as compared with 65 percent of patients prior to device implantation.

TABLE 7-4

OPTIONAL VT DETECTION ENHANCEMENTS

Detection Enhancement Criterion	Variable Measured	Rhythm Differentiation
Sudden onset	Percent of cycle length shortening at onset of tachycardia (e.g., >9% ⇒ VT)	Sinus tachycardia vs. ventricular tachycardia
Rate stability	RR variability (e.g., ≤ 40 ms ⇒ VT)	Atrial fibrillation vs. ventricular tachycardia
Electrogram morphology	Intracardiac electrogram width	SVT with normal His-Purkinje conduction vs. ventricular tachycardia

Ventricular Tachycardia Therapy

In contrast to VF therapy, treatment options in the VT zone(s) include antitachycardia pacing (ATP), cardioversion, and defibrillation. Therapy progresses through a programmable sequence of responses until the episode is terminated. Most sustained monomorphic VTs, particularly in patients with coronary artery disease, are due to reentry and can be terminated by overdrive pacing (ATP). ATP, with backup defibrillation if acceleration occurs, is an attractive, well-tolerated treatment that avoids high-energy shock therapy, which is painful and diminishes battery life. ATP successfully terminates over 90 percent of spontaneous VTs.

Cardioversion, in contrast to defibrillation, is a synchronized low-energy shock that reduces the time to therapy and conserves battery life. Cardioversion and ATP are equally efficacious.

Dual-Chamber Devices

Bradycardia ventricular demand pacing is a standard feature in all single-chamber ICDs. Dual-chamber ICDs provide not only improved diagnostic specificity but also the benefits of dual-chamber pacing, dual-chamber cardioversion, and dual-chamber defibrillation in patients with paroxysmal supraventricular and ventricular tachyarrhythmias. Approximately 20 percent of ICD recipients need antibradycardia pacing; most of these would benefit from a dual-chamber device. If one includes patients with poor ejection fraction and patients who would benefit from dual-chamber sensing, it is possible that up to 50 percent of ICD recipients might benefit from implantation of a dual-chamber ICD. In addition ICDs that incorporate biventricular pacing are also available.

DEVICE IMPLANTATION

ICDs are implanted in the pectoral region using techniques similar to those employed in permanent pacemaker implantation. An integrated lead consisting of pace/sense electrodes and high-energy defibrillation coils (RV and SVC coils) is inserted, preferably via the cephalic vein to avoid the risks of subclavian puncture and subclavian crush syndrome.

In dual-chamber devices, a separate atrial lead is inserted. Anesthesia may be local or general and pulse generator implantation may be prepectoral (subcutaneous) or subpectoral (submuscular). The titanium case of the pulse generator acts as a large surface area defibrillation electrode ("active can"). The usual defibrillation pathway is RV coil to active can/SVC coil. As a result the position of the pulse generator affects the defibrillation wavefront and should, when possible, be implanted in the left pectoral region.

DEVICE TESTING

The ability to reproducibly defibrillate VF is fundamental to the success of ICD therapy in preventing sudden cardiac death. Accomplishing this goal requires meticulous testing at the time of implantation. VF is induced by the device intraoperatively. The relationship between defibrillation energy and success is best described as a sigmoidal dose-response curve, the probability of success increasing steadily with each increase in energy until a 100 percent success plateau is reached (Fig. 7-4). To ensure future efficacy, even if there is a rise in defibrillation threshold (DFT), a safety margin of at least 10 J must exist between the measured DFT and the maximum energy output of the device. Today it is relatively uncommon to encounter DFTs so high that implantation criteria are not met (Table 7-5). Prior to discharge, the pace-sense characteristics of the ICD system are assessed and a chest x-ray is reviewed to rule out lead dislodgment. In the majority of ICD recipients, empiric programming of ATP therapy for VT should be considered.

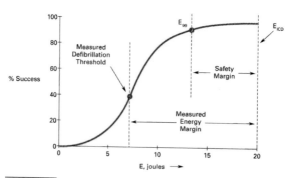

FIGURE 7-4

Percent probability for successful defibrillation versus shock energy. The measured ICD energy margin is the energy difference between the lowest conversion success [defibrillation threshold (DFT)] and the programmed ICD energy. The ICD safety margin is the energy difference between the lowest energy required for consistent defibrillation success (E_{99}) and the programmed ICD energy. The more inductions and successful defibrillations performed, the more closely the measured energy margin approximates the device's safety margin.

TABLE 7-5

MANAGEMENT OPTIONS IN PATIENTS WITH HIGH
DEFIBRILLATION THRESHOLDS

Reposition the lead (closer to the right ventricular apex if
  possible)
Rule out pneumothorax
Reverse shock polarity, pulse duration, or waveform
Add additional defibrillation electrode (e.g., subcutaneous
  coil)
Implant a higher-output device
Stop drugs such as amiodarone and repeat DFT testing
  after washout period

LONG-TERM FOLLOW-UP

The ICD is generally well tolerated, but factors that adversely affect
quality of life include frequent or inappropriate shocks, device malfunction, and/or product recall. As shock delivery has a major impact
on quality of life, it is appropriate to consider measures such as concomitant drug therapy, empiric programming of ATP for VT, and use
of detection enhancement algorithms to minimize the risk of shock
delivery during long-term follow-up. Driving restrictions should be
discussed with patients prior to device implantation. The period of
greatest risk for ICD discharge is within the first 6 months following
implantation. Patients receiving implantable defibrillators comprise a
heterogeneous population. Published guidelines from the American
Heart Association and the North American Society of Pacing and
Electrophysiology recommend that patients who receive an ICD because of a previously documented episode of VT or VF should be
prohibited from all driving for the first 6 months. After 6 months,
if an ICD discharge has not occurred, patients may resume driving.
Patients who have a prophylactic ICD implant and who have never
had a documented episode of spontaneous ventricular tachyarrhythmia are allowed to resume driving.

COMPLICATIONS

ICD therapy is associated with well-known risks (Table 7-6). Lead-
related problems remain a significant problem despite the advances

TABLE 7-6
COMPLICATIONS ASSOCIATED WITH ICD IMPLANTATION

Procedure-related
Short-term
  DFT testing (inability to defibrillate, worsening systolic
    function, electromechanical dissociation)
  Subclavian stick complications (pneumothorax,
    hemothorax, air embolism, subclavian artery puncture)
  Venous thromboembolism
  Phrenic nerve stimulation
  Right ventricular perforation
  Pericardial effusion/tamponade
  Hematoma (pulse generator pocket)
  Seroma (pulse generator pocket)
  Hypotension
  Myocardial infarction
  Cerebrovascular accident
  Proarrhythmia (atrial fibrillation, increased frequency of
    ventricular tachyarrhythmia—"electrical storm")
Long-term
  Infection
  Erosion
  Migration
  Venous thromboembolism
  Endocarditis
  Shoulder-related problems
System-related
  Lead dislodgment (gross dislodgment, microdislodgment,
    Twiddler's syndrome)
  Lead conductor fracture
  Lead insulation defect
  Lead perforation (+/− diaphragmatic pacing)
  Loose set screw
  Exit block (high pacing threshold)
  Inappropriate shock delivery
  Premature battery depletion
  Device recall

in lead technology. In most series, approximately 5 percent of patients have a serious procedure or device related complications requiring surgical intervention in the first 6 months. If one includes mild device-related complications (e.g., inappropriate therapy delivery), approximately 50 percent of patients experience an adverse event within the first year.

One of the most devastating complications is infection of the ICD system. Infection resembles that observed with permanent pacemakers. Direct intraoperative contamination is the usual source; however, due to the low virulence of some organisms, infection may not become obvious for a considerable time. In general, explantation of the entire ICD system is required. After a regimen of intense antibiotic therapy and if all clinical evidence of infection is resolved, reimplantation at a different site may be performed, but the risk of reinfection is higher than that following a primary implant.

Troubleshooting

The differentiation of appropriate from inappropriate device function in a patient who has received an ICD discharge is a challenging problem (Table 7-7). Stored intracardiac electrograms, real-time measurements, system x-rays, device manipulations, and VF induction under anesthesia may all be required to determine the cause of inappropriate device function. Accurate diagnosis is essential in order to institute the appropriate action, which may include device reprogramming, activation of VT detection enhancement algorithms, alteration of antiarrhythmic drug therapy, or surgical revision of the system.

FUTURE DIRECTIONS

ICD technology is evolving rapidly. Advances in battery and capacitor technology, improved lead systems, and more efficient defibrillation waveforms will hopefully enable the ICD of the future to more closely approach the size of permanent pacemakers. Increased battery longevity will reduce the morbidity associated with pulse generator replacements and will improve the cost-effectiveness of ICD therapy. The incorporation of a reliable hemodynamic sensor to differentiate hemodynamically stable from hypotensive tachyarrhythmias would help identify the most appropriate therapy for each arrhythmia. Most important will be a clearer understanding of the role of noninvasive risk stratification and of ICD therapy in the primary prevention of sudden cardiac death. Careful patient selection to reduce overall mortality will ensure that both patients and society benefit.

TABLE 7-7

TROUBLESHOOTING THE CAUSES OF ICD THERAPY

1. Analyze stored intracardiac electrograms
   —Electrogram morphology (near-field electrograms)
     Identical to sinus rhythm (sinus tachycardia? atrial fibrillation?)
     Different to sinus rhythm (ventricular tachyarrhythmia)
   —Atrial activity (far-field electrograms)
     AV dissociation (ventricular tachyarrhythmia)
     Atrial rate > ventricular rate (SVT)
2. Real-time measurements
   Pacing/sensing thresholds (? lead dislodgment)
   Lead impedance (? insulation break, lead fracture)
3. X-ray system (PA and lateral "overpenetrated" views)
   ? Lead fracture, lead displacement
4. Device manipulation during real-time telemetry
   ? noise, ? intermittent defects (loose set screw, lead fracture, etc.)
5. Noninvasive programmed stimulation (NIPS)
   VF induction via device under anesthesia to assess DFTs

SUGGESTED READING

Buxton AE, Lee KL, Fisher JD, et al for the Multicenter Unsustained Tachycardia Trial Investigators: A randomised study of the prevention of sudden death in patients with coronary artery disease. *N Engl J Med* 1999; 341:1882–1890.

Connolly SJ, Gent M, Roberts RS, et al: Canadian Implantable Defibrillator Study (CIDS): A randomised trial of the implantable cardioverter defibrillator against amiodarone. *Circulation* 2000; 101:1297–1302.

Fogoros RN: The impact of the implantable defibrillator on mortality: The axiom of overall implantable cardioverter-defibrillator survival. *Am J Cardiol* 1996; 78:57–61.

Gregoratos G, Cheitlin MD, Epstein AE, et al: ACC/AHA guidelines for implantation of cardiac pacemakers and antiarrhythmic devices: A report of the American College of Cardiology/American Heart Association Task Force on Practice Guidelines

(Committee on Pacemaker Implantation). *J Am Coll Cardiol* 1998; 31:1175–1209.

Moss AJ, Hall WJ, Cannom DS, et al for the Multicenter Automatic Defibrillator Implantation Trial Investigators: Improved survival with an implanted defibrillator in patients with coronary artery disease at high risk for ventricular arrhythmia. *N Engl J Med* 1996; 335:1933–1940.

O'Callaghan PA, Ruskin JN: The implantable cardioverter defibrillator. In: Fuster V, Alexander RW, O'Rourke RA, et al (eds): *Hurst's The Heart*, 10th ed. New York: McGraw-Hill; 2001: 945–962.

The Antiarrhythmics versus Implantable Defibrillators (AVID) Investigators: A comparison of antiarrhythmic-drug therapy with implantable defibrillators in patients resuscitated from near-fatal ventricular arrhythmias. *N Engl J Med* 1997; 337:1576–1583.

CHAPTER

8

CARDIAC PACEMAKERS

Raul D. Mitrani
Robert J. Myerburg
Agustin Castellanos

INTRODUCTION

Pacemakers are coded by a specific abbreviation according to the type of pacemaker and mode of pacing. The first letter refers to the chamber(s) being paced and the second to the chamber(s) being sensed. The letters A and V indicate atrial or ventricular pacing and/or sensing. If dual chambers are paced and/or sensed, the designation D is used. The third letter refers to the response to a sensed event. The pacemaker inhibits (I) pacing output from one or both of its leads, or triggers (T) pacing at a programmable interval after the sensed event. If a pacer can inhibit atrial output and trigger a ventricular paced complex after a sensed atrial complex, then the third letter is designated by D. A fourth letter [R] denotes rate responsiveness.

For an electrical signal from a pacer to cause electrical depolarization, a minimal threshold of current is necessary, which is a function of the pacer lead, longevity, and other clinical factors. The current delivered is a function of the pacemaker voltage and pulse width, which is generally programmed to deliver two to four times the threshold current in order to have an adequate safety margin.

A pacemaker senses intrinsic cardiac activity by measuring intracardiac electrograms. The range for atrial and ventricular electrograms is 1 to 5 mV and 5 to 20 mV, respectively; therefore pacemaker sensitivities are programmed at 0.25 to 2 mV in the atrial channel and 2 to 4 mV in the ventricular channel in order to have an adequate safety margin for sensing.

TEMPORARY PACING

Temporary pacing is used when patients experience intermittent or persistent hemodynamically relevant bradyarrhythmias or when standby pacing is required for patients at increased risk for sudden and complete heart block. Occasionally, temporary pacing is used to control sustained atrial or ventricular tachyarrhythmias. The endpoint for temporary pacing is either resolution of a temporary indication for pacing or implantation of a permanent pacemaker for a continuing indication.

Transcutaneous pacing is a common, rapid method for noninvasively pacing patients who require a prophylactic temporary pacer or emergent pacing. The unit incorporates two large pads placed in the anterior and posterior positions. The main drawback is the high energy requirement (50 to 100 mA at 20 to 40 ms), which causes skeletal muscle stimulation and pain.

INDICATIONS FOR PERMANENT PACEMAKERS

Pacemakers are generally implanted for control of bradyarrhythmias due to chronic or intermittent atrioventricular (AV) conduction system disease, sinus nodal dysfunction, or one of the neurocardiac syndromes (Table 8-1). Many indications for pacemaker implantation are predicated on the presence of symptoms. However, many symptoms—such as fatigue or subtle symptoms of congestive heart failure—may be recognized only in retrospect, after placement of a permanent pacemaker.

Pacing for Specific Causes and Patterns of AV Block

In general, complete heart block, permanent or intermittent, at any anatomic level associated with symptoms such as dizziness, lightheadedness, congestive heart failure, and confusion is an indication for permanent pacemaker. In asymptomatic patients, a ventricular rate <40 beats per minute or pauses >3.0 s are also considered indications for pacemaker implantation.

Asymptomatic third-degree or type II second-degree AV block is generally an indication for permanent pacemaker placement. Asymptomatic type I second-degree AV block is generally not seen as calling for permanent pacing unless there is electrophysiologic evidence that such block is in the His-Purkinje system. First-degree AV block is also not considered to be an indication for permanent pacing unless there are symptoms associated with marked PR prolongation (usually in the setting of left ventricular dysfunction).

In the setting of an acute myocardial infarction (MI), pacemakers are indicated for high-grade or complete block in the His-Purkinje system (see also Chap.15). In the setting of inferior infarction, AV block typically occurs at the level of the AV node and may be due to reversible injury and/or poor autonomic tone; therefore AV block usually subsides if one waits a sufficient time. Transient advanced infranodal AV block with associated bundle branch block is also an indication for pacing; however, electrophysiology studies may be required to determine the level of block.

In the presence of bifascicular or trifascicular block, intermittent third-degree or type II second-degree AV block usually indicates the need for a permanent pacemaker. When these patients present with syncope, a pacemaker may be required.

Pacing in Congenital AV Block

The site of AV block in congenital heart block is usually at the level of the AV node. However, congenital AV block is associated with serious and possibly fatal complications, including syncope and sudden death. Cardiac pacing is indicated in all symptomatic patients. Due to an increased mortality risk from persistent brady-cardia, pacing is now indicated in most adults, even in the absence of symptoms.

Pacing in Sinus Nodal Dysfunction

Sinus nodal dysfunction has become the most common indication for pacing in the United States, especially in the presence of symp-toms correlating with bradyarrhythmias. However, it may be difficult to correlate electrocardiographic (ECG) findings with symptoms, which tend to be nebulous. Fatigue and dyspnea may be due to a bradyarrhythmia but also to lack of conditioning or other cardiac dysfunction.

Therefore, pacing is indicated for symptomatic sinus nodal dys-function when bradycardia or pauses are documented that may be secondary to essential long-term drug therapy. Patients with asymptomatic bradyarrhythmias should be evaluated carefully prior to placement of a pacemaker. Athletes commonly have physiologic bradycardia, even with heart rates <40 beats per minute, due to en-hanced vagal tone. Other etiologies, such as sleep apnea, can also cause asymptomatic nocturnal bradyarrhythmias.

Pacing for Carotid Sinus Syndrome

The diagnosis of carotid sinus syndrome is typically made by demon-strating asystolic pauses of >3 s with carotid sinus massage or a

TABLE 8-1

INDICATIONS FOR PERMANENT PACEMAKER

	Class I	Class II	Class III

Acquired AV block	—Third-degree AV block with:
	  * Bradycardia and symptoms due to AV block
	  * Requirement of drugs that result in symptomatic bradycardia
	  * After catheter ablation of the AV junction or after postoperative AV block not expected to resolve
	  * Neuromuscular diseases with AV block
	  * Escape rhythm <40 bpm or asystole > 3 s in awake symptom free patients
	  * Second-degree AV block, permanent or intermittent, with symptomatic bradycardia
		Class IIa
		—Asymptomatic complete AV block with average awake ventricular rate >40 bpm
		—Asymptomatic type II second-degree AV block (permanent or intermittent)
		—Asymptomatic type I second-degree AV block at or below the bundle or His (documented by electrophysiologic studies)
		—First-degree AV block with symptoms suggestive of pacemaker syndrome and documented alleviation of symptoms with temporary pacing
			—Asymptomatic first-degree AV block
			—Asymptomatic type I second-degree AV block above the level of the bundle of His
			—AV block expected to resolve

After myocardial infarction	—Persistent second- or third-degree AV block in the His-Purkinje system or Transient advanced infranodal AV block and associated BBB —Symptomatic second- or third-degree AV block at any level	*Class IIb* —Marked first-degree AV block in patients with congestive heart failure *Class IIb* —Persistent advanced AV block at the AV node level	—Transient AV conduction disturbances without intraventricular conduction defects or with isolated left anterior fascicular block —Acquired left anterior fascicular block —Persistent first-degree AV block in the presence of old or age indeterminate BBB —Fascicular block without AV block or symptoms —Fascicular block with first-degree AV block without symptoms
Bifascicular or trifascicular block	—Intermittent complete heart block associated with symptoms —Type II second-degree AV block	*Class IIa* —Bifascicular or trifascicular block with syncope not proven to be due to AV block but other causes of syncope not identifiable —HV interval >100 ms or pacing induced infra-Hisian block	

(Continued)

Table 8.1
(*Continued*)

	Class I	Class II	Class III
Sinus node dysfunction	—Sinus node dysfunction with documented symptomatic bradycardia (in some patients, this will occur as a result of long-term essential drug therapy of a type and dose for which there is no acceptable alternative) —Symptomatic chronotropic incompetence	*Class IIa* —Sinus node dysfunction, occurring spontaneously or as a result of necessary drug therapy, with heart rates <40 bpm without clear association between significant symptoms and bradycardia. *Class IIb* —In minimally symptomatic patients, chronic heart rate <30 bpm while awake	—Sinus node dysfunction in asymptomatic patients, including those in whom substantial sinus bradycardia is a consequence of long-term drug treatment —Sinus node dysfunction in patients in whom symptoms suggestive of bradycardia are clearly documented not to be associated with a slow heart rate —Sinus node dysfunction with symptomatic bradycardia due to nonessential drug therapy

| Hypersensitive carotid sinus and neurocardiac syndromes | —Recurrent syncope associated with clear, spontaneous events provoked by carotid sinus stimulation; minimal carotid sinus pressure induces asystole of >3 s duration in the absence of any medication that depresses the sinus node or AV conduction | *Class IIa*
—Recurrent syncope without clear, provocative events and with a hypersensitive cardioinhibitory response
Class IIb
—Syncope with associated bradycardia reproduced by head-up tilt (with or without provocative maneuvers or isoproterenol) | —A hyperactive cardioinhibitory response to carotid sinus stimulation in the absence of symptoms
—Vague symptoms (dizziness or light-headedness) with a hyperactive cardioinhibitory response to carotid sinus stimulation
—Recurrent syncope, light-headedness, or dizziness in the absence of a cardioinhibitory response |

NOTE: Class I refers to conditions where there is agreement that pacer therapy is beneficial, useful, and effective. Class II refers to conditions where there is conflicting evidence and/or divergence of opinion about usefulness of pacer therapy. Class IIa refers to conditions where opinion is in favor of usefulness. Class IIb indicates conditions where evidence and opinion are less well established. Class III refers to conditions for which evidence and agreement that a pacer is not indicated and would possibly be harmful.

141

vasodepressor response of >50 mmHg associated with clear symptoms provoked by carotid sinus stimulation, such as wearing a tight shirt or turning one's head. Improvement of symptoms and suppression of syncope has been demonstrated by treating patients with cardiac pacing, particularly dual-chamber pacing.

Cardiac Pacing in Neurocardiogenic Syncope

Cardiac pacing plays little role for most patients with neurocardiogenic syncope because they still experience hypotension, vasodilatation, and other associated symptoms despite cardiac pacing. However, dual-chamber pacing has been shown to reduce recurrences of syncope in patients who have a prominent cardioinhibitory component.

Pacing in Hypertrophic Cardiomyopathy

DDD pacing with a short AV interval reduces left ventricular outflow tract gradients and improves symptoms in patients with obstructive hypertrophic cardiomyopathy (see also Chap. 31), However, recent randomized studies have yielded conflicting results regarding the long-term hemodynamic benefits of pacing for hypertrophic cardiomyopathy. Therefore pacing in these patients remains controversial. Patients with nonobstructive symptomatic hypertrophic cardiomyopathy do not benefit from DDD pacing.

Pacing in Dilated Cardiomyopathy and Congestive Heart Failure

In the absence of standard indications for a pacer, there is no role for standard dual-chamber pacing in patients with congestive heart failure due to ischemic or nonischemic dilated cardiomyopathy. Recent data suggest that biventricular pacing, an investigational pacing technique employing a left ventricular pacing lead in the coronary sinus system, can improve hemodynamic function in patients with dilated cardiomyopathy and a wide QRS duration (i.e., left bundle branch block). Studies examining the long-term effects of biventricular pacing in these patients are ongoing.

PACEMAKER HARDWARE

Pacemaker leads can be unipolar or bipolar. Unipolar leads use a distal electrode in the catheter as the cathode and the shell of the pacemaker generator as the anode. Therefore the myocardium and adjacent tissue complete the circuit. A bipolar lead consist of two separate conductors and electrodes within the lead. Since the electrodes for sensing in a bipolar lead are much closer together, bipolar signals are sharper, with less extraneous noise.

There are several disadvantages to unipolar lead systems. Because the unipolar lead uses body tissue to complete the circuit, there is the possibility of causing muscle stimulation. Unipolar sensing is far more likely to detect extracardiac signals, including myopotentials, remote cardiac potentials (far-field sensing), and electromagnetic interference. Finally, unipolar pacing is generally contraindicated in patients who have a concomitant implantable defibrillator.

PACEMAKER FUNCTION AND MODES

Magnet Mode

Magnets cause asynchronous pacing in virtually all pacemakers. The magnet response varies according to manufacturer and pacemaker model. In patients who are pacemaker-dependent and experiencing oversensing, thereby inhibiting pacemaker output, a magnet is a convenient short-term method of ensuring pacing. Pacemakers usually have different magnet rates for a battery with adequate charge compared to a battery that is nearing depletion (elective replacement index).

VVI mode

VVI mode ensures that a minimum ventricular rate is maintained by ventricular pacing at the pacemaker rate unless there is an intrinsic ventricular rate greater than the pacemaker's lower rate. This is useful in patients with atrial fibrillation or for those who need backup pacing.

Hysteresis is a programmable function in which the ventricular escape interval is longer after a sensed ventricular event than after a paced ventricular event. This feature is intended to conserve battery life and maintain an intrinsic rhythm, because the effective rate at which a pacer begins to pace is lower than the actual lower rate of the pacemaker.

AAI Pacing

AAI pacing is similar to VVI pacing except that the pacemaker is stimulating the atrium. AAIR is an excellent mode of pacing in a patient with sinus node dysfunction and normal AV nodal and His Purkinje function.

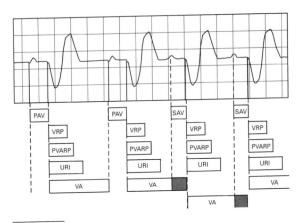

FIGURE 8-1

Schematic diagram of DDD pacing with selected timing cycles and refractory periods. After a paced atrial complex, the paced atrioventricular interval (PAV) begins. If there is no ventricular depolarization before this interval expires, the pacemaker response is to output a ventricular impulse. After a paced ventricular output, several refractory periods and timing cycles are initiated. The ventricular refractory period (VRP) is the time during which a ventricular event will not reset the timing intervals. The postventricular refractory period (PVARP) represents the time during which an atrial event will not be sensed or will not reset the timing intervals. The upper rate interval represents the shortest interval (maximum rate) that a pacemaker will ventricular pace corresponding to the programmed upper tracking rate. The ventricular-atrial escape interval (VA) represents the time during which, if there is no sensed atrial electrogram, atrial pacing occurs. The programmed lower rate corresponds to the AV interval and the VA interval. During the first two complexes, there were no sensed atrial complexes; therefore, the VA interval expired and atrial pacing occurred. During the third and fourth complexes, there were sensed atrial electrograms following the PVARP and before the VA interval expired (shaded area in the VA bar). Note that atrial sensing usually occurs after the start of the P wave, representing the atrial conduction time to the atrial electrodes. The programmed AV interval following a sensed atrial complex (SAV) may be programmed at a value lower than the PAV to obtain equivalent PR intervals.

DDD Pacing

DDD pacing is the most common pacing mode for dual-chamber pacemakers. The timing sequences for DDD pacing are described in Fig. 8-1. This mode is used for patients with AV node and/or sinus node dysfunction.

1. *DDD pacing in patients with sinus node dysfunction.* These patients may have intermittent or chronic sinus bradycardia requiring intermittent or continuous atrial pacing. If patients have intact AV conduction, the pacemaker functions as an AAI pacer. However, because patients with sinus node dysfunction frequently have AV nodal or His-Purkinje disease, patients with DDD pacemakers frequently demonstrate fused ventricular complexes originating from ventricular stimulation and passing through the natural AV conduction system. If the QRS complex appears normal with a pacing spike in the middle or end of the QRS complex, this is still consistent with normal pacemaker function and is termed "pseudofusion."

2. *Patients with AV block and normal sinus node function.* In the DDD mode, if the lower rate of the pacer is programmed at a sufficiently low value to permit atrial tracking, the pacemaker stimulates the ventricle synchronously with intrinsic P waves. If a patient does not require atrial pacing, it may be reasonable to implant a dual-chamber pacer with a single tripolar or quadripolar lead that allows atrial sensing as well as ventricular pacing and sensing. These VDD pacing systems allow for ease of implant and for bipolar atrial sensing.

DDI Pacing

This is a useful mode for pacing in patients with a tachycardia-bradycardia pattern of sick sinus syndrome who have intact AV conduction. During atrial tachyarrhythmias, a pacer in the DDI mode will pace the ventricles at the lower rate. During episodes of bradyarrhythmia, the pacer functions in an atrial or AV pacing mode. DDI pacing is inappropriate for patients with permanent or intermittent AV block.

USE OF PACEMAKERS IN DIFFERENT CLINICAL SITUATIONS

Paroxysmal Atrial Fibrillation, Flutter, and Other Tachyarrhythmias

In order to prevent inappropriate upper tracking behavior during atrial tachyarrhythmias, a pacer can be reprogrammed to DDI or DDIR if the patient has intact AV conduction. Alternatively, a pacer feature, the *automatic mode switch,* automatically changes the pacer mode from DDD[R] to VVI[R] or DDI[R] when the atrial rhythm changes from sinus rhythm to a atrial fibrillation or flutter or another type of tachycardia.

Patients with Complete or Intermittent Third-Degree AV Block

Patients with complete or intermittent third-degree AV block generally receive a DDD pacemaker. If such a patient has intact sinus function, a VDD pacer utilizing a single lead may be a reasonable alternative.

Patients with Carotid Sinus Syndrome and Vasovagal Syncope

Patients with one of the neurally mediated syncope syndromes generally require intermittent AV pacing during their episodes. Additionally, they generally benefit from an interventional pacing rate of 75 to 100 beats per minute during these episodes. In order to avoid chronic pacing at such an elevated rate, certain pacemakers offer interventional pacing at increased rates for short periods of time triggered by a precipitous drop in a patient's intrinsic heart rate.

COMPLICATIONS

Infections related to pacemaker implantation are rare. Early infections may be caused by *Staphylococcus aureus* and can be aggressive. Late infections are commonly related to *Staphylococcus epidermidis* and may have a more indolent course. Signs of infection include local inflammation and abscess formation, erosion of the pacer, and fever with positive blood culture but without an identifiable focus of infection. Transesophageal echocardiography may help to determine whether vegetations are present on the pacemaker lead. If the pacemaker is infected, removal of the pacemaker leads and generator is usually required.

The insulation of pacer leads may break or leads may fracture, leading to problems with oversensing (due to electrical noise), undersensing, and failure to capture (due to current leak). This problem often manifests itself intermittently and may be difficult to detect during a routine pacer check. The patient may complain of pectoral muscle stimulation due to current lead around an insulation break.

Pacemaker Syndrome

The pacemaker syndrome is a constellation of signs and symptoms representing adverse reaction to VVI pacing. The basis for pacemaker syndrome is not only loss of AV synchrony but also the presence of VA conduction. Most of the symptoms relate to loss of AV synchrony and also to retrograde conduction. These include orthostatic hypotension, near syncope, fatigue, exercise intolerance, malaise, weakness, cough, awareness of heartbeat, chest fullness, neck fullness, headache, chest pain, and other symptoms, which may be nonspecific. On exam, these patients may have intermittent or persistent cannon A waves and possible liver pulsation. The management of pacemaker syndrome in patients with sick sinus syndrome usually requires restoration of AV synchrony.

Electromagnetic Interference (EMI) with Pacemaker Function

Unipolar pacemakers are usually more susceptible to EMI interference than bipolar pacemakers because the sensing circuit encompasses a larger area. Magnetic resonance imaging is contraindicated in patients with pacers, and cellular phones can adversely affect pacemaker function. It is therefore recommended that patients use analog cellular phones or keep digital cellular phones (with power outputs <3 W) at least 20 cm away from their pacemakers.

PACEMAKER MALFUNCTION

Pacemaker malfunction can be categorized as loss of capture, abnormal pacing rate, undersensing, oversensing, or other erratic behavior. The approach to diagnosing pacemaker malfunction is to carefully inspect the ECG, interrogate the pacemaker, check pacing and sensing thresholds, lead impedances, battery voltage/magnet rate, and a chest x-ray.

Abnormal Pacing Rates

Abnormal pacing rates can be due to normal or abnormal pacing function. Failure of the pacemaker output is usually due to oversensing (Fig. 8-2). Occasionally, the pacemaker output is not visible because bipolar pacing produces pacing artifacts of very low amplitude (artifacts from digital ECG recording are commonly difficult to visualize). Conversely, absence of pacing stimuli may be due to interruption of current flow from a lead fracture, insulation break, or a loose set screw.

Abnormally fast pacing rates usually are due to normal pacing function. They may occur in response to rate-adaptive sensors. In DDD pacing, upper-rate pacing may be due to sinus tachycardia, atrial tachyarrhythmias, or pacemaker-mediated tachycardia. Application of a magnet can terminate pacemaker-mediated tachycardia.

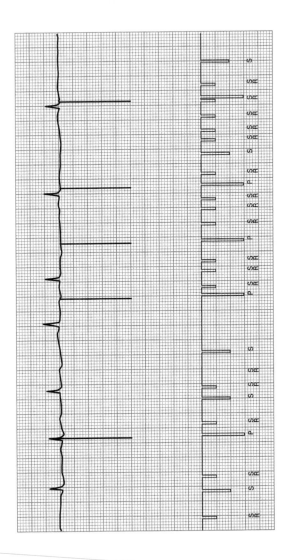

Loss of Capture

Loss of pacemaker capture occurs when there is a visible pacing stimulus and no atrial or ventricular depolarization (Fig. 8-2). This may be intermittent or persistent. Etiologies include elevation of pacing threshold, lead dislodgment, lead fracture or insulation break, and loose set screws. Battery depletion also leads to pacing failure.

Oversensing

This problem leads to inappropriate pauses. The cause can be intra-cardiac or extracardiac or due to EMI. Analysis of the ECG, especially with pacemaker interrogation and pacemaker marker channels, may help to determine the cause. Oversensing due to lead fracture, insulation break, or other electrode problems will be random and erratic. With early lead problems, the malfunction is intermittent and may be exacerbated by certain body positions or motions. In later stages, the combination of oversensing, undersensing, and failure to capture is almost always diagnostic of a lead-related problem. Myopotential oversensing is usually a problem in unipolar but not bipolar systems. This problem can usually be solved by reprogramming pacer sensitivity.

Undersensing

An inadequate intracardiac signal can lead to undersensing. Etiologies include inflammation or scar formation at the tissue-lead

---

FIGURE 8-2

Electrocardiogram and marker channels are shown for a patient with a ventricular lead break. Note that based on the ECG there is failure to sense, as manifested by the second and fourth pacing outputs coming very shortly after the QRS complex. There is failure to capture, demonstrated by the second and third pacing outputs, which should capture the ventricle. There is also evidence of oversensing, as demonstrated by the long pause between the fourth and fifth pacing outputs during a diastolic period that exceeds the interval between the previous two pacing outputs. In general, when there is evidence of oversensing, undersensing, and failure to capture, then the likely etiology is either a lead insulation break, lead fracture, or other mechanical problem. The marker channels confirm the above ECG findings. There are sensed ventricular events (S or SR) that do not correspond to surface QRS complexes, consistent with oversensing. Additionally, the erratic pattern of sensed ventricular events is consistent with electrical noise. There are also lack-of-sense markers corresponding to QRS complexes; finally, there are ventricular pace markers (P) that fail to capture the ventricle.

interface, drugs, electrolyte abnormalities, infarction, ischemia, lead fracture or insulation breaks, and cardiac defibrillation. Usually, undersensing is a greater problem in the atrium than in the ventricle. The optimal solution is to program an enhanced sensitivity (decrease the sensing level).

Other etiologies for undersensing arise when intrinsic atrial or ventricular complexes fall within one of the programmed refractory periods. Undersensing can also result when a pacer functions in an asynchronous mode (as occasionally happens with battery depletion or resetting of the pacemaker generator).

SUGGESTED READING

Gregoratos G, Cheitlin MD, Conhill A, et al: ACC/AHA Guidelines for Implantation of Cardiac Pacemakers and Antiarrhythmia Devices: A report of the ACC/AHA Task Force on Practice Guidelines (Committee on Pacemaker Implantation). *J Am Coll Cardiol* 1998; 31:1175–1206.

Mitrani RD, Myerburg RJ, Castellanos A: Cardiac pacemakers. In : Fuster V, Alexander RW, O'Rourke RA, et al (eds): *Hurst's The Heart*, 10th ed. New York: McGraw-Hill; 2001: 963–992.

Mitrani RD, Simmons JD, Interian A Jr, et al: Cardiac pacemakers: Current and future status. *Curr Probl Cardiol* 1999; 6:341–420.

CHAPTER

9

DIAGNOSIS AND MANAGEMENT OF SYNCOPE

Harisios Boudoulas
Steven D. Nelson
Stephen F. Schaal
Richard P. Lewis

Syncope is defined as a sudden and transient loss of consciousness. Patients with a transient episode of altered consciousness (presyncope) and those with complete loss of consciousness (syncope) can be classified into three broad categories: *cardiac syncope, noncardiac syncope,* and *syncope of undetermined cause.* Clearly, the highest mortality occurs among those with cardiac syncope, and in them the risk of sudden death is high.

NONCARDIAC SYNCOPE (TABLE 9-1)

Neurocardiogenic Syncope

The syndrome of *neurocardiogenic syncope,* the common faint (also referred to as *neurally mediated hypotension, vasovagal syncope,* or *vasodepressor syncope*), is one of the most often seen causes of syncope. It is considered to be an abnormality in the complex neuro-cardiovascular interactions responsible for maintaining systemic and cerebral perfusion. The classic syncopal spell is often preceded by a constellation of prodromal symptoms occurring several seconds prior to the syncopal event. These may include nausea, headache, diaphoresis, dizziness, chest pain, palpitations, and dyspnea. Usually the spell occurs when the patient is upright; it is less likely when he or she is seated. *Syncope while the patient is supine should prompt the search for etiologies other than neurocardiogenic syncope.* During the syncopal episode, patients typically appear pale and diaphoretic, with a slow, diminished pulse. Occasionally, seizure-like activity may occur during hypotension. The syncopal spell classically resolves

151

TABLE 9-1

CLASSIFICATION OF NONCARDIAC SYNCOPE[a]

Neurocardiogenic
Orthostatic
Cerebrovascular
Seizure disorders
Carotid sinus hypersensitivity
Situational
    Cough
    Swallowing
    Valsalva
    Micturition
    Defecation
    Postprandial
Other forms of syncope or conditions mimicking syncope
    Hypoxia
    Hypoglycemia
    Hyperventilation, panic attacks
    Vertigo
    Migraine
    Psychiatric

[a]Source: Boudoulas H, Nelson SD, Schaal SF, Lewis RP, with permission.

spontaneously once the patient is in the supine position but may recur if he or she stands or sits soon after the initial spell. *If the patient experiences a prolonged period of confusion after the syncopal event, etiologies other than neurocardiogenic syncope should be considered.* Neurocardiogenic syncope may occur as a single isolated event, as a cluster of spells over weeks to months, or may be a recurrent lifetime problem. The prognosis in patients with neurocardiogenic syncope is quite favorable as compared with arrhythmic or left ventricular outflow obstructive forms of cardiac syncope. Head-up tilt testing has become a useful diagnostic study for the identification of patients with neurocardiogenic syncope. The management of recurrent neurocardiogenic syncope is challenging and sometimes unsatisfactory. First-line therapy includes counseling the patient to avoid dehydration, prolonged periods of standing motionless, and situations known to trigger syncope. Increased fluid and salt intake is usually beneficial. Patients should be educated to recognize premonitory symptoms and, if they are present, to assume a recumbent position and cough to maintain cerebral perfusion. *Cardiac pacing should be reserved for those patients who have documented episodes of prolonged bradycardia associated with the syncopal spell.*

Orthostatic Syncope (Orthostatic Hypotension)

Orthostatic hypotension is a disorder in which assumption of the upright posture is associated with a fall in arterial pressure associated with light-headedness, blurring of vision, and a sense of weakness and unsteadiness. If the fall in perfusion pressure to the brain is profound, syncope occurs. If the individual assumes the recumbent posture, arterial pressure rapidly normalizes and consciousness is restored. From the diagnostic viewpoint, orthostatic hypotension is conveniently classified under three major causes: *venous pooling and/or blood volume depletion, pharmacologic agents,* and *neurogenic causes* (Table 9-2). Effective therapy of postural hypotension is closely linked to an accurate diagnosis. Primary emphasis must be placed on treatable causes, in particular, pharmacologically induced postural hypotension, blood volume loss, venous pooling, and reversible disease entities. A summary of treatment modalities currently applied among patients with chronic orthostatic hypotension is presented in Table 9-3. The wide variety of recommended approaches reflects the frequently disappointing therapeutic response to each of these modalities. Commonly, multiple therapies are necessary to achieve optimum control of postural hypotension. Of singular importance is the need to have the patient avoid experiences such as dehydration that accentuate postural hypotension and to restrict the use of pharmacologic agents that induce blood volume depletion and vasodilation. *Patients should be instructed about simple adaptive maneuvers, including slow rising from a recumbent or sitting position, flexing of the calf muscles during assumption of the upright posture, and avoidance of prolonged immobility during standing.* The use of erythropoietin to expand red blood cell mass and blood volume has been used to maintain pressure in the upright posture in certain cases of orthostatic hypotension.

Cerebrovascular Syncope

Syncope in the *subclavian steal syndrome* is caused by major occlusive disease of the subclavian artery proximal to the origin of the vertebral artery. With lesser degrees of cerebral occlusive disease, as with atherosclerotic narrowing, transient lowering of arterial pressure—such as that immediately following assumption of the upright posture—may be followed by vague symptoms suggesting

TABLE 9-2

CAUSES OF ORTHOSTATIC SYNCOPE[a]

Venous pooling or volume depletion
   Prolonged bed rest
   Prolonged standing
   Pregnancy
   Venous varicosities
   Blood loss
   Dehydration
Pharmacologic agents
   Antihypertensive
   Sympathetic blocking agents
   Calcium channel blockers
   Converting enzyme inhibitors
   Nitrates
   Diuretics
   Antidepressants, antipsychotics
   Phenothiazides
   Tranquilizers
   Antiparkinsonian agents
   Central nervous system depressants
Neurogenic agents
   Diabetes mellitus
   Alcoholic neuropathy
   Spinal cord disease
   Amyloidosis
   Multiple sclerosis
   Multiple cerebral infarcts
   Parkinsonism
   Tabes dorsalis
   Syringomyelia
   Idiopathic orthostatic hypotension
   Shy-Drager syndrome (multiple system atrophy)
Circulating endogenous vasodilators
   Hyperbradykinism
   Mastocytosis
   Carcinoid syndrome

[a] SOURCE: Boudoulas H, Nelson SD, Schaal SF, Lewis RP, with permission.

TABLE 9-3

TREATMENT OF CHRONIC ORTHOSTATIC HYPOTENSION[a]

Evaluation for reversible and accentuating disease entities
Specific modalities for irreversible orthostatic hypotension
Mechanical measures
    Head-up position of bed
    Lower-body compression garment
    Slow motion and calf muscle flexing on arising
Volume expansion
    High-salt diet
    Fludrocortisone acetate
Pharmacologic agents
    Sympathomimetics
    Vasoconstrictors

[a]SOURCE: Boudoulas H, Nelson SD, Schaal SF, Lewis RP, with permission.

impaired cerebral blood flow. In patients with cerebrovascular occlusive disease, a transient decrease in cardiac output and arterial pressure may provoke syncope at levels of arterial pressure that would otherwise be tolerated. Syncope is rarely due to carotid or vertebrobasilar insufficiency. The treatment of recurrent syncope with cerebrovascular disease is predicated on an accurate diagnosis. In this regard, it is essential to segregate the potential contribution of cardiac and vascular factors and their interplay. Anticoagulants and/or platelet antiaggregant agents are recommended for the prevention of embolic disease stemming from the heart or central vessels. Surgical endarterectomy should be considered in carotid arterial occlusive disease.

Carotid Sinus Hypersensitivity

Stimulation of the carotid sinus by manual compression may produce profound slowing of heart rate and/or a marked diminution of arterial pressure. This disorder is referred to as *carotid sinus hypersensitivity*. Carotid sinus syncope is well established as a complication of carotid body and parotid tumors. Anticholinergic and sympathomimetic agents may be tried, but inadequacy of drug therapy and the occurrence of side effects usually necessitate AV sequential pacemaker therapy.

Situational Syncope

The term *situational syncope* has been applied to a group of syndromes that is defined by the circumstances that precipitate the event. In the past, the syncope in these disorders has been attributed mainly to mechanical factors. Recent observations suggest that, at least in part, neurocardiogenic factors contribute to the syncope. *Cough syncope* is associated with loss of consciousness following a paroxysm of vigorous coughing. In the treatment of cough syncope, the patient should be informed of the deleterious effects of vigorous coughing. Cessation of smoking and initiation of bronchodilator and anti-inflammatory therapy for associated bronchitis are mandatory for the prevention of cough-induced syncope. *Swallowing syncope* has been reported in association with tumor, diverticulum, achalasia, stricture, and spasm of the esophagus. In some patients, no abnormality can be identified radiologically or endoscopically. Syncope is usually associated with sinus bradycardia, sinus arrest, or high-degree atrioventricular (AV) block. *Micturition syncope* is often seen in adult men with nocturia. During or immediately following voiding, there is a loss of consciousness, often without premonitory symptoms. The ingestion of large quantities of alcoholic beverages before retiring is common among such patients. *Defecation syncope* occurs most commonly in the elderly, usually after arising from bed at night or during manual disimpaction of the rectum. It has been attributed to sudden decompression of the rectum. *Postprandial hypotension* is not an uncommon cause for presyncope and/or syncope, usually in the elderly. Therapy of situational syncope should be individualized and should be addressed to the specific associated circumstance.

Other Forms of Syncope or Conditions Mimicking Syncope

In normal persons, anxiety is accompanied by varying degrees of *hyperventilation*. Although mentation is impaired, complete loss of consciousness rarely occurs in hyperventilation. Typical neurocardiogenic syncope may be superimposed, making identification of the syndrome more difficult. *The induction of a typical episode by voluntary hyperventilation is helpful in distinguishing this syndrome and aids in educating the patient regarding the prevention and control of attacks.* Symptoms suggesting syncope are unusual in ordinary types of *migraine*. The unconsciousness is slow in onset and may be preceded by a dreamlike state. This form of migraine usually afflicts young women and has a strong association with the menstrual cycle. Altered consciousness of circulatory origin may be mimicked by *hysteria*. Hysterical episodes occur most frequently in young adults, often with severe emotional illness, and generally in the presence of an audience.

TABLE 9-4

COMMON DISORDERS ASSOCIATED WITH
CARDIAC SYNCOPE[a]

Obstruction of cardiac output
Left-sided heart
    Aortic stenosis
    Hypertrophic cardiomyopathy
    Prosthetic valve malfunction
    Mitral stenosis
    Left atrial myxoma (rare)
Right-sided heart
    Eisenmenger syndrome
    Tetralogy of Fallot
    Pulmonary embolism
    Pulmonary stenosis
    Primary pulmonary hypertension
    Cardiac tamponade
Cardiac arrhythmia
    Sinoatrial disease
    Atrioventricular block
    Supraventricular tachycardia
    Ventricular tachycardia/fibrillation
Pacemaker-related

[a]SOURCE: Boudoulas H, Nelson SD, Schaal SF, Lewis RP, with permission.

CARDIAC SYNCOPE

Either severe obstruction of cardiac output or disturbances of cardiac rhythm can produce syncope of cardiac origin. Obstructive lesions and arrhythmias frequently coexist; indeed, one abnormality may accentuate the other. Common disorders associated with cardiac syncope are listed in Table 9-4.

Syncope Related to Obstruction of Cardiac Output

Obstruction to cardiac output sufficient to cause syncope may occur on the left or right side of the heart. Syncope, particularly that occurring with effort, is a major symptom of aortic stenosis and hypertrophic cardiomyopathy. Transient arrhythmias can also induce syncope in these conditions. The obstruction of left ventricular inflow in atrial myxoma may be posturally induced. Mitral stenosis can produce cardiac syncope but usually does so only when tachycardia or other arrhythmias supervene. Pulmonary hypertension may be complicated by syncope, particularly effort-related syncope. In a young patient without a cardiac murmur who presents with syncope during or shortly after exertion, primary pulmonary hypertension should be considered. Pulmonary embolism as a cause of syncope should also be suspected in paraplegic patients.

Syncope Related to Cardiac Arrhythmia

Arrhythmias are a common cause of syncope and must be considered in any patient, particularly when cardiac disease is present. Either extreme of ventricular rate—bradycardia or tachycardia—can depress cardiac output to the point of critical hypotension with cerebral hypoperfusion and syncope. Additionally, a neurocardiogenic reaction may be precipitated by the hemodynamic effects of arrhythmias. Although arrhythmias occur in the absence of demonstrable underlying cardiac disease, they are usually secondary to such disorders as ischemic heart disease, cardiomyopathy, valvular heart disease, and primary conduction system disease. Primary degenerative disease of the sinus node and the specialized conduction tissue is the most common cause of sinoatrial disease (*sick sinus syndrome*). The presence of sinus bradycardia or sinoatrial block with paroxysmal supraventricular tachycardia of diverse types is quite common and is referred to as the *bradycardia-tachycardia syndrome*. High-grade AV block may be due to disease of either the AV node or the His–bundle branch system. Block of the AV node is usually associated with a functional junctional pacemaker and a normal QRS complex, while AV block due to disease of the His–bundle branch system is usually associated with a wide complex idioventricular escape rhythm, which may be quite slow. Paroxysmal supraventricular tachycardias usually do not produce syncope in young individuals. Syncope, however, may occur in individuals who have accessory AV pathways, as in Wolff-Parkinson-White syndrome, wherein supraventricular tachycardia is associated with a very rapid ventricular response. Paroxysmal ventricular tachycardia may produce syncope at any age. The tachycardia is usually a manifestation of cardiac disease typified by structural abnormalities and/or ischemia. Ventricular tachycardia is the most common arrhythmic cause of syncope in most series. In patients with an implanted pacemaker, syncope may be secondary to pacemaker malfunction or to the pacemaker syndrome. Improvements in technology have reduced the incidence of this complication.

While the history and physical examination often establish the diagnosis of obstructive cardiac syncope, laboratory studies are usually required for the determination of the severity of the disorder. Cardiac catheterization is required when corrective cardiac surgery is contemplated. By far the most challenging diagnostic evaluation occurs when arrhythmic cardiac syncope is suspected. Such patients often have evidence of underlying cardiovascular disease, which, when present, portends a poor prognosis. Thus, diagnostic studies directed to the nature and severity of the underlying cardiac disease must be pursued in addition to evaluation of the arrhythmia. An implantable long-term monitoring device is useful for establishing a diagnosis when symptoms are recurrent but too infrequent for conventional monitoring techniques. For the patient with syncope caused by obstructive heart disease, cardiac surgery, if possible, is often the treatment of choice. Treatment of arrhythmic syncope requires accurate definition of the arrhythmia. The bradycardic rhythm disturbances responsible for syncope usually require the implantation of a pacemaker. The patient with bradycardia-tachycardia syndrome usually requires pacemaker therapy because the antiarrhythmic agents needed to control the tachycardia will often further suppress sinoatrial function. Patients with syncope due to supraventricular tachycardia associated with an accessory pathway are most often approached with catheter ablation of the accessory pathway. Catheter ablation is also a successful mode of therapy in the patient with AV nodal reentry supraventricular tachycardia or other supraventricular tachycardias associated with a rapid heart rate. Except for amiodarone, empiric drug therapy for ventricular tachycardia causing syncope offers little benefit. Other modalities of therapy for ventricular tachyarrhythmias include antitachycardia pacing, use of an automatic internal cardioverter/defibrillator, catheter ablation, and surgical ablative techniques guided by catheter mapping. Antitachycardia pacing with defibrillation capability is an effective approach to the termination of tachycardia and prevention of sudden death. Polymorphic ventricular tachycardia in the setting of a long QT interval (torsades de pointes) is often secondary to drug therapy, particularly antiarrhythmic drug use. The potential offending drug should be stopped. Acute therapy includes intravenous magnesium and measures to increase the heart rate (intravenous isoproterenol or cardiac pacing).

SYNCOPE OF UNDETERMINED CAUSE

Despite careful diagnostic evaluation, the cause of syncope occasionally cannot be defined. Unexplained syncope probably has a broad spectrum of etiologies. The varying mortality in patients with syncope of undetermined cause probably reflects the varying incidence of undetected cardiac syncope. A certain number of these patients probably have experienced syncope of multiple causes.

SPECIAL PROBLEMS IN SYNCOPE

Syncope in the Elderly

Elderly persons are particularly prone to develop syncope or presyncope. The aging process can result in diminished cerebral oxygen delivery by a variety of physiologic mechanisms. Physiologic defenses against a fall in blood pressure may also be impaired. Carotid sinus hypersensitivity is relatively common in the elderly, as is postprandial syncope; these entities should be evaluated. Neurocardiogenic syncope is also commonly identified as the cause of syncope in the elderly. *The elderly frequently have multisystem disease and are likely to be taking several medications, sometimes in excessive amounts, that may aggravate the tendency to syncope (e.g., antihypertensive drugs, diuretics, vasodilators, antiarrhythmic drugs, or psychoactive drugs).* Arrhythmias are common in elderly individuals, especially in those presenting with syncope. Syncope is a significant contributor to unexplained automobile accidents among the elderly and should be suspected when external causes are not apparent.

Multifactorial Syncope

In many instances, syncope requires that a constellation of events occur, either simultaneously or in sequence. Without the full complex, the patient may note only light-headedness or perhaps no definable symptoms. A careful history is required to elucidate such complex presentations. Transient abnormalities such as fever, fatigue, hypoglycemia, or drug ingestion may increase the likelihood of syncope. Coexisting diseases may decrease the patient's physiologic defenses for maintaining adequate cerebral perfusion to sustain consciousness. A cardiac arrhythmia that ordinarily would not produce syncope may become a contributory factor when other predisposing factors are present, particularly when the patient is upright (Fig. 9-1).

Syncope and Sudden Death

Patients with cardiac disease and syncope have a high incidence of sudden death, suggesting that in such patients syncope can be a harbinger of sudden death.

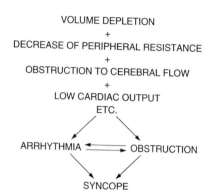

FIGURE 9-1

Frequently, multiple factors must be present simultaneously or in sequence for syncope to occur as a result of an arrhythmia or obstruction to cardiac output. [From Boudoulas H, Lewis RP: Cardiac syncope: Diagnosis, mechanism, and management. In: Hurst JW (ed): *The Heart*, 6th ed. New York: McGraw-Hill; 1986:321–329, with permission.]

Recurrent Syncope

In up to one-third of all patients, syncope is a recurring event. For most patients, the persistence of syncope increases morbidity from trauma but does not increase mortality. Such recurrences most often reflect a lack of effective therapy and/or a failure to establish the correct diagnosis. Unexplained syncope in patients with negative preliminary investigations has a broad spectrum of etiologies, the most common of which is bradycardia. In patients with recurrent syncope, advice regarding the avoidance of certain activities, such as working with dangerous equipment, is needed and, in some cases where public safety is involved, a change in jobs is required (e.g., pilots or bus drivers).

Diagnostic Evaluation of Syncope: An Overview

In the approach to the diagnosis of syncope, it is essential to distinguish the underlying cause. This differentiation is accomplished in a majority of patients by a history, physical examination (Fig. 9-2), and electrocardiogram (Fig. 9-3) and is supplemented by routine laboratory studies, including echocardiography. These tests provide a useful framework for initiating a diagnostic evaluation of syncope

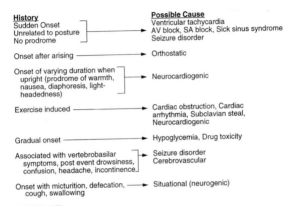

FIGURE 9-2

Differential diagnosis of syncope based on history. AV = atrioventricular; SA = sinoatrial. (From Boudoulas H, Nelson SD, Schaal SF, Lewis RP, with permission.)

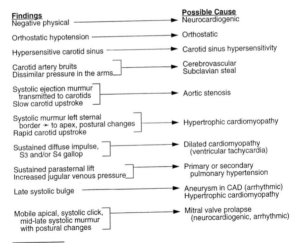

FIGURE 9-3

Differential diagnosis of syncope based on physical examination: CAD = coronary artery disease. (From Boudoulas H, Nelson SD, Schaal SF, Lewis RP, with permission.)

based on age and in situations when syncope is induced with physical activities. Complete evaluation is required for patients with suspected arrhythmic syncope. The diagnostic evaluation of the patient with syncope of unknown cause presents a perplexing problem, particularly when syncope recurs and the risk of sudden death exists. As the understanding of the mechanisms and the breadth of causes of syncope improves (particularly the role of multiple causes), it is reasonable to suspect that the incidence of syncope of unknown cause will be further diminished in the future. In certain cases, devices with extended monitoring capabilities should be used.

SUGGESTED READING

Boudoulas H, Nelson SD, Schaal SF, Lewis RP: Diagnosis and management of syncope. In: Fuster V, Alexander RW, O'Rourke RA, et al. (eds): *Hurst's The Heart,* 10th ed. New York: McGraw-Hill; 2001:995–1014.

Boudoulas H, Weissler AM, Lewis RP, et al: The clinical diagnosis of syncope. *Curr Probl Cardiol* 1982; 7:6–40.

Connolly SJ, Sheldon R, Roberts RS, et al: The North American Vasovagal Pacemaker Study (VPS): A randomized trial of permanent cardiac pacing for the prevention of vasovagal syncope. *J Am Coll Cardiol* 1999; 33:16–20.

Furlan R, Jacob G, Snell M, et al.: Chronic orthostatic intolerance: A disorder with discordant cardiac and vascular sympathetic control. *Circulation* 1998; 98:2154–2159.

Kapoor WN: Workup and management of patients with syncope. *Med Clin North Am* 1995; 79:1153–1170.

CHAPTER

10

SUDDEN CARDIAC DEATH

Duane S. Pinto
Mark E. Josephson

DEFINITION OF SUDDEN CARDIAC DEATH

Sudden cardiac death describes the unexpected natural death due to a cardiac cause within a short time period from the onset of symptoms in a person without any prior condition that would appear fatal. It is most often due to a sustained ventricular tachyarrhythmia. The definition of sudden cardiac death should include the time interval from onset of the symptoms leading to collapse and then to death, the unexpected nature of the event, and the specific cause of death. Though many cardiovascular disorders increase the risk of sudden cardiac death, the presence or absence of preexisting cardiovascular disease is not necessary. Intervals of ≤ 1 h identify populations experiencing sudden cardiac death, including a high proportion of arrhythmic deaths. Processes such as malignant arrhythmias, pump failure, and coronary ischemia, which initiate the cascade of events leading to cardiovascular collapse, can be modified and the episode of sudden cardiac death often averted.

EPIDEMIOLOGY

Incidence

Sudden cardiac death accounts for approximately 300,000 to 400,000 deaths yearly in the United States. When its definition is restricted to death less than 2 h from onset of symptoms, 12 percent of all natural deaths are sudden and 88 percent of these are due to cardiac disease. Sudden cardiac death is the most common and often the first manifestation of coronary heart disease (CHD) and is responsible for half the mortality from cardiovascular disease.

The World Health Organization reported an annual incidence of sudden cardiac death of 1.9 in men and 0.6 in women, again accounting for nearly half the deaths from CHD in a surveillance study of 3.5 million men and women aged 20 to 64 years. Sudden cardiac death rates in developing countries are considerably lower, paralleling the rates of ischemic heart disease as a whole. In the United States, the incidence of sudden cardiac deaths caused by CHD has declined since the early 1980s.

Influence of Age, Race, and Gender

AGE

The incidence of sudden cardiac death increases with age, in men and women as well as whites and nonwhites, because of the higher prevalence of ischemic heart disease in older age groups. Among patients with CHD, however, the proportion of coronary deaths that are sudden decreases with age.

RACIAL DIFFERENCES

The annual age-adjusted incidence of sudden cardiac death is higher in blacks than in whites: 3.4 percent versus 1.6 percent per 1000 population ($p < 0.001$). Not only is the sudden cardiac death rate higher but the overall survival is also lower in blacks than in whites (10.2 percent versus 16.7 percent). The differences in outcome cannot be accounted for by differences in emergency medical team response time or administration of advanced cardiac life support. Blacks are also prescribed diuretics more often than whites, leading to an increased risk of hypokalemia and possibly sudden cardiac death. Societal and socioeconomic factors may play a role in these findings, and they warrant further study.

GENDER

Sudden cardiac death has a much higher incidence in men than in women, reflecting gender differences in the incidence of CHD. The annual incidence of sudden cardiac death in men is overall three to four times higher than in women. As is the case with coronary disease, however, this disparity decreases with advancing age, with a male/female ratio for sudden cardiac death of 7:1 in 45- to 64-year-olds and 2:1 in 65- to 74-year-olds.

A higher percentage of sudden cardiac death in women than in men occurs in patients without prior evidence of coronary heart disease. Among survivors of cardiac arrest, women are more likely than men to have "normal" hearts, valvular heart disease, or idiopathic dilated cardiomyopathy and less likely to have CHD.

SUDDEN CARDIAC DEATH IN THE YOUNG

Sudden cardiac death accounts for 19 percent of sudden deaths in children between 1 and 13 years of age and for 30 percent in those aged 14 to 21 years of age. Structural cardiac abnormalities can be identified in over 90 percent of young victims of sudden cardiac death, and about 40 percent of sudden cardiac deaths in the pediatric population occur in patients with surgically treated congenital cardiac abnormalities. In the majority of young victims, however, sudden cardiac death is often the first manifestation of underlying cardiac disease in otherwise healthy-appearing individuals.

The most common underlying pathologic conditions in people who die of sudden cardiac death in the first three decades of life are myocarditis, hypertrophic cardiomyopathy, congenital anomalies of the coronary arteries, atherosclerotic coronary heart disease, conduction system abnormalities, congenital arrhythmogenic disorders, arrhythmias associated with mitral valve prolapse, and aortic dissection. Among young people with sudden death and known congenital disease, aortic stenosis and primary or secondary pulmonary vascular obstruction are the most common. Patients with surgically corrected tetralogy of Fallot and transposition of the great vessels are at increased risk for sudden cardiac death.

Risk Factors for Sudden Cardiac Death

More than 80 percent of sudden cardiac deaths occur in patients with underlying coronary disease, and the risk factors for sudden cardiac death largely reflect those for CHD (Table 10-1). Left ventricular dysfunction and CHD confer the highest risk for sudden cardiac death. Despite the strong relationship between risk factors for coronary heart disease and sudden cardiac death, there is no single set of risk factors that is specific for sudden cardiac death. The inability to determine a profile based on coronary risk factors that is specific for sudden cardiac death reflects the fact that these factors are manifestations of chronic disease processes which create the structural basis for sustained arrhythmia. These structural abnormalities may be necessary but are not sufficient to cause an episode of sudden cardiac death. Triggers such as acute ischemia, alterations in hemodynamic status, electrolyte abnormalities, transient drug or toxin effects, or circadian variations in vasoconstriction, plaque stability, and thrombosis may precipitate an arrhythmic event in predisposed individuals (Fig. 10-1). Strategies aimed at eliminating or reducing the triggers of arrhythmias may prove to be efficient short- and medium-term

TABLE 10-1

RISK FACTORS FOR SUDDEN CARDIAC DEATH

Left ventricular ejection fraction ≤35%
Congestive heart failure
More than one previous myocardial infarction
Active or provocable ischemia
Inducible ventricular tachycardia
Autonomic dysfunction
  Reduced heart rate variability
  Decreased baroreceptor sensitivity
Complex ventricular ectopy
Positive family history of sudden cardiac death
Syncope in the presence of heart disease
Left ventricular hypertrophy
Cigarette smoking

solutions, since many of the structural abnormalities cannot be cured or require long-term risk-factor modification to prevent their development. Investigation is currently under way to further characterize these triggers.

Lifestyle Factors

ALCOHOL

Individuals who consume large amounts of alcohol (more than 5 drinks per day) have an increased risk of ventricular arrhythmia and sudden cardiac death. The relationship is less clear for drinkers of light-to-moderate amounts. A recent study demonstrated a decreased risk of sudden cardiac death among men who consumed light-to-moderate amounts of alcohol (two to six drinks per week); these individuals had a significantly reduced risk of sudden cardiac death compared with those who rarely or never consumed alcohol.

CIGARETTE SMOKING

Smoking is one of the few coronary risk factors that has been associated with a disproportionate number of sudden deaths as compared with coronary deaths. Smoking has been shown to induce physiologic changes that predispose to sudden cardiac death, such as increases in thrombogenesis, myocardial oxygen demand, and a decrease in coronary blood flow. The annual incidence of sudden cardiac death increases from 13 per 1000 in nonsmokers to 31 per 1000 in those

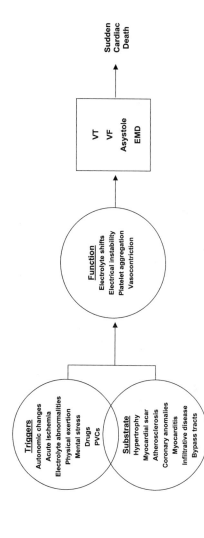

FIGURE 10-1

Interaction between structural cardiac abnormalities, functional changes, and triggering factors in the pathophysiology of sudden cardiac death. The role of triggering factors, such as physical exertion or drugs, is being increasingly recognized. KEY: PVCs = premature ventricular beats; EMD = electromechanical dissociation; VF = ventricular fibrillation; VT = ventricular tachycardia.

smoking more than 20 cigarettes per day. People who stop smoking have a prompt reduction in CHD mortality compared with those who continued to smoke, irrespective of the duration of prior smoking habits.

STRESS AND SOCIOECONOMIC STATUS

There are many reports linking stress, particularly emotional stress, to sudden cardiac death. For instance, in the hours following an earthquake in California, there was a more than fourfold increase in sudden cardiac death in patients with known or unknown CHD. Based on the difference of average and actual daily sudden cardiac death rates in that period, it was estimated that as many as 40 percent of sudden cardiac deaths are precipitated by emotional stress.

PHYSICAL ACTIVITY

There is increasing evidence that regular physical activity may help prevent CHD and its complications. On the other hand, the value of vigorous exercise in patients with known CHD is controversial. An increased risk of cardiac arrest due to ventricular fibrillation during or after exercise is evident in cardiac rehabilitation programs and exercise stress testing in patients with heart disease, where cardiac arrests rates have been reported which are at least six times higher than the general incidence of sudden cardiac death. Although these studies are of selected patients with known heart disease who are already at risk for sudden death, these observations do support the concept that vigorous physical activity can trigger cardiac arrest due to ventricular fibrillation. On the other hand, there is increasing experimental evidence that regular exercise may prevent ischemia-induced ventricular fibrillation and death. It appears that regular participation in moderate-intensity activities is associated with a reduced risk of cardiovascular morbidity and mortality, while the risks of sudden cardiac death and myocardial infarction (MI) are transiently increased during acute bouts of high-intensity activity.

Sudden Cardiac Death in Competitive Athletes The majority of the few cases of sudden cardiac death in athletes occur in those with underlying cardiac disease, and sudden death may be the first manifestation of the disease. In athletes below 35 years of age, sudden cardiac deaths arise most often from a variety of congenital cardiovascular diseases, most commonly hypertrophic cardiomyopathy and congenital anomalies of the coronary arteries. Arrhythmogenic right ventricular dysplasia, myocarditis, aortic dissection, arrhythmias associated with mitral valve prolapse, and the Wolff-Parkinson-White syndrome are much less common. Coronary artery disease is present in only about 10 percent of athletes in this age group, compared with 80 percent in those older than 35 years of age.

MECHANISM OF SUDDEN CARDIAC DEATH

The Relationship between Structure and Function in Sudden Cardiac Death

The vast majority of patients who have experienced sudden cardiac death have had cardiac structural abnormalities. In the adult population, these consist predominantly of coronary heart disease, cardiomyopathies, valvular heart disease, and abnormalities of the conduction system. These structural changes provide the substrate for ventricular tachyarrhythmias, which represent the cause of sudden cardiac death in most cases. As mentioned, triggering factors play an important role in the initiation of ventricular arrhythmia in those who are predisposed.

Tachyarrhythmias versus Bradyarrhythmias in Sudden Cardiac Death

Ventricular fibrillation is the first recorded rhythm in approximately 70 percent of patients who have cardiac arrest. Sustained ventricular tachycardia is only rarely (<2 percent) documented as the initial rhythm, but it is unknown how often it precedes and precipitates ventricular fibrillation. Electromechanical dissociation and asystole are found in about 30 percent of patients experiencing cardiac arrest, and this finding is usually related to the time interval from collapse to first monitoring of the rhythm, suggesting that it is a later manifestation of cardiac arrest. While bradycardia and asystole may be the final manifestations of end-stage pump dysfunction, we believe that bradycardias reflect the failing heart and are not a significant cause of sudden death unless the bradyarrhythmia allows for the development of a tachyarrhythmia. Therefore, treatment of bradycardia may prevent the onset of tachyarrhythmias and is an important consideration in the prevention of sudden cardiac death.

Electrophysiologic Effects of Ischemia

Rapid polymorphic ventricular tachycardias and ventricular fibrillation are the characteristic arrhythmias during the early stages of ischemia and are the cause of sudden cardiac death. A second peak of ventricular arrhythmias coincides with a peak in catecholamine release. Automatic and triggered rhythms have also been implicated in these arrhythmias. Ventricular arrhythmias can be a sign of reperfusion after thrombolysis, percutaneous revascularization, or spontaneous reperfusion, and it appears that the rate, time, and degree of reperfusion influence the incidence, rate, and duration of these arrhythmias.

In the subacute phase of MI (within the first 3 days), sudden cardiac death may occur due to ventricular fibrillation initiated by early, frequent premature ventricular complexes (PVCs) (see also Chap. 15). These PVCs have been shown to be predominantly due to abnormal automaticity and are manifest as accelerated idioventricular rhythm and idioventricular tachycardia. These arrhythmias appear to arise, for the most part, from surviving Purkinje fibers in the subendocardial border zone of a transmural infarction. They have no prognostic significance for development of late arrhythmias and usually subside after 2 to 3 days at about the same time that the resting membrane potential and action potential duration of Purkinje fibers normalize. In the late phases, when the infarction is healed, reentrant excitation appears to be the principal mechanism of ventricular arrhythmias. Critical areas of the reentrant circuit are formed by surviving myocardial cells in the epicardial and endocardial border zone of a healed infarction as well as surviving intramural fibers within the infarct zone.

Mechanoelectrical Feedback

Despite the clinical recognition that acute heart failure can precipitate ventricular tachyarrhythmias, the mechanism by which this occurs is incompletely understood. Besides mechanisms related to acute and chronic ischemia, it has been shown that acute changes in the mechanical state of the heart related to altered preload and contractility can have direct electrophysiologic effects that may precipitate arrhythmias; this relationship is usually referred to as *mechanoelectrical feedback*. The cellular mechanism by which this occurs is unknown, but there is some evidence that these changes might be mediated by fluctuation of intracellular calcium.

Role of the Autonomic Nervous System in the Genesis of Arrhythmias

There is increasing evidence that cardiac abnormalities associated with a high risk of sudden cardiac death are accompanied by changes in autonomic innervation of the heart. MI has been shown to cause autonomic heterogeneity, which may predispose to arrhythmia by creating dispersion of refractoriness and/or conduction.

Sensitivity to sympathetic activation favors the onset of life-threatening cardiac arrhythmias, while vagal activation has been shown to have a protective effect in the presence of tonic sympathetic stimulation. The sinus node has been used as a surrogate to measure autonomic influences on the heart, using indices of heart rate variability (reflecting primarily tonic vagal activity) and baroreflex sensitivity (a measure of reflex vagal activity). A transient (<3 months) decrease in baroreflex sensitivity following MI has been demonstrated in humans and may identify a population with an increased susceptibility to ventricular fibrillation and sudden cardiac death provoked by ischemia.

CARDIAC DISEASES ASSOCIATED WITH SUDDEN CARDIAC DEATH (TABLE 10-2)

Ischemic Heart Disease

CORONARY ATHEROSCLEROSIS

In survivors of cardiac arrest, CHD is present in 40 to 86 percent of patients, depending on age and gender. There is ample evidence to support the concept that the electrical instability caused by acute ischemia is more important than infarction in the pathogenesis of sudden cardiac death. Although the majority of patients who suffer sudden cardiac death have severe multivessel coronary disease, fewer than half of the patients resuscitated from ventricular fibrillation evolve evidence of MI by elevated cardiac enzymes, and less than 20 percent have Q-wave MI. Detailed pathologic studies have confirmed the presence of acute coronary arterial lesions (plaque fissure, plaque hemorrhage, and thrombosis) in up to 95 percent of patients dying suddenly, but only a fraction had total occlusion. Thus, the important observation is that sudden cardiac death can occur in the absence of infarction but usually happens in the presence of diffuse coronary disease.

The incidence of sudden cardiac death in the first 2 years after acute MI ranges from 11 to 18 percent. Patients with both nonsustained ventricular tachycardia and left ventricular dysfunction have the worst prognosis. Few variables, mainly frequent premature ventricular contractions (PVCs) (>10/h), nonsustained ventricular tachycardia, reduced left ventricular ejection fraction (<40 percent), and use of digitalis are independent risk factors for sudden versus nonsudden cardiac death following MI (see also Chap. 15).

The variables identified to predict sudden cardiac death following MI are better in selecting a low-risk population for sudden cardiac death than in predicting who will go on to die suddenly. In the absence of frequent PVCs and with a normal left ventricular ejection fraction following MI, the risk of sudden cardiac death is low (less than 2 percent in the first year), while even when all clinical risk factors for sudden cardiac death are present following MI, the reported risk

TABLE 10-2

CARDIAC ABNORMALITIES ASSOCIATED
WITH SUDDEN CARDIAC DEATH

Ischemic Heart Disease
Coronary atherosclerosis
Acute myocardial infarction
  Chronic ischemic cardiomyopathy
  Anomalous origin of coronary arteries
  Hypoplastic coronary artery
  Coronary artery spasm
  Coronary artery dissection
  Coronary arteritis
  Small vessel disease
Nonischemic heart disease
  Cardiomyopathies
    Idiopathic dilated cardiomyopathy
    Hypertrophic cardiomyopathy
    Hypertensive cardiomyopathy
    Right ventricular cardiomyopathy
Infiltrative and inflammatory heart disease
  Sarcoidosis
  Amyloidosis
  Hemochromatosis
  Myocarditis
Valvular heart disease
  Aortic stenosis
  Aortic regurgitation
  Mitral valve prolapse
  Infective endocarditis
Congenital heart disease
  Tetralogy of Fallot
  Transposition of the great vessels
    (post-Mustard/Senning)
  Ebstein's anomaly
  Pulmonary vascular obstructive disease
  Congenital aortic stenosis
Primary electrical abnormalities
  Long-QT syndrome
  Wolff-Parkinson-White syndrome
  Congenital heart block
  Idiopathic ventricular tachycardia
    death (Brugada syndrome)
    Syndrome of RBBB, ST-elevation, and sudden
    nocturnal death in Southeast Asian men

(continued)

TABLE 10-2

(Continued)

Drug-Induced and Other Toxic Agents
  Antiarrhythmic drugs (class Ia, Ic, III)
  Erythromycin
  Clarithromycin
  Astemizole
  Terfenadine
  Pentamidine
  Ketoconazole
  Trimethoprim-sulfamethoxazole
  Psychotropic drugs (tricyclic antidepressants,
  haloperidol, phenothiazines, haloperidol, chloral
  hydrate)
  Probucol
  Cisapride
  Cocaine
  Chloroquine
  Alcohol
  Phosphodiesterase inhibitors
  Organophosphates
Electrolyte abnormalities
  Hypokalemia
  Hypomagnesemia
  Hypocalcemia
  Anorexia nervosa and bulimia
  Liquid protein dieting
  Diuretics

varies between only 10 and 40 percent. Risk-stratification models incorporating other methods (heart rate variability, baroreflex sensitivity, nonlinear dynamics, T-wave alternans) assessing triggers of sudden cardiac death, such as autonomic fluctuations and electrical instability, are currently in development.

NONATHEROSCLEROTIC DISEASE OF THE CORONARY ARTERIES

Several nonatherosclerotic diseases of the coronary arteries are associated with increased risk of sudden cardiac death precipitated by cardiac ischemia. Congenital coronary artery anomalies, found in approximately 1 percent of all patients undergoing angiography and in 0.3 percent of those undergoing autopsy, can be complicated by sudden cardiac death in up to 30 percent of patients, often exercise-related. Origin of the left main coronary artery from the right aortic sinus or origin of the right coronary artery from the left coronary sinus is most frequently the cause.

Life-threatening ventricular arrhythmias and sudden cardiac death have been described in patients with coronary artery spasm (e.g., Prinzmetal's angina, variant angina). Significant arrhythmias during attacks of variant angina have been documented in about 40 percent of patients and appear to be associated with a higher risk of sudden cardiac death. Calcium channel blockers are effective in many patients in preventing coronary spasm and appear also to protect from malignant ventricular arrhythmias if the attacks can be completely abolished.

Sudden cardiac death has been described as a rare complication of coronary artery dissection in Marfan's syndrome, after labor and delivery, secondary to trauma or coronary catheterization, as a consequence of syphilitic aortitis, or as an extension of aortic dissection. Myocardial bridges have been reported in association with sudden cardiac death during exercise, but they are also an incidental finding at autopsy in up to 25 percent of patients dying of other causes. Coronary arteritis and subsequent infarction have been reported in Kawasaki's disease, giant cell arteritis, Behçet's disease, systemic lupus erythematous, and Churg-Strauss syndrome.

Cardiomyopathies

IDIOPATHIC DILATED CARDIOMYOPATHY

Idiopathic dilated cardiomyopathy is the substrate for approximately 10 percent of sudden cardiac deaths in the adult population. Mortality in idiopathic dilated cardiomyopathy is high, reaching 10 to 50 percent annually, and seems most closely tied to the severity of pump dysfunction (see also Chap. 30). Mortality is higher in patients with advanced heart failure, but the proportion of sudden cardiac deaths is not increased. Sudden cardiac death in idiopathic dilated cardiomyopathy is usually attributed to both polymorphic and monomorphic ventricular tachyarrhythmias that occur in the setting of a high frequency of complex ventricular ectopy. The terminal event can, however, also be asystole or electromechanical dissociation, especially in patients with advanced left ventricular dysfunction. Often, the classification of the terminal event as being due to pump failure or sudden cardiac death is difficult.

Risk stratification of patients with idiopathic dilated cardiomyopathy is difficult because there are few clinical predictors specific for sudden cardiac death. The only clinical variable that identifies patients with a higher risk of sudden cardiac death is unexplained syncope, and these patients should undergo further evaluation. Patients with idiopathic dilated cardiomyopathy have a very high incidence of simple and complex PVCs and nonsustained ventricular tachycardia, limiting their prognostic value by a low specificity. It is clear that induction of polymorphic ventricular tachycardia or fibrillation during electrophysiologic testing is nonspecific and that the absence of inducible ventricular tachyarrhythmias in this population does not accurately predict a low risk of sudden cardiac death. Nevertheless, electrophysiologic study may be beneficial in some instances, since up to 40 percent of patients with nonischemic dilated cardiomyopathy have an inducible monomorphic ventricular tachycardia or bundle-branch reentry that is potentially amenable to catheter ablation. Prospective trials are currently under way to identify categories of patients with nonischemic cardiomyopathy who will benefit from treatment with implantable cardioverter/defibrillators (ICDs) and/or antiarrhythmic drugs.

HYPERTROPHIC CARDIOMYOPATHY

The incidence of sudden cardiac death in patients with *hypertrophic cardiomyopathy* (HCM) is 2 to 4 percent per year in adults and 4 to 6 percent per year in children and adolescents (see also Chap. 31). The mechanism of sudden cardiac death in HCM is not clear. Primary arrhythmias, hemodynamic events with diminished stroke volume, and/or ischemia have been implicated. It must be emphasized that atrial arrhythmias can lead to ischemia and hemodynamic compromise and eventually to sudden death in these patients.

There are few predictors of sudden cardiac death in patients with HCM. A clinical history of spontaneous, sustained monomorphic VT or sudden death in family members indicates a worse prognosis, as does onset of symptoms in childhood. Hemodynamic and echocardiographic variables such as left ventricular wall thickness or the presence of outflow tract obstruction are not useful in identifying patients at high risk for sudden cardiac death. The prognostic value of electrophysiologic study (EPS) in the absence of spontaneous, sustained ventricular tachycardia is limited; in fact, the study itself may be dangerous. Sustained ventricular tachyarrhythmias, predominantly rapid polymorphic ventricular tachycardia, can be induced in 27 to 43 percent of patients with HCM at EPS, but their prognostic significance is controversial. Ambulatory electrocardiographic (ECG) monitoring has been reported to be of some value in identifying patients with HCM at risk for sudden cardiac death; however, the positive predictive value of asymptomatic nonsustained ventricular tachycardia is also limited. One variable, which shows promise, is paced electrogram fractionation, which may be helpful in identifying patients who are at risk for ventricular fibrillation. Patients without inducible, sustained monomorphic ventricular tachyarrhythmias, nonsustained ventricular tachycardia on ambulatory ECG, a family history of sudden cardiac death, or history of "impaired consciousness" (i.e., cardiac arrest or syncope) identifies a subset (22 percent) of patients with HCM with a low (<1 percent) risk for sudden cardiac death.

HYPERTENSIVE CARDIOMYOPATHY

Left ventricular hypertrophy has been identified as one of the strongest blood pressure–independent risk factors for sudden death. Hypertensive patients with left ventricular hypertrophy have a significantly greater prevalence of premature ventricular contractions and complex ventricular arrhythmias than do patients without left ventricular hypertrophy or normotensive patients (see also Chaps. 12 and 18). In the Framingham study, ECG evidence of left ventricular hypertrophy doubled the risk of sudden cardiac death. It remains to be shown whether the reduction of hypertrophy or concomitant ventricular ectopy confers a clinical benefit that exceeds the benefit from the reduction of arterial pressure alone.

ARRHYTHMOGENIC RIGHT VENTRICULAR DYSPLASIA

Arrhythmogenic right ventricular dysplasia (ARVD) is predominantly right ventricular cardiomyopathy characterized by fatty or fibrofatty replacement of myocardium associated with recurrent ventricular tachycardia with multiple left bundle-branch block morphologies (see also Chap. 5). It is a rare cause of sudden cardiac death except in a few endemic regions. The annual incidence of sudden cardiac death in ARVD has been estimated to be about 2 percent despite various treatments. It is a familial disorder in approximately 30 percent of cases, with an autosomal dominant mode of inheritance, and the gene defect has been localized to chromosomes 1, 3, and 14. In patients with ARVD, particularly at early stages of the disease, ventricular tachycardia is often precipitated by exercise, and its induction is usually catecholamine-sensitive at EPS. The course and prognosis of ARVD is highly variable and difficult to predict. The left ventricle and ventricular septum can be involved later in the course of the disease and confers poor prognosis. The arrhythmias generally arise from one of three sites of fatty degeneration. Called the "triangle of dysplasia," these sites are the right ventricular outflow and inflow tracts and apex.

Valvular Heart Disease

The risk of sudden cardiac death in asymptomatic patients with aortic stenosis or regurgitation appears to be low. In contrast, in the presurgical era, sudden cardiac death was one of the three most common types of death in symptomatic patients with aortic stenosis, the other two being bacterial endocarditis and congestive heart failure (CHF). There appears to be an increased risk of sudden cardiac death following aortic valve replacement for aortic stenosis or regurgitation. Malignant tachyarrhythmias have been suggested as the cause of sudden cardiac mortality in these patients, since PVCs are more common in patients who die suddenly than in those who die of other causes. Transient complete heart block is relatively common following both aortic and mitral (13 percent) valve replacement, pointing to bradyarrhythmias as the potential precipitating factor for sudden cardiac death.

MITRAL VALVE PROLAPSE

Whether *mitral valve prolapse* (MVP) is a cause of sudden cardiac death is controversial (see also Chap. 24). The prevalence of MVP is so high (4 to 5 percent of the general population and up to 17 percent of young women) that it may just be a coincidental finding in victims of sudden cardiac death and not causally related. The overall 8-year probability of survival of asymptomatic or minimally symptomatic patients with echocardiographically documented MVP is not significantly different from that for a matched control population. On the other hand, MVP may not always be benign. MVP is the only structural cardiac disease found in a significant number of victims of sudden cardiac death, especially in the young female population. Ambulatory electrocardiography in patients with mitral valve prolapse who experienced sudden cardiac death suggests that, based on the increased incidence of complex ventricular ectopy, the cause of sudden cardiac death in patients with MVP is a ventricular tachyarrhythmia. Of course, these patients may have had a primary electrical disease unrelated to mitral valve prolapse.

Patients with MVP associated with mitral regurgitation and left ventricular dysfunction are clearly at higher risk for complications such as infective endocarditis, cerebroembolic events, and sudden cardiac death. A prolonged QTc interval and changes in autonomic tone have also been related to sudden cardiac death in patients with MVP. Several risk factors for sudden cardiac death have been identified in asymptomatic or mildly symptomatic MVP patients without significant mitral regurgitation, including increased mitral valve annular circumference, unusual thickness of the anterior and posterior mitral valve leaflets, presence and extent of endocardial plaque, and redundant mitral valve leaflets on M-mode echocardiography. In addition, some victims of sudden cardiac death with MVP, mild mitral regurgitation, and normal left ventricular function have been treated with antiarrhythmic agents, raising the possibility of proarrhythmia as the cause of death.

Inflammatory and Infiltrative Myocardial Disease

Any inflammatory disease can cause sudden cardiac death due to either ventricular tachyrrhythmias or complete heart block (see also Chaps. 32 and 33). Histologic findings suggestive of *myocarditis* have been reported in many young victims of sudden cardiac death. In adults, the diagnosis of myocarditis is made much less frequently, perhaps because of concurrent structural heart disease or because the late manifestations of the disease are indistinguishable from idiopathic dilated cardiomyopathy. In South America, however, myocarditis due to specific pathogens, such as *Chagas' disease,* is the most frequent cause of cardiomyopathy and related sudden cardiac death. Patients with infective endocarditis may also be at risk for sudden cardiac death due to acute coronary emboli from valvular vegetations. More often, sudden cardiac death is caused by acute hemodynamic deterioration due to valvular failure. Intramyocardial abscesses can also precipitate ventricular tachycardia and lead to sudden cardiac death.

Infiltrative cardiomyopathies, such as primary or secondary *amyloidosis, hemochromatosis,* or *sarcoidosis,* have been associated with predominantly cardiac conduction defects but also ventricular tachyrrhythmias and sudden cardiac death. Ventricular tachycardia is sometimes the mode of presentation of sarcoidosis; it can usually be reproduced by programmed electrical stimulation and is associated with a high rate of recurrent arrhythmia and sudden cardiac death.

Congenital Heart Disease

An increased risk of sudden cardiac death due to an arrhythmia has been found predominantly in four congenital conditions: *tetralogy of Fallot, transposition of the great vessels, aortic stenosis, and pulmonary vascular obstruction.* Patients who have undergone reparative surgery for *tetralogy of Fallot* have a reported risk of sudden cardiac death of 6 percent before age 20. A QRS duration ≥ 180 ms has been found to be the most sensitive predictor of sudden cardiac death and ventricular tachyrrhythmias in adults after repair of tetralogy of Fallot and correlates with other parameters of right ventricular volume overload. *Transposition of the great vessels* (post-Mustard/Senning) is associated with a 2 to 8 percent rate of late sudden cardiac death, which is due in some cases to sinus node dysfunction and in others to ventricular tachyrrhythmias. Sudden cardiac death is often the mode of death in patients with primary or secondary pulmonary hypertension. Death is often precipitated by general anesthesia, dehydration, exertion, or pregnancy. The sudden cardiac death risk in *congenital aortic stenosis* is estimated to be 1 percent. Such deaths occur predominantly in symptomatic patients with severe left ventricular hypertrophy. *Ebstein's anomaly* is frequently (up to 25 percent) associated with the presence of accessory pathways and the Wolff-Parkinson-White syndrome, which carries a small risk of sudden cardiac death. Congenital heart block without associated structural heart disease occurs in 1 of 20,000 infants, and a moderate decrease in heart rate is usually well tolerated. As previously noted, however, patients with severe bradycardia have a tendency to develop ventricular arrhythmias; pacemaker therapy has virtually eliminated the risk of sudden cardiac death in this population (see also Chap. 29).

Primary Electrical Abnormalities

LONG-QT SYNDROME

Sudden cardiac death is one of the hallmarks of the idiopathic long-QT syndrome (LQTS), a group of genetically distinct disorders each resulting from a mutation in one of six genes encoding cardiac ion channels or auxiliary ion-channel subunits. The prolonged QT interval reflects abnormal prolongation of repolarization. Other characteristics of this disorder, in addition to the prolonged (>460 ms) QT interval, include abnormal T-wave contours, relative sinus bradycardia, a family history of early sudden death, and a propensity for recurrent syncope and sudden cardiac death due to polymorphic ventricular tachycardia (torsades de pointes) and ventricular fibrillation. Over 90 percent of the congenital forms of LQTS have been linked to specific chromosomal defects, resulting in a genetically based classification (LQTS 1 through 6) with important functional and prognostic implications. Carriers of the LQT gene have been reported to have a 5 percent incidence of aborted sudden cardiac death and a 63 percent incidence of recurrent syncope (see also Chap. 28).

Multivariate analysis in the registry population identified female gender, congenital deafness, history of syncope, and a documented episode of torsades de pointes or ventricular fibrillation as independent risk factors for syncope or sudden cardiac death. Exercise-related cardiac events dominate the clinical picture of LQTS1 patients and auditory stimuli tend to trigger arrhythmic events in LQTS2 patients. Echocardiography has also been reported to reveal specific wall motion abnormalities associated with an increased risk of syncope and sudden cardiac death. In the future, genetic typing may facilitate risk stratification, providing valuable information not only about the underlying abnormality but also about the expected severity of the disease and the preferred therapy.

WOLFF-PARKINSON-WHITE SYNDROME

The risk of sudden cardiac death in patients with Wolff-Parkinson-White (WPW) syndrome is less than 1 per 1000 patient-years of follow-up. Although a rare event, it is an important one to consider, since it usually occurs in otherwise healthy individuals; in the era of catheter ablation of accessory pathways, it is a curable cause of sudden cardiac death. Almost all survivors of sudden cardiac death with WPW have had symptomatic arrhythmias prior to the event, but up to 10 percent have sudden cardiac death as their first manifestation of the disease. The mechanism of sudden cardiac death in most patients with the WPW syndrome is presumably the development of atrial fibrillation (AF) with rapid ventricular rates due to conduction over an accessory pathway and subsequent degeneration into ventricular fibrillation. Survivors of sudden cardiac death tend to have a higher prevalence of AF, multiple bypass tracts, and atrioventricular nodal reentrant tachycardia (AVNRT).

There are no good predictors during sinus rhythm for the development of sudden death in these patients. Spontaneous or exercise-induced intermittent loss of preexitation is helpful in identifying patients who will have a slower ventricular response in atrial fibrillation. Loss of preexitation due to enhanced conduction through the atrioventricular node or other causes of antegrade block in the accessory pathway must be excluded for this finding to be reliable. The best predictor for development of ventricular fibrillation during AF is the spontaneous occurrence of a rapid ventricular response over the accessory pathway, with the shortest interval between preexcited ventricular beats (i.e., those conducted over the accessory pathway) being <220 ms. Although this short RR interval is a highly sensitive marker, identifying virtually 100 percent of patients at high risk for ventricular fibrillation, its specificity is low, since this finding is present in approximately 20 percent of asymptomatic patients with WPW syndrome and 50 percent of those with mild to moderate symptoms due to AVNRT. In symptomatic patients, an EPS offers the opportunity to assess conduction properties of the accessory pathways, the propensity to develop tachyarrhythmias, and the possibility of curing the patient with catheter ablation at minimal risk. There is no evidence that measurements of the refractory period predict sudden death in asymptomatic or symptomatic patients.

IDIOPATHIC VENTRICULAR TACHYCARDIA

Several distinct clinical or electrophysiologic patterns in patients with idiopathic monomorphic ventricular tachycardia have been described. Sudden cardiac death rarely occurs in these populations.

These tachycardias include a reentrant form, known as verapamil-sensitive ventricular tachycardia or idiopathic left ventricular tachycardia, typically located in the region of the left posterior fascicle; an automatic form that may originate from either ventricle; and paroxysmal or repetitive forms that originate from the right ventricular outflow tract. Origin from the left ventricular outflow tract is uncommon. Origin from the right ventricular outflow tract accounts for 80 percent of idiopathic ventricular tachycardias and typically has a pattern of left bundle branch block with an inferior axis. This arrhythmia can be sensitive to vagal maneuvers such as adenosine and can be provoked by isoproterenol. The reentrant form of idiopathic ventricular tachycardia generally arises from the left inferior septum posteriorly and has a right bundle-branch block pattern with left-axis deviation, but it can arise more apically, in which case the axis will be right and superior. Calcium channel blockers are effective in suppressing this arrhythmia, and vagal maneuvers, beta blockers, and lidocaine are usually ineffective.

In contrast, several types of idiopathic polymorphic ventricular tachycardias have been described; these are associated with an unfavorable prognosis. They include idiopathic ventricular fibrillation (see below), torsades de pointes with a short coupling interval, and catecholaminergic polymorphic ventricular tachycardia. They can occur in sporadic or familial forms and are frequently associated with catecholamine release during physical or emotional stress, though not uniformly. Patients with catecholaminergic polymorphous ventricular tachycardia have a favorable response to beta-blocker therapy, while those with idiopathic ventricular fibrillation and short-coupled torsades de pointes may not.

IDIOPATHIC VENTRICULAR FIBRILLATION

Although the list of potential causes of sudden cardiac death continues to grow, a definite cause cannot be established in approximately 1 percent of patients dying suddenly or after successful resuscitation from cardiac arrest. These instances of sudden cardiac death without evident cause are presumed to be due to idiopathic ventricular fibrillation. The incidence of idiopathic ventricular fibrillation is higher in selected populations, such as younger patients or female survivors of sudden cardiac death unrelated to MI. The risk of recurrent ventricular fibrillation in this young and otherwise healthy patient population ranges between 22 and 37 percent at 2 to 4 years. In survivors of cardiac arrest due to idiopathic ventricular fibrillation, the diagnosis is made by exclusion if an extensive cardiac workup (including physical examination, laboratory tests for acute MI and electrolyte abnormalities, ECG, exercise test, echocardiography, cardiac catheterization, and EPS to exclude significant conduction system abnormalities or accessory pathways) reveals no abnormality that is thought to account for the ventricular fibrillation episode. Non-invasive evaluation including exercise testing and ambulatory ECG monitoring may help confirm the diagnosis of idiopathic ventricular fibrillation in selected patients in whom rapid, nonsustained runs of polymorphic ventricular tachycardia can be documented. Unfortunately, such markers are present in less than half the patients with this disorder. The prognostic role of EPS in these patients is controversial. Although sustained rapid polymorphic ventricular tachycardia or ventricular fibrillation is inducible in a majority, these arrhythmias are generally considered a nonspecific finding, and noninducibility of ventricular fibrillation in this patient population does not predict a more favorable outcome.

The syndrome of sudden cardiac death associated with right bundle branch block and persistent ST-segment elevation in leads V_1 through V_3 in patients without demonstrable structural heart disease is known as the Brugada syndrome. Symptomatic patients and those in whom ventricular tachycardia or ventricular fibrillation is inducible at the time of electrophysiologic study have a high incidence of sudden cardiac death. A sudden, unexpected nocturnal death syndrome is described in young, apparently healthy males from Southeast Asia. This syndrome is known among Asian/Pacific populations and has several names. The Thai describe it as *Lai Tai* (death during sleep). In the Philippines, it is known as *Bangungut* (to rise and moan in sleep followed by death), and the Japanese know it as *Pokkuri* (unexpected sudden death at night). A majority of these patients have been found to have the ECG manifestations of the Brugada syndrome. With the development and validation of new diagnostic tools, many forms of "idiopathic" sudden cardiac death in "structurally normal" hearts may have to be reclassified.

Drugs and Other Toxic Agents

PROARRHYTHMIA

The apparent paradox that antiarrhythmic agents can cause arrhythmias has been recognized since introduction of quinidine in 1918. The results of the Cardiac Arrhythmia Suppression Trial (CAST) showed an increased mortality in postinfarction patients treated with encainide, flecainide, and moricizine as compared with placebo, despite effective antiarrhythmic efficacy as documented by the suppression of PVCs. Besides antiarrhythmic drugs, many other agents with diverse actions have been implicated in the induction of tachyarrhythmias. Among commonly used drugs associated with the risk of producing ventricular arrhythmias leading to sudden cardiac death are erythromycin, terfenadine, hismanal, pentamidine, and certain psychotropic drugs, such as tricyclic antidepressants and chlorpromazine, which generally affect repolarization. Phosphodi-esterase inhibitors and other positive inotropic agents that increase intracellular calcium loading have also been shown to be proarrhyth-mic and to increase the risk of sudden cardiac death, despite their beneficial effects on hemodynamic parameters. Several studies in pa-tients with hypertension who received treatment with diuretics have suggested an increased risk of sudden cardiac death due to therapy with *non-potassium sparing diuretics*. Drug-induced potassium or magnesium depletion leading to cardiac arrhythmias has been sug-gested as the underlying mechanism.

COCAINE AND ALCOHOL

The widespread use of cocaine in the United States has led to the re-alization that this drug can precipitate life-threatening cardiac events, including sudden cardiac death. Cocaine causes coronary vasocon-striction, increases cardiac sympathetic effects, and precipitates car-diac arrhythmias irrespective of the amount ingested, prior use, or whether there is an underlying cardiac abnormality. The combina-tion of increased oxygen demand due to sympathetic stimulation and diminished coronary flow due to vasoconstriction may precipitate ischemia-induced arrhythmias and sudden cardiac death.

ELECTROLYTE ABNORMALITIES

Hypokalemia is often found in patients during and following re-suscitation from a cardiac arrest. Although it is often a secondary phenomenon due to catecholamine-induced potassium shift into the cells, primary hypokalemia can also be arrhythmogenic. There is an almost linear inverse relationship between serum potassium concen-tration and the probability of ventricular tachycardia in patients with acute MI. A decrease in extracellular potassium hypopolarizes the resting membrane potential, shortens the plateau duration, prolongs the phase of rapid repolarization in ventricular fibers, and causes an increase in pacemaker activity in Purkinje cells, triggering ventric-ular arrhythmias. These changes in repolarization may increase the dispersion of the recovery of excitability and facilitate reentrant ven-tricular arrhythmias. Many of the electrophysiologic effects of hy-pokalemia are similar to those caused by digitalis and catecholamine stimulation, explaining the high risk of ventricular arrhythmias when a combination of these factors is present.

An association between *magnesium deficiency* and sudden car-diac death has been reported in humans, especially as a cofactor in drug-induced torsades de pointes. Hypomagnesemia in humans is generally associated with CHF, digitalis use, chronic diuretic use, hy-pokalemia, and hypocalcemia, making it difficult to establish whether the hypomagnesemia alone precipitates arrhythmias causing sud-den cardiac death. Acute administration of magnesium has been successfully used in the treatment of drug-induced torsades de pointes, although hypomagnesemia is not usually documented in this situation.

Changes in the intracellular concentration of calcium may also be arrhythmogenic. An *increase in intracellular calcium* concentration causes oscillatory release of calcium from the sarcoplasmic reticulum and gives rise to delayed afterdepolarizations, which may subsequently lead to ventricular arrhythmias due to triggered activity. Increases in intracellular calcium are believed to play a significant role in arrhythmias associated with digitalis glycosides, catecholamine-induced ventricular tachycardia, reperfusion arrhythmias, and the proarrhythmic effect seen with phosphodiesterase inhibitors and other positive inotropic agents.

CLINICAL PRESENTATION AND MANAGEMENT OF THE PATIENT WITH CARDIAC ARREST

Out-of-Hospital Cardiac Arrest

Cardiac arrest is characterized by abrupt loss of consciousness, which would uniformly lead to death in the absence of an acute intervention, although spontaneous reversions rarely occur. About 75 percent of cardiac arrests occur at home and about two-thirds are witnessed. The average age of cardiac arrest victims is around 65 years, and 70 to 80 percent are men.

The most important determinant of successful resuscitation is the time interval from cardiovascular collapse to initial intervention. The importance of early intervention is reflected in the "chain of survival" concept of emergency cardiac care systems: early access, early cardiopulmonary resuscitation (CPR), early defibrillation, and early advanced cardiac life support. Initiation of bystander CPR by people trained in basic cardiac life support is another important element of early intervention and improves the chances of successful resuscitation. The association between early CPR and improved survival appears to be related to the beneficial effects of CPR on ventricular fibrillation. The earlier CPR is performed, the greater the proportion of patients who are found in ventricular fibrillation as opposed to bradycardia or asystole. Further, successful defibrillation is more likely when early CPR is performed.

Since most patients are found in ventricular fibrillation, the time to successful defibrillation is a key element in the acute management of the cardiac arrest victim. The widespread use of automatic external defibrillators has the potential to improve significantly the availability of early defibrillation. The devices are relatively simple and inexpensive and have an automatic detection and treatment algorithm for ventricular tachyarrhythmias, but whether widespread use of these devices will translate into improved overall mortality and quality of life remains to be determined.

Survival and Prognosis after Cardiac Arrest

The in-hospital mortality following successful resuscitation outside the hospital remains high, in the range of 30 to 50 percent. The most important factors associated with increased in-hospital mortality after out-of-hospital cardiac arrest are cardiogenic shock after defibrillation, age ≥60 years, requirement of four or more shocks for defibrillation, absence of an acute MI, and coma on admission to the hospital.

Survival depends largely on the initial recorded rhythm. Some 40 to 60 percent of patients who are found in ventricular fibrillation are successfully resuscitated, but only about one-fourth of patients survive to be discharged from the hospital. The outcome is much better in the small (<7 percent) group of patients in whom ventricular tachycardia is the initial documented rhythm; 88 percent survive to the hospital and 76 percent are discharged alive. Bradycardias and electromechanical dissociation as the presenting rhythms are associated with the worst prognosis, and very few (<5 percent) of these patients survive to discharge from the hospital.

MANAGEMENT OF CARDIAC ARREST SURVIVORS AND RISK STRATIFICATION FOR SUDDEN CARDIAC DEATH

Establishing the Underlying Cardiac Pathology

After successful resuscitation from cardiac arrest and a period of hemodynamic and respiratory stabilization, every effort should be made to establish the cause of cardiac arrest and likelihood of recurrence. Underlying cardiac disease should first be investigated, using the history and physical examination. MI should be excluded by serial cardiac enzymes and ECG. Echocardiography can help determine left ventricular function, regional wall motion abnormalities, valvular heart disease, or cardiomyopathies. Stress imaging studies can demonstrate inducible ischemia. Cardiac catheterization is often recommended to evaluate the coronary anatomy and right and left ventricular hemodynamic parameters. Other tests—such as radionuclide studies, magnetic resonance imaging, or cardiac biopsy—may be necessary in selected patients. As discussed above, an underlying cardiac disease can be found in nearly all patients.

PRIMARY VERSUS SECONDARY CARDIAC ARREST

One of the important questions is whether a cardiac arrest was primarily due to acute circulatory or respiratory failure or to an arrhythmia. While several clinical and historical clues help to answer this question, the distinction sometimes cannot be made with certainty. Separating primary from secondary cardiac arrest has important prognostic and therapeutic consequences. Patients who present with cardiac arrest secondary (and within 48 h) to an acute transmural MI have a similar prognosis as those who have an acute MI without an arrhythmia. Specific antiarrhythmic therapy is therefore usually not recommended if cardiac arrest occurs during or within 2 days of an acute Q-wave MI. In contrast, if the arrhythmia is the primary event and MI developed secondary to the acute hemodynamic deterioration during the arrhythmia, antiarrhythmic therapy with a drug or device is recommended unless a transient or reversible cause is identified.

Every effort should be made to exclude potentially reversible causes of sudden cardiac death, including transient ischemic episodes in patients who are candidates for complete revascularization and in whom the onset of the arrhythmia is clearly preceded by ischemic ECG changes or symptoms Other reversible etiologies for cardiac arrest include transient, severe electrolyte disturbances and proarrhythmic effects of antiarrhythmic drugs and other pharmacologic agents (Table 10-3).

TABLE 10-3

POTENTIALLY REVERSIBLE CAUSES OF CARDIAC ARREST DUE TO VENTRICULAR FIBRILLATION

Myocardial ischemia
Prinzmetal's angina
Proarrhythmia
    Antiarrhythmic agents
    Other drugs
Electrolyte abnormalities
Hypoxia
Acute congestive heart failure

Risk Stratification for Sudden Cardiac Death

Four independent prognostic variables for sudden cardiac death related to *clinical history* have been identified in patients who suffered from ventricular fibrillation or sustained ventricular tachycardia following MI: (1) cardiac arrest at the time of the first documented episode of arrhythmia, (2) New York Heart Association (NYHA) class III or IV, (3) ventricular fibrillation or ventricular tachycardia occurring early after MI (3 days to 2 months), and (4) history of multiple previous MIs. Risk stratification for sudden cardiac death using these four variables can identify subgroups with an incidence of sudden cardiac death ranging from 0 to 28 percent. Syncope in patients with a left ventricular ejection fraction below 30 percent is associated with increased risk of sudden cardiac death (about 50 percent at 3 years) irrespective of finding an arrhythmic cause.

Left ventricular dysfunction is a major independent predictor of total and sudden cardiac mortality in patients with ischemic as well as nonischemic cardiomyopathy. In survivors of cardiac arrest who have a left ventricular ejection fraction below 30 percent, the risk of sudden cardiac death exceeds 30 percent over 1 to 3 years despite therapy with drugs that suppress the inducible arrhythmias or with empiric amiodarone. Assessment of left ventricular function by clinical history and by noninvasive or invasive means is essential in the evaluation of a patient at risk for sudden cardiac death. Unfortunately, severe left ventricular dysfunction is a better predictor of total cardiac mortality and does not distinguish patients who will die suddenly from those who will die of progressive CHF. Selected patients with left ventricular dysfunction have been shown to benefit from antiarrhythmic (drugs or devices) therapy (Table 10-4).

Several ECG parameters have been reported to be associated independently with an increased risk of sudden cardiac death. In survivors of out-of-hospital cardiac arrest, the presence of atrioventricular block or intraventricular conduction defects on ambulatory ECG (72 h) is associated with a higher recurrence rate of cardiac arrest. Prolongation of the QT interval (in the absence of inherited or acquired long-QT syndrome), increased dispersion of the QT interval, and an increase of resting heart rate above 90—particularly in men without a history of coronary artery disease—also identify populations at increased risk.

Detection of nonsustained ventricular arrhythmias by ambulatory ECG monitoring has been reported to be of value in the risk stratification of patients for sudden cardiac death. The incidence of sudden cardiac death in the 2 years following MI in patients enrolled in the Multicenter Post-Infarction Research Group increased with the frequency of PVCs detected during 24-h ECG monitoring from

TABLE 10-4

SELECTED STUDIES IDENTIFYING SUBGROUPS OF PATIENTS WITH LEFT VENTRICULAR DYSFUNCTION WHO BENEFIT FROM DEFIBRILLATOR IMPLANTATION

	N	Population	Follow-up (months)	Therapy	Findings	Comment
Primary prevention						
MADIT (1996)	196	LVEF < 35%, CAD, NSVT Inducible VT/VF	27	ICD vs. conventional therapy	12% Mortality (ICD) vs. 39% (control), ($p = 0.009$)	Terminated prematurely because of significant ICD benefit
MUSTT (1999)	704	LVEF < 40%, CAD, NSVT Inducible VT/VF	60	EPS-guided antiarrhythmic drugs or ICD vs. no therapy	24% mortality (ICD) vs. 55% mortality (EP guided antiarrhythmic), RR 60% ($p < 0.001$) vs. 48% mortality (control)	EPS-guided therapy with ICDs, but not antiarrhythmic drugs, reduced the risk of SCD in high-risk patients with CAD
Fonarow et al. (2000)	147	LVEF < 35%, syncope, NYHA Class III or IV	24	ICD vs. conventional therapy	14% mortality (ICD) vs. 33% mortality (medical)	Appropriate shocks occurred in 40% of ICD patients

190

Secondary prevention						
AVID (1997)	1016	LVEF < 40%, near fatal VF or symptomatic or hemodynamically compromising SMVT	36	IVD vs. antiarrhythmic drugs	25% mortality (ICD) vs. 36% (medical), RR 31% ($p < 0.02$)	Mortality benefit was seen particularly in those with EF 20–34%
CIDS (2000)	659	Prior cardiac arrest or hemodynamically unstable ventricular tachycardia	60	ICD vs. amiodarone	8% (ICD) vs. 10% mortality (medical), RR 20% ($p = $ NS)	50% risk reduction in those with LVEF < 35%, Age > 70 and NYHA Class III or IV ($p < 0.0009$)
CASH (2000)	407	Prior cardiac arrest and documented ventricular arrhythmias	57	ICD vs. amiodarone vs. metoprolol vs. propafenone (discontinued)	36% (ICD) vs. 44% (amiodarone/metoprolol), RR 23% ($p = 0.081$)	Interim analysis showed a 61% higher all-cause mortality rate in Propafenone arm which was discontinued

KEY: CAD = coronary artery disease; EF = ejection fraction; EPS = electrophysiologic study; ICD = implantable cardioverter-defibrillator; NS = not significant; NSVT = nonsustained ventricular tachycardia; RR = risk reduction; SCD = sudden cardiac death; VF = ventricular fibrillation. See text for clinical trial abbreviations.

191

3 percent for <1 per hour to 14 percent for >30 per hour. Similarly, patients with nonsustained ventricular tachycardia had a 17 percent incidence of sudden cardiac death, compared to 6 percent for those with single PVCs. The prognostic value of ambulatory ECG monitoring in patients with CHF is limited by the high incidence of these arrhythmias in this population, resulting in the low specificity of this parameter.

Reduced *baroreflex sensitivity,* reflecting mainly an impairment in the vagal efferent component of the baroreceptor reflex and another noninvasive measure of sympathovagal balance, is *heart rate variability;* beat-to-beat variations of RR intervals and their mathematically derived parameter may help to predict cardiovascular mortality and arrhythmic events. Several measures of heart rate variability have been reported to be associated with an increased risk of sudden and total cardiac death following MI. The sensitivity, specificity, positive predictive value, and relative risk in the prediction of arrhythmic events following MI have been reported to be 60, 94, 55, and 10.4 for reduced heart rate variability [standard deviation of RR intervals (SDNN), <50 ms] and 80, 91, 44, and 23.1 for decreased baroreflex sensitivity (<3.0 ms/mmHg). The prognostic significance of baroreflex sensitivity is not diminished in patients with reduced left ventricular function and carries the highest relative risk for arrhythmic events, superior to that of other prognostic variables including left ventricular function.

Macroscopic T-wave changes with an alternating pattern have been observed in patients with long-QT syndrome prior to onset of ventricular fibrillation as well as in the setting of mechanical alternans, as is sometimes present during cardiac tamponade. Recent studies have indicated that *T-wave alternans,* discernible only by computer averaging techniques, may be a common phenomenon that can identify patients at risk for ventricular arrhythmias. Techniques for computer-assisted analysis of T-wave alternans are being developed and may provide a quantitative, noninvasive method for assessing susceptibility to ventricular fibrillation. T-wave alternans assessed by computer analysis has been shown to predict arrhythmia-free survival over 20 months with a nearly 90 percent sensitivity and specificity. The positive predictive accuracy of this test appears to be similar to others with a very high negative predictive value.

Late potentials, microvolt waveforms extending the duration of a filtered QRS complex detected by *signal-averaging electrocardiography* (SAECG), have been shown to be helpful in the risk stratification of patients following MI. Several studies have reported a 17 to 29 percent incidence of sudden cardiac death, ventricular fibrillation, or sustained ventricular tachycardia in patients with an abnormal SAECG, in contrast to 0.8 to 3.5 percent in those without. Although the negative predictive value of a normal SAECG is good, the application of SAECG in risk stratification for sudden cardiac death is limited by a low positive predictive value in patients following MI as well as by its low sensitivity in patients with nonischemic cardiomyopathies. The sensitivity, specificity, and positive predictive value of SAECG are all improved when used in patients with known left ventricular dysfunction after MI and/or nonsustained ventricular tachycardia.

Electrophysiologic studies (EPSs) have advanced our understanding of life-threatening ventricular arrhythmias and facilitated the development of new therapies for their prevention and treatment. Induction of sustained monomorphic ventricular tachycardia is the generally accepted endpoint for programmed stimulation, whereas induction of nonsustained ventricular arrhythmias, polymorphic ventricular tachycardia, or ventricular fibrillation may be a nonspecific finding depending on the aggressiveness of the stimulation protocol. Information obtained during the EPS—such as ventricular tachycardia rate, morphology, origin, mechanism, and hemodynamic stability—is crucial to determine whether the patient is a candidate for serial drug testing, catheter ablation therapy, surgical therapy, or an implantable defibrillator. In patients who present with sustained monomorphic ventricular tachycardia, ventricular tachycardia is reproducibly inducible in the vast majority, especially in those with coronary artery disease. EPS is also useful in patients with structural heart disease who present with unexplained syncope. Ventricular tachycardia is the most common abnormal finding in these patients, but demonstration of His-Purkinje conduction disease or hemodynamically unstable supraventricular tachycardia can also be important. In survivors of cardiac arrest due to ventricular fibrillation, the prognostic value of electrophysiologic testing is less clear. Since sustained ventricular tachycardia or ventricular fibrillation is inducible in less than half the patients, suppression of induction of ventricular fibrillation by antiarrhythmic therapy is an unreliable endpoint, and even patients with no inducible ventricular arrhythmias remain at a high risk for recurrent cardiac arrest. Nevertheless, in survivors of cardiac arrest, EPS may reveal the mechanism of arrest, have prognostic significance, and be of help in the selection of an appropriate therapy.

TREATMENT OPTIONS FOR PATIENTS AT RISK FOR SUDDEN CARDIAC DEATH

Pharmacologic Therapy

BETA BLOCKERS

Of all the therapies currently available for the prevention of sudden cardiac death, none is more established or effective in patients with coronary heart disease than beta blockers. Although beta blockers are less effective in suppressing spontaneous or induced ventricular ectopy as compared with other membrane-active antiarrhythmic agents, both nonselective beta blockers (timolol, propranolol) and cardioselective agents such as metoprolol have been shown, in placebo-controlled randomized trials, to reduce total mortality, in large part because of a >40 percent reduction of sudden cardiac death. The benefits of beta blockade are additive to standard treatment for CHF.

In a review of 19,000 post-MI patients who were randomized to beta blockers or placebo, active treatment was associated with a decrease in total mortality of 20 percent, of sudden cardiac death rate of 30 percent, and of reinfarction by 35 to 40 percent. Beta blockers are effective in the setting of ventricular arrhythmias provoked by a high sympathetic tone, as in patients with congenital long-QT syndrome, arrhythmogenic right ventricular dysplasia, or CHF. Importantly, the beneficial effects of beta blockers on cardiac mortality are most pronounced in patients who are at higher risk for sudden cardiac death, such as those with CHF, atrial and ventricular arrhythmias, post MI, and diabetes.

ANGIOTENSIN-CONVERTING ENZYME INHIBITORS

Vasodilator therapy is an effective treatment in patients with CHF and has been shown to reduce mortality by up to 40 percent in the first year. The effect of angiotensin-converting enzyme (ACE) inhibitors on sudden cardiac death in established heart failure is less clear. In studies of patients with Class I to IV CHF treated with ACE inhibitors or placebo, more than 20 percent died suddenly, without a significant difference in sudden death mortality rate.

The situation is somewhat different in patients without CHF in the post-MI setting. Several trials have demonstrated a significant reduction in overall deaths in post-MI patients (ejection fraction <35 percent) with or without mild heart failure. These studies have sometimes demonstrated a significant or trend toward a significant decrease in sudden cardiac death. A recent meta-analysis analyzed 15 trials that included 15,104 post-MI patients treated with ACE inhibitors. There were 900 sudden cardiac deaths in these studies and a trend toward significant reduction in sudden cardiac death in all of the larger trials.

ANTIARRHYTHMIC DRUGS

With the exception of amiodarone and possibly sotalol, the efficacy and safety of antiarrhythmic drugs in preventing sudden death has been disappointing (Table 10-5). The role of antiarrhythmic drug therapy in the prevention of sudden cardiac death has changed considerably since placebo-controlled trials such as CAST demonstrated that suppression of spontaneous nonsustained ventricular arrhythmias with certain drugs does not necessarily result in improved survival (Table 10-5). In CAST, type IC antiarrhythmic drugs such as encainide, flecainide, and moricizine were associated with excess mortality from arrhythmias in asymptomatic post-MI patients with frequent ventricular ectopy despite effective suppression of spontaneous ventricular ectopy. These results were interpreted as being due to an excessive proarrhythmic effect, which outweighed the lower mortality risk of these patients.

There is no evidence that other class I antiarrhythmic drugs can prolong survival in any patient group studied; they may even be harmful. Results of a meta-analysis of empiric long-term antiarrhythmic therapy after MI with mostly class I antiarrhythmic agents (mexiletine, phenytoin, tocainide, flecainide, encainide, procainamide, aprindine, imipramine, and moricizine) showed either no beneficial effects or detrimental effects on mortality despite effective reduction of PVCs. A metanalysis of lidocaine in acute MI suggested an increase in in-hospital mortality despite a reduction in the prevalence of ventricular fibrillation. Empiric use of these drugs in survivors of cardiac arrest has been associated with a very high rate of sudden cardiac death. In a randomized trial between electrophysiologically guided conventional (i.e., class I drugs) therapy versus empiric amiodarone in survivors of cardiac arrest (CASCADE), overall survival was lower in the conventional arm. The propafenone arm was stopped early in the Cardiac Arrest Study Hamburg (CASH) because of excess mortality in cardiac arrest survivors compared with amiodarone, beta blockers, and implantable defibrillators.

Sotalol, a racemic mixture of the d- and l-stereoisomers, is a potent class III antiarrhythmic agent with nonselective beta-blocking effects. Sotalol has been reported to suppress inducible ventricular tachycardia in 30 to 40 percent of patients who present with sustained ventricular arrhythmias. One trial compared d-l-sotalol to placebo for 1 year in 1456 patients with recent MI. It demonstrated a decrease in mortality from 8.9 to 7.3 percent, which did not reach statistical significance. The Electrophysiologic Study Versus Electrocardiographic Monitoring (ESVEM) protocol was a randomized trial comparing sotalol to class I antiarrhythmic agents and enrolled patients with hemodynamically tolerated sustained monomorphic ventricular tachycardia (85 percent), syncope, or cardiac arrest and then used EPS or Holter monitoring to evaluate the efficacy of the various class I antiarrhythmic agents and sotalol. These patients tolerated sotalol well, and the arrhythmic death rate as well as the rate of death from any cause was half of that with class I agents ($p = 0.004$). These results, however, were biased in favor of sotalol, since almost two-thirds of the patients studied had previously failed therapy with class I agents.

TABLE 10-5
SELECTED TRIALS FOR PRIMARY PREVENTION OF SUDDEN CARDIAC DEATH

	N	CAD	Low EF	PVCs	NSVT	Therapy	Follow-up (months)	Findings	Comments
Coronary artery disease									
Class IC:									
CAST (1989)	1498	+	+	+	–	Encainide or flecainide vs. placebo	10	7.7% mortality (treatment) vs. 3.0% (placebo)	Terminated prematurely due to excess mortality in treatment group
Amiodarone:									
BASIS (1990)	312	+	–	+	–	Amio vs. mexiletine or Quinidine vs. no therapy	72	5% mortality (amio) vs. 10% (Class I) vs. 13% (placebo), RR 61% ($p = 0.048$)	Amio improved survival primarily in the first year after MI
EMIAT (1997)	1486	+	+	–	–	Amio vs. placebo	21	7.2% mortality (both groups), 35% RR in arrhythmic death ($p = 0.05$)	Subgroup analysis showed RR > 50% in total mortality with decreased HRV and first MI, beta blocker use, or heart rate > 75 bpm

	N								Mortality	Comments
CAMIAT (1997)	1202	+	−	+	−	Amio vs. placebo	−	21	4.4% mortality (amio) vs. 5.4% (placebo), RR 21% (p = NS)	Amio reduced arrhythmic death rate without affecting total survival
ICD:										
MADIT (1996)	196	+	+	+	+	ICD vs. conventional therapy	+	27	15.7% mortality (ICD) vs. 38.6% (placebo), RR 46% (p = 0.009)	Terminated prematurely because of significant ICD benefit
CABG-PATCH (1997)	900	+	+	−	−	ICD vs. no ICD	−	36	No difference in all-cause mortality	All patients had abnormal SAECG; no benefit of prophylactic ICD
MUSTT (1999)	704	+	+	+	+	EP-guided antiarrhythmic drugs or ICD vs. no therapy	+	60	24% mortality (ICD) vs. 55% mortality (EP guided antiarrhythmic), RR 60% (p < 0.001) vs. 48% mortality (control)	EPS-guided therapy with ICDs, but not antiarrhythmic drugs, reduced the risk of SCD in high-risk patients with CAD
Sotalol:										
Julian et al. (1982)	1456	+	−	−	−	d,l-Sotalol vs. placebo	−	12	7.3% mortality (sotalol) vs. 8.9% (placebo), RR 18% (p = NS)	d,l-Sotalol may reduce mortality by up to 25%

(continued)

TABLE 10-5
(Continued)

	N	CAD	Low EF	PVCs	NSVT	Therapy	Follow-up (months)	Findings	Comments
SWORD (1996)	3121	+	+	−	−	d-Sotalol vs. placebo	5	5.0% mortality (sotalol) vs. 3.1% (placebo) ($p = 0.006$)	Trial terminated due to excess mortality in the treatment group
CHF trials GESICA (1994)	516	≅ 1/3	+	−	−	Amio vs. standard therapy	24	33.5% mortality (amio) vs. 41.4% (control), RR 28% ($p = 0.024$)	Amio improved survival in symptomatic heart failure
CHF-STAT (1995)	674	≅ 2/3	+	−	−	Amio vs. placebo	45	30.6% mortality (amio) vs. 29.2% (placebo) ($p = $ NS)	No survival benefit with amio; trend to improved survival in DCM
DIAMOND-CHF (1999)	1518	≅ 2/3	+	−	−	Dofetilide vs. placebo	18	41% mortality (dofetilide) vs. 42% (placebo) ($p = $ NS)	Dofetilide reduced recurrent atrial fibrillation and the risk of hospitalization for worsening heart failure

KEY: + = inclusion criterion; − = not inclusion criterion; amio = amiodarone; CAD = coronary artery disease; CHF = congestive heart failure; DCM = dilated cardiomyopathy; EF = ejection fraction; EPS = electrophysiologic study; HRV = heart rate variability; ICD = implantable cardioverter/defibrillator; MI = myocardial infarction; NS = not significant; NSVT = nonsustained ventricular tachycardia; PVCs = premature ventricular contractions; RR = risk reduction; SCD = sudden cardiac death; VF = ventricular fibrillation. See text for clinical trial abbreviations.

SOURCE: Adapted from: Welch PJ, Page RL, Hamdan MH: Management of ventricular arrhythmias: A trial-based approach. *J Am Coll Cardiol* 1999; 34:621–630.

The beta-blocking effect of sotalol seems to be essential for its benefit, since the Survival with Oral d-Sotalol (SWORD) trial of the d-isomer (class III antiarrhythmic effect only, devoid of beta-blocking effect) in patients with prior MI was associated with increased mortality (Table 10-5). The most serious side effect encountered with sotalol is proarrhythmia (mostly torsades de pointes), which has been reported to occur in up to 8 percent of treated patients. In survivors of cardiac arrest, sotalol therapy was less effective than an ICD.

Amiodarone is widely considered the most effective antiarrhythmic agent for therapy of supraventricular and ventricular arrhythmias. It is a class III antiarrhythmic agent with additional class I, II, and IV properties and has unusual pharmacokinetics, with a delayed onset of action and an elimination half-life of up to 53 days after chronic therapy. In contrast to that of other antiarrhythmic agents, the long-term clinical efficacy of amiodarone is poorly predicted by the results of electrophysiologic evaluation. Uncontrolled trials in patients with sustained ventricular tachycardia or ventricular fibrillation demonstrated a relatively low incidence of sudden cardiac death in those treated with amiodarone, despite a high recurrence rate of ventricular arrhythmias. Again, the most important predictor of sudden cardiac death in patients treated with amiodarone for sustained ventricular tachycardia or ventricular fibrillation is left ventricular ejection fraction. In a series of 122 such patients with mostly coronary artery disease, the actuarial probability of sudden cardiac death at 5 years was 5 percent when the ejection fraction was ≥ 40 percent and 49 percent when the ejection fraction was <40 percent.

Amiodarone has been shown to reduce sudden cardiac death rates significantly following MI in several placebo-controlled randomized studies, but its effects on total mortality are inconsistent (Table 10-5). The Basel Antiarrhythmic Study of Infarct Survival (BASIS)—a prospective randomized trial of empiric amiodarone, ambulatory ECG-guided conventional antiarrhythmic therapy, or placebo in patients with complex ventricular ectopy following MI—showed that amiodarone significantly reduced total mortality at 1 year from 13 percent in the placebo group to 5 percent in amiodarone-treated patients ($p < 0.05$). On the other hand, amiodarone therapy did not reduce total mortality but was shown to be safe compared with placebo in nearly 2700 post-MI patients enrolled in the Canadian Amiodarone Myocardial Infarction Arrhythmia Trial (CAMIAT) and the European Myocardial Infarction Amiodarone Trial (EMIAT), despite a 50 percent risk reduction in the arrhythmic mortality. In both EMIAT and CAMIAT, the addition of beta blockers to amiodarone led to a nonsignificant trend toward improved total mortality.

In patients with CHF, who are at high risk for sudden cardiac death, prophylactic therapy with amiodarone has been shown to decrease mortality (by 28 percent) in the Argentinean Grupo de Estudio de la Sobrevida en la Insuficiencia Cardiaca en Argentina (GESICA) trial but not in the Survival Trial of Antiarrhythmic Therapy in Congestive Heart Failure (CHF-STAT). Comparison of the two patient populations and subgroup analysis suggested that prophylactic amiodarone might be more beneficial in patients with nonischemic cardiomyopathy, who were found in greater numbers in the GESICA study (Table 10-5). The Danish Investigators of Arrhythmia and Mortality on Dofetilide in Congestive Heart Failure (DIAMOND-CHF) trial showed no mortality difference in patients with CHF randomized to dofetilide or placebo. The drug was effective in converting and maintaining atrial fibrillation as well as in decreasing hospitalizations for CHF.

The consequence of the amiodarone and dofetilide trials is that these drugs can be used safely in patients with left ventricular dysfunction and, in contrast to some class I agents, that they do not increase mortality. Therefore amiodarone or dofetilide are the drugs of choice when antiarrhythmic drug treatment is indicated in patients with left ventricular dysfunction.

In patients who survived cardiac arrest not associated with MI, empiric amiodarone therapy has been shown to be superior to electrophysiologically guided conventional therapy. Survival free of cardiac death, resuscitated cardiac arrest, and defibrillator shocks associated with syncope at 1, 3, and 5 years was 91 percent, 76 percent, and 63 percent, respectively, in the amiodarone-treated patients, compared with 77 percent, 56 percent, and 46 percent in the conventionally treated patients. The efficacy of amiodarone in reducing total mortality in patients with ventricular fibrillation or hemodynamically unstable ventricular tachycardia compared with ICD treatment has been evaluated prospectively in the randomized Amiodarone Versus Implantable Defibrillator (AVID) study, which reported a survival benefit in the patients randomized to ICD therapy. Prospective, randomized trials addressed a similar question in cardiac arrest survivors in the Canadian Implantable Defibrillator Study (CIDS) and the Cardiac Arrest Study Hamburg (CASH).

In the United States, intravenous amiodarone remains a powerful parenteral drug for the acute treatment of patients with life-threatening ventricular arrhythmias. The efficacy of intravenous amiodarone in patients with recurrent, hemodynamically unstable ventricular tachycardia refractory to lidocaine, procainamide, and bretylium is approximately 40 percent in prospective studies, and about 80 percent of the arrhythmias are suppressed within the first 48 h. Compared with bretylium, intravenous amiodarone was at least as effective as bretylium and caused significantly less hypotension in patients with recurrent or incessant ventricular arrhythmias refractory to lidocaine and procainamide.

The use of intravenous amiodarone in out-of-hospital cardiac arrest was recently studied. Intravenous amiodarone was compared to placebo in patients suffering out-of-hospital cardiac arrest that was refractory to three or more precordial shocks. Patients receiving 300 mg of intravenous amiodarone had an improved rate of survival to admission to the hospital as compared with placebo. Whether use of intravenous amiodarone confers a survival benefit remains to be determined.

DEVICE THERAPY

Automatic Implantable Cardioverter-Defibrillator

ICDs have the ability to sense lethal ventricular arrhythmias and to deliver therapy to terminate them (see Chap. 7).

ICDs are very effective in detecting and terminating ventricular tachyarrhythmias. They can effectively protect against both tachycardic and bradycardic sudden cardiac death regardless of the underlying heart disease or various triggers of arrhythmias. Since their mode of action is therapeutic rather than preventive, ICD therapy might effectively be combined with other antiarrhythmic strategies, such as drugs or catheter ablation, to prevent frequent recurrences of tachyarrhythmias. Defibrillator therapy has been shown to effectively reduce the annual incidence of sudden cardiac death in patients with severe underlying cardiac disease as well as those without significant structural heart disease. Nevertheless, overall cardiac mortality in patients with severe CHF is more closely tied to the severity of pump dysfunction rather than the risk of sudden death.

To investigate the potential benefit of ICD therapy compared with antiarrhythmic drug treatment in *secondary prevention,* the AVID study, CIDS, and CASH have been conducted, in which patients with documented sustained ventricular arrhythmia were randomized to one of these two treatment strategies (see Chap. 7).

CIDS enrolled 659 patients, randomizing 328 patients to ICD therapy and 331 patients to therapy with amiodarone. Results after 3 years of follow-up showed a 20 percent reduction in mortality and a 33 percent reduction in arrhythmic death with ICDs, but the reduction did not reach statistical significance. CASH enrolled patients with cardiac arrest secondary to a ventricular arrhythmia regardless of the underlying disease or ventricular function. A nonsignificant 23 percent reduction of all-cause mortality at 2 years in the ICD arm compared with the drug arm (metoprolol/amiodarone) was reported.

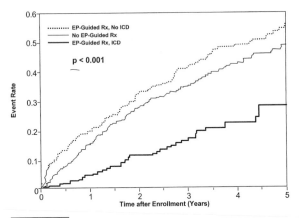

FIGURE 10-2

Overall survival in the Multicenter UnSustained Tachycardia Trial (MUSTT). For CAD patients with EF ≤ 40, asymptomatic NSVT and inducible VT, ICD therapy significantly reduces the total mortality while EP-guided pharmacologic antiarrhythmic therapy provides no survival benefit ($p < 0.001$). (Reprinted with permission from Multicenter Unsustained Tachycardia Trial Investigators: A randomized study of the prevention of sudden death in patients with coronary artery disease. *N Engl J Med* 1999; 16;341: 1882–1890.)

Several studies looking at the *primary prevention* or prophylactic use of defibrillators in high-risk populations have been completed (Table 10-5) (see also Chap. 7). Electrophysiologically guided antiarrhythmic therapy with implantable defibrillators but not antiarrhythmic drugs reduced the risk of sudden death in high-risk patients with coronary disease (Fig. 10-2).

The Coronary Artery Bypass Graft (CABG) Patch Trial enrolled patients with coronary artery disease scheduled for elective CABG who also had a left ventricular ejection fraction of less than 30 percent and an abnormal SAECG (Table 10-5). A total of 900 patients were randomized to receive either an ICD at the time of CABG or usual care and were followed for a mean of 32 months. This study found no significant difference in the primary endpoint of total mortality at 30 days and a mean of 32 months. The findings were not surprising in view of the known benefit of revascularization in preventing sudden cardiac death and the poor positive predictive value of the SAECG.

Permanent Pacemaker

Permanent pacing appears to have a beneficial effect on survival in patients with congenital long-QT syndrome (see also Chap. 8). The beneficial effects of permanent pacing may be related to prevention of bradycardia and pauses, potentially contributing to a more homogeneous repolarization as well as rate-dependent shortening of the QTc interval in patients with mutation in the sodium-channel gene. This is an unreliable approach and is unlikely to be used in the future due to the development of small, dual-chambered ICDs.

Patients with obstructive hypertrophic cardiomyopathy at increased risk for sudden cardiac death may also benefit from pacemaker implantation (see also Chap. 37). While most studies have shown a decrease in left ventricular outflow tract gradient, pacing may have deleterious effects on other hemodynamic parameters, and there are no controlled trials demonstrating improved survival. In a series of 84 patients who had severe, drug-refractory symptoms, half of whom had a history of syncope, only two sudden cardiac deaths during the 2.5-year follow-up period occurred after pacemaker implantation. This annual mortality of approximately 1 percent compares favorably with estimates of 2 to 4 percent per year in adults and 4 to 6 percent per year in children and adolescents for the annual incidence of sudden cardiac death in hypertrophic cardiomyopathy.

Surgical Therapy

There is a reduced prevalence of sudden cardiac death after CABG. Among the 13,476 patients in the Coronary Artery Surgical Study (CASS) registry, all of whom had significant coronary artery disease, operable vessels, and no significant valvular disease, the mean incidence of sudden cardiac death during the 4.6-year average follow-up was 5.2 percent in patients treated medically and 1.8 percent in those treated surgically. The beneficial effect of CABG was even more pronounced in the subgroup of patients with reduced left ventricular ejection fraction and multivessel disease, where survival free from sudden cardiac death at 5 years was 91 percent for the surgical group versus 69 percent in the medical group. CABG also seems to be beneficial in patients with cardiac arrest prior to hospitalization. In an uncontrolled study of 265 survivors of cardiac arrest, 32 percent underwent CABG and 68 percent were treated medically. After adjusting for differences in baseline variables between the two treatment groups, the use of CABG was associated with a significant risk reduction in recurrent cardiac arrest (risk ratio 0.48, CI 0.24 to 0.97). The protective effect of CABG from recurrent cardiac arrest appears to be best in patients with ischemia as the underlying trigger of arrhythmia. Critical coronary artery disease, significant regions of myocardium at risk for ischemia, and no inducible monomorphic ventricular arrhythmias at EPS characterize these patients. Despite the encouraging results of CABG in survivors of cardiac arrest, it should be noted that only a minority of these patients are candidates for operative revascularization and that monomorphic ventricular tachycardia, which is often associated with ventricular scars from healed MIs, is usually not controlled by myocardial revascularization alone.

Electrophysiologically guided subendocardial resection and cryoablation are potentially curative surgical options in patients with recurrent monomorphic ventricular tachycardia. The best candidates are those who require coronary revascularization and have a well-defined left ventricular aneurysm. Catheter ablation of arrhythmias is another curative option for a few specific forms of ventricular tachycardia. The future role of these therapies remains to be defined.

SUGGESTED READING

Bigger JT Jr: Prophylactic use of implanted cardiac defibrillators in patients at high risk for ventricular arrhythmias after coronary-artery bypass graft surgery. Coronary Artery Bypass Graft (CABG) Patch Trial Investigators. *N Engl J Med* 1997; 337:1569–1575.

Buxton AE, Lee KL, Fisher JD, et al: A randomized study of the prevention of sudden death in patients with coronary artery disease. Multicenter Unsustained Tachycardia Trial Investigators. *N Engl J Med* 1999; 341:1882–1890.

Cairns JA, Connolly SJ, Roberts R, et al: Randomised trial of outcome after myocardial infarction in patients with frequent or repetitive ventricular premature depolarisations: CAMIAT. Canadian Amiodarone Myocardial Infarction Arrhythmia Trial Investigators. *Lancet* 1997; 349:675–682.

Connolly SJ, Gent M, Roberts RS, et al: Canadian implantable defibrillator study (CIDS): A randomized trial of the implantable cardioverter defibrillator against amiodarone. *Circulation* 2000; 101:1297–1302.

Fonarow GC, Feliciano Z, Boyle NG, et al: Improved survival in patients with nonischemic advanced heart failure and syncope treated with an implantable cardioverter-defibrillator. *Am J Cardiol* 2000; 85:981–985.

Goldstein S, Hjalmarson A: The mortality effect of metoprolol CR/XL in patients with heart failure: Results of the MERIT-HF Trial. *Clin Cardiol* 1999; 22 (Suppl 5):V30–5.

Julian DG, Camm AJ, Frangin G, et al: Randomised trial of effect of amiodarone on mortality in patients with left-ventricular dysfunction after recent myocardial infarction: EMIAT. European Myocardial Infarct Amiodarone Trial Investigators. *Lancet* 1997; 349:667–674.

Kuck KH, Cappato R, Siebels J, et al: Randomized comparison of antiarrhythmic drug therapy with implantable defibrillators in patients resuscitated from cardiac arrest: The Cardiac Arrest Study Hamburg (CASH). *Circulation* 2000; 102:748–754.

Moss AJ, Hall WJ, Cannom DS, et al. Improved survival with an implanted defibrillator in patients with coronary disease at high risk for ventricular arrhythmia. Multicenter Automatic Defibrillator Implantation Trial Investigators. *N Engl J Med* 1996; 335:1933–1940.

Pinto DS, Josephson ME: Sudden cardiac death. In: Fuster V, Alexander RW, O'Rourke RA, et al (eds): *Hurst's The Heart,* 10th ed. New York: McGraw-Hill; 2001:1015–1048.

Singh SN, Fletcher RD, Fisher SG, et al: Amiodarone in patients with congestive heart failure and asymptomatic ventricular arrhythmia. Survival Trial of Antiarrhythmic Therapy in Congestive Heart Failure. *N Engl J Med* 1995; 333:77–82.

The Antiarrhythmics versus Implantable Defibrillators (AVID) Investigators: A comparison of antiarrhythmic-drug therapy with implantable defibrillators in patients resuscitated from near-fatal ventricular arrhythmias. *N Engl J Med* 1997; 337:1576–1583.

The Cardiac Arrhythmia Suppression Trial (CAST) Investigators: Report: Preliminary effect of encainide and flecainide on mortality in a randomized trial of arrhythmia suppression after myocardial infarction. *N Engl J Med* 1989; 321:406–412.

The Electrophysiologic Study versus Electrocardiographic Monitoring Investigators: A comparison of seven antiarrhythmic drugs in patients with ventricular tachyarrhythmias. *N Engl J Med* 1993; 329:452–458.

Torp-Pedersen C, Moller M, Bloch-Thomsen PE, et al: Dofetilide in patients with congestive heart failure and left ventricular dysfunction. Danish Investigations of Arrhythmia and Mortality on Dofetilide Study Group. *N Engl J Med* 1999; 341:857–865.

Waldo AL, Camm AJ, deRuyter H, et al: Effect of *d*-sotalol on mortality in patients with left ventricular dysfunction after recent and remote myocardial infarction. The SWORD Investigators. Survival With Oral *d*-Sotalol. *Lancet* 1996; 348:7–12.

Zipes DP, Wellens HJ: Sudden cardiac death. *Circulation* 1998; 98:2334–2351.

CARDIOPULMONARY RESUSCITATION AND THE SUBSEQUENT MANAGEMENT OF THE PATIENT

Nisha Chandra-Strobos
Myron L. Weisfeldt

CHAIN OF SURVIVAL

The concept of a "chain of survival" has been adopted by several agencies and underscores the importance of an integrated public education and health care system if survival from prehospital cardiac arrest is to be optimized. Early access [to emergency medical services (EMS) systems], early cardiopulmonary resuscitation (CPR) (to include bystander CPR), early defibrillation [to include the use of automatic external defibrillators (AEDs)], and early advanced cardiac life support (ACLS) care are the major links in the chain, and any one weak link weakens the whole chain of survival.

If mortality from out-of-hospital arrest is to be reduced from its current level of about 95 percent overall, public education programs to increase awareness of the warning signs of a heart attack and to teach CPR are critical. Despite many years of public education, the performance of bystander CPR nationwide remains low. This may have several explanations, including a lack of training in high-risk populations and poor performance or lack of retention despite training. If an individual is unwilling to do mouth-to-mouth CPR, he or she should be taught to at least activate EMS ("call") and start chest compressions ("pump"). Ventilation ("blow") could then be started by suitably equipped, trained EMS rescuers. The CPR message and training must be kept simple (for example, "call-pump-blow"). Dispatcher-assisted CPR teaches CPR on the telephone to the person who is calling to report the arrest (while professional help is in transit) and has been shown to be effective in improving out-of-hospital survival.

CARDIOPULMONARY RESUSCITATION

In 1960, Kouwenhoven and coworkers developed the present technique of external chest compression in the supine position. Immediate defibrillation without CPR can be lifesaving if performed in the first 3 min following ventricular fibrillation. However, CPR is essential to improving survival if there is any delay in defibrillation or a nonfibrillation cause of cardiac arrest. CPR primarily supplies blood flow to the brain and heart. Especially in situations of prolonged resuscitation, air exchange is also important to provide oxygenated blood and to remove carbon dioxide.

MECHANISMS OF MOVEMENT OF BLOOD

The original hypothesis suggested that blood flow to the periphery during external chest compression resulted from direct compression of the heart between the sternum and the vertebral column. This widely held concept is not, however, consistent with a number of observations in animal models and humans. The rise in intrathoracic pressure (and as a consequence a rise of vascular pressures) during chest compression likely leads to blood flow. The importance of fluctuations in intrathoracic pressure as a means for generating blood flow is supported by the observation that by the continuous and early initiation of coughing, patients in ventricular fibrillation can maintain consciousness as long as cough is continued. The critical ingredient of the cough is clearly a rise in intrathoracic pressure, probably with no cardiac compression. The induced increase in aortic pressure leads to flow to the carotid system and the brain. Although superior vena caval pressure also increases with the rise in intrathoracic pressure, venous valves prevent retrograde blood flow to the brain. Myocardial or coronary blood flow occurs between compressions, when aortic pressure exceeds right atrial pressure. The understanding of this physiology has allowed newer techniques of resuscitation to be developed and routine chest compression techniques to be optimized.

Chest compression is best performed with the patient supine on a hard surface. The sternum is manually compressed $1\frac{1}{2}$ to 2 in. at 100 per minute, interrupting for ventilation about every 15 compressions.

Several experimental maneuvers and techniques of CPR have been developed. Following clinical evaluation, some are now

TABLE 11-1

EXPERIMENTAL AND ALTERNATIVE TECHNIQUES OF CPR

Name	Manual or Equipment	Survival Benefit
Interposed Abdominal Compression CPR*	Manual	Positive for in-hospital CPR, no benefit in out-of-hospital CPR
Active compression/ decompression CPR†	Equipment	Positive or neutral benefit
With inspiratory resistance valve‡	Equipment	Not tested
Vest CPR§	Equipment	Not tested
Mechanical (piston) CPR	Equipment	Not tested

*Two rescuers alternate sternal and abdominal compression.
†Requires a chest compression ("toilet plunger–like") device on the chest.
‡Requires endtracheal intubation and a special valve.
§Requires a circumferential vest and inflation device.

considered for limited clinical use. Some of these techniques require special equipment, whereas others can be performed by unequipped health care providers. Table 11-1 lists techniques that have recently been evaluated and deemed to be possibly beneficial.

DIAGNOSIS AND IDENTIFICATION OF CARDIAC ARREST

Cardiac arrest is defined as the sudden cessation of effective cardiac pumping function as a result of either ventricular asystole (electrical or mechanical) or ventricular fibrillation. Rapid diagnosis and treatment are essential because (1) more than a few minutes of total cardiac arrest results in permanent cerebral anoxic damage and (2) the success of resuscitative measures is related to the rapidity with which they are instituted following arrest.

PRELIMINARY PATIENT EVALUATION AND TRIAGE

Cardiac arrest should be considered in the differential diagnosis of sudden collapse in any patient. It can be clinically confirmed by pulseless major vessels and absent heart sounds. Although respirations (agonal respirations) may continue for a minute or two, the patient with cardiac arrest rapidly becomes cyanotic and unconscious.

Once the diagnosis of cardiac arrest is made and no trauma is suspected, the unconscious patient should be positioned supine on a firm surface and the airway opened using the head tilt–chin lift technique or alternative strategies and sternal compression at the rate of 100 per minute performed. The patient should receive rescue breathing either with a bag-valve-mask device or with mouth-to-mouth breathing. Simple airway barrier devices, which are easily deployed, can be used to minimize direct patient contact. Recent animal data suggests that ventilation can be deferred for several minutes in witnessed cardiac arrest without changing survival if chest compressions are initiated promptly. In addition, a recent study that randomized patients receiving dispatcher-assisted CPR to ventilation or no ventilation failed to demonstrate any benefit of early ventilation. These and other data have raised several questions regarding the need and benefit of early ventilation in patients in cardiac arrest. Nevertheless, the American Heart Association (AHA) continues to recommend early ventilation for all patients.

If available, an electrocardiogram (ECG) can confirm the diagnosis and identify asystole, ventricular fibrillation, or electromechanical dissociation as the mechanism of arrest. However, cardiopulmonary resuscitation (CPR) should be initiated immediately, as described above, once the clinical diagnosis is made, without delaying to obtain this information. If a defibrillator but not an ECG is immediately available, a 200-J monophasic or 120-J biphasic countershock should be administered without delay in an adult (lower energy for small children and infants). Early in cardiac arrest, the mechanism of arrest is usually ventricular fibrillation; survival in such patients is critically dependent on time to defibrillation. Once ventricular fibrillation has persisted for more than 3 min, results of defibrillation will likely be improved if CPR is performed first for 60 to 90 s. The drugs often used during CPR are listed in Table 11-2.

AUTOMATIC EXTERNAL DEFIBRILLATORS

Given the value of early defibrillation, automatic external defibrillators (AEDs) were developed for use by professional responders and were shown to dramatically improve survival after prehospital arrest. AEDs have a greater than 90 percent sensitivity and specificity for successfully recognized ventricular fibrillation. They are designed

TABLE 11-2
USE OF DRUGS DURING CPR

Drug	Indication	Adult Dose	Frequency	Value
Epinephrine	Routine CPR	1 mg IV	3–5 min	Possible, limited data
	Refractory/fine VF	1 mg IV	3–5 min	Possible, limited data
	Asystole/electromechanical dissociation.	1 mg IV	3–5 min	Possible, limited data
Vasopressin	Routine CPR in place of epinephrine	40 U IV	Once only	Possible, limited data
Amiodarone	Recurrent VT/VF	150–300 mg IV, then 1.0 mg/min IV,	Over 10 min For 6 h	Probable
	Refractory/Fine VF	then 0.5 mg/min IV	For 18–24 h	Possible
Intravenous beta blocker	Recurrent VT/VF ischemia particularly acute	A number of choices of agents		Possible
Sodium bicarbonate	Acidosis	1 meq/kg	Repeat once every 15 min or on restoration of perfusion	Possible
Calcium chloride	Hyperkalemia or calcium blocker toxicity	2–4 mg/kg of 10% solution	Over 1–5 min, repeat as needed 10 min intervals	Probable
Calcium gluconate		10 mL of 10% solution	Same	
Atropine	Asystole/bradycardia	0.5–1.0 mg IV	5 min to a max of 3 mg	Probable

for use by first responders or persons with little medical training (e.g., firefighters, EMS technicians).

AEDs have been successfully used by nontraditional health care professionals (airline crews, police, and security guards) with dramatic improvement in patient survival. Such programs have been termed *public-access defibrillation*. Survival rates of 50 percent are not uncommon with public-access defibrillation programs. The cost of a defibrillator is <$3000.

RESPIRATORY ARREST

Respiratory arrest is the cessation of effective respiratory effort. It can result from airway obstruction (due to a foreign body or other causes), drowning, smoke inhalation, drug overdose, head trauma, cerebrovascular accident, or suffocation. When respiratory arrest occurs suddenly (as with foreign-body obstruction), the patient rapidly becomes cyanotic, though a palpable pulse with blood pressure, consciousness, and ineffective respiratory efforts may be maintained for several minutes. Opening the airway and/or rescue breathing may be all that is necessary to resuscitate such a patient.

The Heimlich maneuver is recommended for relieving foreign-body airway obstruction. It is implemented by standing behind the victim and delivering a series of sharp thrusts to the upper abdomen with a closed fist. Abdominal thrusts can also be used directly in the unconscious, supine patient by the trained health care provider to help dislodge a foreign body mechanically. If incorrectly administered, this maneuver can lead to visceral damage. When properly used, however, the technique is both safe and effective.

Manual removal of a foreign body in the unconscious victim can be achieved by opening the victim's mouth and attempting to dislodge any obvious foreign body with a finger. As a single method, back blows may not be as effective as the Heimlich maneuver in adults.

VENTILATION DURING CARDIOPULMONARY RESUSCITATION

Clearing the airway is of the utmost importance. Foreign bodies, loose dentures, or any other oral obstruction should be removed. Next, the head tilt–chin lift technique, which causes the tongue to move anteriorly, is used to open the airway. With the fingers of one hand supporting the jaw, the chin is lifted forward, and the head is tilted back by the other hand, which rests on the patient's forehead. The head tilt–neck lift method of opening the airway is also commonly employed and is an acceptable technique for use by the skilled rescuer. Here, the rescuer tilts the head back with one hand on the patient's forehead; the other hand is placed behind the patient's neck, lifting it upward to open the airway. If no spontaneous respirations are present, mouth-to-mouth (or mouth-to-nose) ventilation is immediately initiated, with adequacy being judged by the rise and fall of the patient's chest with each breath. To minimize gastric distention, it is necessary to delivery slow (2-s) ventilatory breaths.

Equipped rescuers will use a barrier device or a bag-valve-mask technique of ventilation together with a small plastic oral "airway," which moves the tongue anteriorly. Adequate ventilation is difficult with the bag-valve-mask technique, since a single rescuer often has difficulty maintaining an adequate seal on the face, and rapid bag deflation commonly results in gastric distention and aspiration. Slow (2-s) ventilation must be employed if the bag-valve-mask technique is used.

Endotracheal intubation is considered the ideal technique for ensuring adequate ventilation during CPR. Whenever possible, a nasogastric tube should be inserted following intubation in order to drain the stomach and thus decrease the chances of aspiration. Intubation can be implemented rapidly, but much valuable time can be wasted by repeated unskilled attempts at intubation. If this technique is used, CPR should be discontinued for no more than 20 to 30 s while the tube is being passed into the airway.

The optimal requirements for ventilation during CPR in human beings remain unknown. During the first few minutes of cardiac arrest without prior hypoxia, ventilation is less important than chest compression and defibrillation. Airflow from chest compression alone and air in the lungs at the time of arrest may initially be sufficient.

VENTRICULAR TACHYCARDIA OR FIBRILLATION

With ventricular fibrillation or pulseless unconscious ventricular tachycardia, an attempt at electrical defibrillation should be made as quickly as possible. Successful defibrillation is accomplished by the passage of adequate electrical current (amperes) through the heart. Current flow is dependent on the energy chosen (joules) and the transthoracic impedance (ohms), or resistance to current flow. Factors that affect transthoracic impedance include the energy selected, electrode size, skin-paddle coupling material, the number and time interval of previous shocks, the distance between the electrodes (size of the chest), the phase of ventilation, and paddle electrode pressure. Transthoracic impedance can be reduced by firm pressure on hand-held electrode paddles and a gel/cream or saline-soaked gauze pads between the electrode and the skin. In addition, proper electrode/paddle placement is essential; one electrode should be placed to the right of the upper sternum below the clavicle and the other to the left of the nipple, with the center of the electrode in the midaxillary line. In female patients with large breasts, the electrodes are best placed to the right of the upper sternum and either under or lateral to the left breast. Direct current is employed during defibrillation. The paddles, coated with low-resistance gel, are applied firmly to the chest and then, for monophasic defibrillations, discharged with 200 J, which is repeated at 200 to 300 J if the first shock is unsuccessful. The current AHA standards suggest that a third 360-J shock should be delivered if ventricular fibrillation persists. These three shocks should be delivered in rapid succession. Newer defibrillators have biphasic defibrillatory shock-wave forms and use lower energy levels with greater success.

When the ECG shows fine fibrillation waves, defibrillation efforts are often unsuccessful. It is suggested that the administration of epinephrine (1.0 mg) intravenously (IV) may result in a more vigorous and coarse fibrillation that is more responsive to defibrillation. This effect is possibly due to improved coronary flow following epinephrine administration (see below), although recent data raise the question of epinephrine-induced deleterious myocardial effects, especially at higher doses. If defibrillation fails, it is likely that marked acidosis or hypoxemia is present. Emphasis should be on modest hyperventilation with supplemental oxygen to correct both hypoxemia and metabolic acidosis. It appears that amiodarone may be of some short-term benefit in patients with recurrent ventricular tachycardia/ventricular fibrillation (VT/VF). Amiodarone is usually dosed as a bolus of 150 to 300 mg over 20 min followed by an infusion of 1 to 2 mg/min for 6 to 24 h. For recurrent VT in the setting of ischemia, intravenous propranolol or other intravenous beta blockers may be effective. Beta blockers seem particularly helpful in the setting of primary ventricular fibrillation complicating acute myocardial infarction. In fact, the early benefit of amiodarone has been ascribed by some to its beta-blocking properties.

Hyperkalemia is a readily treated condition that can cause atrioventricular (AV) block, impaired intraatrial and intraventricular conduction, and occasionally ventricular fibrillation or, less commonly, asystole. It can be recognized by the development of tall, peaked T waves with a normal QT interval and sine wave–like ventricular tachycardia. Life-threatening hyperkalemia responds most readily to calcium infusion; 10 to 30 mL of 10% calcium gluconate is infused intravenously over 1 to 5 min under constant ECG monitoring. Calcium counteracts the adverse effects of potassium on the neuromuscular membranes but does not alter plasma potassium. Its effect, though immediate, is transient. Hyperkalemia should subsequently be treated by glucose-insulin or ion-exchange resins. Sodium bicarbonate is also used as an agent to lower potassium.

With VT in an alert, responsive patient, cough may reverse the arrhythmia without defibrillation, and repeated cough may maintain the conscious state as a result of the rise in intrathoracic pressure. The efficacy of the precordial thump (precordial chest blows) has been variably reported in patients with VT and may rarely cause VF. A thump is generally ineffective for terminating prehospital VF. Hence, a precordial thump should not be used in a patient with VT and a pulse unless a defibrillator is immediately available.

ASYSTOLE OR HEART BLOCK

For patients with prehospital cardiac arrest, asystole is an ominous rhythm associated with a very low likelihood of successful resuscitation. On the other hand, asystole due to vagal stimulation is the commonest cause of cardiac arrest associated with induction of anesthesia and surgical procedures. Asystole also occurs as a result of heart block or sinus node disease. Atropine (0.5 mg) given intravenously and repeated in 5 min can be used acutely to prevent or reverse severe bradycardia in many of these settings.

If asystole is witnessed or of short duration, vigorous blows to the precordium may sometimes restart the heart. Rhythmic chest blows may maintain limited perfusion and can be continued, if needed, while palpating the femoral or carotid pulse until other treatment is available. If chest blows fail, CPR should be initiated and intravenous epinephrine (1.0 mg) administered. Possible treatable causes of asystole—such as acidosis, hypoxemia, hyper- or hypokalemia, and hypothermia—should be considered and treated appropriately if suspected. If an overdose of calcium channel blocker is suspected, calcium chloride, 0.5 to 1.0 g, given as an intravenous bolus, may be very effective. Resuscitation measures may result in the return of a slow ventricular rhythm, which can subsequently be supported with atropine (0.5 to 1.0 mg IV) until a temporary pacemaker is placed. Temporary pacing is the optimal treatment for true asystole or profound bradycardia (see also Chap. 8). Obviously, considerable skill and training are required for temporary transvenous pacemaker placement. *Transcutaneous pacing* has been developed as a noninvasive and simple technique that can be implemented rapidly. It uses external surface electrodes with a high-voltage pacing source. Higher voltages are required to overcome transthoracic resistance. As a consequence, this technique is painful and therefore used mainly on unconscious patients. The energy delivered to the heart by this technique is variable, as is its efficacy.

In rare instances, very fine VF may result in an almost straight line on a single-lead ECG and thus be mistaken for asystole. In such cases, where the diagnosis of asystole is in question, it is suggested that a perpendicular ECG lead be viewed. Rotation of "quick look" ECG paddles by 90 degrees easily achieves this. If ventricular fibrillation is present, the perpendicular ECG lead will demonstrate a typical fibrillation pattern; whereas in true asystole a straight line will be seen in all ECG leads. There is little value (but likely little harm) in defibrillating true asystole.

ELECTROMECHANICAL DISSOCIATION

In electromechanical dissociation (EMD), there is evidence of organized electrical activity on the ECG at a reasonable rate but failure of effective perfusion (no pulse or blood pressure). The most treatable causes of this condition are hypovolemia due to severe hemorrhage, pericardial tamponade, tension pneumothorax, hypoxia, hypothermia, acidosis, hyperkalemia, and massive pulmonary embolism. Signs of these problems should be sought and definitive therapy undertaken with fluids and/or blood replacement, pericardiocentesis, placement of a pleural needle or tube, endotracheal intubation, and other maneuvers as deemed necessary. These conditions should also be strongly considered if CPR results in no palpable pulse or evidence of perfusion. Unfortunately, many patients with electromechanical dissociation have primary myocardial failure. Following diagnosis, ventilation should be optimized and epinephrine administered. Calcium chloride has been used for EMD, but prospective studies have not shown it to improve survival. In acute myocardial infarction, sudden electromechanical dissociation is a sign of myocardial rupture. In such cases, pericardiocentesis and surgical repair can rarely result in survival.

ESTABLISHMENT OF AN INTRAVENOUS ROUTE

While external chest compression and artificial ventilation are continued, a plastic catheter should be inserted into a large peripheral vein. If CPR is properly performed, drugs administered through a peripheral line will often reach the arterial circulation within 15 to 30 s. Larger amounts of fluids should be used if drugs are given via a femoral line. Intracardiac injections are unnecessary except when there is no intravenous access. If an intravenous route is unavailable, epinephrine (1.0 mg in 10 mL of sterile distilled water) can be administered by way of the endotracheal tube into the bronchial tree. The drug should be injected through a long catheter passed beyond the tip of the endotracheal tube. Cardiac compression should be withheld, and several insufflations with an "Ambu bag" should immediately follow drug administration to aid drug absorption through aerosolization.

MAJOR DRUGS USED DURING CARDIOPULMONARY RESUSCITATION

Drugs used for the treatment of various arrhythmias are mentioned above (Table 11-2). Catecholamines are used in cardiac arrest to (1) increase arterial and coronary perfusion during and following CPR, (2) stimulate spontaneous contraction during asystole, (3) make fine VF more responsive to defibrillation, and (4) act as an inotropic agent. Epinephrine is effective in achieving several of those goals, although recent data have highlighted its possible deleterious effects on postresuscitation left ventricular function. During conventional CPR, cerebral and myocardial perfusion pressures are low. Epinephrine preferentially reduces blood flow to the external carotid, renal, and splanchnic beds, thereby redirecting flow toward the brain and heart. Most experts would use 1 mg IV uniformly. Higher doses worsen postresuscitation myocardial dysfunction, hence its use is not routinely recommended. The recommended dose is 0.5 to 1 mg IV, and this dose should be repeated at approximately 3- to 5-min intervals unless effective cardiac activity is restored.

The benefits of epinephrine are principally due to the alpha vasoconstriction induced by this agent. The inotropic effects of the drug may not be helpful, since these effects increase myocardial oxygen demand, even during ventricular fibrillation, when supply or blood flow is limited. Consequently, there is some interest in using a pure vasoconstrictor during CPR rather than epinephrine. Animal studies of vital organ perfusion and human survival studies comparing epinephrine and phenylepinephrine (a pure alpha vasoconstrictor) have yielded similar results. Vasopressin (40 U IV) has recently been evaluated as an alterative pressor agent and has shown promising results.

Norepinephrine is a potent vasoconstrictor and generally produces a rise in blood pressure; it is also an inotropic agent. Its disadvantage is renal and mesenteric vasoconstriction. It should not be used in the initial phase of resuscitation. This agent is most useful where severe hypotension is present but where the chronotropic effects of epinephrine are not desirable (as in acute myocardial infarction or severe ischemia). This agent should be administered cautiously, since severe tissue injury results from extravasation around an intravenous site.

Similarly, dopamine (a chemical precursor of norepinephrine) and dobutamine (a synthetic catecholamine) are preferred for use as inotropic agents because of their lesser chronotropic effect. Isoproterenol (as synthetic catecholamine) is a pure adrenergic agonist and effective vasodilator. Therefore *its use during CPR is contraindicated,* since it can significantly decrease vital organ perfusion pressures. In patients with a palpable pulse, however, it is useful for treatment of bradycardia due to heart block or asystole until a temporary pacemaker is placed.

Sodium Bicarbonate

As with other types of metabolic acidosis, if adequate alveolar ventilation is achieved, the metabolic acidosis of arrest is partially corrected through CO_2 excretion. Several deleterious effects of bicarbonate administration—including respiratory acidosis, hypernatremia, and hyperosmolality—have been reported. Ideally, sodium bicarbonate should be given according to the results of measurement of arterial blood pH and, P_{CO_2} determination, followed by calculation of the base deficit. Bicarbonate should be used if at all only after more established interventions such as defibrillation, ventilation with endotracheal intubation, and pharmacologic therapies (epinephrine and antiarrhythmic drugs) have been tried. If needed, 1 meq/kg of sodium bicarbonate may be administered; then no more than half this dose may be repeated every 15 min. Some benefit from the usual bicarbonate solution (7.2%) may occur as the hyperosmolality of the solution temporarily draws fluid into the intravascular compartment.

Bicarbonate may be most useful during the immediate postresuscitation period, when there is a profound metabolic acidosis.

Calcium Chloride

Calcium chloride (5 to 7 mg/kg) enhances the contractile state of the heart and is indicated in treating severe hypotension due to an overdose of calcium channel blocker or hyperkalemia. It is no longer recommended for use in asystole or electromechanical dissociation.

TERMINATION OF CARDIOPULMONARY RESUSCITATION

Despite resuscitative efforts, the patient in cardiac arrest may not regain spontaneous circulation. The decision to end (or even initiate) CPR should be based on a physician's assessment of the patient's prior advance directives (if known) and his or her cerebral, cardiovascular, and general status. Survival is unlikely in patients who have no return of spontaneous circulation after 30 min of acute cardiac life support (ACLS). Persistent deep unconsciousness and absence of respiration, reflex response, or pupillary reaction suggest cerebral death, and resuscitative efforts are usually unproductive. However, these guidelines should be altered in patients with hypothermia, barbiturate overdose, and perhaps following electrocution, where recovery has been seen even after hours of resuscitation.

POSTARREST CARE

Patients who have been successfully resuscitated usually require monitoring in an intensive care setting. These patients are prone to develop cardiac arrhythmias, hemodynamic and ventilatory instability, and ischemic encephalopathy. Ventilatory support with a respirator may well be necessary initially. Serial arterial blood gas determinations should be made to identify hypoxemia and assess the rapidly changing acid-base status. Commonly, hyperventilation was employed postresuscitation to not only treat acidosis but also to help reduce central nervous system (CNS) edema. Recent studies raise the possibility of worsening cerebral ischemia with low P_{CO_2} levels after brain ischemia. Based on these observations, normal ventilation is preferred in the comatose postresuscitation patient.

Several therapeutic strategies have been employed in animal models to help reduce hypoxic encephalopathy after cardiac arrest. None have clearly been shown to be beneficial in humans.

The treatment of encephalopathy after cardiac arrest involves the prevention of further hypoxia and hypotension. For cerebral edema after cardiac arrest, methylprednisolone (60 to 100 mg) or dexamethasone sodium phosphate (12 to 20 mg IV every 6 h) has been recommended, but data to support benefit are limited. Mild to moderate hypothermia appears to be neuroprotective following an ischemic event. Clinical data are limited but suggestive of benefit. The prognosis of the patient with anoxic encephalopathy is related to the depth and continued duration of cerebral dysfunction. Failure to exhibit neurologic improvement 24 to 72 h following resuscitation is usually an ominous sign. Clinical and laboratory evaluations (electroencephalography, sensory evoked potentials) are often employed to help define prognosis and thus guide further care in such individuals.

Other potential life-threatening problems in the postarrest period include acute renal failure, bowel infarction, infection, adult respiratory distress syndrome, and sepsis. Patients regaining consciousness may have postarrest amnesia or may develop psychotic behavior.

Many, however, do recover sufficiently to return to fairly normal lives.

SUGGESTED READING

Chandra-Strobos N, Weisfeldt ML: Cardiopulmonary resuscitation and the subsequent management of the patient. In: Fuster V, Alexander RW, O'Rourke RA et al (eds): *Hurst's The Heart*, 10th ed. New York: McGraw-Hill; 2001:1049–1061.

Cobb LA, Fahrenbruch CE, Walsh TR, et al: Influence of cardiopulmonary resuscitation prior to defibrillation in patients with out-of-the-hospital ventricular fibrillation. *JAMA* 1999; 281:1182–1188.

Guidelines 2000 for cardiopulmonary resuscitation and emergency cardiovascular care international consensus on science. *Circulation* 2000; 102:11–1380.

Hallstrom A, Cobb L, Johnson E, Copass M: Cardiopulmonary resuscitation by chest compression alone or with mouth to mouth ventilation. *N Engl J Med* 2000; 342:1546–1553.

Nichol G, Hallstrom A, Ornato JP, et al: Potential cost-effectiveness of public access defibrillation in the United States. *Circulation* 1998; 97(133):1315–1320.

Paradis N, Martin G, Goetting M, et al: Simultaneous aortic, jugular bulb, and right atrial pressures during cardiopulmonary resuscitation in humans: Insights into mechanisms. *Circulation* 1989; 80:361–368.

CHAPTER

12

DYSLIPIDEMIA AND RISK FACTORS IN THE PREVENTION OF CORONARY HEART DISEASE

Thomas A. Pearson
David J. Maron
Paul M. Ridker
Scott M. Grundy

Identification and management of risk factors are essential for preventing coronary heart disease (CHD) in asymptomatic individuals (*primary prevention*) and for preventing recurrent events in patients with established disease (*secondary prevention*). *Risk factor management should be conceived as prevention or treatment of the atherosclerotic disease process itself and, as such, should be included as an integral part of any management plan for the many acute or chronic manifestations of this disease.* The intensity of risk factor intervention should correspond to the patient's level of risk. The presence of unmodifiable risk factors may necessitate more intense management of modifiable risk factors.

RISK ASSESSMENT

As detailed in this chapter, the efficacy of secondary prevention of CHD using a variety of therapies has been well established. Therefore, an individual with established CHD or other atherosclerotic disease should be considered at highest risk for a CHD event and deserves the most aggressive evidence-based risk-reduction therapy. The therapeutic success achieved in secondary prevention of CHD has generated enthusiasm for extending this success to primary prevention in clinical practice. The essential issues for primary prevention are the selection of patients and selection of appropriate interventions. The first step in patient selection is to estimate a patient's risk. The key parameter for risk assessment for medical intervention

TABLE 12-1

RISK CATEGORIES

Risk Category	10-Year Absolute Risk for Myocardial Infarction (%) (Nonfatal + Fatal)
High	>20
Intermediate	10–20
Low	<10

is the *absolute risk,* i.e., the probability of developing CHD over a finite period.

Categories of Absolute Risk

For the sake of simplicity, absolute risk can be divided into three categories: high, intermediate, and low. Patients at high risk deserve aggressive risk-reduction therapy. Those at intermediate risk also deserve medical intervention to the extent that therapy is efficacious, safe, and cost-effective. Finally, low-risk patients can be encouraged by their physicians to follow public health recommendations for primary prevention of CHD.

Each category of absolute risk can be examined in quantitative terms (Table 12-1). Patients at high risk are those whose absolute risk for CHD equals that of patients who already manifest clinical CHD. Evidence from clinical trials of cholesterol-lowering therapy indicates that patients with a prior history of myocardial infarction (MI) have a 10-year risk for recurrent nonfatal or fatal MI of about 26 percent. Patients with stable angina pectoris have a 10-year risk for acute MI of about 20 percent. Thus, it is reasonable to say that *patients without manifest CHD who have a 10-year risk for MI of greater than 20 percent are at high risk.* These patients also can be said to have a *CHD risk equivalent.* In accord, *intermediate-risk patients have a 10-year risk for MI of 10 to 20 percent.* Assignment of risk category is first made by measurements of standard risk factors. In some patients, however, estimates of absolute risk may require adjustment on the basis of other kinds of risk factors or the presence of subclinical coronary artery disease. *Low-risk patients are those whose 10-year risk for MI is less than 10 percent.*

Identification of High-Risk Patients (Coronary Heart Disease Risk Equivalents)

NONCORONARY FORMS OF CLINICAL ATHEROSCLEROTIC DISEASE

Patients in this group include those with peripheral arterial disease, abdominal aortic aneurysm, and symptomatic carotid artery disease. The absolute risk for MI in patients with noncoronary forms of atherosclerotic disease equals that for recurrent MI in patients with established CHD.

TYPE 2 DIABETES

Patients with type 2 diabetes who do not manifest CHD still appear to carry a risk for major coronary events equivalent to that of nondiabetic patients with established CHD. Moreover, many patients with type 2 diabetes have had a silent MI, and many other asymptomatic patients have silent ischemia. This has led the American Diabetes Association to designate type 2 diabetes as a CHD risk equivalent.

HIGH-RISK PATIENTS WITH MULTIPLE RISK FACTORS

The category of CHD risk equivalents has been extended to include asymptomatic patients who have multiple risk factors (other than diabetes). A modified version of the Framingham score sheet is presented in Table 12-2. Framingham scores are used to estimate the absolute risk for the development of CHD over the next decade. Table 12-2 shows absolute risk for *hard CHD* (nonfatal and fatal MI) and excludes *soft CHD* (stable and unstable angina). Hard CHD seems a better end point for defining CHD risk equivalency because risk-reduction therapy is aimed primarily at reducing risk for MI. When absolute 10-year risk for hard CHD exceeds 20 percent, a CHD risk equivalent is identified.

Intermediate- and Low-Risk Patients

For patients found to be at intermediate risk by Framingham scoring, additional noninvasive evaluation for subclinical atherosclerotic disease may be considered to define their risk status further. Patients at intermediate risk by the Framingham algorithm deserve medical intervention. Primary prevention is for the long run. Even though these patients are not at high absolute risk for the short term, their risk mounts over time. In view of the proven effectiveness of risk-reduction therapies, there is a growing debate over whom among intermediate-risk patients should receive drug therapy for

TABLE 12-2

SCORING FOR GLOBAL RISK ASSESSMENT (ADJUSTED FRAMINGHAM SCORING POINTS FOR RISK FACTORS)

Risk Factor	Risk Points	
	Men	Women
Age		
<34	−1	−9
35–39	0	−4
40–44	1	0
45–49	2	3
50–54	3	6
55–59	4	7
60–64	5	8
65–69	6	9
70–74	7	10
Total Cholesterol (mg/dL)		
<160	−3	−2
169–199	0	0
200–239	1	1
240–279	2	2
≥280	3	3
Blood pressure (mmHg)		
<120	0	−3
120–129	0	0
130–139	1	1
140–159	2	2
>160	3	3
Smoker		
No	0	0
Yes	2	2
HDL cholesterol (mg/dL)		
<35	2	5
35–44	1	2
45–49	0	1
50–59	−1	0
≥60	−2	−3
Plasma glucose (mg/dL)		
<110	0	0
110–126	1	2
>126	2	4

Adding up the Points:

Age_____ Cholesterol_____ Diabetes_____

HDL cholesterol _____ Smoker_____ Blood Pressure_____

Total_____

risk reduction. The issue revolves around efficacy, safety, and cost-effectiveness of drug therapies. Advances in pharmacologic therapy promise to improve safety and to reduce costs; therefore, in the future, it should be possible to extend the benefits of risk-reducing drugs to more patients. In addition, advances in nondrug therapies may also make these options more attractive to many patients.

An important question is how to manage patients with a single categorical risk factor but who are otherwise at low risk. A fundamental principle of primary prevention is that *all categorical risk factors must be treated, regardless of absolute risk.* For example, cigarette smoking can cause cancer and cardiovascular disease even in the absence of other risk factors. Hypertension alone can cause stroke, heart failure, and kidney failure. Therefore, patients with categorical risk factors must not be ignored even if they are found to have a low absolute risk by Framingham scoring (Tables 12-2 and 12-3).

TABLE 12-3

ABSOLUTE RISK ESTIMATES FOR HARD CORONARY HEART DISEASE (CHD) ACCORDING TO FRAMINGHAM POINTS*

Framingham Risk Points	Absolute 10-Year Risk (%) Hard CHD	
	Men	Women
1	2	1
2	3	2
3	4	2
4	5	2
5	6	2
6	7	2
7	9	3
8	13	3
9	16	3
10	20	4
11	25	7
12	30	8
13	35	11
14	45	13
15		15
16		18
17		20

*Hard CHD = nonfatal and fatal myocardial infarction.

RISK FACTORS FOR WHICH INTERVENTIONS HAVE PROVED TO LOWER RISK OF CORONARY HEART DISEASE

Atherogenic Diet

PRACTICE RECOMMENDATIONS

The current dietary recommendations emphasize a well-balanced diet low in saturated fat, cholesterol, and sodium while rich in fruits and vegetables. Very low fat diets are poorly complied with and have little long-term safety and efficacy data to support them. A diet with less than 30 percent of calories from fat is generally recommended, but with caloric content compatible with maintenance of ideal body weight. For patients with vascular disease or hyperlipidemia, less than 7 percent of calories from saturated fat and less than 200 mg of dietary cholesterol per day are suggested. Monounsaturated fats and omega-3 fatty acids from fish may be a beneficial source of calories as compared with carbohydrates. Consultation with a registered dietitian or other nutrition specialist can be recommended as part of a risk-modification program in high-risk patients.

Dyslipidemia

PRACTICE RECOMMENDATIONS FOR LOW-DENSITY LIPOPROTEIN LOWERING

Lowering of low-density lipoprotein (LDL) can be accomplished with nondrug and drug therapies. *The importance of nondrug therapies must not be minimized.* Chief among them are reducing intake of cholesterol-raising fatty acids (saturated and *trans* fatty acids) and dietary cholesterol. The major source of dietary saturated fatty acids are dairy fats (e.g., milk, butter, cream, cheese, and ice cream) and animal fats [e.g., fatty cuts of meat (especially hamburger), fatty processed meats, lard, and tallow]. *Trans* fatty acids are present in shortening, hard margarine, and processed foods containing these forms of fat. Rich sources of dietary cholesterol are eggs, dairy fats, and other animal products. Achieving a desirable body weight will reduce LDL-cholesterol levels in most overweight patients and will decrease risk for CHD in several other ways.

There is growing interest in obtaining further risk reduction by use of dietary adjuncts. A daily intake of 3 g/day of plant stanols will reduce LDL-cholesterol concentration 10 to 15 percent beyond that which can be achieved by reducing cholesterol-raising fatty acids and cholesterol in the diet. High-intakes of dietary fiber will produce another 3 to 5 percent decrease in LDL levels. Unsaturated fatty acids (monounsaturated, n-6 polyunsaturated, and n-3 polyunsaturated fatty acids) will lower LDL and may reduce global risk for CHD via several other mechanisms.

Statins head the list of cholesterol-lowering drugs. Most patients tolerate statins with few side effects. Occasional patients will have a mild rise in liver transaminases, but this change is currently not believed to be an indication of hepatotoxicity. Rare patients will exhibit signs and symptoms of myopathy. This side effect is more likely to occur in patients who have chronic renal failure or liver disease or who are on drugs that utilize or inhibit the cytochrome P450 3A4 pathway. For every doubling of the dose of a statin, the LDL-cholesterol level will fall by about 6 percent; a more efficacious way to enhance LDL lowering is to combine statins with bile acid sequestrants. For patients with borderline elevated triglyercides (200 to 400 mg/dL) and high LDL, niacin or a statin is an acceptable first-line drug. When triglycerides exceed 400 mg/dL, a fibrate or niacin is usually the most appropriate first-line agent.

GOALS OF THERAPY FOR LOWERING LOW-DENSITY LIPOPROTEINS

For patients with established CHD or CHD risk equivalents, the National Cholesterol Education Program (NCEP) recommends an LDL-cholesterol goal of ≤100 mg/dL (Table 12-4). The American Heart Association recommends starting cholesterol-lowering drugs immediately in all CHD patients when the LDL-cholesterol level is >130 mg/dL. Whether to initiate cholesterol-lowering drugs in patients whose baseline LDL cholesterol is in the range of 100 to 129 mg/dL is unsettled. Without question, these patients should receive maximal nondrug therapy, possibly including dietary adjuncts (see above). Such therapy alone will often achieve the LDL-cholesterol goal of ≤100mg/dL. For patients at intermediate risk (Table 12-1),

---

TABLE 12-4

LDL-C THRESHOLDS (mg/dL) FOR DIET AND DRUG THERAPIES AND GOALS FOR LDL CHOLESTEROL BY RISK GROUP

	Initiate Therapy		
	Diet	Drug	Goal
Low (no CHD, <2 RF)	>160	>190	<160
Moderate-high (no CHD, 2+ RF)	>130	>160	<130
CHD or CHD risk equivalent	>100	>130	<100

a reasonable LDL-cholesterol goal is <130 mg/dL. The strategy for achieving an LDL-cholesterol level <130 mg/dL should be initiated with nondrug therapy, but some patients undoubtedly will require LDL-cholesterol-lowering drugs. Finally, for patients who are at low risk (Table 12-2), the LDL-cholesterol goal is <160 mg/dL. This target can be considered to be a minimal goal, but it must be recognized that the desirable LDL in primary prevention is <130 mg/dL. Most low-risk patients, however, are not candidates for cholesterol-lowering drugs. Most patients whose LDL is in this range should achieve an LDL-cholesterol level of <160 mg/dL with maximal nondrug therapy, including dietary adjuncts. Multiple research studies are currently assessing the benefits of lowering the serum LDL to levels below 80 mg/dL.

PRACTICE RECOMMENDATIONS FOR ATHEROGENIC DYSLIPIDEMIA

Although high LDL cholesterol is the primary lipid risk factor, other lipid parameters increase the risk of CHD in persons with or without an elevated LDL cholesterol. Specifically, the combination of *elevated concentrations of triglycerides, small, dense LDL, and low levels of high-density lipoprotein (HDL) is referred to as atherogenic dyslipidemia.* This is a complex dyslipidemia that usually results from a generalized metabolic derangement. Although an elevated LDL cholesterol deserves primary emphasis for management, atherogenic dyslipidemia is assuming increasing importance as a contributor to CHD because of the growing prevalence of obesity in the United States and worldwide. First-line treatment of atherogenic dyslipidemia is weight control and physical activity. Most patients with atherogenic dyslipidemia are either overweight [body mass index (BMI), 25 to 29 kg/m^2] or obese (BMI $\geq$ 30 kg/m^2). Weight reduction in these patients often will improve the lipoprotein abnormalities associated with this form of dyslipidemia. Introduction of regular physical activity will further correct the lipoprotein pattern. Weight control and regular exercise will not only improve atherogenic dyslipidemia but also mitigate the other components of the metabolic syndrome. The primary goal of lipid therapy in patients with atherogenic dyslipidemia is to reduce the LDL-cholesterol concentration to the targets recommended for primary and secondary prevention. In many patients, statin therapy will be required to achieve the LDL target. If abnormalities persist after reaching the LDL goal, renewed efforts at weight control and increased physical activity may be indicated. If these measures are not successful, a second lipid-lowering drug may be added to modify these other lipoproteins. Either a fibric acid or nicotinic acid can be employed as the second agent to achieve the secondary NCEP goals of HDL >35 mg/dL and triglycerides <200 mg/dL. The combination of fibrates with a high dose of a statin should be avoided because of the increased risk of myopathy.

PRACTICE RECOMMENDATIONS
FOR LIPOPROTEIN (a)

It is not yet clear whether lipoprotein (a) [Lp(a)] provides information independent of the conventional lipid profile, and no recommendation for screening can be made. If elevated levels prove clearly to increase risk among hypercholesterolemic individuals, it may be prudent to lower LDL-cholesterol levels even more aggressively in such individuals than current guidelines dictate. Knowledge of Lp(a) levels may also be useful in the selection of LDL-lowering drugs (e.g., niacin) and to identify a possible treatable cause in the occasional patient with CHD and none of the major risk factors. Unfortunately, many commercial assays for plasma Lp(a) are poorly standardized.

Cigarette Smoking

PRACTICE RECOMMENDATIONS

Nothing less than complete cessation of smoking and other tobacco use should be acceptable in patients with cardiovascular disease. Moreover, the home and work environments to which patients return should be smoke-free, both to encourage cessation and to reduce the risk from passive smoking. Cardiovascular specialists often have unique and time-limited opportunities to influence the behaviors of patients. After an acute event, the patient and their family members may be especially receptive to a smoking cessation intervention.

Smoking cessation clinical practice guidelines were first published by the Agency for Health Care Policy and Research in 1996 and form the basis for a successful smoking cessation program. These guidelines emphasize that tobacco use status should be documented in every patient and that every smoker should be offered an effective treatment intervention. Even a brief intervention may be effective and should, at a minimum, be provided to every patient who uses tobacco (Table 12-5). Three elements of a treatment program found to be effective include social support, skills training/problem solving, and nicotine replacement. More intense efforts by the care provider to achieve complete cessation will generally result in a greater success rate. The huge reduction in risk resulting from smoking cessation in the cardiovascular disease patient provides a strong rationale for sustained and intense efforts to be expended.

Hypertension

PRACTICE RECOMMENDATIONS

The Joint National Committee of Detection, Evaluation, and Treatment of High Blood Pressure recommends a treatment goal of <140/90 mmHg. A goal of <130/85 is appropriate for patients with diabetes, renal insufficiency, or congestive heart failure (CHF).

TABLE 12-5

STRATEGIES FOR SUCCESSFUL CESSATION OF CIGARETTE SMOKING: THE FOUR A'S

Ask	Systematically identify all tobacco users at every visit (e.g., include tobacco as a vital sign).
	Determine exposure to environmental tobacco smoke at home or at work.
Advise	Provide a clear, strong, and personalized message, urging every tobacco user to quit.
	Review benefits of quitting and risk of continuing.
	Assess patient's willingness to quit.
Assist	Have the patient develop a quit plan, including setting a quit date, identifying sources of support for cessation for family and friends, removing tobacco and other cues from the home and work environment.
	Provide counseling, information materials and other behavioral interventions.
	Recommend use of pharmacotherapy including bupropion SR, nicotine gum, nicotine inhaler, nicotine nasal spray, or nicotine patch.
Arrange	Provide a reminder on the quit date.
	See the patient shortly after the quit date to assess success.
	In unsuccessful, identify barriers and solutions to their removal.

The reader is referred to Chap. 18 for a complete discussion of the treatment of hypertension.

RISK FACTORS FOR WHICH INTERVENTIONS ARE LIKELY TO LOWER RISK OF CORONARY HEART DISEASE

Insulin Resistance Syndrome: The Basis of Multiple Risk Factors

PRACTICE RECOMMENDATIONS

Diabetes mellitus is an independent risk factor for CHD, increasing risk by two to four times for men and women, respectively. CHD is the leading cause of death among diabetics, and approximately 25 percent of survivors of myocardial infarction (MI) have diabetes. *Diabetic patients without a history of MI have as high a risk of coronary mortality as nondiabetic patients with a history of MI.* Once patients with type 2 diabetes suffer a myocardial infarction, their prognosis for survival is much worse than that for CHD patients without diabetes.

Weight loss and exercise are key therapeutic interventions because they improve the constellation of metabolic abnormalities that accompany diabetes. Although the optimal proportion of dietary fat and carbohydrate is controversial, calories restriction for obesity and avoidance of sugar and saturated fat are definitely recommended. *Beta blockers should not be withheld from diabetic patients following MI unless strong contraindications exist, because diabetic MI survivors have fewer deaths if treated with a beta blocker.* Although there is no consistent evidence to support intensive glycemic control as a strategy to reduce macrovascular end points, aggressive lipid management in patients with diabetes lowers CHD risk. The NCEP and American Diabetes Association guidelines recommend a more aggressive LDL goal (<100 mg/dL) in primary prevention of CHD in diabetics. The American Heart Association (AHA) recommends near-normal fasting glucose and hemoglobin A_{1C} (HgA$_1$c) of <7 percent as treatment goals for patients with diabetes.

Physical Inactivity

PRACTICE RECOMMENDATIONS

Physical inactivity is an independent risk factor for CHD and roughly doubles the risk. There is an inverse dose-response relation between the amount of exercise performed weekly, from 700 to 2000 kcal of energy, and death from cardiovascular disease and all causes. The American College of Sports Medicine and the Centers for Disease Control and Prevention recommend that every adult should accumulate 30 min or more of moderate-intensity physical activity on most, preferably all, days. Only about 20 percent of U.S. adults meet this goal. The AHA recommends a minimal goal of 30 min of moderate-intensity activity three to four times a week for individuals with and without CHD. Exercise testing should be recommended to apparently healthy men over 40 and women over 50 who are sedentary, as well as to younger adults with coronary risk factors, before starting a *vigorous* physical activity program (intensity >60 percent individual maximum oxygen consumption).

Obesity

PRACTICE RECOMMENDATIONS

Body mass index (BMI) has been adopted widely as a measure of adiposity. BMI is calculated as weight (kg)/height squared (m^2) and estimated as [weight (pounds)/height (inches)^2] $\times$ 704.5 *Overweight* is defined as a BMI of 25 to 29.9 and *obesity* as BMI $\geq$ 30. Abdominal obesity adds to the health risks of obesity, and waist circumference correlates positively with abdominal fat content. In adults with a BMI between 25 and 35, increased relative risk is indicated in men with a waist circumference of >102 cm (>40 in.) and in women of >88 cm (>35 in.).

BMI should be listed as a vital sign; it should be used to assess overweight and obesity and to monitor changes in body weight. National Institutes of Health guidelines recommend that waist circumference be measured in patients with a BMI between 25 and 35 because of its incremental predictive power. Treatment of overweight (BMI 25 to 29.9) is recommended only when patients have two or more risk factors, increased waist circumference, or CHD or a CHD risk equivalent. Treatment should focus on diet and exercise to prevent weight gain and to produce moderate weight loss over years. The initial goal of weight-loss therapy is to reduce body weight by approximately 10 percent from baseline in 6 months. For patients with a BMI in the range of 27 to 35, a decrease of 300 to 500 kcal/day will result in this degree of weight loss. Lost weight is usually regained unless a program consisting of dietary therapy is continued indefinitely. Weight-loss drugs approved by the Food and Drug Administration for long-term use may be useful as an adjunct to diet and physical activity for patients with a BMI $\geq$ 30 and for patients with a BMI $\geq$ 27 with CHD or obesity-related risk factors. CHD end point trials with weight-loss drugs, however, have not been conducted. Fenfluramine and dexfenfluramine have been withdrawn from the market because of associated valvular heart disease (see also Chaps. 22 to 25).

Postmenopausal Status

PRACTICE RECOMMENDATIONS

Postmenopausal women with CHD who have not been on estrogen replacement therapy (ERT) should not be started routinely on hormonal therapy for the purpose of preventing CHD events. Those with CHD who have been on ERT for at least 2 years without a CHD event need not have hormone therapy discontinued. For postmenopausal women without known CHD, clinical trial evidence is still lacking and the decision whether to treat must be individualized according to other health risks. Oral estrogen therapy is contraindicated in women with hypertriglyceridemia (e.g., serum triglycerides >400 mg/dL).

RISK FACTORS FOR WHICH INTERVENTIONS MIGHT LOWER RISK OF CORONARY HEART DISEASE

Psychosocial Factors

PRACTICE RECOMMENDATIONS

Optimal comprehensive secondary prevention should include attempts to identify and treat depression and anxiety in patients with CHD. Group support and stress management can be provided in formal cardiac rehabilitation programs.

Total Plasma Homocysteine Level

PRACTICE RECOMMENDATIONS

Measurement of homocysteine may be useful in patients with CHD in the absence of major risk factors or with a history of recurrent arterial thromboses.

Oxidative Stress

PRACTICE RECOMMENDATIONS

Based on randomized trial data, it is impossible to make recommendations for or against supplementation with vitamin C to prevent CHD, although beta-carotene and vitamin E appear to carry no benefit. Given observational evidence suggesting benefit for diets rich in fruits and vegetables, however, it is prudent to continue such diets, which contain several hundred micronutrients that may have chemopreventive properties.

UNMODIFIABLE RISK FACTORS

Age and Sex as Risk Factors for Atherosclerotic Disease

The incidence and prevalence of CHD increase sharply with age, so that age might be considered one of the most potent cardiovascular risk factors. CHD incidence rates in men are similar to those in women 10 years older. Persons at very advanced age (e.g., 75+ years) should have the risks and benefits of preventive cardiology interventions weighed on an individual basis.

Family History of Early-Onset CHD

The family history most predictive of coronary disease is that of a first-degree relative with onset at age 55 or less or a female relative with onset at age 65 or less is defined as a positive family history, the larger the number of relatives with early-onset CHD. That is, the younger the age of CHD in the relative, the stronger the predictive value. *Although considered a nonmodifiable risk factor, a positive family history should result in the careful screening of individual risk factors known to aggregate in families. Such familial aggregations may represent monogenic factors with known phenotypic expressions and inheritance patterns, polygenic factors with less clear modes of expression and inheritance, or shared environments.* Thus, family members of patients with CHD at a younger age represent fruitful targets for risk-factor assessment. *However, risk-factor screening often does not extend beyond the coronary patient. A strong recommendation that siblings and children of early-CHD patients be screened for CHD risk should be delivered to each patient and his or her family members.*

OTHER PHARMACOLOGIC THERAPY

Antiplatelet and Anticoagulant Therapy

PRACTICE RECOMMENDATIONS

The United States Preventive Services Task Force has recommended that low-dose aspirin be considered in men age 40 and over who are at high risk for MI and lack contraindications. Although observational data generally support the use of aspirin in women, the risk-to-benefit ratio in women may differ from that in men, since the average age at first infarction is higher in women. For secondary prevention, 80 to 325 mg of aspirin daily is recommended, with treatment continued indefinitely. If aspirin is contraindicated, clopidogrel and then warfarin are recommended for secondary prevention, with an International Normalized Ratio (INR) goal of 2 to 3.5.

Beta-Adrenergic Blocking Agents

PRACTICE RECOMMENDATIONS

For primary prevention, beta blockers are recommended as first-line therapy for hypertension. For secondary prevention, beta blockers are recommended in post-MI patients with arrhythmias, left ventricular dysfunction, and inducible ischemia. Although specific studies of beta-blocker cessation are not available, it is commonly recommended that beta-blocker therapy be continued indefinitely as long as side effects are not present.

Angiotensin-Converting Enzyme Inhibitors

PRACTICE RECOMMENDATIONS

For secondary prevention, angiotensin-converting enzyme (ACE) inhibitors should be prescribed to patients with CHF and reduced left ventricular function unless contraindicated. The results of the recent HOPE trial suggest that it is reasonable to prescribe ramipril or another ACE inhibitor for patients with CHD or CHD risk equivalent and normal left ventricular function, particularly for diabetics.

THE PRACTICE OF PREVENTIVE CARDIOLOGY

Barriers to Implementation of Preventive Cardiology Services

A number of barriers to the implementation of preventive services can be identified as the patient, physician, health care setting, and community/society levels. The improved implementation of proven interventions therefore requires a variety of strategies targeted at patients, health care providers, inpatient care settings, ambulatory care settings, and health systems. *Professional societies strongly recommend that risk-factor management be part of the optimal care of patients at high risk for cardiovascular disease[2,5] and therefore be the responsibility of all health care providers.*

SUGGESTED READING

Fuster V, Pearson TA. 27th Bethesda Conference: Matching the intensity of risk factor management. *J Am Coll Cardiol* 1996; 27:957.

Grundy SM, Balady GJ, Criqui MJ, et al: Guide to primary prevention of cardiovascular disease: A statement for healthcare professionals from the Task Force on Risk Reduction. American Heart Association Science Advisory and Coordinating Committee. *Circulation* 1997; 95:2329.

Grundy SM, Pasternak R, Greenland P, et al: Assessment of cardiovascular risk by use of multiple-risk-factor assessment. *Circulation* 1999; 100:1481.

Law MR, Wald NJ, Thompson SG: By how much and how quickly
    does reduction in serum cholesterol concentration lower risk of
    ischemic heart disease? *BMJ* 1994; 308:367–373.
Maron DJ, Ridker PM, Pearson TA, Grundy SM: Dyslipidemia, other
    risk factors, and the prevention of coronary heart disease. In:
    Fuster V, Alexander RW, O'Rourke RA, et al (eds): *Hurst's The
    Heart*, 10th ed. New York: McGraw-Hill; 2001:1131–1160.
National Cholesterol Education Program: Second report of the Expert
    Panel on Detection, Evaluation, and Treatment of High Blood
    Cholesterol in Adults (Adults Treatment Panel II). *Circulation*
    1994; 89:1333.
Smith SC, Greenland P, Grundy SM: Beyond secondary prevention:
    Identifying the high-risk patient for primary prevention. Exec-
    utive Summary: American Heart Association Prevention Con-
    ference. *Circulation* 2000; 101:111.

CHAPTER

13

DIAGNOSIS AND MANAGEMENT OF PATIENTS WITH CHRONIC ISCHEMIC HEART DISEASE

Raja Naidu
Robert A. O'Rourke
Robert C. Schlant
John S. Douglas, Jr.

Ischemic heart disease remains a major public health problem. Chronic stable angina is the first indicator of ischemic heart disease in about 50 percent of patients. The number of patients with stable angina in the United States approximates 16.5 million people, not including individuals who do not seek medical attention for their chest pain or who are shown to have a noncardiac cause of chest discomfort. Angina pectoris is a clinical syndrome that consists of recurrent discomfort or pain in the chest, jaw, shoulder, back, or arm associated with myocardial ischemia but without myocardial necrosis. It is typically precipitated or aggravated by exertion or emotional stress and relieved by nitroglycerin. Angina usually occurs in patients with coronary artery disease (CAD) affecting one or more large epicardial arteries. However, angina often is present in individuals with valvular heart disease, hypertrophic cardiomyopathy, and uncontrolled hypertension. It also occurs in patients with normal coronary arteries and myocardial ischemia due to coronary artery spasm or endothelial dysfunction. The symptom of angina is often observed in patients with noncardiac disorders affecting the esophagus, chest wall, or lungs.

ETIOLOGY

Coronary atherosclerosis is the cause of angina pectoris in most patients. Other causes include congenital artery abnormalities, coronary artery spasm, coronary thromboembolism, coronary vasculitis, aortic stenosis, mitral stenosis with resulting severe right ventricular hypertension with pulmonary hypertension, pulmonic stenosis, hypertrophic cardiomyopathy, and systemic arterial hypertension. Disorders in which angina occurs less frequently include aortic regurgitation, idiopathic dilated cardiomyopathy, and syphilitic heart disease. Mitral valve prolapse rarely causes true angina pectoris. Certain conditions may alter the balance between myocardial oxygen supply–demand and precipitate or aggravate angina pectoris, including severe anemia, tachycardia, fever, and hyperthyroidism.

CLASSIFICATION

The Canadian Cardiovascular Society Grading Scale (Table 13-1) is commonly used to classify the severity of angina pectoris, with the most severe symptoms occurring at rest and the least severe only with excessive exercise.

TABLE 13-1

CANADIAN CARDIOVASCULAR SOCIETY FUNCTIONAL CLASSIFICATION OF ANGINA PECTORIS

I. Ordinary physical activity, such as walking and climbing stairs, does not cause angina. Angina results from strenuous or rapid or prolonged exertion at work or recreation.

II. Slight limitation of ordinary activity. Walking or climbing stairs rapidly, walking uphill, walking or stair climbing when under emotion stress. Walking more than two blocks on level ground and climbing more than one flight of ordinary stairs at a normal pace.

III. Marked limitation of ordinary physical activity. Walking one to two blocks on level ground and climbing more than one flight of stairs under normal conditions.

IV. Inability to carry on any physical activity without discomfort—anginal symptoms may be present at rest.

Source: Modified from Campeau L. Letter to the editor. *Circulation* 1976; 54:522. Reproduced with permission from the American Heart Association, Inc., and the author.

DIAGNOSIS OF ANGINA PECTORIS

History and Physical Examination

After a description of the chest discomfort is obtained, the physician makes an integrated assessment of the location, quality, and duration of discomfort; inciting factors; and factors relieving the pain. The most commonly used classification scheme for chest pain divides patients into three groups: *typical angina, atypical angina,* and *noncardiac chest pain* (Table 13-2). Angina is further labeled as stable when its characteristics have been unchanged over the preceding 60 days. The presence of unstable angina predicts a much higher short-term risk of an acute coronary event. Unstable angina is defined as angina that presents in one of three major ways: rest angina, severe new-onset angina, or prior angina increasing in severity.

Usually, the discomfort of chronic stable angina pectoris is precipitated by physical activity, emotions, eating, or cold weather. Certain patients are able to describe accurately the extent and type of exercise at which they reproducibly experience their chest pain. Emotions—particularly anger, excitement, and frustration—often precipitate angina in patients with coronary CAD. Cigarette smoking induces chest discomfort or lowers the exertion threshold for angina in some patients. In most patients anginal discomfort has a characteristic crescendo nature. It develops and increases to a plateau over 10 to 30 s and disappears within minutes if the exertion is discontinued. The discomfort usually lasts a few minutes, occasionally 10 to 15 min. Very rarely, it may last up to 30 min. The discomfort of

TABLE 13-2

CLINICAL CLASSIFICATION OF ANGINA

Typical angina (definite)
(1) Substernal chest discomfort with a characteristic quality and duration that is (2) provoked by exertion or emotional stress and (3) relieved by rest or NTG.
Atypical angina (probable)
Meets two of the above characteristics.
Noncardiac chest pain
Meets one or none of the typical anginal characteristics.

SOURCE: Modified from Diamond GA, Staniloff HM, Fonester JS, et al: Computer-assisted diagnosis in the noninvasive evaluation of patients with suspected coronary disease. *J Am Coll Cardiol* 1983; 1:444–455, with permission.

angina is most often located substernally or just to the left of the sternum. In describing the discomfort, some patients clench their fists over their upper sternum (Levine's sign), a sign of high diagnostic accuracy. Radiation of the pain down the left arm or to the neck or jaw is common. The pain often radiates down the arms or to the neck, jaw, teeth, shoulders, or back. In addition to exertion, drugs that increase heart rate and blood pressure can precipitate angina, as can cocaine.

Patients with stable angina may have many asymptomatic or silent episodes of myocardial ischemia. Also, myocardial ischemia may result in symptoms from either systolic or diastolic left ventricular (LV) dysfunction without the characteristic chest discomfort. Exertional dyspnea or fatigue are two common angina equivalent manifestations that are usually also relieved with rest and nitroglycerin.

During an anginal attack, many patients appear pale and quiet. Diaphoresis and alterations in blood pressure and heart rate are common. A fourth (most common) or third heart sound, mitral regurgitant

TABLE 13-3

PRETEST LIKELIHOOD OF CAD IN SYMPTOMATIC PATIENTS ACCORDING TO AGE AND SEX[*][†]

Age (years)	Nonanginal Chest Pain		Atypical Angina		Typical Angina	
	Men	Women	Men	Women	Men	Women
30–39	4	2	34	12	76	26
40–49	13	3	51	22	87	55
50–59	20	7	65	31	93	73
60–69	27	14	72	51	94	86

[*]Each value represents the percent with significant CAD on catheterization.
[†]Combined Diamond GA, Staniloff HM, Fonester JS, et al; Computer-assisted diagnosis in the noninvasive evaluation of patients with suspected coronary disease. *J Am Coll Cardiol* 1983; 1:444–455; Chaitman BR, Bourassa MG, Davis K, et al: Angiographic prevalence of high-risk coronary artery disease in patient subsets (CASS). *Circulation* 1981; 64:360–367; O'Rourke RA, Hochman JS, Cohen MC, et al: New approaches to diagnosis and management of unstable angina and non-ST-segment evaluation myocardial infarction. 2000. In press; Lange RA, Cigarroa, Yancy CWJ, et al: Cocaine-induced coronary-artery vasoconstriction. *N Engl J Med* 1989; 321:1557–1562.
Source: Modified from Gibbons et al (1999), with permission.

systolic murmur, bibasilar pulmonary rates, or palpable systolic impulse at the apex may be present. Evidence of noncoronary atherosclerotic disease such as a carotid bruit, diminished pedal pulse, or abdominal aneurysm increases the likelihood of CAD.

Clinical Assessment of the Likelihood of Coronary Artery Disease

Clinicopathologic studies have demonstrated that it is possible to predict the probability of CAD on the basis of the history and the physical examination. The most powerful predictors of the probability of CAD are pain type, age, and sex (Table 13-3).

DIAGNOSTIC TESTS

Electrocardiogram and Chest Roentgenogram

A resting 12-lead electrocardiogram (ECG) should be recorded in all patients with symptoms suggestive of angina; however, it will be normal in up to 50 percent of patients with chronic stable angina. Evidence of prior Q-wave myocardial infarction (MI) on the ECG makes CAD very likely. Patients with a completely normal resting ECG rarely have significant LV systolic dysfunction. An ECG obtained during chest pain is abnormal in about 50 percent of patients with angina and a normal resting ECG. ST-segment elevation or depression establishes a high likelihood of angina and indicates ischemia at a low workload, suggesting an unfavorable prognosis. The chest roentgenogram is often normal in patients with stable angina pectoris and is more useful in diagnosing noncardiac causes of chest pain.

Electrocardiographic Exercise Stress Testing

The ECG exercise stress test is the most frequently used test to obtain objective evidence of myocardial ischemia as well as prognostic information in patients with known CAD. While wide variations are seen, the mean sensitivity is 68 percent and the mean specificity about 77 percent. The modest sensitivity of the exercise ECG is generally lower than that of imaging procedures. The diagnostic value of the test is significantly decreased by the presence of abnormalities on the resting ECG such as bundle branch block, ST-T wave changes, or left ventricular hypertrophy. Diagnostic testing is most valuable when the pretest probability of obstructive CAD is intermediate. In these conditions the test result has the largest effect on the posttest probability of disease and thus on clinical decisions.

Rest Echocardiography

Assessment of global systolic function and the presence of regional systolic wall motion abnormalities may help establish the diagnosis of chronic ischemic heart disease. The extent and severity of regional and global abnormalities are important considerations in choosing appropriate medical or surgical therapy. However, most patients undergoing a diagnostic evaluation for angina do not need a resting echocardiogram.

Myocardial Perfusion Imaging

Patients who should undergo cardiac stress testing with imaging for the diagnosis of CAD, as opposed to exercise ECG alone, include those in the following categories: (1) complete left bundle branch block (LBBB), electronically paced ventricular rhythm, and preexcitation syndromes; (2) patients who have >1 mm of resting ST-segment depression, including those with left ventricular hypertrophy (LVH) or taking drugs such as digitalis; (3) patients who are unable to exercise to a level high enough to give meaningful results on routine stress ECG (pharmacologic stress imaging should be considered); and (4) patients with angina who have undergone prior revascularization, in whom localization of ischemia, establishing the functional significance of lesions, and demonstrating myocardial viability are important considerations. Several methods can be used to induce stress, including (1) exercise (treadmill or bicycle) and (2) pharmacologic techniques (dipyridamole, adenosine, or dobutamine). When the patient can exercise to an appropriate level of cardiovascular stress for 6 to 12 min, exercise stress testing generally is preferred to pharmacologic stress. Myocardial perfusion imaging (MPI) is more expensive than exercise ECG testing, but it provides higher sensitivity and specificity. MPI plays a major role in risk stratification of patients with CAD. A normal perfusion scan in patients with CAD indicates a rate of cardiac death and MI of 0.9 percent per year, nearly as low as that of the general population. Incremental prognostic information will be gained from the number, size, and location of perfusion defects in combination with the amount of thallium-201 lung uptake on poststress images.

Stress Echocardiography

Stress echocardiography relies on imaging LV segmental wall motion and thickening during stress compared with baseline. It has a reported sensitivity and specificity similar to those of MPI. If a patient is unable to exercise, pharmacologic stress is achieved most commonly by using dobutamine. To help enhance endocardial border definition, IV contrast agents are frequently used. The choice of stress echocardiography or MPI depends on the available facilities, local expertise, and considerations of cost-effectiveness.

Coronary Angiography

This is considered the "gold standard" for the diagnosis of CAD, although it is invasive and moderately expensive. Direct referral for diagnostic coronary angiography in patients with chest pain possibly due to myocardial ischemia is appropriate when noninvasive tests are contraindicated or likely to be inadequate. Patients with noninvasive tests that are abnormal but not clearly diagnostic often require clarification of an uncertain diagnosis by coronary angiography. In certain cases a second noninvasive test (imaging modality) may be recommended for a patient with a low likelihood of CAD but an intermediate-risk treadmill result. Coronary angiography is likely to be most appropriate for patients with typical anginal symptoms and a high clinical probability of severe CAD or individuals with high-risk noninvasive tests. In diabetic patients, the diagnosis of chronic stable angina can be particularly difficult because of the absence of characteristic symptoms of myocardial ischemia due to autonomic and sensory neuropathy. Thus, a lower threshold for coronary angiography is appropriate. The American College of Cardiology/American Heart Association (ACC/AHA) recommendations concerning the value of coronary angiography are listed in Table 13-4.

Electron beam computed tomography (EBCT) is being used with increasing frequency. However, the specificity of a positive result may be as low as 49 percent and the predictive accuracy is less than 70 percent. The role of EBCT in CAD diagnosis and risk stratification has been controversial. A recent report of an ACC/AHA expert consensus writing group does not recommend EBCT for routine screening of asymptomatic patients for CAD or its use in most patients with chest pain.

DIFFERENTIAL DIAGNOSIS

Table 13-5 lists the differential diagnosis of angina pectoris. Usually the distinction is clear if an accurate history is obtained and a complete physical examination is properly performed.

TABLE 13-4

INVASIVE TESTING—CORONARY ANGIOGRAPHY
RECOMMENDATIONS FOR CORONARY ANGIOGRAPHY
TO ESTABLISH A DIAGNOSIS IN PATIENTS WITH
SUSPECTED ANGINA, INCLUDING THOSE WITH
KNOWN CAD WHO HAVE A SIGNIFICANT CHANGE
IN ANGINAL SYMPTOMS

Class I*
1. Patients with known or possible angina pectoris who have survived sudden cardiac death.

Class IIa†
1. Patients with an uncertain diagnosis after noninvasive testing in whom the benefit of a more certain diagnosis outweighs the risk and cost of coronary angiography.
2. Patients who cannot undergo noninvasive testing due to disability, illness, or morbid obesity.
3. Patients with an occupational requirement for a definitive diagnosis.
4. Patients who by virtue of young age at onset of symptoms, noninvasive imaging, or other clinical parameters are suspected of having a nonatherosclerotic cause of myocardial ischemia (coronary artery anomaly, Kawasaki disease, primary coronary artery dissection, radiation-induced vasculoplasty).
5. Patients in whom coronary artery spasm is suspected and provocative testing may be necessary.
6. Patients with a high pretest probability of left main or three-vessel CAD.

Class IIb
1. Patients with recurrent hospitalization for chest pain in whom a definite diagnosis is judged necessary.
2. Patients with an overriding desire for a definitive diagnosis and a greater than low probability of CAD.

Class III‡
1. Patients with significant comorbidity in whom the risk of coronary arteriography outweighs the benefits of the procedure.
2. Patients with an overriding personal desire for a definitive diagnosis and a low probability of CAD.

*Class I: Conditions for which there is evidence and/or general agreement that a given procedure or treatment is useful and effective.

†Class II: Conditions for which there is conflicting evidence and/or a divergence of opinion about the usefulness/efficacy of a procedure or treatment.

IIa: Weight of evidence/opinion is in favor of usefulness/efficacy.

IIb: Usefulness/efficacy is less well established by evidence/opinion.

‡Class III: Conditions for which there is evidence and/or general agreement that the procedure/treatment is not useful and in some cases may be harmful.

SOURCE: Gibbons et al (1999), with permission.

TABLE 13-5
DIFFERENTIAL DIAGNOSIS OF CHEST PAIN

1. Angina pectoris/myocardial infarction
2. Other cardiovascular causes
   a. Likely ischemic in origin
      (1) Aortic stenosis
      (2) Hypertrophic cardiomyopathy
      (3) Severe systemic hypertension
      (4) Severe right ventricular hypertension
      (5) Aortic regurgitation
      (6) Severe anemia/hypoxia
   b. Nonischemic in origin
      (1) Aortic dissection
      (2) Pericarditis
      (3) Mitral valve prolapse
3. Gastrointestinal
   a. Esophageal spasm
   b. Esophageal reflux
   c. Esophageal rupture
   d. Peptic ulcer disease
4. Psychogenic
   a. Anxiety
   b. Depression
   c. Cardiac psychosis
   d. Self-gain
5. Neuromusculoskeletal
   a. Thoracic outlet syndrome
   b. Degenerative joint disease of cervical/thoracic spine
   c. Costochondritis (Tietze's syndrome)
   d. Herpes zoster
   e. Chest wall pain and tenderness
6. Pulmonary
   a. Pulmonary embolus with or without pulmonary infarction
   b. Pneumothorax
   c. Pneumonia with pleural involvement
7. Pleurisy

PATHOPHYSIOLOGY

A disparity between the supply of coronary blood flow (CBF) and the metabolic demands of the myocardium is the primary factor in ischemic heart disease. This imbalance may result in clinical manifestations of ischemia when myocardial demand exceeds the capacity of the coronary arteries to deliver an adequate supply of oxygen. In normal hearts there is an excess CBF reserve, so that ischemia does not occur even with very vigorous exercise. Atherosclerosis in the epicardial coronary arteries or in the coronary microvasculature may cause an imbalance between supply and demand at even modest levels of exercise. Heart rate, myocardial contractility, and systolic wall tension—which is related to LV systolic pressure and volume— are the major determinants of myocardial oxygen demand. Oxygen supply to the myocardium is dependent upon the oxygen-carrying capacity of blood and the CBF. Narrowing of the large coronary arteries transiently by vasospasm or permanently by obstructive lesions may increase the coronary resistance sufficiently to reduce CBF. Patients with coronary atherosclerosis also have endothelial dysfunction that may manifest itself by a failure of the coronary vasculature to dilate in response to normal vasodilatory stimuli such as increased flow, exercise, tachycardia, acetylcholine, or cold pressor testing. Most patients with angina pectoris due to coronary atherosclerosis have *myocardial ischemia caused by both epicardial coronary obstruction and endothelial dysfunction* of both large and small vessels.

Circadian Rhythm of Coronary Ischemia

The prevalence of MI, unstable angina, variant angina, and silent ischemia is greatest in the morning, during the first few hours after awakening; the threshold for precipitating anginal attacks in patients with stable angina also appears to be lowest in the morning. The diurnal variation in ischemic threshold is attributed to the endogenous rhythms of catecholamine secretion and to the sensitivity to coronary vasoconstrictors, both of which appear to be highest in the morning. The increase in sympathetic nervous system activity is associated with increases in heart rate, blood pressure, contractility, and MV_{O_2}. The lowered morning anginal threshold and the higher morning systolic blood pressure mandate early-morning use of antianginal and antihypertensive medications.

RISK STRATIFICATION OF PATIENTS WITH CHRONIC ISCHEMIC HEART DISEASE

The prognosis for the patient with chronic artery disease is usually related to four patient factors. First, LV performance is the strongest predictor of long-term survival in patients with CAD and the ejection fraction (EF) is the most often used measure of the presence and the degree of LV dysfunction. The second predictive factor is the anatomic extent and severity of atherosclerotic involvement of the coronary arteries. The number of stenosed coronary arteries is the most common measure of this factor. The third patient factor affecting prognosis is evidence of a recent coronary plaque rupture, indicating a much higher short-term risk for cardiac death or nonfatal MI. Worsening clinical symptoms with unstable features is an important clinical marker of a complicated plaque. The fourth prognostic factor is general health and noncoronary comorbidity. Risk stratification of patients with chronic stable angina by stress testing with exercise or pharmacologic agents has been shown to permit identification of groups of patients with low, intermediate, or high risk for subsequent cardiac events. Noninvasive test findings that identify high-risk patients are listed in Table 13-6. Patients identified as high-risk are generally referred for coronary arteriography independent of their symptomatic status. The ACC/AHA Guidelines for Risk Stratification using Coronary Angiography in Patients with Stable Angina are listed in Table 13-7.

TREATMENT OF CHRONIC STABLE ANGINA

There are two major purposes in the treatment of stable angina. The first is to prevent MI and death and thereby *increase the quantity of life*. The second is to reduce symptoms of angina and the frequency and severity of ischemia, which should *improve the quality of life*. The choice of therapy often depends on the clinical response to initial medical therapy although some patients (and many physicians) prefer coronary revascularization in situations where either may be successful. Patient education, cost-effectiveness, and patient preference are important components in this decision-making process.

General

Patients with angina pectoris due to coronary atherosclerosis should be evaluated for risk factors for coronary disease; whenever possible, these risk factors should be corrected. Tobacco should be avoided in all forms. Hypertension and diabetes should be well controlled. Ideal body weight should be achieved. A low-fat, low-cholesterol diet should be instituted and a lipid profile determined.

Antiplatelet Agents

Aspirin, 80 to 325 mg/daily, should be used routinely by all patients with acute and chronic ischemic heart disease with and without clinical symptoms in the absence of contraindications. In those unable to take aspirin, clopidogrel may be used. The efficacy of newer antiplatelet agents such as glycoprotein IIb/IIIA inhibitors in the management of chronic stable angina has not been established.

TABLE 13-6

NONINVASIVE RISK STRATIFICATION

High-risk (greater than 3 percent annual mortality rate)
1. Severe resting left ventricular dysfunction (LVEF < 35%).
2. High-risk treadmill score (score ≤ 11).*
3. Severe exercise left ventricular dysfunction (exercise LVEF < 35%).
4. Stress-induced large perfusion defect (particularly if anterior).
5. Stress-induced multiple perfusion defects of moderate size.
6. Large, fixed perfusion defect with LV dilation or increased lung uptake (thallium 201).
7. Stress-induced moderate perfusion defect with LV dilation or increased lung uptake (thallium 201).
8. Echocardiographic wall motion abnormality (involving more than two segments) developing at low dose of dobutamine (≤10 mg/kg/min) or at a low heart rate (<120 beats per minute).
9. Stress echocardiographic evidence of extensive ischemia.

Intermediate risk (1–3% annual mortality rate)
1. Mild/moderate resting left ventricular dysfunction (LVEF = 35–49%).
2. Intermediate-risk treadmill score (-11<score<5).
3. Stress-induced moderate perfusion defect without LV dilation or increased lung intake (thallium 201).
4. Limited stress echocardiographic ischemia with a wall motion abnormality only at higher doses of dobutamine involving less than or equal to two segments.

Low risk (less than 1% annual mortality rate)
1. Low-risk treadmill score (score ≥ 5).
2. Normal or small myocardial perfusion defect at rest or with stress.
3. Normal stress echocardiographic wall motion or no change of limited resting wall motion abnormalities during stress.

---

*Duke Treadmill score. See Source below.

SOURCE: Gibbons et al (1999), with permission.

TABLE 13-7

RECOMMENDATIONS FOR CORONARY ANGIOGRAPHY FOR RISK STRATIFICATION IN PATIENTS WITH CHRONIC STABLE ANGINA

Class I
1. Patients with disabling [Canadian Cardiovascular Society (CCS) classes III and V] chronic stable angina despite medical therapy
2. Patients with high-risk criteria on noninvasive testing regardless of anginal severity
3. Patients with angina who have survived sudden cardiac death or serious ventricular arrhythmia
4. Patients with angina and symptoms and signs of congestive heart failure
5. Patients with clinical characteristics that indicate a high likelihood of severe CAD

Class IIa
1. Patients with significant LV dysfunction (ejection fraction < 45%), CCS class I or II angina, and demonstrable ischemia but less than high-risk criteria on noninvasive testing
2. Patients with inadequate prognostic information after noninvasive testing

Class IIb
1. Patients with disabling CCS class I or II angina, preserved LV function (ejection fraction > 45%), and less than high-risk criteria on noninvasive testing

Class III
1. Patients with disabling CCS classes I or II angina who respond to medical therapy and have no evidence of ischemia on noninvasive testing
2. Patients who prefer to avoid revascularization

---

*Note: See classes I–III as described in Table 13-4.
Source: Gibbons et al (1999), with permission.

Lipid-Lowering Agents

Recent clinical studies have conveniently demonstrated that lowering of low-density-lipoprotein (LDL) cholesterol with HMG-CoA reductase inhibitors (statins) can decrease the risk of adverse ischemic events in patients with established CAD. Thus, lipid-lowering therapy should be recommended even in the presence of mild to moderate elevations of LDL cholesterol in patients with chronic stable angina. Patients with ischemic heart disease should have LDL cholesterol levels below 100 mg/dL (2.6 mmol/L). It is now known that the statins have many favorable effects on endothelial function beyond their decrease in LDL cholesterol levels and may reverse the endothelial response to chemical or physical stresses causing coronary vasoconstriction.

Nitroglycerin and Nitrates

The standard first-line therapy of angina remains sublingual nitroglycerin (NTG), which usually relieves the symptoms within 1 to 5 min. NTG may be taken acutely either as a sublingual tablet (0.3 to 0.6 mg) or as an oral spray, each puff of which is calculated to deliver 0.4 mg. Monotherapy with sublingual or oral spray NTG is usually not satisfactory unless the episodes are rare.

The American College of Cardiology/AHA–ASIM Guidelines for chronic stable angina recommend long-acting beta blockers and/or calcium antagonists in preference to long-acting nitrates in patients with recurrent angina (see below). Nevertheless, long-acting nitrates are used prophylactically in many patients who have frequent episodes of angina. The many forms of nitrates include a slowly absorbed buccal capsule, a transdermal ointment or patch, and sublingual or oral forms that are more slowly absorbed. In general, it is important to start with a low dosage and to increase the dose progressively. The most common side effects are headache, dizziness, and postural hypotension. It should also be noted that the coadministration of nitrates and sildenafil (Viagra) significantly increases the risk of potentially life-threatening hypotension.

The *major problem* with long-term use of nitroglycerin and long-acting nitrates is the development of *nitrate tolerance*. For practical purposes, the administration of nitrates with an adequate nitrate-free interval (8 to 12 h) appears to be the most effective method of preventing nitrate tolerance. For many patients, this can be from about 9 P.M. to 7 A.M. Nitroglycerin ointments should be removed about 8 or 9 P.M. Isosorbide dinitrate (ISDN; 10 to 60 mg) can be given orally in doses of 30 mg twice a day at 8 A.M. and 5 P.M. or three times a day at 8 A.M., 1 P.M., and 5 P.M. Isosorbide mononitrate (ISMO), a metabolite of ISDN, is administered orally in 20-mg doses at 7 A.M. and 2 P.M. An extended-release form of isosorbide mononitrate (IMDUR) can be taken orally as a single 60-mg dose at 7 or 8 A.M. Patients who have angina at night may need either to plan the nitrate-free period for another time or to use a beta blocker or calcium channel blocker concurrently.

Patients should be instructed that if an anginal episode persists for more than 10 min despite their having taken three sublingual

NTG tablets or an equivalent dose of NTG spray, they should report promptly to the nearest medical facility for further evaluation and management.

Beta Blockers

Beta-adrenergic blocking agents, which reduce heart rate and myocardial contractility both at rest and during exertion, are very effective in the management of patients with angina pectoris. Many beta blockers are available. In general, long-acting cardioselective agents (e.g., metoprolol) are preferred in patients who have a history of bronchospastic disease, diabetes mellitus, or peripheral vascular disease. However, it should be noted that even cardioselective beta blockers can produce bronchospasm in some patients. All beta blockers can worsen heart block or depress LV function and worsen heart failure. Fatigue, inability to perform exercise, lethargy, insomnia, nightmares, worsening claudication, and erectile dysfunction are other possible side effects.

In treating stable angina, it is essential that the dose of beta blockers be adjusted to lower the resting heart rate to 55 to 60 beats/per minute. If discontinued, beta blockers should be tapered over 3 to 10 days, when possible, to avoid a rebound worsening of angina pectoris.

Calcium Antagonists

Calcium channel blockers decrease myocardial oxygen requirements by producing arterial dilation and often by reducing myocardial contractility. In addition, calcium channel blockers produce coronary vasodilation and prevent coronary artery spasm. Drugs such as verapamil and diltiazem also tend to reduce heart rate. Clinical trials comparing calcium antagonists and beta blockers have demonstrated that calcium antagonists are as effective as beta blockers in relieving angina and improving exercise time to onset of angina or ischemia. The calcium antagonists are also effective in reducing the incidence on angina in patients with vasospastic angina. In the International Multicenter Angina Exercises (Image Trial), combination therapy with metaprolol and nifedipine increased the exercise time to ischemic compared to either drug alone.

Thus, long-acting calcium antagonists including slow-release and long-acting dihydropyridines (nifedipine and amlodipine) and nondihydropyridines (verapamil and diltiazem) should be used in combination with beta blockers when initial treatment with beta blockers is not successful or as a substitute for beta blockers when initial treatment leads to unacceptable side effects. Calcium channel blockers are the preferred agents in patients with a history of asthma, chronic obstructive pulmonary disease, or severe peripheral vascular disease. Combined therapy with a long-acting cardioselective beta blocker and a long-acting dihydropyridine calcium channel is particularly beneficial. Some patients may benefit from triple therapy with a long-acting nitrate, beta blocker, and a calcium channel blocker.

MYOCARDIAL REVASCULARIZATION

Some patients with stable angina pectoris are candidates for revascularization either with coronary artery bypass graft (CABG) surgery or percutaneous coronary intervention (PCI). The two general indications for revascularization are (1) the presence of symptoms that are not acceptable to the patient either because of restriction of physical activity and lifestyle or side effects from medications or (2) the presence of coronary arteriographic findings indicating clearly that the patient would have a significantly better prognosis with revascularization than with medical therapy. In general, patients with stable angina should have objective evidence of myocardial ischemia prior to revascularization. Additional major considerations include the age of the patient, presence of other comorbid conditions, grade or class of angina experienced by the patient on maximal therapy, extent and severity of myocardial ischemia on noninvasive testing, degree of LV dysfunction, and distribution and severity of CAD.

CABG provides good symptomatic relief for most patients who have suitable vessels. It is the treatment of choice for patients with severe CAD including greater than 50 percent left main stenosis or three-vessel disease with impaired LV function. It is also indicated in severely symptomatic patients with two-vessel disease that includes a high-grade stenosis of the proximal left anterior descending artery and in patients in whom revascularization is indicated but who have a lesion not amendable to PCI. Vein grafts have a failure rate that approaches 50 percent at 10 years. In contrast, internal mammary grafts have a superior patency and thus should be used whenever possible during the CABG.

With the proliferation of various new debulking techniques and intracoronary stents, PCI can be successfully performed on a wide variety of native vessel and graft lesions. The advantages of PCI for the treatment of CAD include a low level of procedure-related morbidity and mortality, a short hospital stay, early return to activity, and the feasibility of multiple procedures. However, PCI is not possible for all patients; it is accompanied by a significant incidence of restenoses; and there is an occasional need for emergency CABG surgery. The recommendations of the ACC/AHA/ACP–ASIM Chronic Stable Angina Guidelines for revascularization with PCI or CABG in patients with stable angina are listed in Table 13-8.

TABLE 13-8

REVASCULARIZATION FOR CHRONIC STABLE ANGINA*

Class I

1. CABG for patients with significant left main coronary disease.
2. CABG for patients with three-vessel disease. The survival benefit is greater in patients with abnormal LV function (ejection fraction < 50%).
3. CABG for patients with two-vessel disease with significant proximal left anterior descending CAD and either abnormal LV function (ejection fraction < 50%) or demonstrable ischemia on noninvasive testing.
4. PCI for patients with two- or three-vessel disease with significant proximal left anterior descending CAD, who have anatomy suitable for catheter-based therapy, normal LV function, and no treated diabetes.
5. PCI or CABG for patients with one or two-vessel disease CAD without significant proximal left anterior descending CAD but with a large area of viable myocardium and high-risk criteria on noninvasive testing.
6. CABG for patients with one- or two-vessel CAD without significant proximal left anterior descending CAD who have survived sudden cardiac death or sustained ventricular tachycardia.
7. In patients with prior PCI, CABG, or PCI for recurrent stenosis associated with a large area of viable myocardium or high-risk criteria on noninvasive testing.
8. PTCA† or CABG for patients who have not been successfully treated by medical therapy and can undergo revascularization with acceptable risk.

Class IIa

1. Repeat CABG for patients with multiple saphenous vein graft stenoses, especially when there is significant stenosis of a graft supplying the LAD. It may be appropriate to use PTCA for focal saphenous vein graft lesions or multiple stenoses in poor candidates for reoperative surgery.
2. Use of PCI or CABG for patients with one- or two-vessel CAD without significant proximal LAD disease but with a moderate area of viable myocardium and demonstrable ischemia on noninvasive testing.

(continued)

TABLE 13-8

(Continued)

3. Use of PCI or CABG for patients with one-vessel disease with significant proximal LAD disease.

Class IIb

1. Compared with CABG, PCI for patients with two- or three-vessel disease with significant proximal left anterior descending CAD, who have anatomy suitable for catheter-based therapy, and who have treated diabetes or abnormal LV function.

2. Use of PCI for patients with significant left main coronary disease who are not candidates for CABG.

3. PCI for patients with one- or two-vessel disease CAD without significant proximal left anterior descending CAD who have survived sudden cardiac death or sustained ventricular tachycardia.

Class III

1. Use of PCI or CABG for patients with one- or two-vessel CAD without significant proximal left anterior descending CAD, who have mild symptoms that are unlikely due to myocardial ischemia or who have not received an adequate trial of medical therapy and (a) Have only a small area of viable myocardium or (b) Have no demonstrable ischemia on noninvasive testing.

2. Use of PCI or CABG for patients with borderline coronary stenoses (50 to 60% diameter in locations other than the left main coronary artery) and no demonstrable ischemia on noninvasive testing.

3. Use of PCI or CABG for patients with insignificant coronary stenosis (<50% diameter).

4. Use of PCI in patients with significant left main coronary disease who are candidates for CABG.

KEY: CABG = coronary artery bypass graft; CAD = coronary artery disease; LAD = left anterior descending (coronary artery); LV = left ventricular; PCI = percutaneous coronary intervention; PTCA = percutaneous transluminal coronary angioplasty.

*Recommendations for revascularization with PTCA (or other catheter-based techniques) and CABG in patients with stable angina

†PTCA is used in these recommendations to indicate PTCA or other catheter-based techniques, such as stents, atherectomy, and laser therapy.

NOTE: See classes I to III as described at bottom of Table 13-4.

It is important to remember that most patients with chronic angina have not been shown to have an increased survival rate with invasive treatment but require invasive treatment mainly to control their symptoms.

SUGGESTED READINGS

Afridi I, Quinones MA, Zoghbi WA, Cheirif J: Dobutamine stress echocardiography: Sensitivity, specificity, and predictive value for future cardiac events. *Am Heart J* 1994; 127:1510–1515.

Alexander KP, Shaw LJ, Shaw LK, et al: Value of exercise threadmill testing in women. *J Am Coll Cardiol* 1998; 32(6):1657–1664.

Beleslin BD, Ostojic M, Stepanovic J, et al: Stress echocardiography in the detection of myocardial ischemia. Head-to-head comparison of exercise, dobutamine, and dipyridamole tests. *Circulation* 1994; 90:1168–1176.

Blumenthal RS, Cohn G, and Schulman SP: Medical therapy versus coronary angioplasty in stable coronary artery disease: A critical review of the literature. *J Am Coll Card* 2000; 36:668–673.

Cheltin MD, Hutter AM, Brindis RG, et al: ACC/AHA expert consensus documents: Use of sildenafil (Viagra) in patients with cardiovascular disease. *J Am Coll Cardiol* 1999; 33:273–282.

Comparison of coronary artery bypass surgery with angioplasty in patients with multivessel disease: The Bypass Angioplasty Revascularization Investigation (BARI) investigators. *N Engl J Med* 1996; 335 (4):217–225 [published erratum appears in *N Engl J Med* 1997; 336(2):147].

Gibbons RJ, Balady GJ, Beasley JW, et al: AHA guidelines for exercise testing. *J Am Coll Cardiol* 1999, 30:260–311.

Gibbons RJ, Chatterjee K, Daley J, et al: ACC/AHA/ACP–ASIM guidelines for the management of patients with chronic stable angina: A report of the ACC/AHA Task Force on Practice Guidelines (Committee on the Management of Patients with Chronic Stable Angina) *J Am Coll Cardiol* 1999; 33:2097–2197.

Hachamovitch R, Berman DS, Shaw LJ, et al: Incremental prognostic value of myocardial perfusion single photon emission computed tomography for the prediction of cardiac death: Differential stratification for risk of cardiac death and myocardial infarction. *Circulation* 1998; 97(6):533–543 [published erratum appears in *Circulation* 1998; July 14, 98(2):190].

Mark DB, Shaw L, Harrell FE, et al: Prognostic value of a treadmill exercise score in outpatients with suspected coronary artery disease. *N Engl J Med* 1991; 325:849–853.

Muller JE, Stone PH, Turi ZG, et al: Circadian variation in the frequency of onset of acute myocardial infarction. *N Engl J Med* 1985; 313:1315–1322.

Nishimura S, Mahmarian JJ, Boyce TM, Verani MS: Equivalence between adenosine and exercise thallium-201 myocardial tomography: A mulitcenter, prospective, crossover trial. *J Am Coll Cardiol* 1992; 20:265–275.

O'Rourke RA: Optimal medical management of patients with chronic ischemic heart disease. *Curr Probl Cardiol* 2001. In press.

O'Rourke RA, Froelicher VF, Greenland P, et al: ACC/AHA Expert Consensus Document on Electron Beam Computed Tomography for the Diagnosis of Coronary Artery Disease. *J Am Coll Cardiol* 2000; 36:326–341.

O'Rourke RA, Schlant RC, Douglas JS Jr: Diagnosis and management of patients with chronic ischemic heart disease. In: Fuster V, Alexander RW, O'Rourke RA, et al (eds): *Hurst's the Heart*, 10th ed. New York: McGraw-Hill; 2001:1207–1236.

Pryor DB, Shaw L, McCants CB, et al: Value of the history and physical in identifying patients at increased risk for coronary artery disease. *Ann Intern Med* 1993; 18:81–90.

CHAPTER

14

DIAGNOSIS AND MANAGEMENT OF PATIENTS WITH UNSTABLE ANGINA

Jacob M. Mishell
David D. Waters

INTRODUCTION AND DEFINITION

In 1996, a total of 1,367,000 patients were hospitalized in the United States with the diagnosis of unstable angina (UA). UA can be conveniently defined as new-onset or worsening angina within the previous 60 days or postinfarction angina (after the first 24 h from the onset of infarction). It is an acute coronary syndrome, distinguished from non-ST-segment elevation myocardial infarction (NSTSEMI) by the absence of elevated serologic markers of myocardial necrosis. The usual underlying pathophysiologic mechanism involves rupture or erosion of an atherosclerotic plaque, with thrombus formation that severely obstructs the coronary artery lumen. In the past decade, important advances in the diagnosis and risk stratification of patients presenting with UA have been made. New therapies, specifically low-molecular-weight heparins and platelet glycoprotein IIb/IIIa receptor antagonists, improve outcomes in high-risk patients. The introduction of coronary stents has reduced the incidences of acute vessel closure and restenosis. The exact indications for these newer therapies have not yet been completely defined across different strata of risk in UA. Physicians must therefore continue to integrate the results of new trials into their practice and exercise finely tuned judgment in the management of patients with unstable angina.

CLASSIFICATION

Several systems have been proposed for classifying UA. Patients with UA should be classified according to their level of short-term

TABLE 14-1

BRAUNWALD CLASSIFICATION OF UNSTABLE ANGINA

SEVERITY

Class I   New-onset, severe, or accelerated angina (angina of less than 2 months' duration, severe or occurring more than three times/day, or angina that is distinctly more frequent and precipitated by distinctly less exertion; no rest pain within 2 months)

Class II   Angina at rest, subacute (angina at rest within the preceding month but not within the preceding 48 h)

Class III   Angina at rest, acute (angina at rest within the preceding 48 h)

CLINICAL CIRCUMSTANCES

Class A   Secondary unstable angina (a clearly identified condition extrinsic to the coronary vascular bed that has intensified myocardial ischemia—e.g., anemia, hypotension, tachyarrhythmia)

Class B   Primary unstable angina

Class C   Postinfarction unstable angina (within 2 weeks of a documented myocardial infarction)

INTENSITY OF TREATMENT

1. Absence of treatment, or minimal treatment
2. Standard therapy for chronic stable angina (conventional doses of oral beta blockers, nitrates, and calcium channel blockers)
3. Maximal therapy (maximally tolerated doses of all three categories of oral therapy and intravenous nitroglycerin)

SOURCE: Braunwald E, Antman EM, Beasley JW, et al. ACC/AHA guidelines for the management of patients with unstable angina and non-ST-segment elevation myocardial infarction. A report of the American College of Cardiology/American Heart Association Task Force on Practice Guidelines (Committee on the Management of Patients With Unstable Angina). *J Am Coll Cardiol* 2000; 36:970–1062. With permission.

risk. The classification proposed by Braunwald (Table 14-1) includes three levels of severity and three clinical circumstances to yield nine categories in all. Components of the Braunwald classification have been shown to correlate with clinical outcomes. Specifically, a

TABLE 14-2

CONDITIONS WITH THE POTENTIAL TO PROVOKE
SECONDARY UNSTABLE ANGINA

Tachyarrhythmia
Fever
Hypoxia
Anemia
Hypertensive crisis
Thyrotoxicosis

48 h pain-free interval and the absence of electrocardiographic (ECG) changes are associated with decreased risk, while postinfarction UA and the need for maximal medical therapy carry a higher risk.

Distinguishing *primary* from *secondary* UA is of clinical value, since treatment usually differs. Acute worsening of a coronary stenosis causes primary UA by limiting coronary blood flow. Secondary UA arises as a consequence of increased myocardial oxygen demand superimposed upon severe underlying coronary disease. The major determinants of myocardial oxygen demand are heart rate, inotropic state, and the loading conditions of the left ventricle, primarily afterload. Secondary UA should resolve with successful treatment of the precipitating condition (Table 14-2).

Finally, the recognition of three specific forms of primary UA is worthwhile because the pathophysiology, prognosis, and management are different:

1. Variant or Prinzmetal's angina is caused by coronary spasm and can usually be controlled by calcium channel blockers.
2. UA within 6 months after coronary angioplasty is almost invariably caused by restenosis. Since the underlying mechanism is cellular proliferation instead of plaque rupture, antithrombotic drugs are not needed and intravenous nitroglycerin provides effective treatment.
3. UA in a patient with previous coronary bypass surgery often involves advanced atherosclerosis of venous bypass grafts and a lower likelihood of long-term symptomatic relief as compared with other UA patients.

DIAGNOSIS AND RISK STRATIFICATION

Patients with suspected UA must be evaluated rapidly and efficiently to determine whether the chest pain is due to myocardial ischemia.

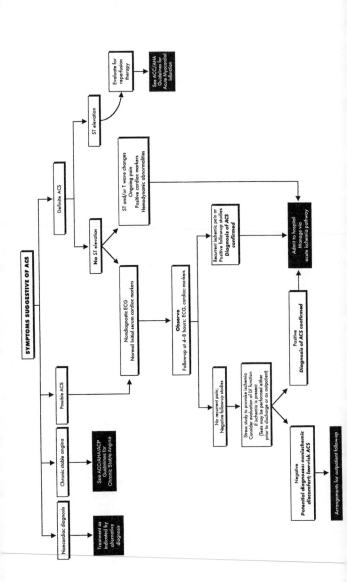

SYMPTOMS SUGGESTIVE OF ACS

Noncardiac diagnosis → Treatment as indicated by alternative diagnosis

Chronic stable angina → See ACC/AHA/ACP Guidelines for Chronic Stable Angina

Possible ACS

Definite ACS

Possible ACS / Definite ACS — No ST elevation

Nondiagnostic ECG
Normal Initial serum cardiac markers

Observe
Follow-up of 4–8 hours: ECG, cardiac markers

No recurrent pain; Negative follow-up studies

Stress study to provoke ischemia
Consider evaluation of LV function
(if ischemia is present
[tests may be performed either
prior to discharge or as outpatient])

Negative
Potential diagnoses: nonischemic discomfort; low-risk ACS

Arrangements for outpatient follow-up

Positive
Diagnosis of ACS confirmed

Recurrent ischemic pain or
Positive follow-up studies
Diagnosis of ACS confirmed

Definite ACS — No ST elevation

ST and/or T wave changes
Ongoing pain
Positive cardiac markers
Hemodynamic abnormalities

Admit to hospital
Manage via
acute ischemia pathway

Definite ACS — ST elevation

Evaluate for reperfusion therapy

See ACC/AHA Guidelines for Acute Myocardial Infarction

A prompt and accurate diagnosis permits the timely initiation of appropriate therapy, which is important, because complications are clustered in the early phases of acute coronary syndromes and appropriate treatment reduces the rate of complications. Patients with chest pain lasting for longer than 20 min, hemodynamic instability, heart failure, or recent syncope or presyncope should be referred to a hospital emergency department. Other patients with suspected UA may be seen initially either in an emergency department or in an outpatient facility where a 12-lead ECG can quickly be obtained.

Initial Evaluation

The initial assessment should be directed toward determining whether the symptoms are caused by myocardial ischemia, and if so, the level of risk (Fig. 14-1). In a patient known to have coronary disease, typical symptoms are highly likely to be caused by myocardial ischemia, particularly if the patient confirms that the symptoms are identical to those experienced during previous episodes with objective documentation. On the other hand, even if the chest pain has some typical features, it is unlikely to be related to myocardial ischemia in a young individual known not to have risk factors for coronary disease. In one prospective multicenter study, older age, male sex, and the presence of chest or left arm pain or pressure as the presenting symptom all increased the likelihood that the patient was experiencing acute myocardial ischemia.

Risk assessment determines the appropriate intensity of therapy, discussed below. At the low end of the risk scale, a patient might be discharged home with aspirin and a beta blocker, to be followed as an outpatient. At the opposite end of the scale, a patient might be hospitalized in a coronary care unit, be treated with multiple drugs, and undergo coronary arteriography urgently as a prelude to revascularization. Finally, when UA is suspected in a patient less than age 50, it is particularly important to ask about cocaine use, regardless of social class or ethnicity.

Symptoms

The sensation of myocardial ischemia is usually located in the retrosternal area, but it may be felt only in the epigastrium, back, arms, or jaw. The description may include adjectives such as *burning*,

---

FIGURE 14-1

Algorithm for the management of patients suspected of having an acute coronary syndrome. (Adapted from ACC/AHA guidelines.)

squeezing, pressure-like, or *heavy* but rarely *sharp, jabbing*, or *knife-like*. The physician should be cautioned that atypical features do not completely rule out the possibility of UA. For example, in one study of patients presenting to the emergency department, acute ischemia was ultimately found to be present in 22 percent of those who used the terms *sharp* or *stabbing* to describe their symptoms and in 7 percent of patients whose pain was reproduced on palpation.

Physical Examination

The physical examination can be normal in patients presenting with UA. However, it is important to evaluate patients suspected of having UA for evidence of left ventricular dysfunction, such as hypotension, mitral regurgitation, basilar rales, or a ventricular gallop. Physical examination may reveal precipitating causes or contributing factors to unstable angina, such as pneumonia or uncontrolled hypertension. Finally, an alternative diagnosis should always be sought, such as pericarditis, suggested by a pericardial friction rub.

The Electrocardiogram

An ECG must be obtained as part of the initial evaluation of a patient with suspected UA. Evidence of existing coronary artery disease, such as q waves or old left bundle branch block, should be identified. The diagnostic yield is greatly enhanced if a tracing can be recorded during an episode of chest pain. A normal ECG during chest pain does not rule out UA as a likely diagnosis; however, it does indicate that an ischemic area, if present, is not extensive or severe enough to induce ECG changes, and thus is a favorable prognostic sign. Conversely, ST-segment elevation of 1 mm or greater in two or more contiguous leads indicates transmural injury and identifies patients who require immediate reperfusion.

Transient ST-segment depression of at least 1 mm that appears during chest pain and disappears with relief represents objective evidence of transient myocardial ischemia. When ST-segment depression is a persistent feature of ECGs recorded with or without chest pain, the finding is less specific. A common ECG pattern of patients with UA is a persistently negative T wave over the involved territory. This usually indicates that a severe stenosis is present in the corresponding coronary artery. Deeply negative T waves are occasionally seen across all of the precordial leads ("Wellens' T waves"), and point to a proximal, severe stenosis of the left anterior descending (LAD) artery as the culprit lesion; these patients should be directed to urgent catheterization.

Serum Cardiac Markers

Biochemical markers of myocardial damage are routinely measured during the evaluation of patients with suspected acute coronary syndromes. Traditionally, elevated serum levels of creatine kinase (CK-MB), CK-MB isoforms, or myoglobin established a diagnosis of MI. Measurement of the cardiac troponins (T or I) is increasingly utilized given the greater sensitivity and specificity of these assays. Initially, elevated troponin levels were considered to indicate more severe UA. However, according to current definitions, an elevated troponin is diagnostic of MI. It is important to remember that UA and NSTEMI are closely related conditions in the spectrum of acute coronary syndromes. Definitions will continue to evolve as further improvements are made in our ability to diagnose myocardial injury.

Elevated troponins are important for risk stratification. Several large studies have demonstrated that elevations of either troponin T or troponin I are independent predictors of adverse events such as recurrent angina, nonfatal MI, or death. Early positivity indicates higher troponin levels and a worse prognosis than when the test is positive later. When the patient presents late after a coronary event, troponin levels remain elevated for 1 week and are thus useful in making a diagnosis.

Acute Echocardiography or Perfusion Imaging

Further testing in the acute setting may be useful in certain clinical scenarios, as when the clinician is still uncertain about the diagnosis of UA. In centers with sufficient expertise, studies have shown that echocardiography obtained at the time of presentation can improve diagnostic accuracy in patients presenting with chest pain. The absence of regional wall abnormalities reduces but does not eliminate the likelihood that symptoms are due to cardiac ischemia. Additionally, patients with reduced ejection fractions are at higher risk for adverse outcomes. Rest nuclear perfusion imaging can also be obtained. Abnormal perfusion defects are associated with a higher risk of further ischemic events.

PROGNOSIS AND RISK STRATIFICATION WITH COMBINATIONS OF PREDICTORS

In clinical practice, several variables are usually integrated into a global assessment of risk (Table 14-3). The combination of ST-segment abnormalities and elevated troponin levels has been shown to be useful. Risk assessment should be updated during hospitalization

TABLE 14-3

SHORT-TERM RISK OF DEATH OR NONFATAL MYOCARDIAL INFARCTION IN PATIENTS WITH UNSTABLE ANGINA

Feature	High Risk (At least one of the following features must be present)	Intermediate Risk (No high-risk feature but must have one of the following features)	Low Risk (No high- or intermediate-risk feature but may have any of the following features)
History	History of accelerating tempo of ischemic symptoms in preceding 48 h	Prior MI, peripheral or cerebrovascular disease, or CABG; prior aspirin use	
Character of pain	Prolonged ongoing (>20 min) rest pain	Prolonged (>20 min) rest angina, now resolved, with moderate or high likelihood of CAD	New-onset CCS class III or IV angina in the past 2 weeks with moderate or high likelihood of CAD
		Rest angina (>20 min or relieved with rest or sublingual NTG)	

	High	Intermediate	Low
Clinical findings	Pulmonary edema, most likely related to ischemia New or worsening mitral regurgitation murmur S_3 or new/worsening rales Hypotension, bradycardia, tachycardia Age >75 years	Age <70 years	
ECG findings	Angina at rest with transient ST-segment changes >0.05 mV Bundle-branch block, new or presumed Sustained ventricular tachycardia	T-wave inversions >0.2 mV Pathologic Q waves	Normal or unchanged ECG during an episode of chest discomfort
Cardiac markers	Markedly elevated (e.g., TnT or TnI >0.1 ng/mL)	Slightly elevated (e.g., TnT >0.01 but <0.1 ng/mL)	Normal

KEY: ECG = electrocardiogram; MI = myocardial infarction; CABG = coronary artery bypass graft; CAD = coronary artery disease; NTG = nitroglycerin.

SOURCE: Adapted from ACC/AHA Guidelines for the Management of Patients with UA and NSTSEMI: Executive Summary and Recommendations. *Circulation* 2000; 102:1193–1209, with permission.

as new information becomes available, so that high-risk patients are not undertreated and low-risk patients are not overtreated. The most important predictors are clinical presentation, ST-segment depression during attacks, elevated troponin levels, and continuing episodes in spite of medical therapy. Continuing angina with ST-segment changes despite medical therapy is an ominous sign that should precipitate urgent coronary arteriography with a view to revascularization, because the risk of MI is high.

Prognosis in UA can be viewed as a composite of the expected prognosis based upon the extent of coronary disease and left ventricular function overlaid with the short-term risk associated with the culprit lesion and the unstable state. The short-term risk is related almost entirely to MI and its complications and to recurrences of UA. Risk is highest in the hours, days, and month after the onset of symptoms. The incremental risk associated with the unstable state dissipates completely by 1 year. For example, 11 percent of UA patients in one series experienced a MI between hospital discharge and 1 year, but the subsequent annual infarction rate was less than 2 percent.

STRESS TESTING AND CORONARY ANGIOGRAPHY

Stress testing is often used in patients with UA as a risk-assessment tool. Low-risk and some intermediate-risk patients whose symptoms stabilize with medical therapy undergo stress testing for advanced risk stratification. Those with high-risk findings such as reversible perfusion defects or ST-segment depression at low exercise levels undergo coronary arteriography, and those with negative or low-risk results are managed medically. This approach has been validated by studies in unstable angina patients demonstrating that these abnormalities correlate with a higher event rate during follow-up. For example, in one study, 60 percent of patients with a reversible perfusion defect as compared with 12 percent of those with a normal exercise sestamibi scan experienced cardiac death, nonfatal infarction, or rehospitalization for UA during a 12-month follow-up. Patients with low exercise tolerance, exercise-induced ST-segment depression, and larger perfusion defects are more likely to have three-vessel coronary disease compared to patients without these high-risk findings. Patients who complete a stay in a chest pain unit without objective evidence of myocardial ischemia can then safely undergo stress testing for diagnostic and prognostic purposes. In patients unable to exercise, dipyridamole or dobutamine can be used as the stress and sestamibi imaging or echocardiography as the method of assessment.

Stress testing is not needed for patients whose clinical features already put them at high risk. Those with continuing angina despite medical therapy, ST-segment depression, or hemodynamic impairment during spontaneous attacks of rest angina or elevated troponin levels should proceed directly to coronary arteriography. Of patients with UA who undergo coronary arteriography, approximately one-quarter will have one-vessel, one quarter two-vessel, and one-quarter three-vessel involvement; 10 percent will have significant left main stenosis and the other 15 percent will have narrowings of less than 50 percent or normal vessels by angiography. Patients with left main stenosis of at least 50 percent or three-vessel disease with left ventricular dysfunction will obtain a survival benefit if they undergo coronary bypass surgery. Although noninvasive testing is sensitive and specific enough to detect many of these patients, the only certain wey to diagnose these conditions is by angiography. At the other extreme, patients without significant lesions at angiography benefit from a reorientation of their management. Noncardiac causes of chest pain should be considered, as well as other potential diagnoses, such as syndrome X and variant angina. Antithrombotic and antiplatelet drugs can often be discontinued and the need for antianginal medication reassessed.

TREATMENT

Once the diagnosis of possible or definite UA has been made, therapy should be instituted without delay. The treatment of UA should be individualized to take into account the specific features of the disease and the particular circumstances of the patient. Nevertheless, recently published algorithms provide a useful framework (Fig. 14-2). In most instances, therapy will be instituted even as the diagnostic workup is under way.

The goals of treatment in UA are to control symptoms and prevent MI. Nitroglycerin, beta blockers, and, to a lesser extent, calcium channel blockers reduce the risk of recurrent ischemic attacks. Revascularization eliminates ischemia entirely in patients with favorable anatomy; in some subgroups, coronary bypass surgery has been shown to prolong life. The risk of MI is reduced by antiplatelet and antithrombotic therapy. In most patients hospitalized with UA, symptoms do not recur after institution of antianginal therapy. Patients with refractory UA have a much higher risk of developing MI than do patients whose angina is controlled with drugs. Patients who are labeled as refractory often become asymptomatic when medical therapy is intensified; for example, in one study, an increase in medical therapy relieved symptoms in 83 percent of patients transferred because their UA was refractory.

The following section discusses the various agents that are currently available in the treatment of UA.

Acute Ischemia Pathway

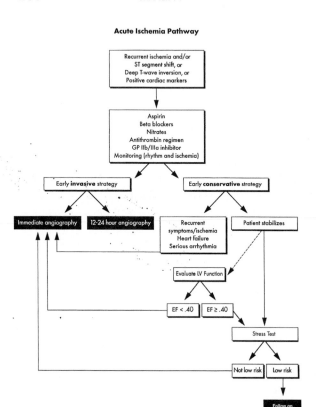

FIGURE 14-2

Algorithm for the treatment of unstable angina. (Adapted from ACC/AHA guidelines.)

Nitroglycerin and Nitrate Therapy

In patients with UA, sublingual nitroglycerin (NTG) usually relieves attacks promptly, although it may be somewhat less efficacious than in stable angina. Patients with UA are often treated initially with 0.4-mg sublingual NTG tablets or NTG spray. The latter is prefered by many patients as "user friendly." An infusion of intravenous NTG to prevent further attacks can then be used. A common starting dose is

10 μg/min. The dose can be increased in 10-μg/min increments until either symptoms are controlled or unwanted side effects develop. The most common adverse effects are headache, nausea, dizziness, hypotension, and reflex tachycardia. NTG is contraindicated in the setting of hypotension or use of sildenafil (Viagra) within the previous 24 h. Most patients will rapidly develop tachyphylaxis with chronic administration of NTG preparations. The evidence that intravenous NTG prevents ischemic attacks or MI in UA patients is sparse.

Beta Blockers

Beta blockers are the most useful category of drug to reduce myocardial oxygen demand, primarily by slowing heart rate but also by decreasing myocardial contractility and afterload. Heart rate and arterial pressure often increase during episodes of rest angina. This unwanted response can be limited by beta-adrenergic blockade. Although it is widely accepted that beta blockers are useful to control ischemic episodes in patients with UA, the data to support this claim are mainly inferential or derived from small trials without placebo-treated controls. These trials date from the early 1980s, an era when patients were not routinely treated with aspirin and heparin.

In the context of UA, it is reasonable to try to achieve beta blockade within hours and not days. Therefore beta blockade should be initiated with intravenous boluses titrated to reduce heart rate to 50 to 60 beats per minute at rest. Early control of heart rate is particularly important in high-risk patients and in those with tachycardia or a high arterial pressure on admission. One regimen is 5 mg of metoprolol slow IV push every 5 min up to 15 mg followed by oral therapy initiated at 25 mg PO bid and titrated upward. In low-risk patients, initiation of therapy with oral agents is appropriate.

The main contraindications to beta blockers in UA are reactive airway disease, sinus node dysfunction or atrioventricular block, severe heart failure, and hypotension. Most patients with chronic obstructive pulmonary disease will tolerate a beta blocker; a beta-selective agent (for example, metoprolol or atenolol) is theoretically less likely to provoke bronchoconstriction. Mild heart failure that is stable is not a contraindication to beta blockers in UA. Diltiazem or verapamil should be considered when a beta blocker cannot be used (see below).

Calcium Channel Blockers

Diltiazem and verapamil both slow heart rate, reduce afterload, and reduce myocardial contractility; they thus reduce myocardial oxygen demand. Diltiazem and verapamil are reasonable choices to treat UA patients for whom beta blockers are contraindicated. The scant evidence discussed above suggests that both drugs reduce the frequency of attacks in UA, but there is no evidence that they prevent infarction. The combination of either diltiazem or verapamil with a beta blocker is not commonly used in UA because the effect of these calcium channel blockers on heart rate and myocardial contractility are additive to the effects of beta blockers. Diltiazem can be started at 30 mg PO tid or qid and verapamil at 80 mg PO tid; both are titrated upward, like beta blockers, for similar heart rate and blood pressure parameters.

Most dihydropyridine calcium channel blockers induce a reflex increase in heart rate in the absence of beta blockade—a feature that is likely to mitigate any beneficial effect on myocardial ischemia. Dihydropyridine calcium channel blockers sometimes worsen myocardial ischemia and may be harmful when used in UA patients not receiving beta blockers, but they may be helpful in controlling angina in patients with an adequate level of beta blockade. Even when the addition of nifedipine does control angina in patients whose UA was previously refractory, the risk of infarction or death over the following few months in the absence of revascularization remains very high. Long-acting formulations of nifedipine and newer dihydropyridines such as amlodipine have not been evaluated in UA trials.

Aspirin

Few treatments in medicine show a cost/benefit ratio superior to that of aspirin in the treatment of UA. The results of several large trials have consistently demonstrated a risk reduction with aspirin for the prevention of death or nonfatal infarction that is relatively large, from one-half to two-thirds. These studies show that the benefit from aspirin begins with the onset of UA and extends for more than 1 year. Other trials have demonstrated that aspirin reduces the risk of infarction in stable coronary patients, so that the drug should be continued for life after an episode of UA.

The dose of aspirin used in trials ranged from 75 to 1300 mg/day. Gastrointestinal side effects increase with increasing dose levels. A dose of 325 mg acutely and 81 mg during chronic treatment is sufficient to maximally inhibit the platelet cyclooxygenase pathway. It is recommended that the first dose be chewed to rapidly achieve platelet inhibition.

Ticlopidine and Clopidogrel

Ticlopidine and clopidogrel are thienopyridines, whose mechanism of action differs from that of aspirin. Both drugs inhibit adenosine diphosphate (ADP)–mediated platelet activation. Because they act independently of the arachidonic acid pathway, the antiplatelet activities of aspirin and either ticlopidine or clopidogrel are synergistic. In the CAPRIE (Clopidogrel versus Aspirin in Patients at Risk of Ischemic Events) Trial, clopidogrel compared with aspirin reduced the combined endpoint of ischemic stroke, MI, or vascular death by 8.7 percent total ($p = 0.043$) for up to 3 years in 19,185 patients with vascular disease. Clopidogrel is preferred over ticlopidine. The usual dose is 75 mg once daily, although 300 mg may be given initially if angioplasty with stent placement is anticipated. Both of these agents have been reported to cause rare but potentially life-threatening hematologic disorders.

Platelet Glycoprotein IIb/IIIa Receptor Inhibitors

Blockade of the platelet glycoprotein (GP) IIb/IIIa receptor is a theoretically attractive concept. Unlike aspirin or clopidogrel, neither of which blocks thrombin-induced platelet aggregation, GP IIb/IIIa inhibitors block aggregation in response to all potential agonists. The first GP IIb/IIIa blocker to be approved and widely used clinically is abciximab. Other GP IIb/IIIa inhibitors are either peptides or smaller molecules. Eptifibatide and tirofiban are examples currently approved for use in the United States (Table 14-4).

Platelet GP IIb/IIIa inhibitors have been evaluated mainly in patients with acute coronary syndromes, patients undergoing coronary angioplasty, or patients in both of these categories. Trials indicate that platelet GP IIb/IIIa inhibition at the time of angioplasty reduces ischemic complications. The benefit with respect to the primary endpoint of the trials was less with eptifibatide and tirofiban (15 to 20 percent) than with abciximab (30 to 60 percent); however, the 95 percent confidence intervals overlap and the drugs have not been compared directly in the same trial. The risk of hemorrhage during angioplasty with GP IIb/IIIa inhibitors can be reduced by early sheath removal, meticulous care of arterial puncture sites, and lower, weight-adjusted doses of heparin than were used traditionally.

Although GP IIb/IIIa inhibitors have firmly established their usefulness in a wide spectrum of patients undergoing coronary angioplasty, their value in unstable angina patients not undergoing intervention is currently incompletely defined. GP IIb/IIIa inhibitors have not been compared to clopidogrel or to low-molecular-weight heparins or studied in patients taking these drugs as background therapy. Current guidelines recommend that eptifibatide or tirofiban should be added to aspirin and heparin in the treatment of patients with some high-risk features or with refractory ischemia. These drugs

TABLE 14-4

ADMINISTRATION OF IIB/IIIA INHIBITORS
IN UNSTABLE ANGINA

Agent	Loading Dose	Infusion
Abciximab (Reopro)	0.25-mg/kg bolus 10–60 min prior to PTCA[a]	10 μg/min IV × 12–24 h
Eptifibatide (Integrilin)	180 μg/kg IV	2 μg/kg/min IV for up to 72 h
Tirofiban (Aggrastat)	0.4 μg/kg/min × 30 min IV	0.1 μg/kg/min IV

[a] Percutaneous transluminal coronary angioplasty.

should be continued during coronary angioplasty, for 12 to 24 h after the procedure for tirofiban, and for 24 to 72 h thereafter for eptifibatide. Abciximab can also be used in patients with unstable angina in whom angioplasty is planned within the following 24 h. However, when abciximab is administered before diagnostic coronary angiography, the prolonged platelet inhibition it induces may force a delay in the urgent coronary bypass surgery that is needed for some patients. When aspirin and unfractionated heparin are used with GP IIb/IIIa inhibitors, the dose of heparin should be conservative during coronary procedures and heparin should be discontinued after the procedure if it is uncomplicated.

Heparin

The principal inhibitory effect of heparin on coagulation is probably via the inhibition of thrombin-induced activation of factors V and VIII. However, several randomized trials have demonstrated that heparin reduces the rate of recurrent UA, nonfatal MI, and death. A metaanalysis of these trials concluded that the addition of heparin to aspirin in the treatment of UA reduces the rate of MI by approximately one-third.

The pharmacokinetics of heparin are complex and the dose-response relationship is nonlinear. Heparin therapy is monitored to maintain the activated partial thromboplastin time (APTT) ratio within 1.5 to 2.5 times normal. The anticoagulant response to a standard dose of heparin varies widely among patients; even when a weight-based nomogram is used in a clinical study, the APTT falls outside the therapeutic range more than one-third of the time. Results in routine clinical practice are probably much worse. Pooled analyses of randomized trials reveal an average incidence of major bleeding of 6.8 percent in the continous infusion groups and 14.2 percent in the intermittent infusion groups (odds ratio 0.42, $p = 0.01$).

Low-Molecular-Weight Heparins

Compared with unfractionated heparin, low-molecular-weight heparins (LMWH) produce a more predictable anticoagulant response because of their better bioavailability, longer half-life, and dose-independent clearance. The main disadvantage of LMWH is that they currently are far more expensive than unfractionated heparin.

Heparin is recommended for the acute treatment of all UA patients except those determined to be at low risk. Unfractionated heparin should be started with an intravenous bolus of 60 to 70 U/kg followed by a constant infusion of approximately 16 U/kg/h adjusted to maintain the APTT at 1.5 to 2.5 times control or to 50 to 70 s. Subcutaneous administration of enoxaparin or dalteparin may be used instead of unfractionated heparin. The dose of enoxaparin is 1 mg/kg twice daily and the dose of dalteparin is 120 IU/kg (maximum 10,000 IU) twice daily. Either standard heparin or LMWH should be continued for 2 to 5 days, until the patient has been stabilized for 24 h, or until revascularization is performed. The dose of unfractionated heparin should be conservative during coronary angioplasty when aspirin and GP IIb/IIIa inhibitors are being administered concomitantly, and heparin should be discontinued after an uncomplicated procedure. Scant information is available on the combined use of LMWH and GP IIb/IIIa inhibitors, particularly during coronary interventions; however, this combination is probably acceptable.

Intraaortic Balloon Pump

Intraaortic balloon counterpulsation prevents myocardial ischemia effectively in patients whose UA is truly refractory. This mechanical approach improves myocardial blood flow and reduces myocardial oxygen demand by collapsing the resistance to left ventricular ejection in early systole. Intraaortic balloon counterpulsation is needed for control of symptoms in less than 1 percent of patients with UA, but it is also used in high-risk cases at the time of coronary angioplasty to provide a margin of safety. Intraaortic balloon counterpulsation causes lower limb ischemia in approximately 10 percent of cases, but this complication almost always resolves with removal of the device.

Thrombolytic Therapy

MI and UA share a common pathophysiologic substrate: plaque rupture or erosion with overlying thrombosis. Thrombolysis effectively reopens occluded culprit arteries and reduces mortality in patients with AMI. It was therefore thought that thrombolytic therapy might prove useful in UA. A metanalysis of nine small, randomized, controlled clinical trials of thrombolysis in UA, with heparin as background therapy, revealed an increased risk of MI with active treatment (odds ratio 2.38; 95 percent confidence interval 1.15 to 4.94). The failure of thrombolytic therapy for UA and non-Q-wave infarction was confirmed in the TIMI-IIIB Trial. Why thrombolytic therapy does not reduce events in UA is uncertain. However, thrombolysis stimulates ongoing thrombin formation and also activates platelets. Thrombolytic therapy should be avoided in patients with UA.

Coronary Revascularization

Coronary bypass surgery and coronary angioplasty are frequently performed in patients with UA; however, the precise indications for revascularization, the choice of procedure, and its timing are controversial. Recent trials of coronary revascularization in UA have compared an "aggressive" approach with a "conservative" approach. The aggressive approach involves early coronary angiography with revascularization by either coronary angioplasty or bypass surgery, depending upon the coronary anatomy. Usually, patients with one or two severe narrowings are treated with angioplasty and those with more extensive disease undergo bypass surgery. The conservative approach limits coronary arteriography, usually to patients who require revascularization to control persistent symptoms, those with very high risk features at presentation, and those who have questionable noninvasive test results when they are risk stratified.

In the TIMI IIIB Trial, 1473 patients with UA or non-Q-wave infarction were randomized within 24 h of chest pain to an early invasive or a conservative strategy. The invasive group underwent coronary arteriography within 18 to 48 h after randomization, followed by a revascularization procedure when possible. Coronary arteriography was done in the conservative group for recurrent chest pain at rest with ischemic ECG changes, episodes of ST-segment depression on ambulatory ECG monitoring, high-risk features on a stress test at the time of hospital discharge, severe angina after discharge, or hospitalization for a recurrence of UA. The TIMI IIIB Trial showed that rapid angiography and revascularization do not produce better outcomes than a more leisurely approach that reserves angiography for patients who exhibit recurrent symptoms or high-risk features.

The Veterans Affairs Non-Q-Wave Infarction Strategies in Hospital (VANQWISH) Trial included no patients with UA, but its results might be relevant to all acute coronary syndromes. The 920 patients were randomly assigned to an invasive or a conservative approach. The composite endpoint of death or nonfatal MI occurred more frequently in the invasive group during the first year: at hospital discharge, the difference was 7.8 versus 3.3 percent ($p = 0.004$); at 1 month, 10.4 versus 5.7 percent ($p = 0.012$); and at 1 year, 24 versus 18 percent ($p = 0.05$). By the end of the 23-month follow-up, the difference between the treatment groups had narrowed and was no longer statistically significant. VANQWISH has been criticized because revascularization was actually performed in only 44 percent of the patients assigned to the invasive strategy but in 33 percent of patients in the conservative group. Additionally, among the invasive patients who underwent bypass surgery, the mortality rate within 1 month of surgery was 11.6 percent, or higher than the norm for this type of patient.

In the FRISC II study, 2457 patients with unstable coronary disease were randomized in a 2×2 factorial design to a dalteparin or placebo and to an invasive or noninvasive treatment strategy. In the invasive arm, coronary angiography was performed within a few days of admission and revascularization shortly thereafter if feasible. An important difference between FRISC II and either TIMI IIIB or VANQWISH is that most of the invasive patients underwent revascularization and most of the noninvasive patients did not, allowing a true comparison between the two approaches. Patients in the invasive group had a reduction in angina by about 50 percent compared with the noninvasive group during the first 6 months of follow-up ($p < 0.001$) and also were significantly less likely to be readmitted to hospital. FRISC II clearly demonstrates that revascularization improves outcomes for UA/NSTEMI patients with ischemic ST changes or elevated troponin levels provided that the procedures can be done with a low rate of complications.

With modern antiplatelet and antithrombotic therapy, revascularization need not be done urgently, within the first day or two after admission, but should be done within the first week or two. The early benefit seen with antiplatelet or antithrombotic drugs tended to dissipate within the first month or two in some of the clinical trials of these drugs. Survey data indicate that UA patients who undergo revascularization outside clinical trial settings may not be obtaining benefit from the procedure. In the OASIS prospective registry of 8000 UA patients treated in 95 hospitals in six countries, the 6-month rates of death or MI did not differ among patients in the three groups, although angina during follow-up was more effectively eliminated in countries with more intervention.

SUGGESTED READING

Antman EM, Tanasijevic MJ, Thompson B, et al: Cardiac specific troponin I levels to predict the risk of mortality in patients with acute coronary syndromes. *N Engl J Med* 1996; 335:1342–1349.

Boden WE, O'Rourke RA, Crawford MH, et al for the Veterans Affairs Non-Q-Wave Infarction Strategies in Hospital (VAN-QWISH) Trial Investigators: Outcomes in patients with acute non-Q-wave myocardial infarction randomly assigned to an invasive as compared with a conservative management strategy. *N Engl J Med* 1998; 338:1785–1792.

Braunwald E, Antman EM, Beasley JW, et al: ACC/AHA guidelines for the management of patients with unstable angina and non-ST-segment elevation myocardial infarction. A report of the American College of Cardiology/American Heart Association Task Force on Practice Guidelines (Committee on the Management of Patients With Unstable Angina). *J Am Coll Cardiol* 2000; 36:970–1062.

Braunwald E, Jones RH, Mark DB, et al: Diagnosing and managing unstable angina. *Circulation* 1994; 90:613–622.

Fuster V, Badimon L, Badimon JJ, Chesebro JH: The pathogenesis of coronary artery disease and the acute coronary syndromes (1 and 2). *N Engl J Med* 1992; 326:242–250, 310–318.

Ohman EM, Armstrong PW, Christenson RH, et al for the GUSTO-IIa Investigators: Cardiac troponin T levels for risk stratification in acute myocardial ischemia. *N Engl J Med* 1996; 335:1333–1341.

PRISM-PLUS Investigators: Inhibition of the platelet glycoprotein IIb/IIIa receptor with tirofiban in unstable angina and non-Q-wave myocardial infarction. *N Engl J Med* 1998; 338:1488–1497.

PURSUIT Investigators: Inhibition of platelet glycoprotein IIb/IIIa with eptifibitide in patients with acute coronary syndromes. *N Engl J Med* 1998; 339:436–443.

Wallentin L, Lagerqvist B, Husted S, et al: Outcome at 1 year after an invasive compared with a non-invasive strategy in unstable coronary artery disease: The FRISC II invasive randomized trial. *Lancet* 2000; 356:9–16.

Waters DD: Diagnosis and management of patients with unstable angina. In: Fuster V, Alexander RW, O'Rourke RA, et al (eds): *Hurst's The Heart*, 10th ed. New York: McGraw-Hill; 2001:1237–1274.

DIAGNOSIS AND MANAGEMENT OF PATIENTS WITH ACUTE MYOCARDIAL INFARCTION

R. Wayne Alexander
Craig M. Pratt
Thomas J. Ryan
Robert Roberts

BACKGROUND AND GENERAL PRINCIPLES

The demonstration in the late 1970s of the role of thrombus formation in the pathogenesis of acute myocardial infarction (AMI) quickly led to the systematic testing of thrombolytic strategies to abort the event. Major multicenter clinical trials on the treatment of AMI demonstrated the efficacy of streptokinase and recombinant tissue plasminogen activator in reducing mortality. Thus, large, adequately powered, randomized studies in the treatment of AMI have helped set a new standard and approach to the goal of treating AMI. The availability of data from clinical trials has permitted the development of practice guidelines for the treatment of AMI. The available data related to each diagnostic and therapeutic alternative have been considered by a panel of experts and graded on the basis of the supporting evidence. The results of these deliberations were expressed in standard format as follows:

Class I: Conditions for which there is evidence and/or general agreement that a given procedure or treatment is beneficial, useful, and effective

Class II: Conditions for which there is conflicting evidence and/or a divergence of opinion about the usefulness/efficacy of a procedure or treatment

Class IIa: Weight of evidence/opinion is in favor of usefulness/
    efficacy
Class IIb: Usefulness/efficacy is less well established by evidence/
    opinion
Class III: Conditions for which there is evidence and/or general
    agreement that a procedure/treatment is not useful/effective and
    in some cases may be harmful

In general, recommendations in this chapter are associated with a
class I, II, or III designation to guide the reader in weighing diagnostic
and therapeutic options.

The progress that has been made in treatment of AMI has resulted in substantial improvement in outcomes. The increased use of
standard CCU procedures—including ECG and hemodynamic monitoring, defibrillation, beta blockers, and, more recently, thrombolytics, coronary interventions, and aspirin—has decreased the mortality,
under the best of circumstances, to 5 percent or less.

CLINICAL ASPECTS

Predisposing Characteristics and Circumstances

The risk factors for the development of coronary artery disease are
dyslipidemia, family history, age, male gender, cigarette smoking,
diabetes mellitus, and hypertension. *Careful consideration of the
probabilities of the presence of coronary artery disease is centrally
important in the initial assessment and evaluation of testing results of
any patient with chest pain.* AMI occurs as a result of the disruption
of a plaque at a site of a high density of inflammatory cells. Thus,
AMI results from the acute exacerbation of a chronic inflammatory
response. This concept has been reinforced by data demonstrating
that patients with elevated C-reactive protein, an acute-phase reac-
tant that is increased by inflammation, have increased rates of acute
coronary events.

Precipitating Events

There is intriguing indirect evidence that external factors might exacerbate the arterial inflammatory response. An association has been
noted between AMI and antecedent mild respiratory syndromes. A
more specific relationship between AMI and an infectious agent has
been posited in the case of *Chlamydia pneumoniae.*

AMI has been associated with emotional or environmental
stresses that activate the sympathetic nervous system, with increases

in catecholamines. Increased sympathetic drive increases cardiac oxygen consumption by increasing contractility and rate and increase stress on vascular lesions by augmenting contraction, torque, and blood pressure. These forces can lead to plaque rupture in an area weakened by inflammation. High catecholamine levels can increase thrombus formation by activating platelets.

Any stressful event can precipitate AMI in a patient with "active," susceptible coronary atherosclerotic lesions. Anesthesia and surgery are well known to enhance the risk of MI, and cardiac events are the leading cause of perioperative morbidity.

Circadian Variation

There is a marked circadian periodicity in the occurrence of MI, with a peak prevalence between 6:00 A.M. and noon (see also Chap. 13). There was a threefold increase in the frequency of infarction at peak (9:00 A.M.) periods, as compared with trough (11:00 P.M.) periods. Sudden death attributed to ischemic heart disease has a similar circadian periodicity. The rhythms both for the occurrence of MI and for deaths from ischemic events are actually bimodal, with a secondary, less pronounced late afternoon or early evening peak (6:00 to 8:00 P.M.). The blunting of the morning peak of AMI by both aspirin and beta-adrenergic blockers emphasizes the contributions of both the sympathetic nervous system and the coagulation pathways to the circadian rhythm of cardiovascular events.

Symptoms

Prodromal symptoms antedating AMI are common and occur in at least 60 percent of patients. Most of these symptoms are anginal or angina-like, especially when assessed retrospectively in the context of the character of the pain of the acute infarct. Considering the general feeling of malaise and fatigue that many patients report having experienced prior to AMI, it is obviously relatively unusual for the event to be totally unheralded.

The *classic symptoms* of AMI involve chest discomfort that is commonly retrosternal or precordial in *location*, and is described as pressure, aching, burning, crushing, squeezing, heavy, swelling, or bursting in *quality*. The location of chest pain is usually of little help in differentiating ischemia/infarction from other causes, but severe chest pain (as opposed to vague discomfort) and the presence of *associated symptoms* (dyspnea, nausea, diaphoresis, and vomiting) are more commonly associated with MI. The discomfort often *radiates* over the anterior chest and frequently into the left or both arms (particularly the medial aspect), and/or into the neck or jaw. In unusual instances, the pain may be in the back, particularly between the scapulae. There may be skip areas with retrosternal pain associated with jaw, antecubital fossa, or wrist pain, or there may be no pain in between the two sites. Moreover, the pain may appear only in the referral area. The *duration* of the pain is prolonged, lasting by definition longer than 15 min. While the intensity of the pain is usually steady following an initial crescendo, there is occasionally some waxing and waning. Sudden relief of pain may accompany reperfusion. Marked apprehension is common. Occasionally, presenting symptoms include syncope, acute confusion, agitation, stroke, or palpitations.

Approximately 23 percent of MIs go unrecognized by patients because of the absence of symptoms or the lack of recognition of the significance of symptoms. The common symptoms in this latter instance are nonclassic or atypical pain, dyspnea, nausea, vomiting, and/or epigastric pain. An MI may also masquerade as the development or worsening of congestive heart failure (CHF), the appearance of an arrhythmia, an overwhelming sense of apprehension, profound weakness, acute indigestion, pericarditis, embolic stroke, or peripheral embolus. Presentation with painless MI is more common in the elderly than in the nonelderly, and this subgroup has an increased frequency of CHF as the initial presenting symptom.

Physical Findings

GENERAL EXAMINATION

The patient is frequently sitting up because of a sense of suffocation or a feeling of shortness of breath. Most patients have some sense of impending doom that is reflected in their facial expression. They may have a grayish appearance, or one of panic or exhaustion. Diaphoresis is frequent. In severe cases, patients may be quite anxious, with an ashen or pale face beaded with perspiration.

It is important to rapidly ascertain the vital signs and the nature, character, and rhythm of the arterial pulse, to observe the jugular venous pulse, to check the peripheral pulses, to palpate the precordium, and to auscultate the chest and precordium. Examination of the extremities should include subjective assessment of the temperature and color of the feet. The presence of very cool feet, especially with acrocyanosis in the setting of tachycardia, suggests low cardiac output.

The heart rate and rhythm in AMI are very important indicators of cardiac function. *A normal rate usually indicates that the patient is not under significant hemodynamic compromise.* In patients with inferior MI, heart rates in the fifties and sixties are very common, especially in the first few hours. The bradycardia may be associated with secondary hypotension resulting from vagal stimulation.

Persistent sinus tachycardia beyond the initial 12 to 24 h is predictive of a high mortality rate. The pulse may be low in volume, reflecting decreased stroke volume. The blood pressure is usually normal but may be increased secondary to anxiety, or it may be decreased from cardiac failure. All peripheral pulses should be examined to exclude current occlusion and to provide a baseline in case of future embolic events. The carotid pulse is most useful in assessing systolic upstroke time and stroke volume, which are decreased in the patient with a low output state. The rhythm of the pulse is very important because of the frequency of ectopic atrial and, in particular, ventricular beats in AMI.

The respiratory rate is usually within the normal range. However, patients who are extremely anxious often exhibit hyperventilation, and those with pulmonary edema and cardiac failure have an increased respiratory rate associated with shallow inspirations.

Examination of the jugular venous pulse is important with AMI, especially in patients with an inferior infarction, because insights can be gained into possible involvement of the right ventricle, which is common in this setting. It may be manifest by elevated jugular venous pressure or by a prominent A wave because of the decreased compliance of the right ventricle. Kussmaul's sign, or an increase in the venous pressure on inspiration, may also be seen in right ventricular (RV) infarction, because of decreased RV compliance (see Chap. 1).

EXAMINATION OF THE LUNGS
Basilar rales are frequently detected in AMI. Cardiac failure diagnosed on the basis of mild signs of pulmonary congestion occurs in 30 to 40 percent of otherwise uncomplicated patients.

CARDIAC EXAMINATION
Palpation of the precordium may reveal evidence of regional wall motion abnormalities and should be performed with the patient initially lying supine; this often is adequate to ascertain whether there is a localized normal apical impulse or dyskinetic impulse. In the left lateral decubitus position, one may palpate a diffuse rather than a localized apical impulse, akinesis, or a paradoxical bulging during late systole, and, in some patients, a palpable atrial contraction corresponding to an audible S_4 gallop may be present (see Chap. 1).

The first and second heart sounds are often soft because of decreased contractility. The second heart sound is usually normal; however, with extensive damage it may be single. Reversed splitting may reflect severe left ventricular (LV) dysfunction. A fourth heart sound is often audible. A third heart sound is heard in probably only about 15 to 20 percent of patients. A pericardial friction rub is heard in only about 10 percent of patients, usually 48 to 72 h after onset.

The crescendo-decrescendo, midsystolic murmur of papillary muscle dysfunction is relatively common early and reflects ischemia of the papillary muscle or the myocardial attachment rather than irreversible injury. This murmur usually disappears after the first 12 to 24 h if soft, but if moderate to loud in intensity, it may persist much longer. Mitral regurgitation is most commonly due to ischemia of the posteromedial papillary muscle.

Diagnosis of Acute Myocardial Infarction

DIFFERENTIAL DIAGNOSIS

MI has typically been diagnosed on the basis of the triad of chest pain, electrocardiographic (ECG) changes, and elevated plasma enzyme activity. Although AMI occurs without chest pain (20 to 25 percent of cases), chest pain is usually responsible for the patient's presentation. It is often impossible on the basis of history alone to distinguish ischemia or infarction from other causes of chest pain. Of patients presenting to the emergency department (ED) with chest pain, only about 14 percent are subsequently documented to have AMI. Most patients at risk for MI will be admitted for evaluation unless definite noncardiac causes of chest pain—such as chest wall pain, hyperventilation, pleurisy, gastrointestinal pain, and so on—that are not imminently dangerous can be identified. Only about 20 percent of patients admitted with chest pain have AMI.

ELECTROCARDIOGRAPHIC DIAGNOSIS

The ECG is very sensitive for detecting ischemia and infarction but is frequently not powerful enough for differentiating ischemia from necrosis. Serial ECGs during AMI will show some evolutionary changes in the majority of patients. An ECG obtained during cardiac ischemic pain frequently exhibits changes in repolarization. The absence of ECG changes during pain provides evidence but not proof that the pain is not ischemic in nature. The early ECG changes of T-wave inversion or ST-segment depression may reflect ischemia or infarction. ST-segment elevation is more specific for AMI and reflects the epicardial injury–associated total occlusion of an epicardial coronary artery. The hallmark of AMI is the development of abnormal Q waves, which appear, on the average, 8 to 12 h from the onset of symptoms but may not develop for 24 to 48 h. Abnormal Q waves usually reflect tissue death and the development of an electrical dead zone. Since abnormal Q waves do not develop immediately, they are not very helpful for initial diagnostic management and therapeutic triage except to signify the presence or absence of prior MI. The diagnostic serial ECG changes consist of ST-segment elevation with the development of T-wave inversion and the evolution of abnormal Q waves. The appearance of abnormal Q waves is very specific to AMI; however, they are present in less than 50 percent of patients with documented AMI. Most of the other patients who have AMI will have ECG changes restricted to T-wave inversion or ST-segment depression or no change at all. These patients represent the group with non-Q-wave infarction.

The evolution of a non-Q-wave infarction is characterized by the appearance of reversible ST-T-wave changes with ST-segment depression, which usually return to normal over a few days but are occasionally permanent. There are major differences in the pathogenesis, clinical manifestations, treatment, and prognosis of Q-wave and non-Q-wave MI. The initiating events are identical—namely, thrombus resulting from disruption of an atherosclerotic plaque superimposed upon vasoconstriction. In non-Q-wave infarction, early spontaneous reperfusion occurs. In contrast, in Q-wave infarction, the coronary occlusion is sustained at least for a period that is long enough to result in extensive necrosis sufficient to result in the development of a large electrical "dead zone."

The ECG criteria for the diagnosis of AMI are the presence, in the setting of chest pain, of any one of the following: (1) new or presumably new Q waves (at least 30 ms wide and 0.20 mV deep) in at least two leads from any of the following: (a) leads II, III, or aV_F; (b) leads V_1 through V_6; or (c) leads I and aV_L; (2) new or presumably new ST-T-segment elevation or depression (≥ 0.10 mV measured 0.02 s after the J point in two contiguous leads of the above-mentioned lead combinations); or (3) new, complete left BBB in the appropriate clinical setting.

The ECG diagnosis of RV infarction offers special challenges. RV infarction occurs in the presence of inferior LV infarction, and the resulting ST-segment elevation is usually overwhelmed in the conventional precordial leads overlying the right ventricle (V_2 and V_3), by the ST-segment elevation in the opposing LV myocardium on the inferior surface. ST-segment elevation must be sought in the right chest leads, V_1, and V_3R through V_6R; when found, it provides reasonably strong evidence for the presence of RV infarction.

In view of a lack of sensitivity and specificity of the chest pain history or of the ECG, confirmation of the diagnosis of AMI is based on elevated plasma levels of cardiac-specific isoenzymes.

DIAGNOSTIC MARKERS IN PLASMA

Myocardial necrosis is associated with the release of a variety of proteins that have been evaluated as diagnostic markers for AMI. The use of CK and MB-CK has become routine, and these markers are highly sensitive, specific, and cost-effective for diagnosing MI (Fig. 15-1). In the adult human heart, 15 percent of total CK activity

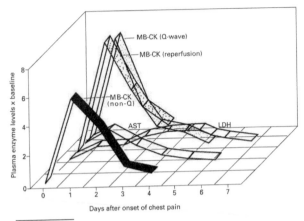

FIGURE 15-1
Typical plasma profiles for the MB isoenzyme of creatine kinase (MB-CK),
aspartate amino transferase (AST), and lactate dehydrogenase (LDH) activities
following onset of acute myocardial infarction.

is MB-CK and the remainder is MM-CK. Myoglobin is ubiquitously
distributed throughout cardiac and skeletal muscles. The cardiac troponin I radioimmunoassay is very specific for myocardial injury. It
is also very sensitive. The assay for plasma cardiac troponin T is also
very specific but may be less sensitive.

**Temporal Profiles of Plasma MB-CK, Myoglobin, Troponin I,
and Troponin T**   Plasma MB-CK activity following MI is significantly elevated, such that reliable diagnostic sensitivity (>90 percent) is reached within 12 to 16 h of the onset of symptoms. Maximal
levels of MB-CK are reached between 14 and 36 h, with a return to
normal levels occurring after 48 to 72 h. Troponin I and troponin T
are released into the plasma, so that reliable diagnostic sensitivity (≥90 percent) is reached by 12 to 16 h and maximal activity
is reached by 24 to 36 h. Plasma myoglobin is increased within
2 h of the onset of symptoms and remains increased for at least 7
to 12 h.

**Early Diagnosis (6 to 10 H of Onset): MB-CK Subforms and
Myoglobin**   Early, rapid diagnosis is required to triage patients with
chest pain in order to reduce costs and to select appropriate therapy
because of the difficulty in distinguishing cardiac ischemia from

infarction based on clinical criteria. The only specific ECG findings of AMI on admission are the recent development of ST-segment elevation or of left BBB. It is estimated that less than 50 percent of patients with AMI will have a diagnostic ECG. The only two plausible candidates as early (<6 h) diagnostic markers are MB-CK subforms and myoglobin.

When MB-CK is released into plasma after myocardial injury, it is converted by proteolytic activity into subforms that can be rapidly separated and detected by electrophoresis. The parent (MB-2) form is converted into MB-1. The total assay can be performed in less than one-half hour. Normally, MB-1 and MB-2 are in equilibrium with a ratio of 1 to 1. *When infarction occurs, MB-2 initially is released into the circulation in minute amounts so that total MB-CK remains within the normal range, but the ratio of MB-2 to MB-1 changes markedly and provides the basis for an early diagnosis of MI.*

MB-CK subforms afford a sensitivity and specificity of about 90 percent for the diagnosis of AMI within 6 h of the onset of symptoms. Myoglobin has a sensitivity of 83 percent. Thus, if a patient has a negative MB-CK subform test at 6 h after the onset of symptoms, one can reliably conclude that the patient does not have infarction. The total MB-CK (activity or mass assay) and troponins T and I have afforded a sensitivity of only 65 percent within the first 6 h (Table 15-1). For the same time intervals, myoglobin had a sensitivity of 83 percent. Total MB-CK and troponins I and T have high sensitivity and specificity for the diagnosis of MI from 10 to 14 h from the onset of symptoms.

Diagnosis of Acute Myocardial Infarction in Patients 48 H or More from the Onset of Symptoms In patients admitted 48 to 72 h after the onset of symptoms, particularly when associated with minimal myocardial damage, the preferred diagnostic marker has become troponin I or T. Both remain elevated for 10 to 14 days.

Noninvasive Imaging in Acute Myocardial Infarction
Chest Roentgenogram The chest roentgenogram (x-ray) provides very important information and may assist in excluding causes of chest pain such as pneumothorax, pulmonary infarction with effusion, aortic dissection, skeletal fractures, and so on. In the patient with AMI, the chest film can be useful in establishing the presence of pulmonary edema, in assessing heart size to assist in determining whether or not cardiomegaly is present, and in deciding whether heart failure or myocardial or valvular disease is acute or chronic.
Echocardiography Two-dimensional and Doppler echocardiography have become very useful tools in the assessment of the patient with suspected AMI. Echocardiography is particularly valuable in assessing the patient with a nondiagnostic ECG. The detection of

TABLE 15-1

DIAGNOSTIC SENSITIVITY AND SPECIFICITY OF MARKERS FOR MYOCARDIAL INFARCTION BASED ON TIME FROM ONSET OF CHEST PAIN

Time, hours	Early Diagnosis				Late Diagnosis			
	2	4	6	10	14	18	22
MARKER							
MB-CK subforms							
Sensitivity (%)	21.1	46.4	91.5	96.2	90.6	80.9	53.1
Specificity (%)	90.5	88.9	89.0	90.2	90.0	89.9	92.2
Myoglobin							
Sensitivity (%)	26.3	42.9	78.7	86.5	62.3	57.5	42.9
Specificity (%)	87.3	89.4	89.4	90.2	88.3	88.8	91.3
Troponin T							
Sensitivity (%)	10.5	35.7	61.7	86.5	84.9	78.7	85.7
Specificity (%)	98.4	98.3	96.1	96.4	96.1	95.7	94.6
Troponin I							
Sensitivity (%)	15.8	35.7	57.5	92.3	90.6	95.7	89.8
Specificity (%)	96.8	94.2	94.3	94.6	92.2	93.4	94.2
Total MB-CK activity							
Sensitivity (%)	21.1	40.7	74.5	96.2	98.1	97.9	89.8
Specificity (%)	100.0	98.8	97.5	97.5	96.1	96.9	96.2
Total MB-CK mass							
Sensitivity (%)	15.8	39.3	66.0	90.4	90.5	95.7	95.7
Specificity (%)	99.2	98.8	100.0	99.6	98.9	99.6	99.1

a regional wall motion abnormality provides strong supportive evidence of acute coronary ischemia; such an abnormality is generally present in transmural or Q-wave MI. Wall motion abnormalities are less common in non-Q-wave infarction but are still present in the majority of cases. Echocardiography also provides an assessment of ventricular function and is useful in predicting the prognosis and in diagnosing RV infarction. It can also provide information concerning alternative diagnoses such as aortic dissection, and, coupled with Doppler, can provide information on such complications as ruptured chordae tendineae with mitral regurgitation and ventricular septal defect. It is useful in detecting ventricular thrombus and pericardial fluid.

Measurement of Myocardial Infarct Size   The major determinant of both an acute and a long-term prognosis following MI is the extent of myocardial damage.

Electrocardiographic Estimates of Infarct Size   The ECG has long been used to obtain a semiquantitative assessment of the extent of MI. In general, it has been found, for example, that patients with anterior infarcts who develop Q waves in leads V_1 to V_6 usually have extensive damage and an unfavorable prognosis. In general, there is a direct relationship between the number of leads showing ST-segment elevation and mortality.

Infarct Size Assessment by Imaging   For practical reasons, echocardiography is the most commonly used imaging modality in the acute evaluation.

PREHOSPITAL CARE

Modern in-hospital care of the AMI patient has resulted in a substantial reduction in mortality. Some 40 to 65 percent of deaths from AMI, however, occur within an hour of the onset of symptoms and prior to arrival at a hospital. Most of these deaths are attributable to ventricular fibrillation. Substantial further reductions in acute mortality rates are likely to require marked improvements in prehospital care and in patient responsiveness to symptoms. The goals for community emergency response services (EMS) have been discussed extensively (see Chap. 42 in *Hurst's The Heart,* 10th ed.) and include the availability of 911 telephone access and of personnel trained in defibrillation and, potentially, in initiation of out-of-hospital thrombolysis.

The major contribution that the physician can make to minimizing delay from the time that a patient first appreciates subjective manifestations of AMI to the time he or she presents at the ED is in educating him or her beforehand as to the proper responses to ischemic coronary symptoms. *The guiding principles are recognition and response.* Thus, the patient should be taught to recognize and appreciate chest pain as potentially representing coronary ischemia, and, if sustained, threatened AMI. Patients should be warned specifically of the dangers of rationalizing the pain as having a noncardiac origin or of trying extensive "diagnostic trials" of home remedies; they should also be instructed in the standard protocol for using nitroglycerin. That is, the patient, at the onset of pain, should immediately use nitroglycerin in a form that is absorbed rapidly from the oral muscosa. If the pain is not relieved within 5 min, the dosing should be repeated. If the discomfort persists for another 5 min, a third dose should be administered. If no relief is obtained at this point, the patient should proceed immediately to the nearest ED. The potential risk of fatal arrhythmia in the early course of AMI should be explained. *Educating patients about this protocol is one of the most important functions of the physician caring for patients with coronary artery disease.*

EVALUATION AND MANAGEMENT OF PATIENTS WITH CHEST PAIN IN THE EMERGENCY DEPARTMENT

Background

The goals of the ED with respect to patients with chest pain are as follows: to rapidly identify those patients with AMI with both typical and atypical presentations so that appropriate therapy can be initiated; to recognize those patients with acute coronary syndromes (unstable angina) but without MI, who thus are at high risk; and to assess accurately those patients at low risk who are candidates for noninvasive evaluation and early discharge. The earlier perfusion therapy is initiated in the subset of patients with diagnostic ST-segment elevation, the more favorable the clinical results.

An important objective, obviously, should be a triage system that minimizes the number of patients at high risk (AMI or unstable angina) who are inadvertently discharged from the ED, while also minimizing the admission of low-risk patients without MI to high-intensity CCUs.

Misdiagnosis of AMI is commonly associated with misinterpretation of the ECG. A major contributing problem to the difficulty of diagnosing AMI is that even experienced clinicians appear to be able to achieve sensitivity and specificity of only about 80 percent in the diagnosis of AMI on clinical grounds alone. The problem extends also to the difficulty of diagnosing unstable angina in the absence of infarction. It is recognized now that there is a continuum between those patients with ischemic symptoms without diagnostic ECG changes and those with unequivocal AMI. As noted, these patients are categorized as having an "acute coronary syndrome"(ACS) and are at high intermediate term risk. *The clinical focus in the ED should not be simply to "rule out" AMI but, taking a proactive approach, to "rule in" either acute infarction or ACS in an expeditious manner. Once these urgent conditions have been excluded or ascertained to be of low probability, the next level of concern is determining the presence of other acute cardiovascular or cardiopulmonary conditions, such as aortic dissection, pulmonary embolus, pericarditis, and so on.*

Initial Approach, Detection, and Assessment of Risk

A major goal in dealing with chest pain patients is establishment of a routine approach that leads to a rapid (10-min) preliminary evaluation, acquisition of a 12-lead ECG, and establishment of intravenous access and continuous ECG monitoring and supplemental oxygen (class I) (Fig.15-2). The initial assessment is guided by the differential diagnosis of chest pain, with the goal of establishing whether or not myocardial ischemia is a likely or possible diagnosis. Blood is drawn for baseline cardiac marker levels, and if coronary ischemia is suspected and there are no contraindications, the patient is given aspirin of 160 to 325 mg to chew and swallow. Also, the patient with suspected coronary ischemia is given sublingual nitroglycerin unless the systolic blood pressure is less than 90 mmHg. This should be avoided with severe bradycardia or tachycardia. The history of chest pain alone usually dictates entry into the system for evaluation. In general, the only chest pain patients not systematically evaluated for myocardial ischemia would be those in whom a clear noncardiac cause, such as chest wall tenderness, can be demonstrated unequivocally to be the etiology of the presenting symptoms. Continuous ECG monitoring is essential because of the propensity of any patient with an acute coronary ischemic syndrome to develop a sudden and potentially lethal ventricular arrhythmia. Intravenous access is essential for therapeutic interventions under such circumstances as well as for more general purposes. Additionally, paroxysmal changes in the ST segment may be recognizable on the monitor. The differential diagnosis of chest pain and the clinical recognition of AMI were discussed previously. The causes of chest pain not due to acute pathologic changes that are compromising the structural integrity of the large coronary arteries are listed in Table 15-2.

As a general rule, one should begin the evaluation of the chest pain patient with the assumption, until proven otherwise, that one is dealing with myocardial ischemia. The three most serious and urgent alternative diagnoses that need to be considered specifically

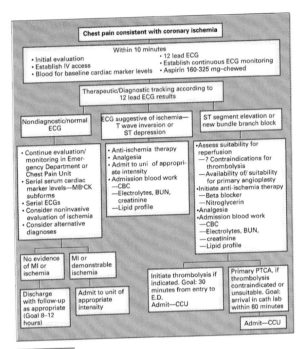

FIGURE 15-2

Algorithm for the initial assessment and evaluation of the patient with acute chest pain in the emergency department. The emergency department should be organized to facilitate the rapid triage of chest pain patients so that the initial evaluation, obtaining a 12-lead ECG, and establishing intravenous access and continuous monitoring are accomplished within 10 min. The path in the decision tree is determined by the results of the 12-lead ECG. The presence of ST-segment elevation diagnostic of AMI or of presumptively new BBB suggestive of this diagnosis should lead to the immediate consideration of the suitability of the patient for reperfusion therapy, which, if indicated, should be initiated within 30 min of the patient's arrival. The primary PTCA option is applicable only in those settings in which it is immediately available and can be performed by highly qualified interventional cardiologists. In general, patients should not be transferred for angioplasty if thrombolysis is an option, especially if significant delays will be incurred. Thrombolysis is not indicated in patients with only ST-segment depression. KEY: BUN = blood urea nitrogen; BBB = bundle-branch block; PTCA = percutaneous transluminal coronary angioplasty.

TABLE 15-2

CAUSES OF CHEST PAIN OTHER THAN ACUTE CORONARY ARTERY SYNDROMES

Cardiovascular
  Aortic dissection
  Aortic stenosis
  Pericarditis
  Mitral valve prolapse
  Microvascular angina
    Hypertrophic cardiomyopathy
    Syndrome X
  Pulmonary embolus
  Arrhythmia/palpitations
Noncardiovascular
  Pleurisy
  Pneumonia
  Pneumothorax
  Costochondritis
  Gastrointestinal
    Esophageal spasm/reflux
    Acid peptic disease
    Cholecystitis
    Gastritis
Psychiatric
  Panic attack
  Cardiac neurosis
  Depression
  Malingering

during the initial evaluation are *aortic dissection, acute pulmonary embolus,* and *acute pneumothorax. Acute pericarditis* and *myopericarditis* need to be considered as well.

Aortic dissection must be considered and ruled in or out during the initial evaluation, since specific intervention can decrease its high mortality. Furthermore, administration of thrombolytic agents in the presence of aortic dissection is associated with high mortality. Suspicion of dissection should be heightened especially in hypertensive patients or in those with marfanoid habitus.

Pulmonary embolus can be life-threatening and should be suspected in anyone with a sudden onset of shortness of breath and chest pressure or pain, especially if there is a history of being sedentary or immobilized and/or a history of deep venous thrombosis.

Acute pericarditis may mimic AMI in that the pain can be substernal and persistent. Frequently, however, there will be a positional component as well as characteristics of pleurisy, with accentuation by deep breathing. Furthermore, the diffuse ST-segment elevation may lead to a misdiagnosis of MI. The key differentiating features in pericarditis include PR depression, the diffuse nature of ST-segment elevation in most leads, and the absence of reciprocal changes.

It should be kept in mind that esophageal disorders are very common in patients presenting with chest pain in whom cardiac ischemia is ruled out. Because of the high frequency of gastrointestinal disease in chest pain patients, "GI cocktails" or antacids have been used as a diagnostic tool to guide triage and disposition. Only 25 percent of patients with esophageal pain, however, have been reported to obtain pain relief with antacids. Furthermore, coincidental, spontaneous relief of ischemic chest pain at the time of administration of the GI cocktail can be misleading. Similarly, administration of nitroglycerin as a diagnostic strategy for ischemic disease can be misleading because it can relieve esophageal spasm. Moreover, it has been found that pain relief after nitroglycerin did not predict unstable angina or AMI in the chest pain patient. The use of these "response-to-treatment" strategies as major decision points in the evaluation of chest pain has been discouraged.

DETECTION

The 12-Lead Electrocardiogram as a Guide to Management Strategy The results of the 12-lead ECG guide the next level of decision making for the patient with chest pain thought to be compatible with myocardial ischemia (Fig 15-2). The ECG interpretation is assigned to one of three categories: (1) ST-segment elevation in two or more leads or a presumptively new BBB implicating acute coronary occlusion, usually thrombotic; (2) ST-segment depression and/or T-wave inversion implying subtotal occlusion and nontransmural ischemia; and (3) normal or nondiagnostic. The group with ST-segment elevation or a left BBB is particularly important to define, as it is this group that has been shown to benefit from thrombolytic therapy. There is no indication as yet of the benefit of thrombolytic therapy or primary angioplasty in those patients without ST-segment elevation or BBB. The ECG also serves as a basis for initial risk assessment. ST-segment elevation or a new left BBB in the patient with chest pain defines a high-risk group; in those with elevated ST segments, the mortality correlates positively with the number of leads with the ST changes. The presence of ST-segment depression or T-wave inversion also defines a high-risk group.

The measurement of serum markers of myocardial damage plays a major role in diagnosis. Measurement of CK-MB is the benchmark laboratory test, and the specificity and sensitivity of samples taken 2 h apart during serial sampling have been reported to be 91 and 94 percent, respectively.

Two-dimensional echocardiography can be useful as an adjunctive modality. It may be especially useful in detecting wall motion abnormalities in the presence of conduction abnormalities on the ECG.

RISK STRATIFICATION

Stratifying risk in the patient with AMI is an essential part of the management strategy during all phases of care.

Predictors of an increased risk of complications include the following: ECG evidence of ST-segment elevation or Q waves in two or more leads that are not known to have been present previously; ST-segment depression or T-wave inversions consistent with myocardial ischemia and not known to be present previously; pain worse than prior angina or the same as that experienced with prior MI; systolic blood pressure of less than 100 mmHg; or rales bilaterally.

Blood levels of cardiac markers are prognostically important, as noted. *In particular, the levels of troponins (I and T) at presentation appear to be strong predictors of risk in patients with acute ischemic syndromes.*

INITIAL MANAGEMENT

As discussed, one frequently does not have a definitive diagnosis of AMI in the chest pain patient in the ED. Nevertheless, the initial general treatment of the ACSs is the same.

Routine General Measures

Oxygen Administration   Hypoxemia is not uncommon in patients with AMI, even with an uncomplicated course. Nasal oxygen should be administered to all AMI patients with pulmonary congestion and Sa_{O_2} of less than 90 percent (class I). O_2 should be administered to all uncomplicated AMI patients for the first 2 to 3 h (class IIa). There appears to be little justification for extending use of oxygen administration in uncomplicated MI with an Sa_{O_2} of greater than 90 percent beyond 2 to 3 h (class IIb). Oxygen administration should be continued in patients with pulmonary congestion and desaturation.
Analgesia   The alleviation of pain and anxiety remains an essential element in the care of the patient with AMI. The pain and accompanying anxiety contribute to excessive activity of the autonomic nervous system and to restlessness. These factors, in turn, increase the metabolic demands on the myocardium.

The approach to pain consists of the dual strategy of relieving ischemia and attacking the pain directly. Anti-ischemic therapy consists of reperfusion, beta blockers (if appropriate), nitrates, and oxygen administration. Narcotics relieve pain not only directly but also indirectly by diminishing the sympathetic nervous system's drive and catecholamine secretion, which will decrease oxygen consumption and ischemia and thus the potential for serious ventricular arrhythmias. Morphine, in most instances, is the drug of choice, since it is well tolerated and offers analgesia without significant cardiac depression. It also relieves anxiety and the feeling of doom commonly described. Morphine sulfate can be given at doses of 2 to 4 mg every 15 min until adequate relief has been obtained, which, in some patients, may require 25 to 30 mg. If the patient's anxiety is not controlled by the administration of narcotics, mild sedation with a benzodiazepine is appropriate. Diazepam in doses of 5 mg orally every 8 to 12 h or alprazolam in doses of 0.25 mg every 8 h is most often used.

Nitroglycerin   Nitroglycerin should be administered for the first 24 to 48 h to AMI patients with congestive heart failure (CHF); large anterior MI; persistent or recurrent angina; hypertension; or persistent pulmonary congestion (class I). Nitroglycerin should be considered beyond 48 h in an oral or sublingual spray form in patients with a large or complicated AMI (class IIb).

Nitroglycerin has become very widely used in the treatment of AMI. It is an anti-ischemic agent not only by virtue of its actions to decrease preload and afterload—and thus to decrease oxygen demand—but also because of its vasodilator actions on epicardial coronary arteries and on coronary collaterals. Both clinical data and animal studies suggest that the early administration of nitroglycerin limits the extent of myocardial damage and favorably affects survival.

COMPLICATIONS AND LIMITATIONS   The most serious complication of nitroglycerin is hypotension. Thus, nitroglycerin should be avoided with a systolic pressure of less than 90 mmHg. Caution should be exercised in the case of inferior wall infarction because of the possibility of RV involvement. Nitroglycerin should be used only with extreme caution, if at all, in RV infarction, because the right ventricle in this circumstance becomes extremely dependent upon preload, which can be diminished by the venodilating properties of the drug.

DOSAGE OF NITROGLYCERIN   Long-acting nitrates should generally not be used as initial therapy in AMI. Intravenous nitroglycerin is preferable because of its rapidity of onset, ease of titration, and ease of removal in case of complications. Dose titration can be assessed by frequent determinations of blood pressure and heart rate. Invasive monitoring is not essential but is probably prudent if high doses are required or if there is hemodynamic instability or uncertainty about the adequacy of ventricular preload.

Treatment should be initiated with a bolus injection of 12.5 to 25 μg and should be followed by infusion by pump of 10 to 20 μg/min, with increases of 5 to 10 μg every 5 to 10 min while the hemodynamic and clinical responses are being assessed. Control of symptoms is a major endpoint; in the case of high LV filling pressure, the objective is a decrease of 10 to 30 percent in pulmonary artery wedge pressure. Limitations of nitroglycerin dosing are as follows: (1) a decrease in mean arterial pressure of 10 percent in normotensive patients; (2) a decrease of 30 percent in hypertensive patients but not below a systolic pressure of 90 mmHg; or (3) an increase in heart rate of 10 beats per minute, not to exceed 110 beats per minute.

Doses of nitroglycerin of greater than 200 μg/min are associated with an increased risk of hypotension. Requirements this high which develop may indicate tolerance, and alternative drugs such as angiotensin-converting enzyme (ACE) inhibitors or nitroprusside should be considered. If tolerance is the issue, responsiveness should return after a 12- to 18-h period off nitroglycerin.

Aspirin   Aspirin reduces the incidence of vascular events in patients with AMI at 1 month; a prior history of MI (2 years); a history of transient cerebral ischemia or stroke; and unstable angina. The patient suspected of having a coronary ischemic syndrome and without contraindication should receive, early in the course, 160 to 325 mg of non–enteric coated aspirin, which is chewed. If coronary artery disease is confirmed, aspirin treatment should be continued indefinitely (class I). In case of true aspirin allergy, other antiplatelet agents such as clopidogrel may be substituted (class IIb).

Management after Triage into Electrocardiographic Subgroups

The initial ECG, as a first approximation, permits the assignment of patients with chest pain into subgroups distinguishable by therapeutic responsiveness and risk, as discussed previously. *It must be kept in mind that these initial categorizations do not necessarily define ultimate outcome. Thus, patients with no ST-segment elevation at presentation may, in fact, have unstable angina and ultimately have no infarction or may progress to have either a Q-wave or a non-Q-wave infarction. Similarly, those presenting with ST-segment elevation may have a non-Q-wave infarction, although the majority of these will develop Q waves* (see also Chap. 14). This potential for variable outcomes provides the underlying rationale for close monitoring and continuous reassessment of clinical course, risk, and therapeutic strategies during the period of observation and for monitoring both in the ED and subsequently in other hospital units.

APPROACH TO THE PATIENT WITH ST-SEGMENT ELEVATION

The approach to the patient with chest pain and ST-segment elevation is guided heavily by the evidence that this subgroup has a high

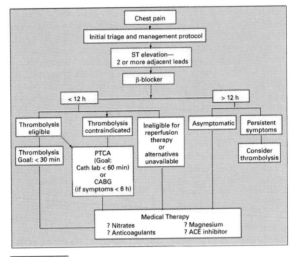

FIGURE 15-3

Evaluation of patients with ST-segment elevation. Algorithm for initial decision making in regard to reperfusion therapy in patients with suspected acute myocardial infarction and ST-segment elevation. Whether or not to administer thrombolytics or to perform primary PTCA is determined by the time from onset of symptoms. When more than 12 h have elapsed since the onset of symptoms, reperfusion should be considered only if there are persistent or recurrent symptoms associated with ST-segment elevation. For patients with ST-segment elevation where the duration of symptoms is between 7 and 12 h, the decision to proceed with a reperfusion strategy requires careful clinical judgment in weighing the risk/benefit issues, as discussed in the text. KEY: PTCA = percutaneous transluminal coronary angioplasty; CABG = coronary artery bypass graft. [Modified from Ryan TJ, Antman EM, Brooks NH, et al: 1999 Update: ACC/AHA guidelines for the management of patients with acute myocardial infarction: A report of the American College of Cardiology/American Heart Association Task Force on Practice Guidelines (Committee on Management of Acute Myocardial Infarction). *J Am Coll Cardiol* 1999; 34:904, with permission.]

frequency of epicardial coronary artery occlusion by a thrombus, and evidence that thrombolytic therapy has shown clinical benefit. Evaluation and management of the patient with ischemic chest pain and ST-segment elevation is focused on the rapid assessment of suitability for reperfusion therapy and its subsequent delivery (Fig. 15-3).

Initial evaluation and management have been discussed. The appropriate next steps are to administer a beta-adrenergic blocker, if not contraindicated, and to initiate evaluation for reperfusion therapy.

The 12-h point defines the time frame in which the risk/benefit ratio is clearly favorable for administering thrombolytic therapy—although, obviously, the earlier the better.

Beta-Adrenergic Receptor Blockers   Beta-adrenergic receptor blockers interfere with the positive inotropic and chronotropic effects of catecholamines; therefore they reduce myocardial oxygen consumption.

The available data strongly support the use of beta blockers early in the course of acute Q-wave M—in the absence of contraindications—irrespective of concomitant thrombolytic therapy or primary angioplasty (class I). Patients with continuing or recurrent ischemic pain or with tachyarrhythmias, such as atrial fibrillation with rapid ventricular response, should also be considered for beta-blocker therapy (class I). Use of beta-blocker therapy in non–ST segment AMI is now recommended (class I). Patients with moderate CHF or other contraindications can receive beta blockers only if they can be monitored very closely (class IIb). Patients with severe LV failure should not receive beta blockers. While metoprolol and atenolol are the only beta blockers approved by the U.S. Food and Drug Administration (FDA) for use in AMI, *therapeutic efficacy is a class effect of beta blockers lacking intrinsic sympathomimetic activity.*

The relative contraindications to beta-blocker therapy are as follows: (1) heart rate less than 60 beats per minute; (2) systolic blood pressure less than 100 mmHg; (3) moderate or severe LV failure; (4) signs of peripheral hypoperfusion; (5) PR interval greater than 240 ms; (6) second- or third-degree atrioventricular (AV) block; (7) severe chronic pulmonary disease; (8) history of asthma; (9) severe peripheral vascular disease; and (10) insulin-dependent diabetes mellitus. Since these contraindications are relative and not absolute, the clinician has the option of assessing the effects of beta blockade with the short-acting intravenous beta-blocker esmolol, which has an onset of action within 5 to 10 min and a half-life of about 30 min.

Thrombolysis

Indications for Thrombolytic Therapy   Reperfusion therapy should be given immediate consideration in all patients presenting with AMI. The primary indication for attempts at reperfusion, given an appropriate history, is the findings on the ECG, as discussed above. Patients with ST-segment elevation in two or more contiguous leads or a bundle branch block (BBB) masking ST-segment changes occurring within 12 h of onset of symptoms are candidates for thrombolytic therapy. *Patients with ongoing symptoms should be repeatedly evaluated by 12-lead ECGs as frequently as every 10 to 15 min in order to identify ST-segment elevation as soon as possible.* Conversely,

ST-segment elevation in the absence of suggestive symptoms should raise such possibilities as early repolarization, pericarditis, and previous infarction with aneurysm formation. Elderly patients with ST-segment elevation should be considered for thrombolytic therapy (class IIa indication for age 75 or older) and should not be excluded primarily because of their age or the perceived increased risk of bleeding.

Large, placebo-controlled clinical trials have consistently demonstrated reduced mortality in patients receiving thrombolytic therapy within 6 h of the onset of an AMI. Because of suggestion of benefit between 6 and 12 h, it has been recommended that the time limit for therapy be up to 12 h from the onset of symptoms. The benefit of thrombolytics given between 6 and 12 h after infarction is greater in patients classified as having high-risk infarctions, such as those with severe heart failure and large infarctions. Thrombolysis can be considered in the case of ongoing pain and marked ST-segment elevation at times between 12 to 24 h from onset, although there is only a trend for benefit under these circumstances in clinical trials (class IIb). Patients with ST-segment depression, T-wave inversion, or no ECG changes have not been shown to benefit from thrombolytic therapy (class III).

The potential for therapeutic benefit of thrombolysis in the setting of a high risk of MI when the blood pressure is markedly elevated (>180 mmHg systolic and/or >110 mmHg diastolic) must be carefully considered against the increased risk of intracranial hemorrhage under these circumstances (class IIb). Lowering of the blood pressure pharmacologically before thrombolytics are administered has been recommended but is of unproven benefit (class IIb). If available, coronary artery bypass grafting (CABG) or primary percutaneous transluminal coronary angioplasty (PTCA) should be considered (class IIb).

Contraindications to Thrombolytic Therapy The absolute and relative contraindications to thrombolytic therapy are summarized in Table 15-3.

Choice of Thrombolytic Agent Four thrombolytic agents have been approved in the United States for routine use: streptokinase (SK), rt-PA, APSAC, and reteplase (r-PA). Each has been shown to limit infarct size, preserve ventricular function, and improve survival rates.

Dose and Administration of Thrombolytic Agents Streptokinase is given in a dose of 1.5 million units intravenously over 30 to 60 min. Since antibodies develop and may persist for several years, a subsequent need for thrombolytic therapy, as for early or late reocclusion, would require the use of rt-PA or r-PA. APSAC is identical to SK as a thrombolytic agent but can be given as a rapid infusion of 30 U over 5 to 10 min. The FDA-approved dose of rt-PA is an initial bolus of 15 mg, followed by an infusion of 50 or 0.75 mg/kg over the next 30 min, and an infusion of 35 mg or 0.50 mg/kg over the subsequent 60 min, for a total of up to 100 mg given over 90 min. Reteplase is

TABLE 15-3

ABSOLUTE AND RELATIVE CONTRAINDICATIONS
TO THROMBOLYTIC THERAPY

Absolute Contraindications	Relative Contraindications
Active internal bleeding	History of nonhemorrhagic cerebrovascular accident in distant past with complete recover
Intracranial neoplasm or recent head trauma	Prolonged traumatic CPR*
Suspected aortic dissection	Recent trauma or surgery >2 weeks previously
Pregnancy	
History of hemorrhagic cerebrovascular accident or recent nonhemorrhagic cerebrovascular accident	Active peptic ulcer disease
	History of severe hypertension with diastolic blood pressure >100
Recorded blood pressure >200/120	
Trauma or surgery that is a potential bleeding source within previous 2 weeks	Bleeding diathesis or concurrent use of anticoagulants
Allergy to SK or APSAC if being considered	Previous treatment with SK or APSAC if being considered (does not apply to rt-PA)

KEY: CPR = cardiopulmonary resuscitation; SK = streptokinase; APSAC = anistreplase; rt-PA = recombinant tissue plasminogen activator.

given as an initial bolus of 15 megaunits (MU), followed by a second bolus of 15 MU in 30 min. Thrombolytic therapy is rapidly evolving, and both the specific agent and various combinations as well as the specific doses and regimens of administration are changing rapidly. *Overall Strategy for Reperfusion of Patients with Acute Myocardial Infarction* The criteria for initiating thrombolytic therapy are outlined in Table 15-4.

1. Patients presenting with chest pain suggestive of myocardial ischemia, having ST-T-segment elevation greater than 1 mm in two contiguous limb leads, greater than 2 mm in two contiguous

TABLE 15-4

CRITERIA FOR INITIATING THROMBOLYTIC THERAPY

Chest pain consistent with angina
ECG changes
    ST ↑ ≥1 mm, ≥2 contiguous limb leads
    ST ↑ ≥2 mm, ≥2 contiguous precordial leads
    New left bundle branch block
Absence of contraindications

precordial leads, or new left BBB and who are within 6 h of the onset of symptoms should receive thrombolytic therapy if there are no contraindications. In patients presenting between 6 and 12 h, the bias should be toward thrombolytic therapy the higher the risk of the AMI. Patients presenting after 12 h are not routinely considered for thrombolytic therapy.

2. Contraindications for thrombolytic therapy are absolute or relative, as discussed earlier (Table 15-3).

3. In patients receiving rt-PA or r-PA, it is recommended that, at the initiation of thrombolytic therapy, heparin be given as a bolus infusion of 60 U/kg, followed by a continuous infusion of 12 U/kg/h (with a maximum of 4000-U bolus) and 1000 U/h for patients weighing >70 kg, adjusted to keep the PTT at one-half to two times the normal control for 24 to 48 h. Heparin should be given in patients who have received SK or APSAC who are at high risk for systemic embolization. Aspirin (160 to 325 mg) should be administered as soon as possible and continued indefinitely. Beta blockers, nitrates, and occasionally calcium channel blockers may be given as indicated with or without thrombolytic therapy.

4. Patients allergic to SK or APSAC who require thrombolytic therapy should receive rt-PA or r-PA. Patients who received SK or APSAC and who again require thrombolytic therapy should receive rt-PA or r-PA.

5. Patients presenting with ST-T-segment depression and chest pain are not candidates for thrombolytic therapy and need to be triaged, as indicated in Fig 15-2.

6. PTCA, as a primary procedure, is an alternative to thrombolytic therapy only if performed in a timely fashion by individuals skilled in the procedure and supported by experience by personnel in high-volume centers (class I). PCI is indicated in patients with a contraindication to thrombolytic therapy or in patients in cardiogenic shock (class IIa).

7. Elective angioplasty should be reserved for patients who develop ischemia or reinfarction or in whom thrombolytic therapy appears ineffective. In patients in whom angioplasty cannot be performed and who develop recurrent ischemia with possible infarction, the possibility of readministering a thrombolytic agent should be considered.

Heparin as Conjunctive or Adjunctive Therapy. Heparin is recommended for patients undergoing percutaneous revascularization (class I). After thrombolysis with either SK or APSAC, it is recommended that heparin not be started immediately but that an activated partial thromboplastin time (aPTT) be drawn at 4 h and that heparin be started when the aPTT returns to less than twice control (about 70 s). Lysis of a thrombus by any thrombolytic agent induces a highly thrombogenic surface. Furthermore, lysis with either rt-PA or SK is associated with marked elevation of plasma levels of thrombin. The use of heparin during the initial 24 to 48 h is critical to prevent rethrombosis and reocclusion.

Heparin is not necessary to achieve reperfusion but is essential in the first 24 h to maintain patency rates with rt-PA. While heparin may be beneficial when SK is used, subcutaneous administration of heparin appears adequate in this circumstance. At present, heparin is recommended as described above to keep the PTT at 1.5 to 2.0 times normal. It is recommended that the PTT not be measured until 4 h after heparin therapy is initiated because it has not yet reached a steady state until then. If the PTT has increased more than twofold over normal, the same dose of heparin should be continued; if the PTT exhibits less than a twofold increase, the infusion rate of heparin should be increased. Initiation of heparin is recommended either during or following completion of thrombolytic therapy and should be maintained in the uncomplicated patient for 24 to 48 h.

The use of heparin has also been recommended conjunctively in patients with AMI who are not being treated with the drug for other reasons, i.e., postthrombolysis or after primary PTCA. Currently, guidelines recommend heparin 7500 U twice daily subcutaneously as prophylaxis against deep venous thrombosis. Given the enhanced risk of stroke after AMI in patients with atrial arrhythmias, those with large and especially anterior and apical infarction, and those with history of previous stroke, guidelines have incorporated this recommendation for broader prophylaxis against systemic embolization. In high-risk patients, the intravenous route is probably preferable. Heparin therapy should be continued for 48 h and judgment should be made at that point about continuation based on individual patient characteristics.

Low-molecular-weight heparin preparations are being evaluated as adjunctive therapy for thrombolysis and are extensively used in non–ST-segment elevation AMI and ACS, as discussed subsequently. They have a class IIa indication (as an alternative to unfractionated heparin) in all AMI patients with ST-segment elevation who are not treated with thrombolytic agents.

Early Coronary Angiography in Patients with ST-Segment Elevation Not Undergoing Primary Percutaneous Transluminal Coronary Angioplasty   Routine immediate or delayed angioplasty is not recommended as a standard mode of therapy following thrombolysis. *At present, the most widely accepted recommendation is to perform cardiac catheterization for possible angioplasty or bypass surgery in patients who develop angina or manifest evidence of myocardial ischemia during submaximal exercise testing or who develop hemodynamic or ischemic instability.* Thus, if intervening with PTCA generally offers no demonstrable benefit after thrombolysis, there is little apparent reason to perform early coronary angiography routinely.

Patients with cardiogenic shock have a very high (>70 percent) mortality with or without thrombolysis, and some studies have provided evidence that outcomes are improved with an aggressive reperfusion strategy. Successful PTCA in conventionally treated patients who had cardiogenic shock reduced mortality from greater than 80 to about 30 percent. *Thus, an aggressive interventional strategy including PTCA seems reasonable, based on available data, in appropriate patients with cardiogenic shock who have failed thrombolytic therapy.*

In patients with evolving large or anterior infarction and evidence that thrombolysis has not resulted in arterial patency and if adjuvant PTCA is planned, early angiography has been advocated by some. This strategy has not produced results that are superior to no intervening after thrombolysis. *Thus, rescue angioplasty as a routine strategy for failed or presumptively failed thrombolysis cannot be recommended (class IIb).*

Emergency or Urgent Coronary Artery Bypass Surgery   In the presence of cardiogenic shock, CABG in patients in whom other strategies have either failed or not been indicated has been associated with mortality rates from about 10 to 40 percent. These results are generally better than those associated with PCI. *Thus, AMI patients with multivessel coronary artery disease or cardiogenic shock who have had unsuccessful thrombolysis and/or PTCA and are within 4 to 6 h of the onset of symptoms should be considered for emergency CABG.* Similarly, AMI patients with hemodynamic instability or persistent pain and suitable anatomy after failed PTCA should be considered for emergency coronary artery bypass surgery, as should those with medically refractory recurrent ischemia who are not candidates for PTCA.

Arrhythmias Early in the Course of Acute Myocardial Infarction

Bradycardia   Bradyarrhythmias are relatively common (30 to 40 percent) early in the course of AMI, especially in inferior infarction, or after reperfusion of the right coronary artery. Atropine, because of its anticholinergic effects, can be very useful in this situation, since it enhances the discharge rate of the sinus node and facilitates AV conduction as well as reversing the peripheral effects of excessive cholinergic activity, such as vasodilation with associated hypotension. Parasympathomimetic effects—with bradycardia, hypotension, and nausea and vomiting—are also produced by morphine and can be reversed by atropine.

SINUS BRADYCARDIA, ATRIOVENTRICULAR BLOCK, OR VENTRICULAR ASYSTOLE   Atropine is indicated for the treatment of type I second-degree AV block, especially with complicating inferior MI, and is useful at times in third-degree AV block at the AV node in restoring AV conduction or for increasing the junctional response rate. Treatment of sinus bradycardia or first- or second-degree AV block is generally not indicated in the absence of hemodynamic compromise, and atropine should seldom be used in the treatment of type II AV block (location of block below the AV node). *Symptomatic bradycardia that is unresponsive to atropine should be treated with pacing.* Atropine should be administered intravenously at a dosage of 0.5 to 1.0 mg and repeated every 3 to 5 min, as necessary, to achieve an adequate heart rate, up to a total maximum dose of 2.5 mg, which provides complete vagal blockade.

HEART BLOCK   Heart block develops in about 10 percent of patients with AMI and is associated with an increased mortality during hospitalization, but it does not predict long-term mortality in those who survive to be discharged. Intraventricular conduction delay or BBB is also associated with increased in-hospital mortality. The increase in mortality associated with heart block reflects the extent of myocardial damage. Thus, heart block in the setting of anterior MI reflects extensive infarction and concomitant destruction of the conduction system and is associated with relatively high mortality. In contrast, heart block with inferior MI may primarily reflect ischemia of the AV node rather than extensive tissue damage and is associated with a more favorable prognosis. Because of the overwhelming effect of the extent of myocardial damage on prognosis, pacing has not been shown to lessen mortality associated with AV block or BBB. *In AMI, the risk of developing heart block is augmented by the presence of any evidence of conduction system abnormality, including first-degree AV block, Mobitz type I or II AV block, left anterior or posterior hemiblock, or a left or right BBB.*

TEMPORARY PACING EARLY IN THE COURSE OF ACUTE MYOCARDIAL INFARCTION   Recent guidelines place increased emphasis on transcutaneous pacing, in view of the availability of new systems that provide standby status for pacing in AMI patients who do not necessitate immediate pacing and are at intermediate risk for developing heart block. These systems use a single pair of multifunctional electrodes, permitting ECG monitoring, transcutaneous pacing, and defibrillation. Transcutaneous pacing does not entail the risk and complications of transvenous pacing and is well suited for use in the patient who has undergone thrombolysis because invasive procedures may thus be avoided or delayed. Percutaneous pacing is painful; if prolonged pacing is required, the patient should be switched to transvenous systems.

The following conditions have class I indications for placement of patches or activation (demand) of transcutaneous pacing: (1) sinus bradycardia (rate less than 50 beats per minute) with symptoms of hypotension unresponsive to drug therapy; (2) Mobitz type II second-degree AV block; (3) third-degree heart block; (4) bilateral BBB (alternating left and right BBB or right BBB with alternating left anterior and posterior fascicular block; (5) newly acquired or age-indeterminate left BBB, right BBB, and anterior or posterior fascicular block; and (6) right or left BBB and first-degree AV block.

As noted, transcutaneous pacing is intended to be temporary; if prolonged pacing is required, transvenous pacing should be instituted (discussed subsequently). In addition, patients with a high probability of requiring pacing should have it instituted early on (see also Chap. 8).

Ventricular Ectopy, Tachycardia, and Fibrillation   Ventricular rhythm abnormalities are common during the early phases of AMI, with an incidence of ventricular fibrillation (VF) within the first 4 h—so-called *primary* VF—of 3 to 5 percent, which declines rapidly thereafter. Primary VF is associated with increased in-hospital mortality, but not with increased long-term mortality for patients who survive and are discharged.

Post-AMI ventricular tachycardia (VT) occurs in about 15 percent of patients and is also most commonly manifest during the relatively early period. VT is classified according to its ECG morphology (*monomorphic or polymorphic*) and by its duration and consequences: *sustained (lasting more than 30 s and/or causing hemodynamic compromise earlier, which requires intervention)* and *nonsustained (not resulting in hemodynamic compromise and lasting less than 30 s)*. Short runs (5 beats or less) of nonsustained VT are very common in the early post-MI period, and do not require specific treatment.

Accelerated idioventricular rhythm normally occurs frequently during the first hours of AMI and occurs after thrombolysis as a reperfusion arrhythmia. In neither case is it a premonitory rhythm for VT/VF. *Accelerated idioventricular rhythm should ordinarily be observed and not treated specifically.*

Formerly, it was common practice, in order to prevent VT/VF, to treat prophylactically with lidocaine. *Routine use of prophylactic lidocaine in AMI in the presence or absence of thrombolysis is not recommended.* Two prophylactic approaches to the prevention of VT/VF, however, are recommended. Routine administration of beta blockers, as described previously, has been shown to reduce the incidence of VT/VF. Also, since evidence suggests that hypokalemia is a risk factor for VT/VF, it is recommended that serum potassium levels be kept above 4.0 meq/L by supplementation as necessary.

TREATMENT OF VENTRICULAR TACHYCARDIA/FIBRILLATION   Electrical cardioversion of VT that is hemodynamically compromising should be performed immediately. Rapid polymorphic VT should be considered the equivalent of VF and cardioverted with an unsynchronized shock of 200 J; monomorphic VT at a rate of greater than 150 beats/min can be treated initially with a synchronized discharge of 100 J. Urgent cardioversion for VT with rates of under 150 beats per minute is usually not needed. VT that is tolerated hemodynamically can be approached initially with trials of lidocaine, procainamide, or amiodarone.

VF should initially be treated with an unsynchronized shock of 200 J, then incrementally at 200 to 300 J, and finally, at 360 J as needed. The Advanced Cardiac Life Support (ACLS) protocol recommends the following hierarchical approach, as needed, to adjunctive therapy of resistant VF: (1) epinephrine (1 mg IV); (2) lidocaine (1.5 mg/kg IV); and (3) bretylium (5 to 10 mg/kg IV). Intravenous amiodarone (150 mg IV bolus over 10 min followed by a constant infusion of 1.0 mg/min for 6 h and then a rate of 0.5 mg/min) may also be used. In the case of resistant or recurrent VT/VF, electrolyte imbalances should be sought and corrected and ongoing ischemia suspected. Beta-adrenergic blockers should be used in recurrent VT or primary VF to decrease sympathetic input to the heart and decrease ischemia. Intravenous amiodarone should be used in these life-threatening ventricular tachyarrhythmias. *If ongoing ischemia is involved, intra-aortic balloon pumping or emergency revascularization should be considered.*

APPROACH TO THE PATIENT WITH ISCHEMIC-TYPE CHEST PAIN AND WITHOUT ST-SEGMENT ELEVATION

As discussed, the initial criterion differentiating patients with symptoms compatible with AMI for therapeutic purposes is the presence or absence of ST-segment elevation; this is a distinction of importance because, in the absence of ST-segment elevation, thrombolysis is of no therapeutic benefit. AMI in which Q waves do not develop is categorized as *non-Q-wave MI (NQWMI)*; most such patients (90 percent) present with ST-segment depression (see also Chap. 14).

NQWMI is precipitated by plaque disruption. Total coronary occlusion demonstrated angiographically is much less common than in Q-wave MI. Thus, NQWMI is associated either with less than total compromise of blood flow or with early spontaneous reperfusion. Because of the residual noninfarcted myocardium at risk distal to a disrupted plaque, moreover, patients with NQWMI have a marked propensity for recurrent ischemia, infarction, and death and present an opportunity for secondary prevention. Two important conclusions can be derived from the available data: *(1) thrombolysis cannot be recommended in AMI patients without ST-segment elevation and (2) in the NQWMI group and based on the admission ECG, there is a graded, decremental spectrum of risk ranging from ST-segment depression to T-wave inversion to normal.*

Management of Non-Q-Wave Myocardial Infarction   Initially, the NQWMI patient, who by definition does not have diagnostic ST-segment elevation, cannot be distinguished from the patient with unstable angina and no myocardial necrosis. These patients are thus characterized as having ACS, as discussed above. Thus, patients are admitted to the CCU and, *other than avoiding thrombolytic therapy, the initial pharmacologic approach is identical* (Fig 15-2). Serial ECGs and cardiac marker measurements should be performed and, in the case of recurrent pain with the development of ST-segment elevation, thrombolysis or primary PTCA should be performed. If the patient has recurrent stuttering symptoms, angiography should be performed.

ANTITHROMBOTIC THERAPY   The role of antiplatelet therapy in NQWMI has evolved rapidly recently. Clinical studies have generally been performed in patients with ACS without separating out the NQWMI subset specifically. Drugs used in trials have included the platelet glycoprotein IIb/IIIa inhibitors (abciximab, eptifibatide, and tirofiban) and low-molecular-weight heparin. An overview of the trials with glycoprotein IIb/IIIa inhibitors shows a reduction in the composite endpoint of death and the need for revascularization procedures. There was no reduction in mortality; when treatment was discontinued, no further beneficial or detrimental effects were observed. Thus, intravenous glycoprotein IIb/IIIa inhibitors are being utilized frequently as treatment in NQWMI to stabilize patients in the acute phase and have a class IIa recommendation for those at high risk and with refractory ischemia who do not have contraindications of risk of bleeding.

The role of low-molecular-weight heparin has been explored extensively in ACS. In patients with unstable angina and NQWMI, low-molecular-weight heparin has been shown to be superior to unfractionated heparin in reducing acute events, with a decrease of relative risk by about 25 percent. Low-molecular-weight heparin subcutaneously or intravenous unfractionated heparin has a class IIa recommendation in NQWMI (see also Chap. 14).

Retrospective analyses have shown significant benefit of aspirin in NQWMI. Aspirin (160 to 325 mg/day has a class I recommendation in this setting.

BETA BLOCKERS IN NON-ST–SEGMENT ELEVATION MYOCARDIAL INFARCTION   No prospective studies of beta blockers have been performed solely in NQWMI, but retrospective studies have previously cast doubt on the efficacy of these drugs in preventing reinfarction in patients recovering from NQWMI. Nonetheless, the efficacy of beta blockers in relieving pain or arrhythmia, as discussed previously for Q-wave MI, as well the general benefit in the ACS has led to their being given a class I indication in NQWMI.

CALCIUM CHANNEL BLOCKERS   The calcium channel blocker diltiazem (immediate-release form) has been shown to be effective in reducing reinfarction in NQWMI patients with preserved LV function and no evidence of CHF (class IIa indication when given to control ongoing ischemia or rapid ventricular response in case of atrial fibrillation when beta blockers are ineffective or contraindicated; class IIb for general prophylaxis and may be added to standard therapy after 24 h and continued for 1 year). Similar results have been seen for verapamil, although it has been studied less extensively than has diltiazem. Both drugs are contraindicated in the presence of significant LV dysfunction or CHF. Dihydropyridine calcium channel blockers have not shown benefit and may be detrimental (class III—not indicated). In a recent trial comparing PCI with conventional therapy, there was a decrease in mortality associated with diltiazem in the arm comparing conventional medical management with diltiazem to that without the drug. Parenthetically, there were more deaths in the invasive than in the conservative arm.

Early Invasive/Interventional Strategy: Early Coronary Angiography and /or Interventional Therapy   There are conflicting data regarding the efficacy of strategies of conservative management versus PTCA in NQWMI. The early data favored the conservative approach over that of proceeding to routine early angiography and PCI. A more recent trial of patients with NQWMI, who were all treated with low-molecular-weight heparin, compared a strategy of routine early angiography within 2 to 7 days versus a strategy of referral for angiography only if the exercise test were positive for ischemia. In this instance the invasive group had a lower rate of MI at 6 months. This issue is still an open one and must be considered further in light of ongoing trials using glycoprotein IIa/IIb inhibitors and low-molecular-weight heparin. Currently, early angiography and/or interventional therapy is indicated (class I) in MI without ST-segment elevation only with spontaneous or induced ischemia.

MANAGEMENT AFTER HOSPITAL ADMISSION

General Approach

The general issues involved in the management of the patient with suspected or manifest AMI in the intensive or moderate care unit areas follows: to provide for adequate monitoring for the detection of arrhythmia, ischemia, and hemodynamic instability; to provide the patient with a calm, supportive, and reassuring environment; to control the level of activity; to begin the education process for a lifetime of living with coronary heart disease; to control pain and inappropriate anxiety; and to treat adverse events promptly. It is assumed, as previously discussed, that oxygen therapy, beta-adrenergic blockers, aspirin, thrombolytics, heparin, and nitroglycerin have been begun or given, as appropriate, in the ED.

ACTIVITY
Minimizing physical exertion is an important approach to decreasing myocardial oxygen demand and thus decrease myocardial ischemia and necrosis. *Prolonged bed rest and a severe limitation of activities such as self-feeding are no longer recommended except in the case of continuing ischemic pain and/or hemodynamic instability.* Constipation should be avoided and stool softeners routinely prescribed. A bedside commode is preferable to a bedpan in all but the most unstable patients.

ANALGESICS AND ANXIOLYTICS
The importance of controlling chest pain and excessive anxiety and the use of morphine and diazepam were discussed. Anxiolytics may be useful in treating symptoms of nicotine withdrawal in smokers. Intravenous haloperidol can be useful and safe in treating intensive care unit (ICU) psychosis, particularly in the elderly.

EDUCATION
Education of the AMI patient, by both the CCU staff and the physician, with information about the management of symptoms and the prevention of the recurrence, provides a sense of empowerment associated with changes in behavior and decreased anxiety. Because of the substantial risk of cardiac arrest in the 18 months after AMI, family members should be taught cardiopulmonary resuscitation (CPR).

Adjunctive Therapy during the Early In-Hospital Period

ANGIOTENSIN-CONVERTING ENZYME INHIBITORS

Angiotensin-converting enzyme (ACE) inhibitors reduce LV dysfunction and dilatation and slow the progression to CHF in patients with LV dysfunction after AMI. Efficacy may be greatest in those at highest risk—i.e., patients with the worst LV function. Oral therapy with low doses should begin within the first 24 h after hemodynamic stabilization whether or not thrombolytic therapy has been administered. There is a class I indication in the presence of MI with ST-segment elevation manifesting in the anterior precordial leads and in AMI patients with a LV ejection fraction of <40 percent, absent contraindications. ACE inhibitors should not be given if systolic blood pressure is below 100 mmHg. If there is no evidence of LV dysfunction at 4 to 6 weeks, therapy can be stopped, although recent evidence suggests that ACE inhibitors reduce the rate of cardiovascular events in high-risk patients (including those with history of MI) even in those with normal LV function. With significant LV dysfunction, therapy clearly should be continued indefinitely (class I). Currently there is a class IIa recommendation for treatment with ACE inhibitors (absent contraindications) in all the remaining AMI patients other than as defined above and in asymptomatic patients with only mildly impaired LV dysfunction (ejection fraction of 40 to 50 percent).

Management of the Low-Risk Patient

The patient with AMI who has an uncomplicated initial course and is at low risk for developing complications is a candidate for transfer out of the CCU within 24 to 36 h. These patients, including those who have had thrombolysis, may be candidates for early discharge at 3 to 4 days. Excessive diagnostic testing in all post-AMI patients, especially those at low risk, should be discouraged.

If AMI is effectively ruled out using serum markers in the low-risk patient (i.e., normal ECG and absence of the characteristics noted above, especially the absence of prolonged initial pain or the recurrence of pain), noninvasive testing can establish the safety of early discharge (3 to 12 h) from the ED or CCU for further evaluation as an outpatient. In general, such patients do not necessarily need to be admitted to the CCU unless noninvasive testing is positive for ischemic heart disease. Patients with ischemic-type chest discomfort and intermediate probabilities of AMI—i.e., duration of chest pain greater than 20 to 30 min and nondiagnostic ECG changes (without significant ST-segment elevation or depression, T-wave inversion, or

BBB) and without known coronary artery disease—should be admitted to an observation unit or to the CCU. They should be placed on a fast track to rule in AMI or unstable angina. If the clinical course is unrevealing and early imaging is negative, stress testing and further evaluation can be planned. Clinical decisions can usually be made within 12 h in this setting.

Management of the High-Risk Patient with Acute Myocardial Infarction

The high-risk AMI patient is defined by the presence of one or more of the following: recurrent chest pain; CHF and low cardiac output; arrhythmias, in particular recurrent or sustained VT or VF; mechanical cardiac complications of AMI, such as a ruptured papillary muscle or intraventricular septum; and/or inducible ischemia and extensive coronary artery disease.

RECURRENT CHEST PAIN

The most common causes of recurrent chest pain after AMI are coronary ischemia and pericarditis.

Recurrent Ischemia   Recurrence of chest pain in the AMI patient is a serious development and requires immediate diagnosis and treatment, especially if the pain represents recurrent ischemia. Postinfarction angina is chest pain occurring at rest or with limited activity during hospitalization 24 h or more after onset of the AMI. Three categories of patients are at high risk: (1) patients with NQWMI, (2) those who have received thrombolysis, and (3) patients with multiple risk factors.

The approach to recurrent ischemia is similar to that for the original episode. Coronary arteriography generally should be performed. If a high-grade stenosis is found, PTCA should be performed if the lesion is suitable or additional thrombolysis administered if there is associate ST-segment elevation and mechanical reperfusion is not feasible or available. If multiple high-grade stenoses are found, CABG should be considered.

Pericarditis

Early Postinfarction Pericarditis   Early postinfarction pericarditis, as reflected by pain and a friction rub, occurs in ~10 percent of patients, usually between days 2 and 4.

The treatment of choice is aspirin (160 to 325 mg daily), although higher doses (650 mg every 4 to 6 h) may be required, but other nonsteroidal anti-inflammatory drugs (NSAIDs) may be used. The use of anticoagulants is relatively contraindicated in AMI complicated by pericarditis.

HEART FAILURE IN ACUTE MYOCARDIAL INFARCTION

Pathophysiology and Hemodynamics Cardiac failure develops when LV function is reduced by 30 percent or more of normal and usually occurs within minutes or hours of onset of a large infarction. Some compromise of cardiac function is associated with perhaps more than two-thirds of cases of AMI and is usually transient. The severity of the failure, its duration, and whether or not it is reversible are predominantly dependent on infarct size.

Right Ventricular Infarction Inferior MI associated with RV infarction defines a high-risk subset with a mortality rate of 25 to 30 percent. This group should be approached aggressively with consideration for reperfusion therapy. *RV involvement should always be considered and should be specifically sought in inferior MI with clinical evidence of low cardiac output because the therapeutic approaches are quite different in the presence of RV involvement from those for predominantly LV failure. All patients with inferior MI should have an ECG with right-sided precordial leads in addition to the standard leads.*

ST-segment elevation in lead V_{4R} is the single most powerful predictor of RV involvement in inferior infarction and identifies a patient subset with a markedly increased in-hospital mortality. All patients with inferior infarction should be screened by recording ECG lead V_{4R}. Echocardiography can also be useful as an adjunctive diagnostic approach.

Treatment of Right Ventricular Ischemia/Infarction The major objectives in treating RV infarction are to maintain RV preload, provide inotropic support, reduce afterload of the right ventricle, and achieve early reperfusion. The recommendations are summarized in Table 15-5.

MANAGEMENT OF CONGESTIVE HEART FAILURE IN ACUTE MI—GENERAL ISSUES

Hemodynamic Monitoring The balloon flotation (Swan-Ganz) catheter fundamentally permits one, in the setting of low cardiac output, to distinguish between inadequate ventricular filling pressures and inadequate systolic function. The former is treated with volume expansion and the latter with inotropic support and frequent afterload reduction. The catheter, even when used correctly, is not totally benign. Class I indications for insertions are severe or progressive CHF or shock and suspected mechanical

TABLE 15-5

TREATMENT STRATEGY FOR RIGHT VENTRICULAR
ISCHEMIA/INFARCTION

Maintain right ventricular preload
   Volume loading (IV normal saline)
   Avoid use of nitrates and diuretics
   Maintain AV synchrony
      AV sequential pacing for symptomatic high-degree heart
         block unresponsive to atropine
   Prompt cardioversion for hemodynamically significant
      SVT
Inotropic support
   Dobutamine (if cardiac output fails to increase after
      volume loading)
Reduce right ventricular afterload with left ventricular
   dysfunction
   Intra-aortic balloon pump
   Arterial vasodilators (sodium nitroprusside, hydralazine)
   ACE inhibitors
Reperfusion
   Thrombolytic agents
   Primary PTCA
   CABG (in selected patients with multivessel disease)

KEY: IV = intravenous; AV = atrioventricular; SVT = supraventricular tachycardia; ACE = angiotensin converting enzyme; PTCA = percutaneous transluminal coronary angioplasty; CABG = coronary artery bypass graft.
SOURCE: Ryan TJ, Antman EM, Brooks NH, et al: 1999 Update: ACC/AHA guidelines for the management of patients with acute myocardial infarction: A report of the American College of Cardiology/American Heart Association Task Force on Practice Guidelines (Committee on Management of Acute Myocardial Infarction). *J Am Coll Cardiol* 1999, 34:904, with permission.

complications (ventricular septal defect, papillary muscle rupture, tamponade).

    Arterial monitoring in AMI is useful (class I) in all hypotensive patients but especially in those in shock. Arterial monitoring is also recommended in patients receiving vasopressor agents. The radial artery is the preferred site, although the brachial and femoral arteries can be used.

Intraaortic Balloon Counterpulsation   The intraaortic balloon pump reduces afterload during ventricular systole, and increases coronary perfusion during diastole. The decrease in afterload and increased coronary perfusion account for its efficacy in cardiogenic shock and ischemia. It is particularly useful as a stabilizing bridge to facilitate diagnostic angiography and revascularization and repair of mechanical complications of AMI (all class I indications).

Diuretics and Positive Inotropic Agents

Diuretics and Cardiac Failure in Acute Myocardial Infarction   Diuretics generally should not be the drugs used initially in the treatment of pulmonary congestion in AMI because intravascular pressure is initially normal (unless there was existing CHF). Their use early in the course should usually be guided by hemodynamic measurements from a Swan-Ganz catheter. Diuretic therapy may become appropriate later if salt and water retention occur and LV filling pressures become excessively high.

Inotropic Agents in Congestive Heart Failure   Digoxin is not the drug of choice in acute heart failure in MI. The primary use of digoxin in AMI is to control heart rate in atrial fibrillation. Dobutamine has favorable pharmacologic properties for use in heart failure in MI. Dopamine has a tendency to increase heart rate more than dobutamine. With higher doses, it may increase peripheral resistance and filling pressures, thus offsetting some of the positive inotropic effects.

Management of Uncomplicated Cardiac Failure after Acute Myocardial Infarction   *In patients with uncomplicated AMI, there is no need to perform invasive monitoring if careful clinical observations are made.*

If cardiac failure is not complicated by mechanical factors—such as mitral valve rupture, ventricular septal rupture, pulmonary embolus, or tamponade—the failure in most patients is transient and of mild to moderate severity. If the cardiac output is normal, aggressive treatment is often not recommended. In patients with rales at the base of the lungs with only minimal increase in heart rate and no other signs of hypoxemia, conventional therapy with morphine; nasal oxygen; intravenous, oral, or transdermal nitrates; and bed rest is adequate. In patients with extensive pulmonary edema who are normotensive and exhibit hypoxia and dyspnea, the treatment of choice is nitroglycerin given intravenously at 0.1 μg/kg/min and increased in increments of 5 to 10 μg/min, stopping at a dose that does not decrease the systolic blood pressure below 100 mmHg. It is preferable that hemodynamics be monitored invasively (Swan-Ganz catheter) when one gives a vasodilator to reduce the ventricular filling pressure to 15 to 17 mmHg. An intravenous inotropic agent may be needed. The inotropic agents are generally dobutamine or dopamine. Dobutamine is the preferred agent. The infusion should be initiated at 2 to 5 μg/kg/min and should be increased such that adequate systemic pressure is maintained and the heart rate does not increase by more than 10 to 15 percent. The ventricular filling pressure should be decreased to a range of 14 to 18 mmHg while maintaining adequate cardiac output and blood pressure.

In patients with borderline blood pressure and evidence of peripheral hypoperfusion, therapy should be initiated with an inotropic agent and not a vasodilator. Low doses of dopamine (2 to 7 μg/kg/min) are usually given and are associated with an increase in stroke volume, cardiac output, renal blood flow, and peripheral resistance to a modest degree. Higher doses of dopamine induce significant vasoconstriction and an increase in LV filling pressure. Diuretics should be used with caution. If high filling pressure (> 18 to 20 mmHg) persists after achieving adequate output with positive inotropic agents and/or vasodilators, diuretics may be added.

Complicated Heart Failure after Myocardial Infarction   In fulminating heart failure, administration of high concentrations (60 to 100%) of oxygen via a face mask is essential and endotracheal intubation may be needed. Invasive hemodynamic monitoring is particularly useful in these patients. The therapy for severe pulmonary edema should include intravenous morphine. If systolic blood pressure is adequate ($\geq$ 100 mmHg), nitroglycerin is administered intravenously. In severe pulmonary edema, nitroprusside may be essential to reduce afterload. If the systolic blood pressure is < 100 mmHg, treatment should be initiated with a positive inotropic agent, with the subsequent addition of a vasodilator if adequate blood pressure is achieved.

Hypotension and Cardiogenic Shock   Due to massive ischemia and necrosis, cardiogenic shock usually occurs within hours of the onset of infarction. Reversible causes must be excluded. These include mitral valve rupture, ventricular septal rupture, RV infarction, pulmonary embolus, and cardiac tamponade.

The approaches to pulmonary congestion include the use of morphine and the maintenance of adequate oxygenation together with endotracheal intubation and mechanical ventilation if necessary. Pulmonary artery and arterial catheters should be placed. Urinary output is monitored using an indwelling catheter. The cornerstones of therapy are inotropic and vasopressor agents. If the systemic arterial vasopressure is below 80 to 90 mmHg, a pressor agent such as dopamine should be infused, as described. If high doses of dopamine are necessary to maintain adequate perfusion (and pressure of 90 to 100 mmHg), a change to norepinephrine infusion should be considered. On occasion, the severity of cardiac pump dysfunction will require the combined use of nitroprusside and dopamine. Stabilization in cardiogenic shock may be achieved by the intra-aortic balloon. Aortic counterpulsation is usually reserved for patients with a potentially reversible condition or in whom cardiac transplantation is being considered.

Restoration of coronary blood flow will probably be the most effective therapy in salvaging patients with cardiogenic shock. Mechanical revascularization appears to improve survival in cardiogenic shock complicating AMI, as discussed previously.

Mechanical Dysfunction Contributing to Cardiac Failure   Papillary muscle rupture is manifest by the sudden appearance of pulmonary edema, usually 2 to 7 days after the infarction. A mid- or holosystolic murmur with wide radiation is usually audible. The diagnosis can be established by Doppler echocardiographic studies.

Immediate recognition and treatment are essential. Intra-aortic balloon counterpulsation alone or with vasodilator and inotropic therapy is frequently required for temporary stabilization. The patient should undergo cardiac catheterization to define coronary anatomy, and surgery for mitral valve replacement or repair and CABG should be performed.

PAPILLARY MUSCLE DYSFUNCTION   The sudden development of an apical systolic murmur after a MI is much more often secondary to papillary muscle dysfunction than to rupture. Papillary muscle dysfunction is frequently compatible with long-term survival.

Echocardiography coupled with Doppler flow studies will confirm the presence of mitral regurgitation, grade its severity, and permit assessment of LV function. Ordinarily papillary muscle dysfunction will require no specific therapy, while the unusual patient with severe regurgitation should be treated like one with papillary muscle rupture. In intermediate cases, afterload reduction with ACE inhibitors should be considered.

VENTRICULAR SEPTAL RUPTURE   There is a higher prevalence of ventricular septal rupture in first infarctions, and the majority occurs within the first week. Ventricular septal rupture is usually manifest by the appearance of a new harsh, holosystolic murmur along the left sternal border (often associated with a thrill) and sudden clinical deterioration with hypotension and pulmonary congestion. Often the event is heralded by a recurrence of chest pain. The diagnosis can be established by two-dimensional and Doppler echocardiographic studies. Results of the Doppler echocardiographic studies and/or the oxygen step-up on right heart catheterization would confirm the presence of septal rupture.

Medical therapy can be expected to be ineffective. Prompt but temporary stabilization can be achieved with intra-aortic balloon counterpulsation alone or in conjunction with vasodilator and inotropic drug therapy. Cardiac catheterization should be performed in an expeditious manner. An aggressive approach of immediate operative repair of these patients results in a short-term survival rate of 42 to 75 percent.

ARRHYTHMIAS AND CONDUCTION
DISTURBANCES COMPLICATING
ACUTE MYOCARDIAL INFARCTION

**Ventricular Ectopy, Ventricular Tachycardia, and Ventricular
Fibrillation**   The management of VT and fibrillation after the first
24 h of hospitalization for AMI is similar to that for the early phase.
The occurrence of symptomatic, sustained VT or of VF in the later
phases of the hospital course, however, suggests that a chronic arrhythmogenic focus may be developing in the damaged ventricle.
These ventricular arrhythmias are classified as *secondary* and are
indicators of increased risk for subsequent sudden cardiac death.

Sinus Tachycardia or Atrial Premature Beats   Sinus tachycardia
following AMI is common and is frequently an unfavorable prognostic sign. Patients with a large area of infarcted myocardium may
have sinus tachycardia on the basis of LV dysfunction, which causes
reflex activation of the sympathetic nervous system. Frequent atrial
premature complexes are relatively common in AMI, and specific
therapy is indicated.

Paroxysmal Supraventricular Tachycardia   Episodes of paroxysmal supraventricular tachycardia occur rather commonly in AMI
and usually are transient. Rate control is essential, and the therapeutic
approaches may include carotid sinus massage, adenosine, digoxin,
verapamil, or diltiazem.

Atrial Flutter and Atrial Fibrillation   Atrial flutter is relatively
uncommon in AMI, whereas atrial fibrillation has an incidence of
10 to 15 percent. Atrial fibrillation is associated with an increased
in-hospital mortality rate. A rapid ventricular response can worsen
ischemia and infarction. Risk of systemic embolization is increased
in AMI in the presence of atrial fibrillation and to a lesser extent in
atrial flutter. Thus, heparin therapy is indicated in patients not already receiving it. If the patient experiences new or worsening pain,
ischemic ST changes, or hemodynamic instability during atrial fibrillation with a rapid ventricular response rate, immediate electrical
cardioversion is indicated.

Heart Block   First-degree block is seen frequently in AMI, espe-
cially in inferior MI. This is attributable to ischemia or enhanced
vagal activity. Treatment is seldom required.
    Second-degree AV block is also relatively common, especially
Mobitz type I or Wenckebach block. It is associated with a narrow
QRS and frequently is the result of AV node ischemia in inferior MI.
It is usually transient, and its presence does not affect the prognosis.

Mobitz type II block is uncommon but is associated with more serious complications and a worse prognosis. It usually occurs with anterior MI and reflects trifascicular block. It is characterized by a wide QRS and a nonvarying PR interval before a nonconducted atrial beat. Heart block may develop suddenly and is an ominous sign, with a mortality of about 80 percent. It is usually permanent.

Third-degree AV block, or complete heart block, occurs in about 5 percent of patients with AMI and is most commonly seen with inferior infarction, usually with block at the AV node. There is some increase in in-hospital mortality rates in this setting, but complete heart block in inferior MI is not an independent predictor of poor long-term prognosis. In contrast, patients with anterior infarction who develop third-degree AV block have a high mortality rate (80 percent).

Indications for Temporary Transvenous Pacing   The indications generally agreed on for temporary pacemaker insertion in AMI include asystole, complete heart block in the setting of anterior MI, new onset of right or left BBB with persistent Mobitz II second-degree AV block in the setting of anterior MI, or other symptomatic bradycardias unresponsive to atropine. BBB in the setting of AMI identifies a population at risk for both electrical and mechanical complications. Such patients must be monitored for evidence of transient high-degree heart block.

Permanent Pacing   The use of permanent pacemakers is reviewed extensively in the ACC/AHA guidelines for pacemaker implantation and is summarized in Chap. 42 of *Hurst's The Heart,* 10th ed. The fact that temporary pacing may have been required in the course of AMI does not necessarily indicate the need for permanent pacing. Patients who have had permanent pacemakers inserted after AMI usually have a relatively unfavorable prognosis primarily related to the extensiveness of the underlying disease and myocardial damage.

DISCHARGE FROM THE CORONARY CARE UNIT

The length of stay in the CCU should be based on the risk of developing VT and VF. The risk of developing primary VF after AMI decreases exponentially, with the majority of arrhythmic deaths occurring within the first 24 h. A patient with an uncomplicated infarction can be transferred from the CCU on the third day. Certain patients need more prolonged cardiac monitoring. Those who are prime candidates for late-hospital sudden deaths manifest, while in the CCU, one or more of the following: (1) the arrhythmias of pump failure (sinus tachycardia, atrial flutter, or atrial fibrillation); (2) the arrhythmias of electrical instability (VT or VF); (3) acute interventricular conduction disturbances; (4) evidence of circulatory failure (CHF, pulmonary edema, or significant hypotension); or (5) large anterior infarction. The effectiveness of prolonged monitoring of this select group of patients in an intermediate-care unit following CCU discharge is evident in a doubling of the rate of successful resuscitations.

In an uncomplicated MI, the patient does not need to be confined to bed for longer than 24 h. Upon transfer from the CCU, the patient should be started on a progressive ambulation program. The speed with which the patient progresses from one stage to the next depends on the severity of the infarction, the presence or absence of complications, his or her age, and the presence of comorbid conditions. The length of hospitalization following an AMI should likewise depend on these same factors. If the patient has not manifested complications during the first 4 days of hospitalization, he or she is very unlikely to do so at any later time. This patient could probably be discharged after 7 days or fewer in the hospital. The last 2 to 3 days of the hospitalization are generally necessary to resolve the questions pertaining to residual ventricular function, the presence or absence of ventricular ectopy, and the adequacy of the remainder of the coronary circulation. In addition, time is needed for instruction in risk-factor modification.

Noninvasive Risk Stratification in Patients Surviving Acute Myocardial Infarction

Survivors of AMI have a substantial risk of facing subsequent cardiovascular events. Noninvasive risk assessment provides useful information to individualize the extent of further workup and therapy, with the aim of (1) targeting specific long-term therapies, (2) identifying high-risk patients requiring aggressive diagnostic tests, (3) counseling the patient on prognosis, (4) developing an exercise program, and (5) planning modifications of lifestyle.

Three interrelated prognostic factors are the focus of predischarge assessment: (1) assessment of LV function, (2) detection of residual myocardial ischemia (jeopardized myocardium), and (3) assessment of the risk of arrhythmic (sudden cardiac) death. High-risk patients can be identified clinically because of the presence of one or more of the following: decompensated CHF, angina associated with ECG changes, in-hospital cardiac arrest, spontaneous sustained VT, or the development of a high-degree heart block. In the majority of patients who have a relatively benign hospital course, noninvasive testing can accurately identify a group at very low risk whose annual mortality is 1 to 3 percent. The practical consequence of identifying a low-risk group is that emphasis is focused on early discharge and lifestyle modification as well as targeted prophylactic medical therapy rather than expensive, invasive diagnostic testing.

Early coronary angiography and aggressive interventional therapy is indicated for patients with recurrent episodes of spontaneous or induced (with low-level exercise testing) angina or ischemia or with evidence of persistent pulmonary congestion, clinical LV dysfunction, or cardiogenic shock. *There is general agreement that there is not adequate evidence to support routine coronary angiography as the initial assessment in asymptomatic patients; therefore the guidelines dissuade its use as the primary tool for diagnostic evaluation.*

ASSESSMENT OF LEFT VENTRICULAR FUNCTION AND LEFT VENTRICULAR EJECTION FRACTION

Ventricular function is an important determinant of long-term survival after AMI regardless of reperfusion status; in general, such patients should be assessed by noninvasive or, if otherwise indicated, angiographic techniques.

ASSESSMENT OF MYOCARDIAL ISCHEMIA

Exercise Testing in Uncomplicated Patients

Clinical Significance of Predischarge Submaximal Exercise Testing Predischarge exercise testing consistently identifies a high-risk group for recurrent cardiac events (MI, unstable angina, etc.) or mortality in the first year after the AMI. Exercise testing also identifies a very low risk group (1 to 3 percent mortality rate for the first year). A negative test should promote early discharge as well as discourage an aggressive diagnostic approach. Submaximal exercise testing in *uncomplicated* patients, including those who have had thrombolysis before discharge, has a class I indication.

The presence of ischemia generally mandates cardiac catheterization to define the coronary anatomy and to consider revascularization. A recommended approach to post-AMI risk stratification is summarized in Fig. 15-4.

ASSESSMENT OF THE RISK OF ARRHYTHMIC (SUDDEN CARDIAC) DEATH

The identification of asymptomatic but high-risk patients for arrhythmic death after AMI has not been associated with the delineation of a successful treatment strategy. Although the presence of asymptomatic spontaneous ventricular arrhythmias as detected on ambulatory monitoring is predictive of increased arrhythmic (sudden) death, the positive predictive value is poor. The dearth of safe and effective

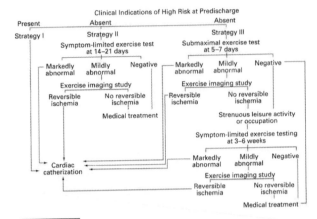

FIGURE 15-4

Strategies for exercise test evaluations soon after myocardial infarction (MI). If patients are at high risk for ischemic events based on clinical criteria, they should undergo invasive evaluation to determine if they are candidates for coronary revascularization procedures (strategy I). For patients initially deemed to be at low risk at time of discharge after myocardial infarction, two strategies for performing exercise testing can be used. One is a symptom-limited test at 14 to 21 days (strategy II). If the patient is on digoxin or if the baseline ECG precludes accurate interpretation of ST-segment changes (e.g., baseline left BBB or left ventricular hypertrophy), then an initial exercise imaging study can be performed. Results of exercise testing should be stratified to determine need for additional invasive or exercise perfusion studies. A third strategy is to perform a submaximal exercise test at 5 to 7 days after myocardial infarction or just befor hospital discharge. The exercise test results could be stratified using the guidelines in strategy I. If exercise test studies are negative, a second symptom-limited exercise test could be repeated at 3 to 6 weeks for patients undergoing vigorous activity during leisure or at work. [From Ryan TJ, Antman EM, Brooks NH, et al. 1999 Update: ACC/AHA guidelines for the management of patients with acute myocardial infarction: A report of the American College of Cardiology/American Heart Association Task Force on Practice Guidelines (Committee on Management of Acute Myocardial Infarction). *J Am Coll Cardiol* 1999; 34:904, with permission.]

antiarrhythmic drugs has limited the usefulness of routinely evaluating the asymptomatic post-AMI patient in this regard.

Assessing Arrhythmic Death: Conclusions   None of the noninvasive (ambulatory monitoring) or invasive (electrophysiologic testing) techniques is generally agreed upon to be beneficial, useful, and effective in the assessment of arrhythmic death. No clinical trial has demonstrated that the use of any one or a combination of these modalities of testing identifies a high-risk population in whom intervention resulted in clinical benefit.

Coronary Angiography and Percutaneous Transluminal Coronary Angioplasty

The selection of patients for cardiac catheterization and coronary angiographic studies prior to hospital discharge should be based on identifying patients at risk for ischemic events and on whether or not the information provided by cardiac catheterization and coronary angiography will change patient management. *In general, studies that have compared acute or early cardiac catheterization to a more conservative approach of performing cardiac catheterization and coronary angiographic studies only for patients with spontaneous recurrent angina or exercise-induced ischemia have demonstrated no benefit to the strategy of routine catheterization.* Patients who have a complicated clinical course characterized by refractory cardiac failure, unstable angina, an episode of sustained VT, or cardiac arrest should be studied.

The recommended algorithm for selecting asymptomatic, uncomplicated post-AMI patients for cardiac catheterization is presented in Fig. 15-4. Decision making focuses on the presence or absence of myocardial ischemia. Where patients have received thrombolytic therapy, it seems reasonable that those who have evidence of residual ischemia are still at increased risk of future ischemic events and should undergo coronary angiography. Consideration of PTCA following coronary angiographic studies should be based on established clinical and anatomic guidelines. CABG should be considered in those groups in whom it has been shown to be of proven benefit: patients with triple-vessel disease, patients with ischemia, and those with significant LV dysfunction.

SECONDARY PREVENTION AND CARDIAC REHABILITATION

Risk-Factor Reduction

There is now abundant evidence that risk-factor reduction decrease coronary events in susceptible patients. Thus, since those who have had AMI are among those at highest risk for recurrence, management strategies to mitigate this risk are very important.

SMOKING

Smoking cessation is an essential goal after AMI, since the recurrence rate and death rates after AMI are doubled by the continuation of smoking and risk associated with smoking declines rapidly, within 3 years, to that of the nonsmoking cohort survivors. The role of the physician in motivating the patient to quit smoking is extremely important, and the likelihood of success appears to be directly related to the extent of his or her involvement.

DYSLIPIDEMIA

Recent large secondary prevention trials have provided compelling evidence that in patients after AMI, therapy with HMG-CoA reductase inhibitors to lower serum cholesterol levels that were either initially elevated, as in the Scandinavian Simvastatin Survival Study (4S), or within the "average" range, as in the Cholesterol and Recurrent Events trial (CARE), was effective in reducing both cardiovascular and total mortality as well as cardiovascular events. The guidelines of the expert panel of the National Cholesterol Education Program provide target goals for patients with manifest coronary artery disease. These goals areas follows: LDL cholesterol at 100 mg/dL (2.59 mmol/L) and HDL cholesterol above 35 mg/dL (0.91 mmol/L). *All AMI patients should have serum lipids evaluated and treated intensely in order to achieve target goals.* Treatment should start in the hospital with initiation of the American Heart Association's step II diet.

INACTIVITY

A sedentary lifestyle is a risk factor for coronary artery disease. Metanalysis of cardiac rehabilitation studies has shown a reduction in mortality in the exercise group as opposed to a control group. *The greatest benefits of exercise are those observed with moderate, regular exercise as contrasted with no exercise.*

Regular aerobic exercise should be prescribed for post-AMI patients in stable condition at an intensity, duration, and frequency as determined by formal testing and clinical judgment. Optimum benefit is achieved in a supervised program, although asymptomatic, stable patients can exercise without direct supervision; the latter, however, should receive regular monitoring by a physician.

Drug Therapy

BETA-ADRENERGIC BLOCKERS

The benefits of beta-blocker therapy given early in the course of AMI were discussed. Multiple clinical trials have also demonstrated the benefits of long-term treatment of post-AMI patients with beta blockers. Mortality is reduced by about 25 to 35 percent. The beneficial effect is highest in high-risk patients with large (usually anterior) MI and compensated LV dysfunction. The beneficial effects in low-risk patients are less clear, but the consensus is that these patients probably should be treated because of the relatively favorable side-effect profile. Beta blockers with intrinsic sympathomimetic activity should not be used in this context.

ASPIRIN

The role of aspirin during the early phases of AMI was discussed. Aspirin use over the long-term after AMI is also associated with a reduction in mortality. Aspirin at relatively low doses (81 to 325 mg/day) is recommended for all patients with AMI in the absence of contraindications.

ANTICOAGULATION

Anticoagulation can reduce mortality, recurrent MI, and stroke after AMI. The role of warfarin is rather limited to those at increased risk for developing mural thrombi. In addition those post-AMI patients with demonstrable LV thrombus and atrial fibrillation should be anticoagulated. The duration of anticoagulation should be limited to 3 months in the case of LV thrombus.

ANGIOTENSIN-CONVERTING ENZYME INHIBITORS

The ACE inhibitors and recommendations for their use early in the course of AMI were discussed. Recent studies have documented their efficacy in secondary prevention. Thus, ACE inhibitors are recommended for chronic use after AMI in patients with significant LV dysfunction; their use should be considered in those with only mild to moderate LV dysfunction (ejection fraction less than 45 percent). The recent evidence that ACE inhibitors may be efficacious in preventing future cardiovascular events in most patients at risk (including those post-AMI patients with normal LV function) was discussed previously.

Modification of Lifestyle and Cardiac Rehabilitation after Acute Myocardial Infarction

Because of the relatively high risk of recurrence and the need for lifelong modification of lifestyles and risk factors, most post-AMI patients should be enrolled in a cardiac rehabilitation program that emphasizes dietary modification, risk-factor reduction, and exercise. The low-risk patient does not require prolonged supervised exercise. All patients, however, can benefit from a structured environment to launch a lifetime of healthy living. Cardiac rehabilitation is discussed in detail in Chap. 50 of *Hurst's The Heart*, 10th ed.

SUGGESTED READING

Alexander RW, Pratt CM, Ryan TJ, Roberts R: Diagnosis and management of patients with acute myocardial infarction. In: Fuster V, Alexander RW, O'Rourke RA, et al (eds): *Hurst's The Heart,* 10th ed. New York: McGraw-Hill; 2001:1275–1359.

Antman EM, Tanasijevic MJ, Thompson B, et al: Cardiac-specific troponin I levels to predict the risk of mortality in patients with acute coronary syndromes. *N Engl J Med* 1996; 335:1342–1349.

Downs JR, Clearfield M, Weis S, et al for the AFCAPS/TexCAPS Research Group: Primary prevention of acute coronary events with lovastatin in men and women with average cholesterol levels. Results of AFCAPS/TexCAPS. *JAMA* 1998; 279:1615–1622.

Falk E, Fuster V: Atherogenesis and its determinants. In: Fuster V, Alexander RW, O'Rourke RA, et al (eds): *Hurst's The Heart,* 10th ed. New York: McGraw-Hill; 2001:1065–1093.

Fibrinolytic Therapy Trialists' (FTT) Collaborative Group: Indications for fibrinolytic therapy in suspected acute myocardial infarction: Collaborative overview of early mortality and major morbidity results from all randomized trials of more than one-thousand patients. *Lancet* 1994; 343:311–322.

GUSTO IIA Investigators, Ohman EM, Armstrong PW, Christenson RH, et al: Cardiac troponin T levels for risk stratification in acute myocardial ischemia. *N Engl J Med* 1996; 335:1333–1341.

Hochman JS, Boland J, Sleeper LA, et al: Current spectrum of cardiogenic shock and effect of early revascularization on mortality: Results of an International Registry. SHOCK Registry Investigators. *Circulation* 1995; 91:873–881.

HOPE Investigators: Effects of an angiotensin-converting-enzyme inhibitor, ramipril, on cardiovascular events in high-risk patients. The Heart Outcomes Prevention Evaluation Study. *N Engl J Med* 2000; 342:145–153.

Kinch JW, Ryan TJ: Right ventricular infarction. *N Engl J Med* 1994; 330:1211–1217.

Pfeffer MA, Braunwald E, Moye LA, et al: Effect of captopril on morbidity and mortality in patients with left ventricular dysfunction after myocardial infarction: Results of the Survival and Ventricular Enlargement Trial. The SAVE Investigators. *N Engl J Med* 1992; 327:669–677.

Puleo PR, Meyer D, Wathen C, et al: Use of rapid assay of subforms of creatine kinase MB to diagnose or rule out acute myocardial infarction. *N Engl J Med* 1994; 331:561–566.

Ryan TJ, Antman EM, Brooks NH, et al: 1999 Update: ACC/AHA guidelines for the management of patients with acute myocardial infarction: A report of the American College of Cardiology/American Heart Association Task Force on Practice Guidelines (Committee on Management of Acute Myocardial Infarction). *J Am Coll Cardiol* 1999; 34:890–911.

Sacks FM, Pfeffer MA, Moye LA, et al: The effect of pravastatin on coronary events after myocardial infarction in patients with average cholesterol levels. Cholesterol and Recurrent Events (CARE) Trial Investigators. *N Engl J Med* 1996; 335:1001–1009.

Scandinavian Simvastatin Survival Study Group: Randomised trial of cholesterol lowering in 4444 patients with coronary heart disease: the Scandinavian Simvastatin Survival Study (4S). *Lancet* 1994; 344:1383–1389.

Wenger NK: Rehabilitation of the patient with coronary heart disease. In: Fuster V, Alexander RW, O'Rourke RA, et al (eds): *Hurst's The Heart,* 10th ed. New York: McGraw-Hill; 2001:1537–1549.

16

PERCUTANEOUS CORONARY INTERVENTION

John S. Douglas, Jr.
Spencer B. King III

DEVELOPMENT OF BALLOON ANGIOPLASTY

Percutaneous transluminal coronary angioplasty (PTCA) was conceived and shepherded into worldwide acceptance and application by Andreas R. Gruentzig. The use of percutaneous revascularization soon increased dramatically, exceeding 130,000 procedures in the United States in 1986. Some 400,000 procedures were completed in 1995, and 600,000 in 1999.

Initially, coronary balloon angioplasty was performed for discrete, proximal, noncalcified subtotal lesions located in one coronary artery. A 10-year follow-up of Gruentzig's early Zurich series revealed an overall survival rate of 90 percent, and 95 percent for those with single-vessel disease.

Recently published observational data from the 1993–1995 New York State Cardiac Procedure Registry of 60,000 coronary artery bypass grafting (CABG) and percutaneous transluminal angioplasty (PTCA) procedures reported better 3-year survival with CABG in patients with three-vessel disease and those with two-vessel/proximal left anterior descending (LAD) disease treated with CABG, while those with one-vessel/no LAD disease had better survival with PTCA. All other patients had similar survival with PTCA and CABG.

RANDOMIZED TRIALS OF BALLOON ANGIOPLASTY

The Angioplasty Compared to Medical Therapy Evaluation (ACME), involving 212 patients with single-vessel disease and abnormal stress tests, revealed greater freedom from angina in the angioplasty group at 6 months (64 versus 46 percent), but there was no difference in rates of death or myocardial infarction (MI). The second Randomized Intervention Treatment of Angina (RITA-2) trial randomized 1018 patients with stable angina and predominantly single-vessel disease to PTCA or medical therapy. Angina relief and treadmill performance were significantly better in the PTCA patients, but death or myocardial infarction occurred in 6.3 percent of PTCA patients compared to 3.3 percent of medically treated patients. In the Veterans Affairs Non-Q Wave Infarction Strategies in Hospital (VANQWISH) trial, 920 patients were randomly assigned to either an invasive strategy or conservative management. There was a higher incidence of a composite endpoint (death or nonfatal infarction) in the invasive group at 1 year (111 versus 85 events, $p = 0.05$). There were no deaths at 30 days in the invasive group treated with PTCA, but an 11.6 percent 30-day mortality occurred in the group treated with CABG. The recently reported larger Fast Revascularization During Instability in Coronary Disease (FRISC II) study strongly supported an invasive approach in patients randomized after 5 days of dalteparin (Fragmin) therapy. Among men at 6 months, the invasive strategy in FRISC II resulted in a 34 percent reduction in death or MI ($p = 0.002$) and a 52 percent reduction in mortality (1.5 versus 3.2 percent, $p = 0.03$).

Percutaneous Transluminal Angioplasty versus Coronary Artery Bypass Grafting

Two trials of patients with multivessel coronary artery disease were sponsored by the National Heart, Lung and Blood Institute (NHLBI) and performed in the United States. The first, the Emory Angioplasty versus Surgery Trial (EAST), was a single-center study, while the larger Bypass Angioplasty Revascularization Investigation (BARI) involved 18 centers. In-hospital mortality was similar for angioplasty and bypass surgery. Long-term survival was similar in both studies. Long-term survival in BARI and EAST is shown in Table 16-1. The difference favoring surgery is completely explained by a striking surgical advantage for the diabetic patients. Repeat revascularization procedures were more common in the angioplasty group. Pending clarification by these trials, caution should be exercised in the use of PTCA in diabetic patients with multivessel disease.

NEW DEVICES AND STRATEGIES FOR CORONARY INTERVENTION

Directional atherectomy, rotational ablation, and intravascular laser therapy have been used for debulking coronary lesions. Although each has niche applications, their use has declined in recent years. Directional atherectomy is sometimes used in bulky bifurcation lesions,

TABLE 16-1
RANDOMIZED COMPARISONS OF PTCA AND CABG

	EAST		BARI	
	PTCA	CABG	PTCA	CABG
Patient characteristics				
Age (years)	62	61	62	61
Ejection fraction, %	61	62	57	58
Heart failure, %	3	4	9	9
Prior MI, %	41	41	54	55
Diseased vessels, %				
Two	60	60	57	58
Three	40	40	41	41
In-hospital outcome, %				
Myocardial infarction	3	10	2.1	4.6
Death	1	1	1.1	1.3
Repeat revascularization				
PTCA	0	0	3.4	0
CABG	10	0	10.2	0.1
Five-year outcome, %				
Death	12.1	8.8	13.7	10.7
Additional PTCA	48.6	15.5	34.0	7.3
Additional CABG	25.1	0.5	31.3	1.1
Any additional revascularization	61.2	16.1	54.5	8.0

KEY: EAST = Emory Angioplasty Surgery Trial; BARI = Bypass Angioplasty Revascularization Investigation; PTCA = percutaneous transluminal coronary angioplasty; CABG = coronary artery bypass graft surgery.

laser therapy for in-stent restenosis, and rotational atherectomy for heavily calcified lesions.

Stents: After a Decade of Use, the Dominant Strategy

Stents were developed for two indications: to reduce restenosis and to solve acute vessel closure after angioplasty; they were first implanted in 1986. On the basis of two carefully conducted randomized trials that showed reduced restenosis compared to balloon angioplasty, stents were approved in 1994 for the elective treatment of de novo

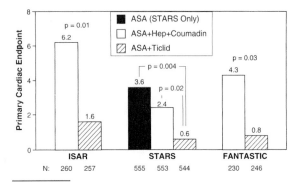

FIGURE 16-1

Results of three trials evaluating antiplatelet versus anticoagulant or aspirin-alone therapy for stent prophylaxis. Aspirin and ticlopidine led to significant reduction of death, MI, or need for urgent revascularization.

lesions in native coronary arteries. The interest in stenting was greatly heightened by a pivotal observation by Colombo that when aspirin and ticlopidine were substituted for warfarin, complete stent expansion by high-pressure balloon inflation confirmed by intravascular ultrasound, yielded a very low rate of thrombosis. A randomized trial of stent placement without ultrasound guidance comparing aspirin and ticlopidine with a warfarin derivative revealed a low 30-day incidence of cardiac events and bleeding rates in the aspirin-ticlopidine patients, supporting this simplified antithrombotic strategy (ISAR). This finding was confirmed and extended by the Stent Anticoagulation Restenosis Study (STARS) Investigation and the FANTASTIC trial (Fig. 16-1). Clopidogrel proved as effective as ticlopidine in a randomized investigation, the Clopidogrel Aspirin Stent Interventional Cooperative Study (CLASSICS), and it was observed that a combination of neutropenia, thrombocytopenia, or early discontinuation of drug was more common in the ticlopidine group (9.1 versus 2.9 percent). The use of coronary stents was reviewed extensively in a recent American College of Cardiology Expert Consensus Document.

Stents versus Coronary Artery Bypass Grafting in Multivessel Disease

Intermediate-term data is available from the Arterial Revascularization Therapy Study (ARTS), which randomized 1205 patients with multivessel disease in 68 clinical centers to stent or standard CABG. At 1 year, there was no difference in rates of death or myocardial infarction; however, repeat interventions were higher in the stent group. The occurrence of late events in 26 percent of ARTS stented patients was approximately one-half the incidence seen following balloon angioplasty in multivessel disease in BARI and EAST due to a reduced need for repeat revascularization in stented patients. As in BARI, the mortality rate in ARTS of diabetics treated percutaneously was higher than that of nondiabetics (6.3 versus 3.1 percent).

IIb/IIIa Platelet Receptor Inhibitors

These platelet receptor blockers have been used as an adjunct to coronary intervention. The antibody fragment, abciximab; the peptide, eptifibatide; and the nonpeptide small-molecule agent, tirofiban, each have reduced periprocedural events, most commonly CK-MB elevation. Ongoing studies will help to establish whether there is a clinical difference between the agents. A better understanding of the long-term clinical impact of using these agents is needed.

INDICATIONS FOR CORONARY INTERVENTION

In general, when one is selecting percutaneous coronary intervention (PCI), there should be assurance that the operator can treat, with a high probability of success, the coronary lesion(s) accounting for the symptoms or signs of myocardial ischemia. Further, the associated risk and durability of the revascularization should be acceptable—as compared with bypass surgery or medical therapy—during both early and long-term follow-up. The latter estimate requires consideration of the likelihood and consequences of abrupt vessel closure, restenosis, and incomplete revascularization. The American College of Cardiology/American Heart Association Guidelines for Percutaneous Transluminal Coronary Angioplasty and Coronary Bypass Surgery provide a detailed analysis of many of these issues.

Selection of Patients

SINGLE-VESSEL DISEASE

Percutaneous revascularization is an attractive option for many symptomatic patients who are anatomically suitable, having single-vessel coronary disease. It is important, however, to remember that there are no large studies comparing angioplasty with surgery in this group of patients and none that show a statistically significant survival benefit of angioplasty compared with surgery or medical therapy.

MULTIVESSEL DISEASE

Rational selection of patients requires a careful analysis of multiple issues, including a risk-benefit assessment of each ischemia-producing lesion, a projection of the possible completeness and durability of the physiologic revascularization, and an estimate of resource consumption compared with surgery and medical therapy. In the experience of EAST, 71 percent of index segments were revascularized in PTCA patients. Culprit-lesion angioplasty is clearly an accepted strategy, but care must be taken to avoid significant residual ischemia after intervention. Recently published data from BARI indicated that planned incomplete revascularization was unrelated to 5-year risk of cardiac death or death/MI but was related to risk of CABG.

The risks of percutaneous coronary intervention are increased in the presence of unstable angina, advanced age, poor left ventricular function, extensive coronary disease, comorbid conditions, and female gender.

Selection of Lesions

LESION CHARACTERISTICS

The importance of coronary stenosis angiographic morphology in predicting the outcome of coronary angioplasty is reflected in the American College of Cardiology/American Heart Association PTCA Guidelines. In an effort to update this classification based on results of contemporary coronary intervention using stents and IIb/IIIa platelet inhibitors, Ellis and colleagues analyzed results from 10,907 lesions and proposed a new classification scheme for risk stratification (see Table 16-2). Nine preintervention variables were independently correlated with adverse outcome.

PREDICTORS OF RESTENOSIS

Lesion characteristics that were associated with increased restenosis rates following balloon angioplasty alone or after stent implantation include length, total occlusion, vessel size < 3 mm, ostial location, previous angioplasty to the same site, and saphenous vein grafts.

IN-STENT RESTENOSIS

One of the most vexing lesions confronting the interventionalist is in-stent restenosis. This lesion is solely the result of neointimal proliferation as opposed to a combination of negative remodeling and intimal proliferation seen with nonstented lesions. Recurrence rates after repeat angioplasty have ranged from 20 to 80 percent, depending on the length and severity of the in-stent restenosis process.

TABLE 16-2
NEW RISK-ASSESSMENT SCHEMA*

Strongest correlates	Nonchronic total occlusion
	Degenerated saphenous vein graft (SVG)
Moderately strong correlates	Length $\geq$ 10 mm
	Lumen irregularity
	Large filling defect
	Calcium + angle $\geq$ 45 degrees
	Eccentric
	Severe calcification
	SVG age $\geq$ 10 years
Highest risk	Either of strongest correlates
High risk	$\geq$3 moderate correlates and the absence of strong correlates
Moderate risk	1–2 moderate correlates and the absence of strong correlates
Low risk	No risk factors

*Based on analysis of 10,907 lesions treated in the stent and IIb/IIIa era.
SOURCE: Ellis SG, Guetta V, Miller D, et al: Relation between lesion characteristics and risk with percutaneous intervention in the stent and glycoprotein IIb/IIIa era: An analysis of results from 10,907 lesions and proposal for new classification scheme. *Circulation* 1999; 100:1971–1976.

Debulking with atherectomy and laser techniques has been advocated, and although safe and associated with a larger postprocedure minimal lumen diameter (MLD), it has not been shown to be superior to balloon angioplasty. The investigational use of radiation to inhibit neointimal proliferation has produced the most promising strategy for its potential use in the treatment of this difficult problem.

SELECTION OF DEVICES
Table 16-3 outlines the various technologies compared with balloon dilatation.

PRIMARY STENTING
In our hospital, stents are usually selected for primary treatment of complex lesions, aortoostial sites, shelf-like lesions, early recurrence, total occlusions, and lesions with high restenosis rates (proximal LAD and saphenous vein grafts).

TABLE 16-3

NEW CORONARY INTERVENTIONAL STRATEGIES COMPARED WITH BALLOON ANGIOPLASTY

Technique	Indications	Contraindications	Advantages and Limitations
Balloon angioplasty	Focal stenosis	Insignificant narrowing, no ischemia, unimportant artery	Broad applicability, lower cost; poor outcome in thrombotic, ostial, and calcified lesions; significant restenosis
Stents	Focal stenosis	Heavy calcification or thrombus, vessel diameter <2.5 mm	Reduced emergency CABG and restenosis; more expensive, rare stent thrombosis
Directional atherectomy	Focal noncalcified	Diffuse disease, severe tortuosity or bend	Debulks, reduced restenosis; more frequent non-Q-wave MI, more expensive, technically difficult
Rotational atherectomy	Focal calcified stenosis, ostial site	Thrombus, large plaque burden, severe tortuosity or bend	Effective in calcified lesions, reduced elastic recoil; more expensive, similar restenosis, transient left ventricular dysfunction
Laser	Ostial lesion, SVG, in-stent restenosis	Severe calcification, tortuosity or bend	Debulks effectively; increased cost, similar restenosis
Transluminal extraction atherectomy	Thrombotic lesion, bulky SVG lesion	Severe tortuosity or bend, calcification	Thrombus and plaque removed; high complication rate in native vessels, distal embolization
Rheolytic thrombectomy	Thrombus	No thrombus	Effective thrombus removal; no plaque removal

KEY: SVG = saphenous vein graft; CABG = coronary artery bypass grafting; MI = myocardial infarction.

ATHERECTOMY

Suitable lesions are generally proximal in vessels ≥ 3 mm in diameter and have features that predict poor outcome with primary stenting, such as high-bulk stenoses, ostial site, proximal LAD and protected left main coronary lesions, including carefully selected bifurcation lesions. In general, moderate angiographic calcification and significant superficial calcification on intracoronary ultrasound are predictors of failure. Rotational atherectomy has proved useful in the presence of calcium, in the treatment of aortoostial and branch ostial lesions, and in nondilatable lesions.

Transluminal extraction atherectomy, which is unique in its ability to cut and aspirate plaque and thrombus, is occasionally used in saphenous vein grafts containing thrombus.

LASER ANGIOPLASTY

Some continue to use laser angioplasty to debulk in-stent restenosis lesions, but its use is not widespread.

PERFORMANCE OF CORONARY INTERVENTION

Current guidelines recommend that cardiologists who wish to become competent in coronary intervention receive special training in diagnostic and therapeutic catheterization during an additional year after the standard fellowship training program and maintain skills by performance of a minimum of 75 procedures per year. Adequate case mix is an important aspect of a physician's training in interventional cardiology.

Interventional Laboratory

Most studies also suggest that laboratory procedural volume is important and inversely related to adverse procedural outcomes.

The Coronary Interventional Procedure

Prior to coronary intervention, patients receive an explanation of the procedure, including the operator's estimate of success, possible complications, risks, and benefits.

Antiplatelet therapy is used routinely. The therapy most widely used is aspirin, 160 to 325 mg daily. Patients in whom stenting is planned also receive clopidogrel, usually in a 300- to 525-mg loading dose, unless pretreatment for several days has been performed. The platelet glycoprotein IIb/IIIa receptor blockers are frequently used, and patients with a high risk of thrombotic events are targeted. Patients selected for use of a low-osmolar contrast agent include those with renal insufficiency or severe left ventricular dysfunction. Nonionic agents are generally used for patients with known allergy to the available ionic agents or with a history of severe bradycardia with ionic agents.

RESULTS OF CORONARY INTERVENTION

The technical performance of balloon angioplasty, atherectomy, and stenting is beyond the scope of this handbook. Experienced interventional cardiologists should offer the best insight to the performance of the procedure and should be valuable consultants in the process of determining which patients are expected to benefit from interventions. Experienced operators should achieve primary success rates in excess of 95 percent in ideal proximal lesions, compared with a reduced success rate of approximately 75 percent in recent (<3 months) total occlusions or in attempts to treat fibrotic, calcified, eccentric stenoses located distally in tortuous coronary arteries. In all techniques, including stenting, lesion characteristics are a major determinant of the outcome of the procedure. Selection for interventional procedures should always include the expected long-term as well as the acute outcomes.

Complications

Patients undergoing PCI are subject to the same complications encountered with the performance of coronary arteriography. In addition, because instrumentation of the atherosclerotic lesion takes place, coronary artery dissection, thrombus formation, and coronary artery spasm may occur, leading to acute occlusion of the coronary artery or of side branches arising from it. Atheroembolism may occur and lead to myocardial infarction in an otherwise successful procedure. Occlusion of the treated artery is the most common serious complication of coronary angioplasty and accounts for most of the morbidity and mortality related to the procedure.

The use of stents in the course of a failing angioplasty and prospectively in patients with unfavorable anatomy has significantly reduced the risk of urgent bypass surgery and Q-wave myocardial infarction (MI). New complications specifically related to the use of nonballoon devices include coronary perforation, distal atheroembolization, arterial access complications increased by the use of GP IIb/IIIa blockers, and "domino stenting" (additional stents to treat end-of-stent dissections).

FUTURE DIRECTIONS

The future of coronary intervention is bright indeed. Restenosis, which has been reduced by stenting of de novo and restenotic lesions, remains a challenge that is currently being addressed on multiple fronts with good prospects for meaningful solutions.

SUGGESTED READING

Douglas JS Jr, King SB III: Percutaneous coronary intervention. In: Fuster V, Alexander RW, O'Rourke RA, et al (eds): *Hurst's The Heart,* 10th ed. New York: McGraw-Hill; 2001:1437–1469.

Eagle KA, Guyton RA, Davidoff R, et al: ACC/AHA guidelines for coronary artery bypass graft surgery: executive summary and recommendations. A report of the American College of Cardiology/American Heart Association Task Force on Practice Guidelines (Committee to Revise the 1991 Guidelines for Coronary Artery Bypass Graft Surgery). *Circulation* 1999; 100: 1464–1480.

Fischman DL, Leon MB, Baim DS, et al: A randomized comparison of coronary-stent placement and balloon angioplasty in treatment of coronary artery disease. *N Engl J Med* 1994; 331: 496–501.

Fragmin and Fast Revascularization during InStability in Coronary artery disease Investigators. Invasive compared with noninvasive treatment in unstable coronary-artery disease: FRISC II prospective randomised multicentre study. *Lancet* 1999; 354:708–715.

Hannan EL, Racz MJ, McCallister BD, et al: A comparison of three-year survival after coronary artery bypass graft surgery and percutaneous transluminal coronary angioplasty. *J Am Coll Cardiol* 1999; 33:63–72.

Holmes DR, Hirshfeld J, Faxon D, et al: ACC expert consensus document on coronary artery stents: Document of the American College of Cardiology. *J Am Coll Cardiol* 1998; 32:1471–1482.

King SB III, Kosinski AS, Guyton RA, et al: Eight-year mortality in the Emory Angioplasty versus Surgery Trial (EAST). *J Am Coll Cardiol* 2000; 35:1116–1121.

Ryan TJ, Bauman WB, Kennedy JW, et al: Guidelines for percutaneous transluminal coronary angioplasty: A report of the American Heart Association/American College of Cardiology Task Force on Assessment of Diagnostic and Therapeutic Cardiovascular Procedures (Committee on Percutaneous

Transluminal Coronary Angioplasty). *Circulation* 1993; 88: 2987–3007.

Serruys PW, de Jaegere P, Kiemeneij F, et al: A comparison of balloon expandable stent implantation with balloon angioplasty in patients with coronary artery disease. *N Engl J Med* 1994; 331:489–495.

The BARI Investigators: Seven-year outcome in the Bypass Angioplasty Revascularization Investigation (BARI) by treatment and diabetic status. *J Am Coll Cardiol* 2000; 35:1122–1129.

CHAPTER

17

MECHANICAL INTERVENTIONS IN ACUTE MYOCARDIAL INFARCTION

William O'Neill
Bruce R. Brodie

INTRODUCTION

In the last two decades there have been extraordinary advances in the emergency management of patients with ST-segment elevation and acute myocardial infarction. In 1985, those patients presenting within 12 h of symptom onset had 13 percent in-hospital mortality with conventional care. Currently, in-hospital mortality rates of 7 percent are reported with modern thrombolytic treatment, and even more impressive 2.5 percent mortality rates are achieved with balloon angioplasty–mediated reperfusion. These heartening outcomes have reestablished mechanical reperfusion therapy as an attractive treatment option for patients with acute myocardial infarction, especially where logistics allows this approach. This chapter summarizes the randomized clinical trials that serve as the scientific basis for recommending mechanical reperfusion therapy.

PRIMARY ANGIOPLASTY

Comparison of Outcomes with Thrombolytic Therapy

RANDOMIZED TRIALS

In 1997, Weaver and colleagues published a metanalysis of ten randomized trials comparing thrombolytic therapy with primary angioplasty and comprising a total of 2606 patients. The largest of these trials were the PAMI-1 Trial, the Zwolle Trial, and the GUSTO IIb

Trial. In the Weaver metanalysis, primary angioplasty was associated with a lower in-hospital mortality (4.4 versus 6.5 percent, $p = 0.02$), a lower incidence of nonfatal reinfarction (2.9 versus 5.3 percent, $p = 0.002$), and a lower incidence of death or nonfatal reinfarction (7.2 versus 11.9 percent, $p = 0.001$). Primary angioplasty was also associated with a significantly lower incidence of stroke (0.7 versus 2.0 percent, $p = 0.007$) and hemorrhagic stroke (0.01 versus 1.1 percent, $p = 0.0005$). The survival benefit of primary angioplasty compared with thrombolytic therapy reported in this metanalysis was substantial (21 lives saved per 1000 patients treated) and compared favorably with the survival benefit of thrombolytic therapy compared with placebo reported by the Fibrinolytic Therapy Trialists' (FTT) Collaborative Group (19 lives saved per 1000 patients treated).

IMPORTANCE OF TIMI FLOW

The importance of achieving timely restoration of normal blood flow in the infarct artery in patients with acute myocardial infarction was convincingly demonstrated in the GUSTO Trial. Patients with normal (TIMI-3) antegrade flow in the infarct artery at 90 min after treatment had the greatest left ventricular function at follow-up catheterization and the lowest 30-day mortality (Table 17-1). Patients with slow (TIMI-2) flow had a left ventricular ejection fraction and 30-day mortality significantly worse than that of patients with TIMI-3 flow and similar to that of patients with no flow (TIMI 0-1). A similar relationship between TIMI flow and mortality has been found with primary angioplasty (Table 17-1). These data indicate that only restoration of TIMI-3 flow is associated with optimal outcomes and that only TIMI-3 flow should be regarded as "true patency." A comparison of the rates of TIMI-3 flow with various reperfusion strategies in the GUSTO Trial and with primary angioplasty from the PAMI-1

TABLE 17-1

RELATIONSHIP BETWEEN TIMI FLOW AND 30-DAY
MORTALITY AFTER REPERFUSION THERAPY FOR
ACUTE MYOCARDIAL INFARCTION

	30-Day Mortality	
TIMI Flow	GUSTO-1 (Lytic Therapy)	PAMI-1 and PAMI-2 (Primary PTCA)
TIMI 0–1	8.9%	17.2%
TIMI 2	7.4%	7.6%
TIMI 3	4.4%	2.1%

and PAMI-2 Trials are shown in Fig. 17-1. The ability of primary angioplasty to achieve significantly higher TIMI-3 flow rates than thrombolytic therapy probably explains most of the mortality advantage seen with primary angioplasty. Indeed, there appears to be a tight inverse relationship between short-term mortality and the ability to achieve TIMI-3 flow with various thrombolytic regimens and with primary angioplasty (Fig. 17-2). Newer thrombolytic strategies combining low-dose thrombolytics with platelet glycoprotein IIb/IIIa inhibitors have shown improved TIMI-3 flow rates, but these rates are still well below the TIMI-3 flow rates achieved with primary angioplasty. These strategies remain to be tested in large clinical trials.

LATE CLINICAL AND ANGIOGRAPHIC OUTCOMES

A comparison of late clinical outcomes of patients with acute myocardial infarction (AMI) treated with primary angioplasty versus thrombolytic therapy has been provided by the PAMI investigators. The initial benefit of primary angioplasty in reducing death and reinfarction was maintained out to 2 years with event-free survival curves that remain nearly parallel after hospital discharge. Primary angioplasty was also associated with lower hospital readmission rates (59 versus 69 percent, $p = 0.035$) and lower rates of target vessel revascularization with either angioplasty or bypass surgery (33 versus 54 percent, $p = 0.001$) compared with tissue plasminogen activator (t-PA). More recently, the Zwolle group has demonstrated that the early mortality and reinfarction benefit is maintained over 5 years' follow-up.

The restenosis rate at the 6-month follow-up angiography after primary angioplasty is similar to that after elective angioplasty and occurs in 24 to 46 percent of patients. While this remains a significant clinical and economic problem with primary angioplasty, only about one-half of patients with restenosis require repeat target vessel revascularization, and restenosis does not interfere with recovery of left ventricular function as long as the infarct artery remains patent. The use of stents with primary angioplasty, like elective angioplasty, has significantly reduced restenosis rates. The Stent PAMI Trial showed a reduction in restenosis rates from 34 percent with angioplasty to 20 percent with stenting.

ADJUNCTIVE THERAPY

Stents

Numerous studies have now documented the safety of stent deployment in the setting of AMI. Several studies with first-generation stents have documented superior outcomes with stenting as compared

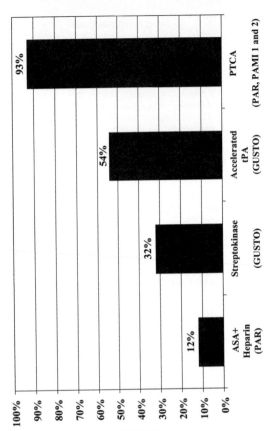

FIGURE 17-1
Frequency of achieving TIMI-3 flow in the infarct artery with aspirin and heparin thrombolytic therapy (measured 90 min after treatment) and primary percutaneous transluminal coronary angioplasty (PTCA) (measured immediately after intervention).

FIGURE 17-2

Relationship between in-hospital or 30-day mortality and the frequency of achieving TIMI-3 flow measured acutely in the infarct artery with several thrombolytic strategies from the GUSTO Trial and several primary percutaneous transluminal coronary angioplasty (PTCA) trials.

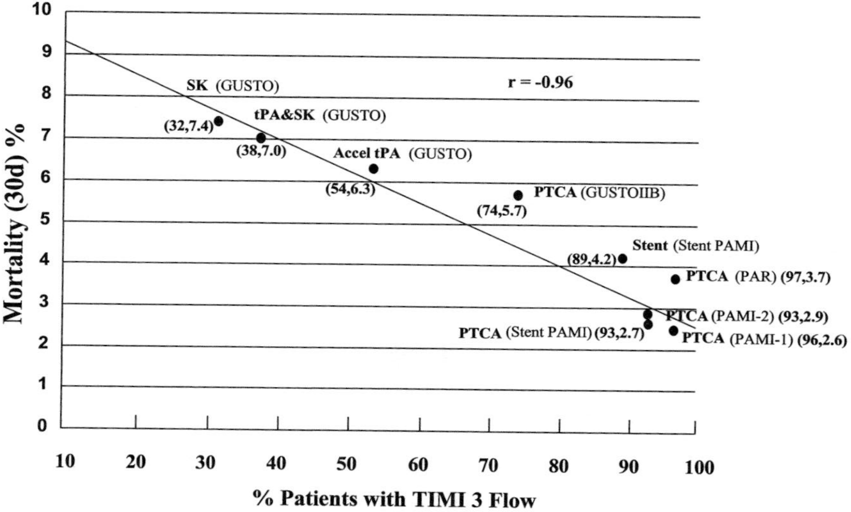

TABLE 17-2

RANDOMIZED TRIALS COMPARING PRIMARY STENTING
WITH PRIMARY PERCUTANEOUS TRANSLUMINAL
CORONARY ANGIOPLASTY IN ACUTE
MYOCARDIAL INFARCTION[a]

	PTCA (%)	Stent (%)	p Value
Zwolle Trial ($N = 227$)			
Death	2.7	1.7	NS
Reinfarction	7.0	0.9	0.04
TVR[b]	17.4	3.6	0.002
Composite	20.0	5.4	0.001
GRAMI Trial ($N = 104$)			
Death	7.6	3.8	NS
Reinfarction	7.6		NS
Recurrent	11.5	0	0.05
Ischemia			
Composite	19.2	3.8	0.03
FRESCO Trial ($N = 150$)			
Death	0	1.3	NS
Reinfarction	2.7	1.3	NS
TVR	25.3	6.7	0.002
Composite	28.0	9.3	0.003
Stent PAMI Trial ($N = 900$)			
Death	2.7	4.2	NS
Reinfarction	2.2	2.4	NS
Ischemic TVR	17.0	7.7	0.0001
Composite	20.1	12.6	0.01

[a]Outcomes are at 6 months in all trials except the GRAMI Trial, which lists
in-hospital outcomes. The Gianturco-Rubin stent was used in the GRAMI and
FRESCO Trials, the Palmaz-Shatz stent in the Zwolle Trial, and the heparin-
coated Palmaz-Shatz stent in the Stent PAMI Trial.
[b]Target vessel revascularization.

with angioplasty alone, with lower composite endpoints due primarily to less target vessel revascularization or less recurrent
ischemia (Table 17-2). The largest randomized trial, the Stent PAMI
Trial with 900 patients, has documented lower restenosis rates
(20 versus 34 percent, $p = 0.001$), including less reocclusion

(5 versus 9 percent, $p = 0.04$) and less ischemia-driven target vessel revascularization (8 versus 17 percent, $p = 0.0001$) with stenting versus angioplasty alone, but there was no difference in mortality or reinfarction (Table 17-2). Currently, stenting cannot be recommended for routine use with primary angioplasty, but should be used in selected patients especially when there are suboptimal results or dissection following angioplasty. The results of large ongoing trials with newer stents may provide data that will extend these indications.

Platelet Inhibitors

Several trials have documented the efficacy of glycoprotein IIb/IIIa platelet inhibition during elective coronary intervention. The RAPPORT Trial evaluated platelet inhibition with abciximab in patients with AMI undergoing primary angioplasty and found a significant reduction in the 30-day composite endpoint (Table 17-3). However, by 6 months, there was no difference in outcomes (Table 17-3). Also, the use of high-dose heparin in concert with prolonged sheath dwell times resulted in an excess of major bleeding episodes. Two European trials, the ADMIRAL Trial and the Munich Trial, have evaluated abciximab in patients with AMI undergoing primary stenting, and both have found a significant reduction in composite endpoints with abciximab compared with placebo. The CADILLAC Trial has evaluated the efficacy of abciximab in 2000 patients with AMI undergoing either primary angioplasty or primary stenting. Preliminary analysis suggests that no mortality benefit is achieved by the addition of abciximab therapy. This study should provide efficacy as well as cost data that will help to define the role of platelet inhibition with primary angioplasty for acute myocardial infarction.

Intraaortic Balloon Counterpulsation

Clinical studies have shown that the use of intraaortic balloon counterpulsation results in augmentation of systemic pressure, reduction in preload and afterload, and an increase in coronary blood flow velocity. This has given hope that intraaortic balloon counterpulsation may improve outcomes in patients with AMI. Unfortunately, randomized trials in high-risk patients with AMI have shown little or no benefit when intraaortic balloon counterpulsation is used alone without concomitant reperfusion or revascularization. Several studies have evaluated the prophylactic use of intraaortic balloon counterpulsation after reperfusion with primary or rescue angioplasty in high-risk patients. Initial studies suggested benefit in terms of less infarct artery reocclusion and less recurrent ischemia, but larger, more

TABLE 17-3

RANDOMIZED TRIALS COMPARING ABCIXIMAB VERSUS
PLACEBO WITH PRIMARY ANGIOPLASTY OR PRIMARY
STENTING FOR ACUTE MYOCARDIAL INFARCTION[a]

	Abciximab (%)	Placebo (%)	p Value
RAPPORT Trial (30 day) ($N = 483$)			
Death	2.5	2.1	NS
Reinfarction	3.3	4.1	NS
Urgent TVR[b]	1.7	6.6	0.006
Composite	5.8	11.2	0.03
RAPPORT Trial (6 month) ($N = 483$)			
Death	4.1	4.5	NS
Reinfarction	6.6	7.4	NS
Any TVR	20.7	21.9	NS
Composite	28.2	28.1	NS
ADMIRAL Trial (30-day) ($N = 300$)			
Death	3.3	4.4	
Reinfarction	2.0	4.7	
Urgent TVR	4.7	10.0	
Composite	10.0	19.3	0.03
Munich Trial (30-day) ($N = 401$)			
Death	2.5	6.0	0.08
Reinfarction	0.5	1.5	NS
TLR[c]	3.0	5.0	NS
Composite	5.0	10.5	0.04

[a] Patients in the ADMIRAL and Munich Trials were treated with primary stenting.
[b] Target vessel revascularization.
[c] Target lesion revascularization.

recent studies—including the large PAMI-2 Trial—have shown little or no benefit. The results of these trials and the advent of coronary stenting, which has reduced the incidence of reocclusion and recurrent ischemia, have diminished the role of intraaortic balloon counterpulsation after primary angioplasty in hemodynamically stable patients. Intraaortic balloon counterpulsation still has a role in hemodynamically unstable patients with congestive heart failure or shock prior to primary angioplasty and in patients with mechanical complications of acute infarction or anatomy that is unsuitable for percutaneous coronary intervention as a bridge to surgery. There may also be a role for prophylactic intraaortic balloon pumping before primary angioplasty in selected high-risk patients to prevent hemodynamic deterioration.

RESCUE ANGIOPLASTY

In the early 1990s, intravenous thrombolytic therapy became the overwhelmingly preferred reperfusion strategy. Unfortunately, with current fibrinolytic regimens, successful reperfusion after thrombolytic therapy is achieved in only 54 to 81 percent of patients, and TIMI-3 flow is achieved in only 29 to 54 percent of patients. Rescue angioplasty, the mechanical reopening of an occluded infarct artery after failed thrombolysis, has been used as adjunctive therapy in an attempt to improve outcomes in patients with failed thrombolysis. Despite the intuitive benefit of this approach, the value of rescue angioplasty remains controversial, especially given the disappointing results of the TAMI, TIMI-IIa, and European cooperative studies.

Numerous observational studies have documented that rescue angioplasty can achieve successful reperfusion in 82 to 92 percent of patients with occluded infarct arteries after failed thrombolysis, but reocclusion of the infarct artery has been common (18 percent in Ellis's meta-analysis), and recovery of left ventricular function has been variable. Mortality associated with unsuccessful rescue angioplasty has been very high, and mortality associated with all rescue angioplasty (successful and unsuccessful) has been no better than in patients with failed thrombolysis who do not undergo rescue angioplasty and has been higher than in patients with successful thrombolysis. The lack of benefit in these observational studies with rescue angioplasty may be related to selection bias, since rescue angioplasty is often selected for higher-risk patients. It is not clear whether the particularly high mortality in patients with failed rescue angioplasty is due to additional associated high-risk features or if there may be harmful effects from the rescue angioplasty procedure itself.

Two moderately sized randomized trials have evaluated the efficacy of rescue angioplasty. The TAMI-5 Trial randomized 575 patients with acute infarction treated with t-PA, urokinase, or both to emergency angiography with rescue angioplasty for failed thrombolysis versus conservative care. Rescue angioplasty was performed in 18 percent of the emergency catheterization group, with a success rate of 83 percent. At hospital discharge, the emergency catheterization group had a slightly higher infarct artery patency rate (94 versus 90 percent, $p = 0.07$), better regional wall motion, and less recurrent ischemia, but there was no difference in mortality, reinfarction, or global left ventricular ejection fraction.

The Randomized Evaluation of Salvage Angioplasty with Combined Utilization of Endpoints (RESCUE) Trial studied 151 patients with first anterior wall MI treated with thrombolytic therapy who had an occluded infarct artery within 8 h of the onset of chest pain. These patients were randomized to rescue angioplasty versus conservative care. There was no difference in left ventricular ejection fraction at 30 days (40 versus 39 percent, $p = $ NS), but the rescue angioplasty group had a lower mortality (5.1 versus 9.6 percent, $p = 0.18$), less congestive heart failure (1.3 versus 7.0 percent, $p = 0.11$), a lower composite of death and congestive heart failure (6.4 versus 16.6 percent, $p = 0.05$), and better exercise left ventricular ejection fraction (43 versus 38 percent, $p = 0.04$). These benefits occurred despite what the authors felt was a strong investigator bias not to randomize patients presenting very early in the course of their infarction.

Rescue angioplasty is associated with lower angiographic success rates and higher reocclusion rates than primary angioplasty, especially after tPA, and this limits its effectiveness. Recent studies using coronary stenting with rescue angioplasty have reported high procedural success rates and low reocclusion rates. The largest of these studies reported a success rate of 98 percent in 167 patients, a reocclusion rate of only 1.2 percent, and combined endpoint of death or reinfarction of 1.4 percent at 30 days in nonshock patients. Glycoprotein IIb/IIIa platelet inhibitors may also potentially enhance outcomes with rescue angioplasty, but this has not been well studied, and the risk of bleeding when aspirin, heparin, ticlopidine, or clopidogrel and glycoprotein IIb/IIIa platelet inhibitors are used in conjunction with thrombolytic therapy may be high.

Based on the available data, acute angiography with rescue angioplasty should be considered in patients with anterior or large MI who are thought to have failed thrombolysis, as evidenced by persistent chest pain, lack of resolution of ST segment elevation, or hemodynamic compromise at greater than 90 min after treatment.

SUGGESTED READING

Grines CL, Brown KF, Marco J, et al: A comparison of immediate angioplasty with thrombolytic therapy for acute myocardial infarction. *N Engl J Med* 1993; 328:673.

Grines C, Cox D, Stone G, et al: Coronary angioplasty with or without stent implantation for acute myocardial infarction. Stent Primary Angioplasty in Myocardial Infarction Study Group. *N Engl J Med* 1999; 341:1949.

GUSTO Angiographic Investigators: The effects of tissue plasminogen activator, streptokinase, or both, on coronary artery patency, ventricular function, and survival after acute myocardial infarction. *N Engl J Med* 1993; 329:1615.

O'Neill W, Brodie BR: Mechanical interventions in acute myocardial infarction. In: Fuster V, Alexander RW, O'Rourke RA, et al (eds): *Hurst's The Heart*, 10th ed. New York: McGraw-Hill; 2001:1471–1488.

Stone GW, Marsalese D, Brodie BR: A prospective, randomized evaluation of prophylactic intra-aortic balloon counterpulsation in high risk patients with acute myocardial infarction treated with primary angioplasty. *J Am Coll Cardiol* 1997; 29:1459.

The CADILLAC Trial, presented at the Annual Scientific Session of the American Heart Association, 1999.

The Global Use of Strategies to Open Occluded Coronary Arteries in Acute Coronary Syndromes (GUSTO IIb) Angioplasty Substudy Investigators: A clinical trial comparing primary coronary angioplasty with tissue plasminogen activator for acute myocardial infarction. *N Engl J Med* 1997; 336:1621.

Weaver WD, Simes RJ, Betriu A, et al: Comparison of primary coronary angioplasty and intravenous thrombolytic therapy for acute myocardial infarction: A quantitative review. *JAMA* 1997; 278:2093.

Zijlstra F, Jan de Boer M, Hoorntje JCA, et al: A comparison of immediate coronary angioplasty with intravenous streptokinase in acute myocardial infarction. *N Engl J Med* 1993; 328:680.

CHAPTER

18

HYPERTENSION: DIAGNOSIS, EVALUATION, AND TREATMENT

Henry R. Black
William J. Elliott
George L. Bakris

INTRODUCTION

Hypertension is the most common disease-specific reason that Americans visit a physician. Hypertension is expected to have an even greater impact on the health of the public as more of the world becomes westernized. Hypertension [or high blood pressure (BP)] is among the leading causes of morbidity and mortality throughout the world and is a powerful risk factor that increases the risk of a wide variety of cardiovascular diseases.

DEFINITION

BP is a continuous variable; whatever cutoff value we use to define hypertension is arbitrary. In the past several decades, the definition of hypertension changed from $\geq 160/95$ mmHg to $\geq 140/90$ mmHg. Most authorities agree on several important principles:

- Hypertension is defined by either systolic or diastolic BP.
- Office BPs have traditionally been the basis for diagnosis, although other techniques are sometimes helpful (see below).
- Assessing the level of BP is insufficient, since the BP should be interpreted in the context of the absolute risk of the individual, which is most easily estimated by evaluating target-organ damage (TOD) and comorbidities (Tables 18-1 and 18-2).

351

TABLE 18-1

STRATIFICATION OF RISK GROUPS IN HYPERTENSIVE PATIENTS

	Group A	Group B	Group C
Number of risk factors	None	More than one but not diabetes mellitus	Diabetes mellitus
Target-organ damage	Absent	Absent	Present
Cardiovascular disease	Absent	Absent	Present

DIAGNOSIS OF HYPERTENSION

Currently, the terminology introduced by Korotkoff is used: systolic BP is recognized when clear and repetitive tapping sounds are heard; diastolic BP is recorded when the sounds disappear. Exceptions to

TABLE 18-2

INITIAL TREATMENT RECOMMENDATIONS IN HYPERTENSIVE PATIENTS

Blood Pressure Stage	Blood Pressure, mmHg	Group A	Group B	Group C
High normal	130–139/ 85–89	LM* only	LM only	LM + drug therapy
Stage 1	140–159/ 80–99	LM × 12 months	LM × 6 months	LM + drug therapy
Stage 2	160–179/ 100–109	LM + drug therapy	LM + drug therapy	LM + drug therapy
Stage 3	≥180/ ≥110	LM + drug therapy	LM + drug therapy	LM + drug therapy

*Lifestyle modification.

these general rules are still recognized for patients who have audible sounds even down to 0 mmHg or in obstetrics: in both situations, the "muffling" of the sounds (Korotkoff phase IV) is recorded, either in addition to the phase V measurement or as the diastolic BP, respectively.

Techniques of Measuring Blood Pressure

The proper technique of accurate BP measurement is typically taught very early during medical training but then seldom followed. Many expert panels have made recommendations regarding methodology of BP measurement and these frequently do not agree in all details, but several general principles can be distilled:

- The cuff size appropriate for the patient's arm circumference should be used. The deflation rate of the column of mercury should be 2 to 3 mmHg/s.
- Multiple measurements should be made on different occasions to decide whether a person should have his or her BP lowered.

BP measurements have much intrinsic variability. Several steps can be taken to minimize this variability, including:

- Taking multiple measurements, especially when the pulse is irregular.
- Centering the bladder of the cuff over the brachial artery, with its lower edge within 2.5 cm of the antecubital fossa. The subject should be resting silently and comfortably (with back support if seated) for at least 5 min prior to the measurement.
- The subject should abstain from drinking caffeine- or alcohol-containing beverages or tobacco use within 30 min prior to a BP measurement.
- BP should be measured when the rectum and bladder are not full. The arm should be supported at the level of the heart.
- To listen, the stethoscope is placed over the brachial artery, with minimal pressure exerted by the bell of the stethoscope on the skin. The cuff is inflated to 20 mmHg higher than the pressure at which the palpable pulse at the radial artery disappears. A properly calibrated sphygmomanometer should be used.
- "Terminal digit preference" (more than 20 percent of measurements ending with a specific even digit) is best avoided.
- BP should be measured in both arms initially and in the arm with the higher BP thereafter if the difference is greater than 10/5 mmHg.

Home Blood Pressure Measurements

There are now many devices available for obtaining accurate and reproducible BP measurements outside the traditional medical environment. Home BP readings are typically lower (by an average of 12/7 mmHg) and correlate better with TOD and risk of future mortality than office measurements. Home BP readings should be interpreted cautiously, carefully, and conservatively. Several preliminary reports show benefit to supplementing office BP measurements with home readings, but clinical trial and insurance industry data are all based on BPs measured by trained observers.

Ambulatory Blood Pressure Monitoring

Automatic BP recorders that measure BP throughout the day and night are now widely available and have been carefully studied. The use of these devices by healthcare practitioners in the United States has been extremely limited, mostly due to lack of reimbursement by third-party payers. Ambulatory BP readings correlate better than home or office readings with TOD, left ventricular hypertrophy (LVH), and the incidence of cardiovascular events. Outcome studies from Italy, Ohasama (Japan), and Europe have all demonstrated the excess risk defined by abnormal ambulatory blood pressure monitoring (ABPM) profiles (e.g., "nondipping" of BP at night).

"White-Coat Hypertension"

About 20 percent of the hypertensive population have BP readings that are considerably higher in the doctor's office or hospital than those measured in other settings. The consequences of this phenomenon are unclear: one school of thought suggests that the stimuli of a clinical setting raise BP only transiently and reversibly; the opposing view is that "white-coat hypertensives" will all eventually develop sustained hypertension. How and when to treat such individuals is even less clear. Lifestyle modifications are recommended, but monitoring of drug therapy with yearly ambulatory BP measurements is unlikely to be cost-effective.

EVALUATION OF THE HYPERTENSIVE PATIENT

There are six key issues that must be addressed during the initial office evaluation of a person with elevated BP readings:

- Documenting an accurate diagnosis of hypertension (see above).
- Defining the presence or absence of TOD related to hypertension.

- Screening for other cardiovascular risk factors that often accompany hypertension.
- Stratifying risk for cardiovascular disease (e.g., according to risk group A, B, or C in Joint National Committee VI; see Table 18-1).
- Assessing whether the person is likely to have an identifiable cause of hypertension (secondary hypertension) and should have further diagnostic testing to confirm or exclude the diagnosis.
- Obtaining data that may be helpful in choice of therapy.

Routine Evaluation of All Hypertensive Patients

The recommendations of JNC VI and other expert panels limit the initial evaluation of a hypertensive patient to physical examination, BUN/creatinine, electrolytes, urinalysis, and an electrocardiogram (ECG). A directed physical examination searches for clues that might indicate an identifiable secondary cause of hypertension—for example, an abdominal bruit suggesting renal artery stenosis or an abdominal mass that could be a pheochromocytoma. Direct ophthalmoscopy can assess both the severity and duration of hypertension. Antihypertensive drug therapy reduces vision loss, retinal hemorrhages, and the need for laser photocoagulation, particularly among diabetic hypertensives.

Cardiac Evaluation

Although physical examination of the heart is useful in detecting valvular disorders or an atrial gallop (S_4) associated with hypertensive heart disease, a key part of the laboratory evaluation is testing for LVH. The ECG is recommended primarily because of the high cost of echocardiography, a more sensitive and specific test. A "limited echo" has been recommended as one way around this problem but is not widely available in the United States. LVH is often thought of as the "hemoglobin A_{1c} of BP," since it is an objective measure of both the severity and duration of elevated BP. In the Framingham Heart Study, ECG-evidence of LVH was associated with an approximately threefold increase in incidence of cardiovascular events. LVH detected by echocardiogram appears to be even a better predictor of future cardiovascular events. One reason echocardiography is not recommended for routine evaluation is the high intrinsic variability of a single echocardiogram (about 10 to 15 percent in left ventricular myocardial infarction). The important unanswered question about LVH is the best way to reverse it. Several meta-analyses have suggested that, with the exception of direct vasodilators, any drug therapy that reduces BP is likely to have a beneficial effect on reducing LVH.

Renal Evaluation

Current recommendations for evaluation of renal function include a measurement of blood urea nitrogen (BUN) and creatinine and a dipstick to detect red or white cells, casts, or proteinuria. Some authorities recommend the special dipstick for microalbuminuria (protein excretion between 30 and 300 mg/day) because microalbuminuria is an independent risk factor for cardiovascular events, especially in diabetics. Like LVH, microalbuminuria may also be a marker for previous BP control, since all agents except dihydropyridine (DHP) calcium antagonists (CAs), and central or peripheral sympathetic blockers reduce albuminuria.

Evaluation of the Vasculature

Currently, palpation of the peripheral pulses is the only examination of the vascular tree for most hypertensive patients, despite the nearly universal finding of reduced arterial compliance in hypertensive people over 40 years of age. "Pseudohypertension" occurs mostly in heavily calcified arteries that cannot be compressed using the usual BP cuff. Because making the diagnosis requires a potentially dangerous and expensive intra-arterial measurement, few clinicians routinely check for and diagnose pseudohypertension. This does not diminish the importance of treating older individuals with decreased vascular compliance (a hallmark of isolated systolic hypertension), as clinical trials have shown impressive benefits of drug therapy in this condition.

Evaluation for Secondary Causes of Hypertension (see Table 18-3)

RENOVASCULAR HYPERTENSION

Patients with renovascular hypertension often have stage 3 disease, considerable TOD, and are at risk of losing renal function. The 90 percent with atherosclerotic disease typically are ≥50 years old and have other vascular disease as well as a history of cigarette smoking. The other 10 percent are typically young white women with fibromuscular dysplasia. Except in specialized centers, imaging studies are routinely used for screening for renovascular hypertension. Most experienced centers have good results with the captopril renal scan, but renal artery ultrasound is sometimes useful. Magnetic resonance imaging (MRI)/angiography is a newer and more expensive technique that is becoming more widely available. Angiography (using digital subtraction techniques) is usually recommended when the pretest probability of renal artery stenosis is very high

TABLE 18-3

COMMON SECONDARY CAUSES OF HYPERTENSION

Diagnosis	Prevalence	Physical Sign(s)	Recommended Screening Test	Localization or Confirmatory Test
Renovascular hypertension	3–10%	Renal bruit	Captopril renogram	Renal arteriogram
Primary aldosteronism	1–5%	None	24-h urine for aldosterone (salt loaded) or serum aldosterone/PRA ratio	CT of adrenals
Pheochromocytoma	<1%	Phakomatoses; abdominal mass	24-hour urine for VMA, metanephrines	MRI of abdomen (usually)
Hypercortisolism	<1%	Moon facies, buffalo hump, abdominal striae	Morning cortisol level	Dexamethasone suppression tests (low and high doses)
Coarctation of aorta	<1%	Elevated arm BP	Thigh BP; radiofemoral delay	Echocardiogram
Hypothyroidism	<1–7%	Nonspecific	Thyroid-stimulating hormone	

KEY: PRA = peripheral renin activity; VMA = vanillylmandelic acid; CT = computed tomography; MRI = magnetic resonance imaging.

(based on clinical and noninvasive laboratory criteria); otherwise it follows a suggestive screening test. When renal artery stenoses are found, most radiologists insert a stent after angioplasty, but this practice has recently been questioned. *Most clinicians search for renal artery disease only when there is difficult-to-control hypertension or a diminution in renal function; otherwise, for most patients, medical therapy with multiple antihypertensive pills is preferred.*

PHEOCHROMOCYTOMA

Most pheochromocytoma patients are very symptomatic. The three most common symptoms of pheochromocytoma are headache, diaphoresis, and palpitations, but other symptoms—particularly anxiety, weakness, and tremulousness—are also frequently found. Screening for pheochromocytoma requires demonstration of an overproduction of catecholamines. Because of their lower cost and wider availability, we prefer 24-h urinary collections for total catecholamines, vanillylmandelic acid, and metanephrines, although plasma testing is also occasionally useful, particularly in conjunction with pharmacologic testing with clonidine or glucagon. After elevated catecholamine levels have been demonstrated, the T2-weighted MRI scan is probably the most readily available and useful imaging test because the pheochromocytoma tissue "lights up" with this technique. A nuclear scan using meta-iodo-benzylguanidine (MIBG) is also occasionally helpful, especially when a metastatic tumor is suspected. Computed tomography (CT) may be more sensitive than MRI in finding small tumors but is probably less specific. Surgery to remove the tumor should be attempted after a suitable period of alpha blockade. Occasionally a beta blocker is also required, but this should be added only *after* alpha blockade is established. Although most patients do not have a heredofamilial reason for their pheochromocytoma, a skin examination and screening for other tumors (related to multiple endocrine neoplasia syndromes) is recommended.

PRIMARY ALDOSTERONISM

Hypokalemia and symptoms related to it are the hallmark of this disease. The single best test in people with normal renal function for identifying patients with primary aldosteronism is the measurement of 24-h urinary aldosterone excretion during salt loading. An aldosterone excretion rate of $>14 \ \mu g/24$ h following 3 days of salt loading (>200 meq/day) distinguishes most patients with primary aldosteronism from those with essential hypertension. Because there are a substantial number of patients with primary aldosteronism who do not present with hypokalemia, the plasma aldosterone:renin ratio has been used to define the appropriateness of peripheral renin activity for the circulating levels of aldosterone. Some authorities recommend this calculation as an initial screening tool.

The most common cause of primary aldosteronism is an aldosterone-producing adenoma (50 to 60 percent of cases). Although some authorities recommend a number of hormonal tests to distinguish adenomas from bilateral adrenal hyperplasia, we typically perform a thin-cut adrenal CT scan instead. It is noninvasive, and all adenomas ≥ 1.5 cm in diameter can be located in this way. The sensitivity of high-resolution CT for adenomas exceeds 90 percent. Adrenal venous aldosterone levels should be measured when the biochemical findings are highly suggestive of an adenoma but the adrenal CT scan is ambiguous.

Chronic medical therapy is indicated in patients with adrenal hyperplasia, in those with adenomas who are poor surgical risks, and in patients with bilateral adrenal adenomas that may require bilateral adrenalectomy. Typically potassium-sparing diuretics and calcium antagonists are most useful. In the majority of patients, surgical excision of an aldosterone-producing adenoma reverses hypertension and the biochemical defects. One year postoperatively, about 70 percent of patients are normotensive, but 5 years postoperatively, only 53 percent remain normotensive. The restoration of normal K^+ homeostasis is permanent. Patients undergoing surgery should receive drug treatment for at least 8 to 10 weeks, both to decrease BP and to correct metabolic abnormalities. These patients have significant K^+ deficiency that must be corrected preoperatively because hypokalemia increases the risk of cardiac arrhythmias during anesthesia.

TREATMENT OF HYPERTENSION

The patient with JNC VI stage 2 or 3 hypertension [systolic blood pressure (SBP) ≥ 160 mmHg or diastolic blood pressure (DBP) ≥ 100 mmHg] and those in risk group C [with either diabetes mellitus (DM), TOD, or clinical cardiovascular disease] (see Tables 18-1 and 18-2) should receive drug therapy in addition to lifestyle modifications once hypertension has been diagnosed and confirmed. The length of time given to lifestyle modifications alone (before starting drug therapy) is based on absolute risk estimates, not just on the level of BP. Individuals with stage 1 hypertension (SBP 140 to 159 mmHg and/or DBP 90 to 99 mmHg) in risk group A (see Table 18-2) can be treated with lifestyle modifications alone for up to 1 year, even if goal BP is not reached, before drug therapy becomes necessary. Since male gender and age >60 years are risk factors, only women under 60 years of age can fall into risk group A.

Patients with stage 1 hypertension who are in risk group B (other cardiovascular risk factors but no diabetes mellitus, TOD, or concomitant cardiovascular disease) should receive pharmacologic therapy after only a 6-month trial of lifestyle modifications unless the goal

BP is achieved without drugs. Those in risk group C (TOD, clinical cardiovascular disease, and/or DM) should be treated with pharmacologic agents *and* lifestyle modifications even if they have high-normal BP (SBP 130 to 139 mmHg and/or DBP 85 to 89 mmHg).

Lifestyle Modifications

JNC VI recommended weight loss for obese hypertensive patients, modification of dietary sodium intake to ≤ 100 mmol/day, and modification of alcohol intake to no more than two drinks per day. Physical activity was also advised for all hypertensives without a specific condition that would make it unsafe. Yet for many of our patients, these suggestions are either not practicable or are already being acted on. For such patients, drug therapy may be indicated even sooner than the 6 to 12 months recommended for group A and B hypertensives. Smoking cessation is also recommended to improve cardiovascular health rather than because of a proven direct relationship between smoking and hypertension. A direct relationship between smoking and BP, in fact, has not been demonstrated in epidemiologic studies, and often the opposite (BP lower in smokers) has been observed. Perhaps the greatest role of lifestyle modification will be in preventing hypertension, although some patients are able to reduce the number and dose of antihypertensive medications in the long-term by adopting lifestyle modifications.

PHARMACOLOGIC THERAPY

The primary goal of BP reduction is to reduce cardiovascular morbidity and mortality using the *least intrusive means possible*. The term *intrusive* has several interpretations—economic, office visits, adverse effects, and convenience. There is a strong and direct relationship between achieving the goal BP and reducing cardiovascular morbidity and mortality, so achieving the BP goal becomes the short-term objective of antihypertensive treatment. The initial choice of drug therapy is probably the most important decision the clinician must make when treating hypertensive patients. Approximately *half* of the patients we treat will respond to our first choice and can tolerate most of our rational options. If we choose wisely, our first choice will be successful in getting BP to goal in many patients, and that will be the drug those patients remain on indefinitely. Since the remainder will need additional treatment, the choice of the first drug must be made with an eye toward what can be added to achieve the goal BP.

Before 1997, only diuretics and beta blockers had been shown to reduce morbidity and mortality in clinical trials in hypertension. Dihydropyridine (DHP) CAs and angiotensin converting-enzyme (ACE) inhibitors were added to the list after the Syst-EUR trial was completed. This trial used the DHP CA nitrendipine, followed by enalapril and hydrochlorothiazide if needed, to get BP to goal. It was only in 1999, when the Captopril Prevention Project (CAPP) was published, that the ability of an ACE inhibitor to reduce morbidity and mortality in hypertensive subjects was demonstrated. CAPP showed that a regimen starting with the ACE inhibitor captopril, was not significantly different from one starting with either a diuretic or beta blocker ("conventional therapy") in reducing morbidity and mortality. Three more recently completed active comparative studies of newer versus conventional drug regimens [the second Swedish Trial of Hypertension in Older Persons (STOP-2), the Nordic Diltiazem Study, and the International Nifedipine Study: Intervention as a Goal in Hypertension Treatment (INSIGHT)] also demonstrated that ACE inhibitors, DHP CAs, and non-DHP CAs reduce morbidity and mortality as well as (but no better than) diuretics and/or beta blockers.

In the next few years, approximately 35 more outcome trials will be completed. When some or all of these trials are published, we should know with some degree of certainty whether lowering BP is all that matters or whether a particular class of drugs prevents hypertension-related events more effectively. The largest of these trials (with 42,448 subjects), the Antihypertensive and Lipid Lowering (to Prevent) Heart Attack Trial (ALLHAT), is due to be completed in 2003. This study compares a diuretic with a DHP CA, ACE inhibitor, and an alpha blocker, with acute myocardial infarction as the primary endpoint. In February of 2000, the alpha blocker arm of ALLHAT was stopped, despite no difference in the rate of primary endpoints, because of a 25 percent higher cardiovascular mortality and twofold increase in heart failure (HF) with the alpha blocker as compared with the diuretic. The chlorthalidone group had a 3/0-mmHg lower BP throughout the study compared with those getting doxazosin. So the question of whether it is more important to lower BP or to choose a specific drug therapy remains open.

Matching the Goal Blood Pressure to the Level of Cardiovascular Risk

According to several guidelines committees, hypertensive patients should have their SBP lowered to below 140 mmHg and DBP below 90 mmHg; higher-risk patients should go even lower. Diabetics should have SBP < 130 mmHg and DBP < 85 mmHg; some authorities suggest <130/80 mmHg. JNC VI recommended <130/85 mmHg for diabetics without the support of clinical trial evidence. The Hypertension Optimal Treatment (HOT) study and the United Kingdom Prospective Diabetes Study (UKPDS) provided solid evidence to support this recommendation. In patients with renal disease and at least 1 g/day of proteinuria, JNC VI recommended an even lower goal (SBP < 125 mmHg and DBP < 75 mmHg). This too was not an "evidence-based" recommendation but predicated on the expectation that a much lower BP would be helpful in preventing morbidity and mortality in this special hypertensive population. The African-American Study of Kidney Disease (AASK) will provide definitive evidence for or against this very stringent goal. Whether this lower goal should also be extended to other subpopulations, such as those with prevalent cardiovascular disease, remains to be proven.

One of the perceived limitations to accepting this lower target for BP control was the fear that lowering BP too far might be harmful (the concept of the "J" curve). In some studies, subjects treated to a diastolic BP level below 85 mmHg had higher rates of myocardial infarction than those whose on-treatment diastolic BP was between 85 and 90 mmHg. Yet an increased risk associated with a low diastolic BP is also evident in other epidemiologic studies and in the placebo groups of several trials. Furthermore, MIs were successfully prevented in the Systolic Hypertension in the Elderly Program (SHEP) among the individuals treated to an average diastolic BP of 67 mmHg compared with the placebo group, who finished the study with an average DBP of 71 mmHg. The HOT and UKPDS trials also showed that lowering BP beyond 85 mmHg diastolic was not harmful, especially in high-risk diabetics.

The cost-analysis of the UKPDS data showed that the lower BP goal was associated with an overall savings of £1047 ($1507) per year of life saved without diabetic complications and £720 ($1036) saved per year of extended life. Similar conclusions were reached using American epidemiologic and clinical data: treating diabetic hypertensives above age 60 years to a goal of <130/85 mmHg saves both lives and money, compared with treatment to only 140/90 mmHg. The lower BP goal lowers both direct and indirect costs (e.g., hospitalization for the greater number of events and time lost from work, respectively) more than the cost of the additional antihypertensive drugs, adverse reactions, and extra visits to health care providers necessary to achieve it.

Tailoring Antihypertensive Drug Therapy to Specific Clinical Situations

Perhaps because hypertension is a condition with few characteristic symptoms, patients rarely present to the physician with only hypertension on their standardized problem list. It is often possible to choose specific antihypertensive drug therapy that will have a positive impact on the prognosis in the patient's other conditions. In JNC VI, a "compelling" reason to choose a specific antihypertensive agent exists when one drug or class is known to improve morbidity and mortality in another disease (e.g., an ACE inhibitor in heart failure);

a "clinical indication" is recognized when a drug or class improves symptoms but perhaps not prognosis (e.g., beta blocker for migraine headache prophylaxis). This section reviews and extends these special uses of antihypertensive drugs in common clinical scenarios.

HYPERTENSIVES WITH DIABETES MELLITUS

The combination of hypertension and DM confers much more risk for cardiovascular events and renal failure than either risk factor alone. ACE inhibitors, diuretics, and beta blockers have been consistently shown to reduce cardiovascular and renal risk. There are very few outcome studies using other classes of antihypertensive agents, although there are some preliminary results with angiotensin receptor blockers (ARBs) and CAs. In JNC VI, only type 1 DM was listed as a "compelling reason" to prescribe an ACE inhibitor, because, at that time, the only randomized clinical trial demonstrating that ACE inhibitors reduce clinical events was done in a group of type 1 diabetic patients with hypertension. Although there are no long-term events trials yet completed that have proven the value of ACE inhibitors in patients with type 2 DM, many feel that the benefits shown for type 1 diabetics can also be extrapolated to type 2 diabetics. Others argue that if the appropriate goal BP is achieved, it does not matter what drug or drugs are used. In UKPDS, the group that initially received the ACE inhibitor captopril did no better than the group that received atenolol, which lends some support to the argument that it is BP control and not how it is accomplished that is the key factor in reducing events in type 2 diabetics. Although some experts have raised concerns about the safety of DHP CAs in type 2 diabetics, the Syst-EUR study, in which these drugs were the initial therapy, demonstrated that the benefit accrued was greater in diabetics than in non-diabetics.

Trials of cardiovascular mortality involving non-DHP CAs in high-risk hypertensives have not yet been completed. However, non-DHP CAs reduce cardiovascular mortality following myocardial infarction and slow the progression of diabetic nephropathy. Moreover, in combination with ACE inhibitors, non-DHP CAs reduce urinary protein excretion and, unlike DHP CAs, they can reduce proteinuria independent of BP reduction. The combination of non-DHP CAs and ACE inhibitors is particularly useful in diabetics with nephropathy and proteinuria.

LEFT VENTRICULAR HYPERTROPHY

LVH is a robust and independent risk factor for cardiovascular disease and premature mortality. It is common in the elderly, especially women, and is often associated with diastolic dysfunction. All antihypertensive agents recommended for initial therapy reduce left ventricular mass. Data from meta-analyses suggest that agents that block the renin-angiotensin-aldosterone system reduce left ventricular mass better or more quickly than other antihypertensive agents. However, the Treatment of Mild Hypertension Study (TOMHS) and the Veterans Administration (VA) study of monotherapy showed no difference among antihypertensive agents in reducing LVH. Moreover, in TOMHS, nutritional-hygienic measures such as weight loss, sodium and alcohol restriction, and exercise were effective by themselves in regressing left ventricular mass. Perhaps the most important factor responsible for left ventricular mass regression is the prolonged reduction of systolic BP.

HEART FAILURE

Hypertension has recently been identified as a major risk factor for the subsequent development of heart failure (HF), the onset of which typically occurs many years later. For many untreated or undertreated hypertensives, LVH is an important intermediate step, resulting in "hypertensive heart disease" with impaired LV filling and increased ventricular stiffness. This type of HF (which has been seen in up to 40 percent of hospitalized patients with an antecedent history of hypertension) is commonly called *diastolic dysfunction*. The more common type of *systolic dysfunction,* characterized by a reduced left ventricular ejection fraction, is most often due to previous myocardial infarction (for which hypertension is also an important risk factor). In a recent meta-analysis of clinical trials in hypertension, there was a 42 percent reduction in HF incidence among hypertensives randomized to either a low-dose diuretic or beta blocker.

Distinguishing between the two subtypes of HF is most easily done by quantitating of the LV ejection fraction; the results dictate therapy. Patients with low ejection fractions ("systolic HF") improve both their BP and long-term prognosis with an ACE inhibitor and diuretics, to which a beta blocker, spironolactone, and/or other drugs are sometimes added. The role of ARBs is controversial unless cough or other adverse effects preclude an ACE inhibitor. In the first direct comparative study of captopril and losartan [Evaluation of Losartan In The Elderly (ELITE)], a survival benefit (a tertiary hypothesis) was attributed to the ARBs, which the larger study (ELITE 2), with exactly the same protocol, did not confirm. Ongoing research may define the benefit of using both an ACE inhibitor and an ARB simultaneously in systolic HF. The role of DHP CAs and/or direct-acting vasodilators (e.g., hydralazine in combination with isosorbide dinitrate) remains controversial. Most authorities recommend these drugs as second- or third-line therapy (after maximum doses of ACE inhibitor and/or ARBs) if BP is still elevated. In the Randomized Aldactone Evaluation Study (RALES), spironolactone, an aldosterone antagonist, in doses that do not lower BP, reduced morbidity and mortality in patients with HF, most of whom were already taking an ACE inhibitor, aspirin, and diuretics. Many were also on a beta blocker.

Treatment of hypertensive patients with diastolic dysfunction and HF has not been as well studied, but most authorities recommend using beta blockers or non-DHP CA, which reduce the HR, increase diastolic filling time, and allow the heart muscle to relax more fully. While these options make physiologic sense, there are no randomized clinical trials with outcome data to demonstrate their efficacy long-term.

VALVULAR HEART DISEASE

A murmur of aortic sclerosis is found in approximately 21 to 26 percent of adults over 65 years of age. In the Cardiovascular Health Study, echocardiograms found that 29 percent of the 5621 subjects aged 65 and over had this valvular abnormality; those with high BP and LVH had a higher prevalence. "Aortic sclerosis" was associated with a 50 percent increased risk of cardiovascular events over an average of 5 years of follow-up, but this risk estimate decreased on multivariate analysis. Calcific aortic stenosis is about 10 times less common but often must be more extensively evaluated, usually with an echocardiogram. Aortic regurgitation in hypertensives is almost exclusively found in patients having isolated systolic hypertension and is most easily recognized by the murmur and several peripheral signs. Unloading the left ventricle with arteriolar vasodilators (e.g., nifedipine) improves the time to valve replacement.

Mitral valvular disease is less common now than in decades past, primarily due to treatment of streptococcal pharyngitis. Mitral stenosis is still occasionally seen in developing countries but is uncommonly associated with systemic hypertension. Since digoxin is typically used to control the ventricular rate in atrial fibrillation, antihypertensive drugs that interfere with the excretion of digoxin should be used cautiously.

MICROALBUMINURIA

Although lowering BP itself reduces microalbuminuria (MA), ACE inhibitors and ARBs most consistently reduce proteinuria, including MA. Even in the absence of hypertension, these agents prevent the usual progression of MA to proteinuria. Non-DHP CAs (diltiazem and verapamil) also reduce urinary protein excretion (and MA) in hypertensive patients with kidney disease and have additive effects on MA when combined with ACE inhibitors. Since we have so much more data, including outcomes, about ACE inhibitors than any other class, including ARBs, they should be the initial choice for hypertensives with MA and included in all multidrug antihypertensive regimens in such patients if tolerated.

RENAL DYSFUNCTION

Any agent or group of agents that adequately lowers BP to levels <130/85 mmHg will slow progression of nephropathy. Intensive BP reduction (<125/75 mmHg) is needed to maximally slow the progression of renal disease, especially among patients with an elevated serum creatinine. ACE inhibitors will slow progression of diabetic and nondiabetic nephropathy if the BP is reduced to levels below 140/90 mmHg.

Many clinicians are fearful of using ACE inhibitors in patients with renal impairment because serum creatinine increases up to 25 percent over baseline after the ACE inhibitor is begun. *This acute apparent reduction in renal function plateaus within a month and is reversible on stopping the ACE inhibitor*. If serum creatinine increases less than 25 percent, however, we recommend continuing the ACE inhibitor, because these agents do prevent progression of renal impairment in the long-term. If the increase is larger than 25 percent, evaluations for volume depletion and/or renovascular hypertension are appropriate. Hyperkalemia after initiating an ACE inhibitor in patients with renal dysfunction is worrisome only if the serum potassium rises by ≥0.5 meq/L, which is unusual.

Whether ARBs delay nephropathy and reduce cardiovascular events as well or better than ACE inhibitor is still uncertain. All animal studies and one completed clinical trial in patients with HF suggest that these agents will be as good as ACE inhibitors in slowing the progression of renal disease and reducing proteinuria and cardiovascular events. Whether ARBs may be useful when added to ACE inhibitors remains to be demonstrated. There are two ongoing clinical trials in subjects with diabetic nephropathy scheduled to be completed by 2002 that will answer these important questions.

While any antihypertensive agent may be used to achieve the recommended BP target to preserve renal function, certain principles should be kept in mind:

- BP will rarely be adequately controlled in patients with significant renal impairment (serum creatinine >1.8 mg/dL) without a loop diuretic, typically furosemide or bumetanide twice daily or torsemide once daily.
- Combinations of antihypertensive medications are needed to achieve the BP target, and one of these drugs should be an ACE inhibitor. If side effects are noted with the ACE inhibitor, an ARB may be substituted.
- Because most patients with renal impairment eventually die of coronary heart disease, beta blockers also have a role, especially after a myocardial infarction.

CORONARY ARTERY DISEASE

The coexistence of coronary artery disease (CAD) and hypertension influences both the choice of drug(s) used and the BP goal to be achieved. Because both beta blockers and calcium antagonists (CA) are effective antihypertensive and antianginal agents, these drugs are preferred. The recent Heart Outcomes Prevention Evaluation (HOPE) study indicates that an ACE inhibitor (added to other drugs such as aspirin, beta blockers, CAs, and/or statins) prevents cardiovascular events. The issue of how far to reduce the BP in the setting of CAD is controversial. The "J-shaped curve" arose from studies of patients with CAD, suggesting that if the BP was <85 to 90 mmHg diastolic, patients had a higher risk of death and recurrent myocardial infarction. Theoretically, since coronary artery filling occurs during diastole, a reduction of perfusion pressure during this time increases coronary ischemia. Although the HOT study did not support this construct, caution is still advised in lowering BP beyond 85 mmHg in patients with angina and/or known CAD. In such patients, we use beta blockers, calcium channel blockers, ACE inhibitors, and perhaps nitrates; attain a slightly lower than usual BP target; and recommend aspirin and intensive treatment of dyslipidemia [to achieve or exceed a low-density lipoprotein (LDL)-cholesterol target of <100 mg/dL].

POST-STROKE

Optimal BP management in this setting depends on the nature, cause, and chronology of the neurologic symptoms. In acute ischemic stroke, the optimal level of BP is controversial. If BP is reduced acutely, there may be a reduction in blood flow to "watershed" areas of the brain that are already poorly perfused. Acute worsening of cerebrovascular function and evolving neurologic deficits have been observed when BP is reduced "too much" or "too quickly." Most physicians, therefore, are uncomfortable in reducing BP to <180/100 mmHg. Many do not institute treatment until mean arterial pressure is >130 mmHg (e.g., BP >200/100 mmHg) except in the setting of concomitant hemorrhagic transformation or other hypertensive emergency (see below). The inclusion/exclusion criteria for the National Institutes of Heath (NIH)-sponsored trial of rt-PA in acute stroke supports this recommendation. Optimal drug therapy for acute stroke–related hypertension is also ill-defined, but most authorities prefer intravenously administered short-acting agents because they can be discontinued quickly if the patient's neurologic condition deteriorates acutely.

BLACKS AND OTHER ETHNIC MINORITIES

Some classes of drugs have different efficacy across various ethnic groups. Thiazide diuretics are more effective in lowering BP among blacks than whites, whereas ACE inhibitors, ARBs, and beta blockers are effective at lower doses in whites. Many blacks *do* respond to agents that block the renin-angiotensin-aldosterone system, but higher doses may be needed. If a black hypertensive patient would benefit from special properties of a drug (e.g., ACE inhibitor in diabetes or HF), a putatively less effective drug should be used even if additional agents will be needed to achieve the goal BP. Calcium antagonists, alpha/beta blockers, and alpha blockers are equally effective across ethnic groups. Response rates to antihypertensive drugs in Hispanics are intermediate between those of whites and blacks, while East Asians though not necessarily South Asians (e.g., from the Indian subcontinent) often need smaller doses than whites.

THE ELDERLY

All classes of antihypertensive agents lower BP effectively in older persons, although the doses needed to reach goal are often lower than the doses necessary in younger patients. Certain drugs, however, should be used with caution in older hypertensives. The alpha blockers can exacerbate the postural fall in BP in older individuals with baroreceptor dysfunction. Non-DHP CAs and beta blockers may aggravate subtle or subclinical conduction defects or precipitate systolic dysfunction and HF. Verapamil may cause constipation. Cough from ACE inhibitor is more common in older women. Diuretics and DHP CAs have both been shown to reduce morbidity and mortality in older persons with stage 2 or 3 isolated systolic hypertension, making them excellent choices in such patients. The absolute benefit of lowering BP is greater in older hypertensives; drug therapy should not be withheld for fear of toxicity or lack of efficacy in the elderly.

HYPERTENSIVE URGENCIES AND EMERGENCIES

Hypertensive urgencies are situations in which the BP must be reduced within hours (e.g., after vascular surgery). With the exception of nifedipine capsules, which are *not* indicated, any of a number of oral antihypertensive medications is likely to be effective, reasonably well tolerated, and safe. We typically recommend labetalol, clonidine, or captopril, with careful and frequent monitoring of BP for the first few hours after initial treatment and a quick outpatient follow-up appointment to assure adherence to chronic antihypertensive medication.

Hypertensive emergencies occur when BP must be reduced within minutes lest ongoing acute target-organ damage progresses. Table 18-4 summarizes the preferred antihypertensive agent and goal BP for the most common hypertensive emergencies.

Safety (Adverse Reactions and Side Effects)

Recent clinical trials have added ACE inhibitors and both DHP CAs and non-DHP CAs to diuretics and beta blockers as antihypertensive drug classes that reduce cardiovascular morbidity and mortality.

TABLE 18-4

TYPES OF HYPERTENSIVE CRISES, WITH SUGGESTED DRUG THERAPY AND BLOOD PRESSURE TARGETS

Type of Crisis	Drug of Choice	BP Target
Neurological		
Hypertensive encephalopathy	Nitroprusside*	25% reduction in mean arterial pressure over 2–3 h
Intracranial hemorrhage or acute stroke in evolution	Nitroprusside* (controversial)	0–25% reduction in mean arterial pressure over 6–12 h (controversial)
Acute head injury/trauma	Nitroprusside*	0–25% reduction in mean arterial pressure over 2–3 h (controversial)
Subarachnoid hemorrhage	Nimodipine	Up to 25% reduction in mean arterial pressure in previously hypertensive patients, 130–160 systolic in normotensive patients
Cardiac		
Ischemia/infarction	Nitroglycerine or nicardipine	Reduction in ischemia
Heart failure	Nitroprusside* or nitroglycerin	Improvement in failure (typically 10–15% decrease in BP)
Aortic dissection	Beta blocker + nitroprusside*	120 mmHg systolic in 30 min (if possible)
Renal		
Hematuria or acute renal impairment	Fenoldopam	0–25% reduction in mean arterial pressure over 1–12 h
Catecholamine excess states		
Pheochromocytoma	Phentolamine	To control paroxysms of BP
Drug withdrawal	Drug withdrawn	Typically only one dose necessary
Pregnancy-related		
Eclampsia	MgSO₄, methyldopa, hydralazine	Typically <90 mmHg diastolic but often lower

* Some physicians prefer an intravenous infusion of either fenoldopam or nicardipine, neither of which has potentially toxic metabolites, over nitroprusside. Recent studies have also shown improvements in renal function during therapy with the former as compared with nitroprusside.

SOURCE: Updated from Elliott WJ, Black HR: Hypertensive crises. In: Parrillo E, Bone RC (eds): *Critical Care Medicine: Principles of Diagnosis and Management.* Philadelphia: Mosby–Year Book; 1995:565–576.

When the WHO-ISH Collaborative Clinical Trialists complete their analyses of the roughly 270,000 hypertensive patients in ongoing clinical trials, we may know if there are major differences across commonly used drug classes for hypertension.

SIDE EFFECTS

Most symptomatic side effects with commonly used antihypertensive drugs can be minimized by stopping the drug (e.g., cough with ACE inhibitors), reducing the dose (e.g., constipation with high-dose verapamil), or encouraging the patient to continue until the symptom abates (e.g., dry mouth with low-dose clonidine). ARBs have the lowest incidence of symptomatic side effects, but their higher cost and limited outcomes data put them in second place to ACE inhibitors in many formularies. Biochemical side effects are less common with the drugs and doses used currently. They may also be less important as harbingers of future problems: although beta blockers do increase triglycerides, they still reduce recurrent rates of myocardial infarction among people with CAD. Similarly, the alpha blocker in ALLHAT had a more favorable biochemical profile than the diuretic (lower total cholesterol, triglycerides, and glucose, and a higher serum potassium), yet the latter was more effective in reducing cardiovascular events. It is still reasonable to monitor patients for hypokalemia with loop or high-dose thiazide diuretics, but this seldom requires discontinuation of these drugs.

DRUG INTERACTIONS

Because many hypertensive patients require multiple agents to achieve goal BP, adverse drug-drug interactions are always possible. Besides the general caution about agents competing for the same elimination pathway (e.g., cytochrome P450 subfamilies or the renal anion excretory pump), verapamil and a beta blocker together can cause cardiac conduction abnormalities and precipitate HF. Some combinations of antihypertensive agents are synergistic. Several fixed-dose combinations of diuretics and drugs that interfere with the renin-angiotensin-aldosterone system are available; adding an ACE inhibitor to a DHP CA reduces the incidence and severity of pedal edema. Several publications attest to the efficacy of simultaneous ACE inhibitor and ARB as well as a non-DHP and a DHP CA. Nonsteroidal anti-inflammatory agents can interfere with all antihypertensive agents and raise BP.

Cost

Many health care administrators believe that the antihypertensive drug with the lowest purchase price is the best, but this view overlooks the costs due to extra visits to health care providers, laboratory testing, and side effects that result in emergency department visits or hospitalization. Generically available drugs are usually less expensive to purchase than their branded counterparts and are strongly favored in most managed care pharmacy plans. Some plans insist that, for the first month of antihypertensive therapy, a low-dose thiazide diuretic always be prescribed, because of its proven efficacy and low cost, unless there is a "compelling condition" for which another agent would be justified.

Many authorities are concerned that achieving the new, lower target BPs for diabetic and renally impaired hypertensives will cost more, as it will require more visits to health care providers and more antihypertensive medications. These increases in short-term expenditures are likely, however, to be offset by a lower future incidence of expensive outcomes, including heart attack, stroke, end-stage renal disease, and HF, as seen in UKPDS 40 and for diabetic patients over age 60 in the United States.

Many proposals for reducing the high cost of antihypertensive therapy have been advanced. JNC VI has suggested withholding drug therapy for 6 to 12 months from those at low risk (risk groups A and B) with stage 1 hypertension and giving it instead to patients in risk group C, with BP $\geq 130/85$ mmHg. In stage 2 to 3 hypertension, wider use of combination drug tablets has been advocated, since the total cost of these is typically less than two separate prescriptions for the same doses of individual agents. Some formularies and pharmacy benefits managers prefer agents that have all doses priced identically, with the theory that a pill splitter can then be used to cut up one tablet for 2 or more days of treatment. Aggressive health care plans have implemented strategies that prohibit use of more expensive medications (e.g., ARBs) unless two physicians independently ascribe an adverse effect to a less expensive drug (e.g., an ACE inhibitor), and others require that three separate ACE inhibitors to be administered sequentially before an ARB can be dispensed. Until a universal pharmacy benefits program is instituted, wide variations in the pricing and cost of antihypertensive agents are likely. While it is difficult for physicians to stay abreast of fluctuations in these costs, it is important that all health care providers attempt to provide tolerable antihypertensive medications at the lowest possible cost for the benefit of the patient, the health plan, and the national budget.

SUGGESTED READING

ALLHAT Collaborative Research Group: Major cardiovascular events in hypertensive patients randomized to doxazosin vs chlorthalidone: The Antihypertensive and Lipid-Lowering Treatment to Prevent Heart Attack Trial (ALLHAT). *JAMA* 2000; 283:1967–1975.

Bakris GL, Williams M, Dworkin L, et al for the National Kidney Foundation Hypertension and Diabetes Executive Committee Working Group: Preserving renal function in adults with hypertension and diabetes: A consensus approach. *Am J Kidney Dis* 2000; 35:646–661.

Black HR, Bakris GL, Elliott WJ: Hypertension: Epidemiology, pathophysiology, diagnosis, and treatment. In: Fuster V, Alexander RW, O'Rourke RA, et al (eds): *Hurst's The Heart,* 10th ed. New York: McGraw-Hill; 2001:1553–1604.

Brown MJ, Palmer CR, Castaigne A, et al: Morbidity and mortality in patients randomised to double-blind treatment with a long-acting calcium-channel blocker or diuretic in the International Nifedipine GITS study: Intervention as a Goal in Hypertension Treatment (INSIGHT). *Lancet* 2000; 356:366–372.

Elliott WJ, Weir DR, Black HR: Cost-effectiveness of the lower treatment goal (of JNC VI) in hypertensive diabetics. *Arch Intern Med* 2000; 160:1277–1283.

Hansson L, Hedner T, Lund-Johansen P, et al for the NORDIL Study Group: Randomised trial of effects of calcium antagonists compared with diuretics and β-blockers on cardiovascular morbidity and mortality in hypertension: The Nordic Diltiazem (NORDIL) Study. *Lancet* 2000; 356:359–365.

Hansson L, Lindholm L, Ekbom T, et al: Randomised trial of old and new antihypertensive drugs in elderly patients: Cardiovascular mortality and morbidity in the Swedish Trial in Old Patients with Hypertension-2 Study. *Lancet* 1999; 354:1751–1756.

Hansson L, Zanchetti A, Carruthers SG, et al on behalf of the HOT Study Group: Effects of intensive blood pressure lowering and low-dose aspirin in patients with hypertension: Principal results of the Hypertension Optimal Treatment (HOT) randomised trial. *Lancet* 1998; 351:1755–1762.

Ramsay LE, Williams B, Johnston GD, et al: British Hypertension Society guidelines for hypertension management 1999: Summary. *Br Med J* 1999; 319:630–635.

The Heart Outcomes Prevention Evaluation Study Investigators: Effects of an angiotensin-converting enzyme inhibitor, ramipril, on death from cardiovascular causes, myocardial infarction, and stroke in high-risk patients. *N Engl J Med* 2000; 342:145–153.

The Sixth Report of the Joint National Committee on The Detection, Evaluation, and Treatment of High Blood Pressure (Joint National Committee VI). *Arch Intern Med* 1997; 157:2413–2446.

The World Health Organisation/International Society of Hypertension Guidelines for the Management of Hypertension. *J Hypertens* 1999; 17:151–185.

Turner R, Holman R, Stratton I, et al for the United Kingdom Prospective Diabetes Study Group: Tight blood pressure control and risk of macrovascular and microvascular complications in type 2 diabetes: UKPDS 38. *Br Med J* 1998; 317:707–713.

19

PULMONARY HYPERTENSION

Lewis J. Rubin

INTRODUCTION

Pulmonary hypertension, a hemodynamic abnormality common to a variety of conditions, is characterized by increased right ventricular afterload and work. The clinical manifestations, natural history, and reversibility of pulmonary hypertension depend on the nature of the pulmonary vascular lesions and the etiology and severity of the hemodynamic disorder. The degree of pulmonary hypertension that develops is a function of the amount of the pulmonary vascular tree that has been eliminated. Pulmonary hypertension is usually secondary to cardiac or pulmonary disease. Although primary pulmonary hypertension (PPH) is uncommon, it has attracted considerable attention as a distinctive clinical entity in which intrinsic pulmonary vascular disease is free of the complicating features of secondary pulmonary hypertension contributed by diseases of the heart and/or lungs. Mild or even moderate pulmonary hypertension can exist for a lifetime without becoming evident clinically. When pulmonary hypertension does become manifest clinically, the symptoms tend to be nonspecific.

Definitions

This chapter deals with *chronic* pulmonary arterial hypertension. Acute pulmonary arterial hypertension is usually a result of either pulmonary embolism or the adult respiratory distress syndrome. Pulmonary *venous* hypertension is usually encountered clinically as a consequence of left ventricular failure or mitral valvular disease. Occasionally it may occur in the course of fibrosing mediastinitis. Only rarely is the entity known as pulmonary venoocclusive disease (PVOD) encountered. The hallmarks of pulmonary venous hypertension are pulmonary congestion and edema. Pulmonary venous hypertension is said to exist when pulmonary venous (or left atrial) pressure rises above 15 mmHg.

Cor pulmonale signifies the presence of pulmonary hypertension in the setting of chronic respiratory disease. The degree of pulmonary hypertension that develops in patients with chronic lung disease tends to be less severe than in connective tissue diseases, chronic thromboembolic disease, or primary pulmonary hypertension. Pulmonary hypertension may be severe, however, in some patients with interstitial lung disease.

Hemodynamics

At *sea level,* a cardiac output of 5 to 6 L/min is associated with a pulmonary arterial pressure of about 20/12 mmHg, with a mean of about 15 mmHg. At an altitude of 15,000 ft, the same level of blood flow is associated with somewhat higher pressures. Pulmonary arterial pressures also tend to increase somewhat with age.

A pressure drop of only 5 to 10 mmHg between the pulmonary artery and left atrium accompanies the cardiac output of 5 to 6 L/min. Determination of pulmonary vascular resistance, calculated as the ratio of the difference in mean pressure at the two ends of the pulmonary vascular bed (pulmonary arterial minus left atrial pressures divided by the cardiac output) is a practical clinical tool for assessing the hemodynamic state of the pulmonary system. In practice, since the left atrium is not readily accessible, pulmonary wedge pressure is generally substituted for left atrial pressure.

PULMONARY HYPERTENSION: GENERAL FEATURES

Clinical Manifestations

Pulmonary hypertension is a final common hemodynamic consequence of multiple etiologies and diverse mechanisms. Most cases of pulmonary hypertension are secondary. Among the underlying causes of pulmonary hypertension are mechanical compression and distortion of the resistance vessels of the lungs, hypoxic vasoconstriction (e.g., in severe obstructive airway or diffuse parenchymal diseases), intravascular obstruction (e.g., thromboemboli or tumor emboli), and combinations of mechanical and vasoconstrictive influences. The significance of pulmonary hypertension, however, is that, if uncontrolled, it leads to right ventricular failure. Once pulmonary arterial pressures reach systemic levels, right ventricular failure becomes inevitable.

Special Studies

The "gold standard" for the diagnosis of pulmonary hypertension is right-sided heart catheterization. This technique enables the direct determination of right atrial and ventricular pressures, pulmonary arterial pressure, pulmonary wedge pressure (as an approximation of pulmonary venous pressure), pulmonary blood flow (cardiac output), and the responses of these parameters to interventions (vasodilators, oxygen, exercise). From the measurements and samples obtained during cardiac catheterization, pulmonary vascular resistance can be calculated. As a rule, noninvasive methods are less reliable and less informative.

CHEST RADIOGRAPHY

The characteristic findings of pulmonary hypertension are enlargement of the pulmonary trunk and hilar vessels in association with attenuation (pruning) of the peripheral pulmonary arterial tree. Right-sided heart enlargement can be best detected radiographically on the lateral view as fullness in the retrosternal air space. In secondary pulmonary hypertension, changes in the lungs (e.g., hyperinflation, fibrosis) and in the position of the heart and diaphragm often mask the radiologic changes of pulmonary hypertension.

THE ELECTROCARDIOGRAM

The electrocardiogram (ECG) can disclose hypertrophy of the right ventricle and is more reliable in respiratory disorders that do not involve the parenchyma of the lungs (e.g., alveolar hypoventilation and sleep apnea) than in obstructive airways disease or parenchymal lung disease.

ECHOCARDIOGRAPHY

Echocardiographic techniques have proved useful in providing a measure of right ventricular thickness as an index of right ventricular hypertension. In some clinics, reliable estimates of the level of pulmonary hypertension have been obtained by determining regurgitant flows across the tricuspid and pulmonic valves using continuous-wave Doppler echocardiography.

LUNG SCANS

Ventilation/perfusion scans are of most value in the diagnosis and exclusion of pulmonary thromboembolic disease.

LUNG BIOPSY

The sampling of lung tissue by thoracotomy or thoracoscopy is occasionally helpful in identifying the etiology of the pulmonary hypertension—for example, in the setting of suspected pulmonary vasculitis. However, the procedure carries substantial risk in these hemodynamically compromised individuals.

SECONDARY PULMONARY HYPERTENSION

Cardiac and/or respiratory diseases are the most common causes of secondary pulmonary hypertension. Pulmonary thromboembolic disease ranks third. Cardiac disease leads to pulmonary hypertension by increasing pulmonary blood flow (e.g., large left-to-right shunts) or by increasing pulmonary venous pressure (e.g., left ventricular failure). In respiratory disease, the predominant mechanism for the pulmonary hypertension is an increase in resistance to pulmonary blood flow arising from perivascular parenchymal changes coupled with pulmonary vasoconstriction due to hypoxia. In pulmonary thromboembolic disease, clots in various stages of organization and affecting pulmonary vessels of different sizes increase resistance to blood flow.

Acquired Disorders of the Left Side of the Heart

Left ventricular failure is the most common cause of pulmonary hypertension. Among the various etiologies, myocardial disorders and lesions of the mitral and aortic valves predominate. Both categories of lesions lead to an increase in pulmonary venous pressure that, in turn, evokes an increase in pulmonary arterial pressure. The medical management of myocardial failure is considered elsewhere. The treatment of congenital heart disease and of mitral valvular disease is usually mechanical (e.g., surgical or balloon mitral valvuloplasty). The prospect for relief of the pulmonary venous hypertension, as by mitral valve commissurotomy or replacement, depends on the reversibility of the pulmonary vascular and perivascular lesions.

Congenital Heart Disease

Pulmonary hypertension is part of the natural history of many types of congenital heart disease and is often a major determinant of the clinical course, feasibility of surgical intervention, and outcome. Congenital defects of the heart associated with large left-to-right shunts (e.g., atrial septal defect) or abnormal communications between the great vessels (e.g., patent ductus arteriosus) are commonly associated with pulmonary arterial hypertension. The major cause of pulmonary hypertension in congenital heart disease is an increase in blood flow, an increase in resistance to blood flow, or, most often, a combination of the two.

Caution is required in administering vasodilator agents to patients with congenital heart disease because of the potential to increase right-to-left shunting by reducing systemic vascular resistance to a greater degree than its pulmonary counterpart. Phlebotomy, with replacement of fluid (e.g., plasma or albumin), is helpful in congenital cyanotic heart disease in which severe hypoxemia has evoked a large increase in red cell mass.

Thromboembolic Disease

Thromboembolic disease is a form of occlusive pulmonary vascular disease. It may be acute or chronic. Tumor emboli to the lungs from extrapulmonary sites (e.g., the breast) can cause pulmonary hypertension by invading the adjacent minute vessels of the lungs. Intravenous drug use may be associated with talc or cotton fiber embolism to the lungs, which can result in a granulomatous pulmonary arteritis.

CHRONIC PROXIMAL PULMONARY THROMBOEMBOLISM

In some patients who have survived large to massive pulmonary emboli, resolution fails to occur and the clots become organized and incorporated into the walls of the major pulmonary arteries, leading to pulmonary hypertension By the time the diagnosis is made, the obstructing lesions in the central pulmonary arteries have become an integral part of the vascular wall through the processes of endothelialization and recanalization.

The importance of recognizing *proximal* pulmonary thromboembolism as a cause of pulmonary hypertension is in the possibility of relieving the pulmonary hypertension by surgical intervention, i.e., by pulmonary thromboendarterectomy. Ventilation/perfusion lung scanning is the critical diagnostic test. As a rule, patients with proximal pulmonary thromboembolism show two or more segmental perfusion defects. If the perfusion defects are segmental or larger, selective pulmonary angiography is called for to define the location, extent, and number of pulmonary vascular occlusions. Cardiac catheterization for selective pulmonary angiography also enables hemodynamic assessment.

Surgery is advocated for patients with pulmonary hypertension who have persistent clotting in lobar or more proximal pulmonary arteries after at least 6 months of anticoagulation. Thromboendarterectomy is done via a median sternotomy using deep hypothermic cardiopulmonary bypass with intermittent periods of circulatory arrest. Postoperatively, hemodynamic improvement is usually quite dramatic. Reperfusion pulmonary edema can be a severe complication immediately after the obstruction has been relieved. In experienced hands, mortality is of the order of 5 percent. After the operation, patients are placed on lifelong anticoagulants. A filter is usually placed in the inferior vena cava to further prevent recurrence.

RESPIRATORY DISEASES AND DISORDERS

In addition to intrinsic pulmonary diseases, disturbances in respiratory muscle function or in the control of breathing can also lead to pulmonary hypertension. Among the intrinsic lung diseases are those affecting the airways (e.g., chronic bronchitis) as well as those affecting the parenchyma (i.e., emphysema, pulmonary fibrosis). Among the ventilatory disorders are the syndromes of alveolar hypoventilation due to respiratory muscle weakness and sleep-disordered breathing.

Interstitial Fibrosis

Pulmonary sarcoidosis, asbestosis, idiopathic, and radiation-induced fibrosis are common causes of widespread pulmonary fibrosis that culminates in cor pulmonale. Dyspnea and tachypnea generally dominate the clinical picture of interstitial fibrosis; cough is rarely prominent. As a rule, severe pulmonary hypertension occurs toward the end of the illness, when hypoxemia and hypercapnia are present at rest. Right ventricular failure is a common sequel.

Systemically administered vasodilators have no proven place in dealing with the pulmonary hypertension associated with interstitial fibrosis and may worsen intrapulmonary gas exchange. Oxygen therapy, particularly during daily activity or sleep, can be important in attenuating the hypoxic pulmonary pressor response. Glucocorticoids and other potent immunosuppressive agents are the mainstay of therapy and often effect some symptomatic relief. The advent of lung transplantation has widened greatly the therapeutic horizons for dealing with widespread interstitial fibrosis.

Chronic Obstructive Airways Disease

Chronic bronchitis and emphysema [chronic obstructive pulmonary disease (COPD)] are the most common causes of cor pulmonale in patients with intrinsic pulmonary disease. Cystic fibrosis is an example of a mixed airway and parenchymal lung disease in which pulmonary hypertension plays a significant role in outcome.

Cor pulmonale is encountered in two different settings: *acutely* in the setting of decompensation, which is often due to an acute respiratory infection, and *chronically* when progressive lung disease and worsening gas exchange lead to unremitting vascular remodeling.

In the patient with COPD with acute cor pulmonale precipitated by a bout of bronchitis or pneumonia, the goal of therapy is to maintain tolerable levels of arterial oxygenation while waiting for the upper respiratory infection to subside. Supplemental oxygen, such as 28% oxygen delivered by a Venturi mask, generally suffices to relieve arterial hypoxemia and to restore pulmonary arterial pressures toward normal. Considerable improvement may also be accomplished even in the individual who has chronic pulmonary hypertension by sustained (>18 h/day) breathing of oxygen-enriched air.

Arterial blood gas composition is the therapeutic compass to the control of pulmonary hypertension in COPD. The degree of hypoxia may be underestimated by blood sampling while the patient is awake and at rest, since hypoxemia is more marked during sleep and with physical activity. Determinations of the oxygen saturation during sleep or with ambulation, using pulse oximetry, are helpful in optimally prescribing supplemental oxygen.

Vasodilators have recently been tried in various types of secondary pulmonary hypertension, including that due to COPD. The agents tried are the same as those outlined for *primary* pulmonary hypertension. They run the risk of aggravating arterial hypoxemia by exaggerating ventilation/perfusion abnormalities. To date, the safest and most effective approach to pulmonary vasodilatation in obstructive lung disease with arterial hypoxemia is the use of supplemental oxygen.

CONNECTIVE TISSUE DISEASES

Pulmonary vascular disease is an important component of certain connective tissue diseases. Among these, the more common are systemic lupus erythematosus (SLE), the scleroderma spectrum of diseases, and dermatomyositis.

In progressive systemic sclerosis (scleroderma) and its variants, such as the CREST syndrome (*c*alcinosis, *R*aynaud's syndrome, *e*sophageal involvement, *s*clerodactyly, and *t*elangiectasis) and in overlap syndromes (e.g., mixed connective tissue disease), the incidence of pulmonary vascular disease is high. In these patients, pulmonary hypertension is the cause of considerable morbidity and mortality. The pulmonary vascular disease may be independent of pulmonary or other visceral disease. As in the case of SLE, the pathology of these lesions is often indistinguishable from that of primary pulmonary hypertension. Vasodilator therapy has not proved to be highly effective; however, continuous intravenous epoprostenol has recently been shown to improve hemodynamics and exercise tolerance.

Alveolar Hypoventilation in Patients with Normal Lungs

In patients who hypoventilate despite normal lungs (alveolar hypoventilation), the primary pathogenetic mechanism is alveolar hypoxia potentiated by respiratory acidosis. These abnormal alveolar and arterial blood gases play the same role in eliciting pulmonary hypertension in patients with alveolar hypoventilation as in those in whom the abnormal alveolar and blood gases are the result of ventilation/perfusion abnormalities. For the patient with alveolar hypoventilation with combined respiratory and cardiac (right ventricular) failure, the highest therapeutic priority is to improve oxygenation. Assisted ventilation, particularly during sleep, may be particularly helpful in improving oxygenation and reducing hypercapnic [e.g., continuous positive airway pressure (CPAP)] breathing.

PRIMARY PULMONARY HYPERTENSION

Definition

Primary pulmonary hypertension (PPH), a disorder intrinsic to the pulmonary vascular bed, is characterized by sustained elevations in pulmonary artery pressure and vascular resistance that generally lead to right ventricular failure and death. The diagnosis of PPH requires the exclusion on clinical grounds of other conditions that can result in pulmonary artery hypertension. PPH is a rare disease, with an incidence of 1 to 2 per million. Its prevalence is about 0.1 to 0.2 percent of all patients who come to autopsy.

The clinical diagnosis of PPH rests on three different types of evidence: (1) clinical, radiographic, and electrocardiographic manifestations of pulmonary hypertension; (2) hemodynamic features consisting of abnormally high pulmonary arterial pressures and pulmonary vascular resistance in association with normal left-sided filling pressures and a normal or low cardiac output; and (3) exclusion of the causes of secondary pulmonary hypertension.

SPECIAL TYPES

Certain associations of PPH have attracted interest because of their prospects for shedding light on some etiologies. These include so-called anorexigen-induced pulmonary hypertension; familial pulmonary hypertension; human immunodeficiency virus (HIV) associated pulmonary hypertension, and portal-pulmonary hypertension.

In each of these, the clinical findings and the histologic appearance of the lungs at autopsy are identical to those that characterize the sporadic form of PPH. This diversity in associations underscores the likelihood that so-called PPH is the final common expression of heterogeneous etiologies.

As a rule, median survival of patients can be predicted on the basis of the New York Heart Association functional classification: 6 months for class IV; $2\frac{1}{2}$ years for class III; and 6 years for classes I and II. Unless interrupted by sudden death, which occurs in approximately 15 percent of patients, the usual downhill course terminates in intractable right ventricular failure.

The combination of right-sided heart catheterization and vasodilator testing is particularly useful not only for defining the hemodynamic state of the patient but also in providing a hemodynamic baseline for future invasive and noninvasive studies, such as serial echocardiograms.

Treatment

A patient with PPH has several therapeutic options, ranging from oral calcium channel blockers to continuous infusion of prostacyclin to lung transplantation.

In experienced centers, the trial of nifedipine or diltiazem orally is preceded by use of testing of acute vasoreactivity using one or more of three agents: (1) inhaled nitric oxide (NO), in concentrations of 10 to 40 ppm for 5 to 10 min; (2) prostacyclin (PGI_2; epoprostenol, Flolan), administered intravenously in increasing doses—starting dose of 1 to 2 ng/kg/min followed by successive increments every 15 min of 2 ng/kg/min until a maximal dose of 12 ng/kg/min is reached or side effects preclude further increases; (3) adenosine, 50 to 200 ng/kg/min. Only patients who manifest significant reductions in pulmonary vascular resistance (usually greater than 20 to 30 percent), resulting from a fall in pulmonary artery pressure without systemic hypotension and accompanied by an unchanged or increased cardiac output, are considered candidates for chronic therapy with oral calcium channel blockers.

Intravenous epoprostenol (Flolan, prostacyclin, PGI_2), a metabolite of arachidonic acid, and its analogs continue to be a major focus of attention as treatments for a variety of forms of pulmonary hypertension. Success in long-term management has recently been reported using aerosolized iloprost, a stable prostacyclin analog. Currently, its most effective use is for long-term management in patients with severe (NYHA class III or IV) primary pulmonary hypertension or scleroderma who are unresponsive to therapy with calcium channel blockers or are not candidates for it.

The use of anticoagulants has been incorporated into the therapeutic regimen in patients with PPH. The usual goal of anticoagulation is to achieve and maintain an International Normalized Ratio (INR) of 2 to 2.5.

ATRIAL SEPTOSTOMY

Blade-balloon atrial septostomy has been performed in patients with severe right ventricular pressure and volume overload refractory to maximal medical therapy. The goal of this approach is to decompress the overloaded right heart and improve systemic output of the underfilled left ventricle. Improvements in exercise function and signs of severe right heart dysfunction such as syncope and ascites have been observed. Since the creation of an interatrial communication results in an increased venous admixture, worsening hypoxemia is an expected outcome. The size of the septostomy that is created should be carefully monitored in order to achieve the ideal balance of optimizing systemic oxygen transport and reducing right heart filling pressures without overfilling a noncompliant left ventricle or producing extreme degrees of venous admixture.

LUNG TRANSPLANTATION

Only one-third of patients with PPH are responsive to long-term oral vasodilator therapy. Of the remainder, approximately 65 to 75 percent maintain sustained clinical improvement with long-term continuous intravenous therapy using prostacyclin. When pulmonary hypertensive disease has progressed or threatens to progress to the stage of right ventricular failure, the physician and patient are left with few therapeutic options other than lung transplantation. Lung transplantation is currently being done at specialized centers and is almost invariably handicapped by shortage of donor lungs, which can lead to long delays. Single- or double-lung transplantation has largely replaced heart-lung transplantation. Rejection phenomena, notably bronchiolitis obliterans, are the major limiting factor to prolonged survival. The median survival after lung transplantation is approximately 3 years. Recurrence of PPH after transplantation has not been reported.

SUGGESTED READING

Barst RJ, Rubin LJ, Long WA, et al: A comparison of continuous intravenous epoprostenol (prostacyclin) with conventional therapy for primary pulmonary hypertension. *N Engl J Med* 1996; 334:296–302.

D'Alonzo GE, Barst RJ, Ayres SM, et al: Survival in patients with primary pulmonary hypertension. *Ann Intern Med* 1991; 115: 343–349.

Fedullo PF, Auger WR, Channick RN, et al: Chronic thromboembolic pulmonary hypertension. *Clin Chest Med* 1995; 16:353–374.

Olschewski H, Ardeschir H, Walmrath D, et al: Inhaled prostacyclin and iloprost in severe pulmonary hypertension secondary to lung fibrosis. *Am J Respir Crit Care Med* 1999; 160:600–603.

Rich S, Kaufmann E, Levy PS: The effect of high doses of calcium-channel blockers on survival in primary pulmonary hypertension. *N Engl J Med* 1992; 327:76–81.

Rubin LJ: Primary pulmonary hypertension. *N Eng J Med* 1997; 336:111–117.

Rubin LJ: Pulmonary hypertension. In: Fuster V, Alexander RW, O'Rourke RA, et al (eds): *Hurst's The Heart,* 10th ed. New York: McGraw-Hill; 2001:1607–1623.

Voelkel NF, Tuder RM, Weir EK: Pathophysiology of primary pulmonary hypertension: In Rubin LJ, Rich S (eds): *Primary Pulmonary Hypertension.* New York: Marcel Dekker; 1997:83–133.

Weitzenblum E, Oswald M, Mirhom R, et al: Evolution of pulmonary haemodynamics in COLD patients under long-term oxygen therapy. *Eur Respir J* 1989; 2(suppl 7):669S–673S.

20

PULMONARY EMBOLISM

Victor F. Tapson

Approximately 100,000 patients die each year in the United States directly from acute pulmonary embolism (PE). PE contributes significantly to the death of another 100,000 patients with concomitant disease. A substantial number of patients die prior to being diagnosed with PE. Many of these deaths appear to be preventable. Autopsy studies have repeatedly documented the high frequency with which PE has gone unsuspected and undetected. Despite advances in diagnostic technology and therapeutic approaches, PE remains underdiagnosed and prophylaxis continues to be dramatically underutilized. PE nearly always results from deep venous thrombosis (DVT) of the proximal deep veins of the leg—that is, including and proximal to the popliteal veins, although axillary and subclavian vein thrombi may also embolize. Treatment of established PE substantially reduces the mortality from this disease.

DEEP VENOUS THROMBOSIS: RISK FACTORS AND PATHOGENESIS

Virchow proposed that the pathogenesis of DVT was based upon several potential initiating events, including stasis, venous injury, and hypercoagulability. Risk factors for DVT—which may be acquired or inherited—are based upon these processes (Table 20-1). Frequently more than one risk factor is present. Antecedent pulmonary thromboembolism forecasts an appreciable risk of recurrence in the hospitalized patient. Surgery, trauma, immobility, cancer, and pregnancy and the postpartum period are important acquired risks. In addition, several hereditary risk factors have been identified over recent years. These include the factor V Leiden mutation and the prothrombin gene (G20210A) defect. The factor V Leiden mutation is a common genetic polymorphism associated with activated resistance to protein C and appears to be present in approximately 4 to 6 percent of the general population. There has been increasing interest in the potential role of homocysteine in venous

TABLE 20-1

RISK FACTORS FOR VENOUS
THROMBOEMBOLISM

Acquired factors
    Age greater than 40
    Prior history of venous thromboembolism
    Prior major surgical procedure
    Trauma
    Hip fracture
    Immobilization/paralysis
    Venous stasis
    Varicose veins
    Congestive heart failure
    Myocardial infarction
    Obesity
    Pregnancy/postpartum period
    Oral contraceptive therapy
    Cerebrovascular accident
    Malignancy
    Severe thrombocythemia
    Paroxysmal nocturnal hemoglobinuria
    Antiphospholipid antibody syndrome (including lupus
        anticoagulant)
Inherited factors
    Antithrombin III deficiency
    Factor V Leiden (activated protein C
      resistance)
    Prothrombin gene (G20210A) defect
    Protein C deficiency
    Protein S deficiency
    Dysfibrinogenemia
    Disorders of plasminogen

thromboembolism (VTE). In vitro, homocysteine has potentially thrombogenic effects, including injury to vascular endothelium and antagonism of the synthesis and function of nitric oxide. Coexisting hyperhomocysteinemia has been shown to increase the risk for thrombosis in patients with factor V Leiden. The importance of elevated factor XI and factor VIII levels as risk factors have recently been reported.

ACUTE PULMONARY EMBOLISM: PATHOPHYSIOLOGY

Gas Exchange Abnormalities

Hypoxemia develops in the preponderance of patients with PE and has been attributed to various mechanisms. When no previous cardiopulmonary disease is present, lung regions with low ventilation/perfusion ratios and shunting due to perfusion of atelectatic areas appear to be the predominant mechanisms of hypoxemia. Hypoxemia leads to an increase in sympathetic tone, with systemic vasoconstriction, and may actually increase venous return with augmentation of stroke volume, at least initially, if significant underlying cardiac or pulmonary pathology is not already present.

Hemodynamic Alterations

Massive emboli can cause profound hemodynamic compromise. The consequence of the embolic event depends upon the extent of obstruction of the pulmonary vascular bed as well as the presence or absence of underlying cardiovascular disease. The increased pulmonary vascular resistance impedes right ventricular outflow, with a reduction in left ventricular preload. When no underlying cardiopulmonary disease is present, occlusion of 25 to 30 percent of the vascular bed by emboli is associated with a rise in pulmonary artery pressure. As the extent of vascular obstruction increases, hypoxemia worsens, stimulating vasoconstriction and a further rise in pulmonary artery pressure. Greater than 50 percent obstruction of the pulmonary arterial bed is generally present before there is substantial elevation of the mean pulmonary artery pressure (PAP). When the extent of embolic occlusion approaches 75 percent, the right ventricle must generate a systolic pressure in excess of 50 mmHg and a mean PAP of greater than 40 mmHg to preserve pulmonary perfusion. Theoretically, a hypertrophied right ventricle (in an otherwise normal patient) may be capable of achieving pressures this high, but a normal right ventricle is unable to do so and will fail.

THE DIAGNOSIS OF DEEP VENOUS THROMBOSIS AND PULMONARY EMBOLISM

Venous thromboembolism represents the spectrum of one disease. Most clinically significant PEs arise from the prior development of DVT in the lower extremities, with subsequent embolization of at least part of the thrombosis to the lungs. Patients may present with symptoms of either DVT, PE, or both. At the present time, the diagnostic strategy usually involves an imaging study aimed at either the legs or the lungs, depending upon the presentation. The diagnostic approach to acute DVT and PE has recently been exhaustively reviewed and presented in clinical practice guidelines by the American Thoracic Society.

The History and Physical Examination

The clinical diagnosis of both DVT and PE, based upon the history and physical examination, are insensitive and nonspecific. Patients with DVT of the lower extremity may be asymptomatic or may have erythema, warmth, pain, swelling, and/or tenderness. These findings, however, while not specific for DVT, suggest the need for further evaluation. The differential diagnosis of DVT includes cellulitis, edema from other causes, musculoskeletal pain, or trauma (some of these may be concomitant and may or may not be related). Pulmonary embolism must always be considered when unexplained dyspnea is present. Dyspnea as well as pleuritic chest pain and hemoptysis are common in PE but are nonspecific. Anxiety, light-headedness, and syncope are all symptoms that may be due to PE but may also result from a number of other entities that cause hypoxemia or hypotension. Tachypnea and tachycardia are the most common signs of PE but are also nonspecific. Syncope or sudden hypotension should suggest the possibility of massive PE. The cardiac and pulmonary physical examinations are both nonspecific. In spite of the limitations of the history and physical examination for PE, the index of clinical suspicion becomes a more useful parameter when it is considered in conjunction with ventilation/perfusion ($\dot{V}/\dot{Q}$) scanning. Dyspnea, tachypnea, clear lung fields, and hypoxemia may often be attributed to a flare of chronic obstructive pulmonary disease (COPD) or asthma when underlying PE is present. Thus, diagnostic efforts aimed at possible VTE should still be considered despite alternative explanations if risk factors and the clinical setting are suggestive.

Laboratory Testing for Acute Deep Venous Thrombosis and Pulmonary Embolism

Routine laboratory testing is not useful in proving the presence of DVT or PE but may be helpful in confirming or excluding other diagnoses. The utility of plasma measurements of circulating D-dimer, a specific derivative of cross-linked fibrin, as a diagnostic aid in PE has been extensively evaluated. A normal enzyme-linked immunosorbent assay (ELISA) appears to be sensitive in excluding PE. When the D-dimer level is 500 ug/L or greater, the sensitivity and specificity for PE have been shown to be 98 and 39 percent respectively. While the sensitivity of the D-dimer appears high, the specificity is not high enough to be diagnostic. The D-dimer level would appear to be most useful when it is negative and clinical suspicion for DVT or PE is not particularly high (low pretest probability). Rapid "bedside assays" are becoming increasingly available, and additional outcome studies will further define their role. At the present time, plasma D-dimer measurements should be interpreted with caution and in the context of other diagnostic tests.

Hypoxemia is common in acute PE. Some individuals, particularly young patients without underlying lung disease, may have a normal Pa_{O_2}. The diagnosis of acute PE cannot be excluded based upon a normal Pa_{O_2}, and although the alveolar-arterial difference is usually elevated, even this may rarely be normal in patients without preexisting cardiopulmonary disease.

Electrocardiography (ECG) cannot be relied upon to rule in or rule out PE, though electrocardiographic proof of a clear alternative diagnosis, such as myocardial infarction, is useful when PE is among the possible diagnoses. The potential coexistence of PE together with another process must, however, be a consideration. ECG findings in acute PE are generally nonspecific and include T-wave changes, ST-segment abnormalities, and left- or right-axis deviation. The S1Q3T3 pattern, while commonly considered specific for PE, is seen in only a minority of patients. The low frequency of specific ECG changes associated with PE was confirmed in the PIOPED study.

Chest Radiography in Suspected Pulmonary Embolism

Most patients with PE have an abnormal but nonspecific chest radiograph. Common radiographic findings include atelectasis, pleural effusion, pulmonary infiltrates, and mild elevation of a hemidiaphragm. Classic findings of pulmonary infarction—such as Hampton's hump or decreased vascularity (Westermark's sign)—are suggestive but infrequent. A normal chest radiograph in the setting of severe dyspnea and hypoxemia without evidence of bronchospasm or anatomic cardiac shunt is strongly suggestive of PE. Under most circumstances, the chest radiograph cannot be used to conclusively diagnose or exclude PE.

Other Imaging Studies for Suspected Acute Pulmonary Embolism

The $\dot{V}/\dot{Q}$ scan has been the pivotal diagnostic test performed when PE is suspected. Normal and high-probability scans are considered diagnostic. A normal perfusion scan rules out the diagnosis of PE with a high enough degree of certainty that further diagnostic evaluation is unnecessary. Matching areas of decreased ventilation and perfusion in the presence of a normal chest radiograph generally represent a process other than PE. However, low- or intermediate-probability (nondiagnostic) scans are commonly found with PE; in such situations, further evaluation with pulmonary arteriography is often appropriate. In the PIOPED study, when the clinical suspicion of PE was considered very high, PE was found to be present in 96 percent of patients with high-probability scans, 66 percent of patients with intermediate scans, and 40 percent of those with low-probability scans. The diagnosis of PE should be rigorously pursued even when the lung scan is of low or intermediate probability if the clinical scenario suggests PE. Therefore, while the $\dot{V}/\dot{Q}$ scan may sometimes be diagnostic of PE or may exclude the possibility with sufficient certainty, it is often nondiagnostic. Even in such circumstances, however, it may serve as a useful guide for limited pulmonary arteriography.

Spiral (helical) computed tomography (CT) has been increasingly performed at many hospitals instead of $\dot{V}/\dot{Q}$ scanning for suspected PE. Studies to date suggest that spiral CT has a relatively high specificity for PE, but its sensitivity has been more variable. Spiral CT appears sensitive in many clinical trials to the level of segmental pulmonary arteries. An advantage of CT over the $\dot{V}/\dot{Q}$ scan is the potential to diagnose other entities. A prospective, multicenter clinical trial is under way in the United States to better determine the sensitivity and specificity of the spiral CT compared with the $\dot{V}/\dot{Q}$ scan.

Pulmonary arteriography has remained the accepted "gold standard" technique for the diagnosis of PE. It is a very sensitive, specific, and safe test. An alternative to pulmonary arteriography when the $\dot{V}/\dot{Q}$ or CT scan is nondiagnostic is to perform lower extremity studies; if these are positive, treatment may often be instituted based on this result.

Echocardiography is not generally useful for proving the presence of PE, although it may offer compelling clues to its presence in certain clinical settings and it has been suggested as a potential means by which to determine the need for thrombolytic therapy. However, this test can often be obtained more rapidly than either lung scanning or pulmonary arteriography, and it may reveal findings that strongly support hemodynamically significant PE. Studies of patients with documented PE have revealed that more than 80 percent have imaging or Doppler abnormalities of right ventricular size or function that may suggest acute PE. Unfortunately, because patients with PE often have underlying cardiopulmonary disease such as COPD, neither right ventricular dilation nor hypokinesis can be reliably used even as indirect evidence of PE in such settings.

Magnetic resonance imaging (MRI) is also being utilized to evaluate clinically suspected DVT or PE. In a comparison with spiral CT, the average sensitivity of CT for five observers was 75 percent and of MRI 46 percent. The average specificity of CT was 89 percent, compared with 90 percent for MRI. Sensitivity and specificity values for expert readers were higher, however. Helical CT may be somewhat more useful than MRI for detecting PE at the present time, but MRI has several attractive advantages, including excellent sensitivity and specificity for the diagnosis of DVT. This technique may ultimately allow simultaneous accurate detection of both PE and DVT. Future investigations will determine the roles of these modalities in the evaluation of PE.

Imaging Studies for Suspected Deep Venous Thrombosis

The available technology used to pursue the diagnosis of DVT has expanded over the past several decades. Each technique has advantages and limitations. While contrast venography remains the gold standard for the diagnosis of DVT, it has been less commonly performed since the advent of Doppler ultrasonography. Venography should be performed whenever noninvasive testing is nondiagnostic or impossible to perform. Doppler ultrasonography is a portable and accurate diagnostic technique for proximal lower extremity DVT. Its sensitivity and specificity for symptomatic proximal DVT has been well above 90 percent in most recent clinical trials. Limitations include insensitivity for asymptomatic DVT, operator dependence, the inability to accurately distinguish acute from chronic DVT in symptomatic patients, and insensitivity to calf vein thrombosis. Compared to other technology, it is relatively inexpensive and is the most commonly utilized initial diagnostic modality for the straightforward case of symptomatic presumed proximal DVT. Impedance plethysmography (IPG) has been shown to be reliable for the detection of DVT occurring above the knee. Early studies suggested greater than 90 percent sensitivity and 97 percent specificity for DVT involving the proximal lower extremity, although less than 30 percent of isolated calf vein thromboses were detected. Other reports have emphasized the limitations of IPG. The specificity is affected by disorders that obstruct venous outflow, such as tumor or hematoma. External fixation or plaster immobilization of extremities reduces the utility of IPG. This technique is rarely used in the United States. Magnetic resonance imaging (MRI) is being increasingly used at some centers to diagnose DVT and appears to be an accurate, noninvasive alternative to venography. A major advantage of this technique is excellent resolution of the inferior vena cava and pelvic veins. Preliminary experience with this technique suggests that it is at least as accurate as contrast venography and ultrasound imaging.

PRINCIPLES OF MANAGEMENT

Prophylaxis of Deep Venous Thrombosis

A significant reduction in the incidence of DVT can be achieved when patients at risk receive appropriate prophylaxis. Such preventive measures appear to be grossly underutilized. A review of the use of prophylaxis for DVT in 16 Massachusetts hospitals indicates that such therapy is administered to only 44 percent of high-risk patients in teaching hospitals and only 19 percent in nonteaching hospitals. The frequency of prophylaxis ranged from 9 to 56 percent among hospitals. Surgical and medical patients can be stratified according to DVT risk, and certain prophylactic measures are more appropriate for some patients than for others. The American College of Chest Physicians has published guidelines for antithrombotic therapy that offer evidence-based recommendations for the prevention and therapy of venous thromboembolism. These guidelines offer specific preventive recommendations for general, orthopedic, trauma, stroke, spinal cord injury, and medical patients. The low-molecular-weight heparin (LMWH) preparations are being used increasingly for the prevention and treatment of VTE. Certain populations of patients, such as those who have undergone total knee and hip replacement, are at particularly high risk, and the use of LMWH has proven particularly effective as prophylaxis in these individuals. Enoxaparin has been approved for use as prophylaxis in both of these joint replacement groups as well as for general abdominal surgery prophylaxis. Dalteparin, another LMWH, is approved for prevention in patients undergoing total hip replacement and general abdominal surgery. In general medical patients at risk for DVT, subcutaneous heparin at 5000 U every 8 to 12 h is generally adequate. More recently LMWH (enoxaparin 40 mg delivered subcutaneously once daily) has been approved for use in medical patients deemed at moderate risk for DVT. This regimen reduced the risk of DVT compared with either 20 mg of this drug or placebo. It is important to realize that these preparations are not identical, and the results of clinical trials with one agent cannot be extrapolated to another agent. Intermittent pneumatic compression devices should be utilized in medical or surgical patients when prophylactic anticoagulation is contraindicated. Both methods combined are reasonable in patients deemed to be at exceptionally high risk. Recommendations for specific settings can be obtained from the Sixth American College of Chest Physicians Consensus Conference on Antithrombotic Therapy (supplement to *Chest,* January 2001).

Treatment of Established Venous Thromboembolism with Heparin and Low Molecular Weight Heparin

Anticoagulation has been proven to reduce mortality in acute PE. When VTE is diagnosed or strongly suspected, anticoagulation therapy should be promptly instituted unless contraindications exist. Confirmatory testing should always be planned if anticoagulation is to be continued. Heparin and LMWH exert a prompt antithrombotic effect, preventing thrombus growth. While thrombus growth can be prevented, early recurrence can develop even in the setting of therapeutic anticoagulation.

With the institution of continuous intravenous heparin, the activated partial thromboplastin time (APTT) should be aggressively followed at 6-h intervals until it is consistently in the therapeutic range of 1.5 to 2.0 times control values. In general, heparin should be administered as an intravenous bolus of 5000 U followed by a maintenance dose of at least 30,000 to 40,000 U/24 h by continuous infusion. The lower dose is administered if the patient is considered at high risk for bleeding. This aggressive approach decreases the risk of subtherapeutic anticoagulation, and although supratherapeutic levels are sometimes achieved initially, bleeding complications do not appear to be increased. An alternative regimen consisting of a bolus of 80 U/kg followed by 18 U/kg/h has been recommended. Further adjustment of the heparin dose should also be weight-based (Table 20-2). Warfarin therapy may be initiated as soon as the APTT is therapeutic, and heparin should be maintained until a therapeutic International Normalized Ratio (INR) of 2.0 to 3.0 has been overlapped with a therapeutic APTT for 3 consecutive days. While proximal lower extremity thrombus is more likely to result in PE, calf thrombi should either be followed for proximal extension over 10 to 14 days with noninvasive testing or anticoagulation should be instituted. Documented proximal DVT or PE should be treated

TABLE 20-2

WEIGHT-BASED NOMOGRAM FOR HEPARIN THERAPY
IN ACUTE VENOUS THROMBOEMBOLISM

Initial heparin dose = 80-U/kg bolus, then 18 U/kg/h
Subsequent modifications are shown below.

APTT		Heparin Dose Adjustment
(seconds)	(times control)	
<35	<1.2	80-U/kg bolus, then increase by 4 U/kg/h
35 to 45	1.2 to 1.5	40-U/kg bolus, then increase by 2 U/kg/h
46 to 70	1.5 to 2.3	No change
71 to 90	2.3 to 3	Decrease infusion rate by 2 U/kg/h
>90	>3	Hold infusion 1 h, then decrease rate by 3 U/kg/h

SOURCE: Hyers et al. and Raschke et al.

for 3 months. Longer treatment is appropriate when significant risk factors persist.

A number of clinical trials have strongly suggested the efficacy and safety of LMWH for treatment of established acute proximal DVT, using recurrent symptomatic VTE as the primary outcome measure. There are several advantages of these drugs. They have excellent bioavailability and can be administered once or twice daily. No monitoring is required in most patients. Because of the ease of administration of these preparations, home therapy of DVT is being practiced increasingly. In two large randomized (Canadian and European) trials, therapy with LMWH was safely initiated at home or continued at home after a brief hospitalization. Metanalyses have examined the use of LMWH compared with unfractionated heparin in the initial treatment of acute proximal DVT, and these have helped to confirm the efficacy and safety of LMWH for the treatment of established DVT. At the present time, enoxaparin and—more recently—tinzaparin are approved for use in patients presenting with DVT with or without PE. As yet, tinzaparin has no other approved indications. Advantages of LMWH preparations are summarized in Table 20-3 and dosing guidelines are outlined in Table 20-4.

TABLE 20-3

POTENTIAL ADVANTAGES OF LOW-MOLECULAR-WEIGHT HEPARINS OVER UNFRACTIONATED HEPARIN

Comparable or superior efficacy
Comparable or superior safety
Superior bioavailability
Once- or twice-daily dosing
No laboratory monitoring
Less phlebotomy
Subcutaneous administration
Earlier ambulation
Home therapy in certain patient subsets

TABLE 20-4

USE OF FDA-APPROVED LOW-MOLECULAR-WEIGHT HEPARINS FOR TREATMENT OF DEEP VENOUS THROMBOSIS WITH OR WITHOUT PULMONARY EMBOLISM*

LMWH[†]	Dose
Enoxaparin	1 mg/kg subcutaneously every 12 h (inpatient or outpatient) 1.5 mg/kg subcutaneously once daily (inpatient)
Tinzaparin	175 Xa U/kg subcutaneously once daily[‡]

*These two LMWH preparations are the only two that are FDA-approved for treatment of established venous thromboembolism.

[†]Warfarin is initiated within 24 h after the LMWH is started. At least 5 days of therapy with LMWH is appropriate; the International Normalized Ratio (INR) should be 2.0 or greater for two consecutive mornings prior to discontinuing the LMWH.

[‡]FDA approval based upon data derived from hospitalized patients.

NOTE: There are inadequate data from randomized trials to treat symptomatic pulmonary embolism in the outpatient setting.

KEY: Xa = factor Xa measured level.

Novel Anticoagulants and Experimental Models of Thrombosis

Newer agents are being explored. Although heparin is the best-studied antithrombin agent, it works indirectly, requiring antithrombin III as a cofactor. Heparin's effects vary considerably among patients. Hirudin, a direct thrombin inhibitor, has several advantages over heparin, including efficacy against fibrin clot–bound thrombin. It does not require any cofactors and is not inactivated by platelet factor 4 or plasma proteins. Other agents, such as the hirudin analog bivalirudin, await study. As with heparin, these direct thrombin inhibitors have very narrow therapeutic indices.

Complications of Anticoagulation

Complications of heparin include bleeding and heparin-induced thrombocytopenia (HIT). The rates of major bleeding in recent trials using heparin by continuous infusion or high-dose subcutaneous injection are less than 5 percent. When necessary in the setting of bleeding, heparin can be reversed with protamine. Heparin-induced thrombocytopenia (defined as a platelet count less than 150,000 mm^3) typically develops 5 or more days after the initiation of heparin therapy, occurring in 5 to 10 percent of patients. The syndrome is caused by heparin-dependent IgG antibodies that activate platelets via their Fc receptors. It has been demonstrated that these antibodies recognize heparin complexed with platelet factor 4. LMWHs may be considered in this setting, since the formation of heparin-dependent IgG antibodies and the risk of HIT may be lower with this form of heparin. Argatroban, a direct thrombin inhibitor, and lepirudin (hirudin) are approved for use in heparin-induced thrombocytopenia.

Vena Cava Interruption

If anticoagulation therapy cannot be continued, inferior vena cava (IVC) filter placement can be undertaken to prevent lower extremity thrombi from embolizing to the lungs. The primary indications for filter placement include contraindications to or significant bleeding complications during anticoagulation or recurrent embolism while the patient is on adequate therapy. Filters are sometimes placed in the setting of massive PE when it is believed that any further emboli might be lethal. A number of filter designs exist, but the Greenfield filter has been most widely used. In general, anticoagulation is continued when a filter is placed unless this is contraindicated.

Thrombolytic Therapy and Acute Embolectomy

Acceleration of clot lysis in PE using thrombolytic therapy was first documented several decades ago. The National Institutes of Health consensus guidelines for PE thrombolysis, issued in 1980, recommended thrombolytic therapy for patients with obstruction of blood flow to a lobe or multiple pulmonary segments and for patients with hemodynamic compromise regardless of the size of the PE. Specific thrombolytic regimens are listed in Table 20-5. Thrombolytic therapy appears appropriate in patients with hemodynamic instability (hypotension) or severely compromised oxygenation. Stable patients with a significant embolic load are individualized, often receiving treatment in the absence of absolute or relative contraindications. Hemorrhagic complications due to thrombolytic therapy can be minimized when venous cut-downs and unnecessary arterial phlebotomy are avoided. At present, both streptokinase and recombinant tissue plasminogen activator (rt-PA) are approved for use in the treatment of PE. The latter drug is administered as a 100 mg intravenous infusion delivered over 2 h rather than a prolonged continuous infusion, as is the case with streptokinase. Urokinase is not currently available. It is recommended that heparin be withheld until the thrombolytic infusion is completed. The APTT is then determined and heparin is initiated without a loading dose if this value is less than twice the upper limit of normal. If the APTT exceeds this value, the test is repeated every 4 h until it is safe to proceed with heparin. The method of delivery of thrombolytic agents has also been investigated. Intrapulmonary arterial delivery of thrombolytic agents appears to offer no advantage over the intravenous route; *intraembolic* thrombolytic infusions, however, may offer advantages over merely infusing the agents into the pulmonary artery. Such techniques have been applied

TABLE 20-5

THROMBOLYTIC THERAPY FOR ACUTE PULMONARY EMBOLISM: APPROVED REGIMENS

Streptokinase: 250,000 U IV (loading dose over 30 min); then 100,000 U/h for 24 h*

Tissue-type plasminogen activator: 100 mg IV over 2 h

*Streptokinase administered over 24 to 72 h at this loading dose and rate has also been approved for use in patients with extensive deep venous thrombosis.

in both animal models of PE and in patients with enhanced thrombolysis. Larger randomized studies are needed to demonstrate the efficacy, potential advantages, and safety of such techniques. It is reasonable to consider systemic thrombolytic therapy in patients with proximal occlusive DVT associated with significant swelling and symptoms when there are no absolute or relative contraindications. The most devastating complication associated with this form of treatment is the development of intracranial hemorrhage. Clinical trials have suggested that this occurs in significantly less than 1 percent of patients. Bleeding related to thrombolytic therapy requires immediate diagnosis and management. Intracranial bleeding requires immediate discontinuation of thrombolytics or heparin, and emergent neurologic and neurosurgical consultation should be obtained. A noncontrasted brain CT scan should be performed. Patients with severe or refractory bleeding should be transfused with 10 U of cryoprecipitate and 2 U of fresh frozen plasma, and heparin can be reversed with protamine.

Pulmonary embolectomy may be performed in the setting of acute massive PE. While many patients die of PE before surgical embolectomy would be feasible, some deteriorate hours after the initial episode, suggesting that surgery may occasionally be appropriate. This approach is especially useful when there are contraindications to thrombolytic therapy. Transvenous embolectomy via a suction-catheter device has been utilized by some but has not received widespread acceptance. Catheter-directed thrombolytic therapy has been successfully employed in the setting of acute iliofemoral DVT. Further investigation in this area is under way.

Hemodynamic Management of Massive Pulmonary Embolism

Once massive PE associated with hypotension and/or severe hypoxemia is suspected, supportive treatment is immediately initiated. Intravenous saline should be infused rapidly but cautiously, since right ventricular function is often markedly compromised. Dopamine or norepinephrine appears to be the favored choice of vasoactive therapy in massive PE and should be administered if the blood pressure is not rapidly restored. Because death in this setting results from right ventricular failure, dobutamine has been suggested by some as a means by which to augment right ventricular output. However, in view of the potential for hypotension, caution is warranted. A vasopressor such as norepinephrine combined with dobutamine might offer optimal results; further exploration of such combined therapy could prove enlightening. Oxygen therapy is administered and thrombolytic therapy is considered, as described above. Intubation and institution of mechanical ventilation are instituted as needed to support respiratory failure.

CHRONIC THROMBOEMBOLISM

Although the vast majority of acute PEs resolve with treatment, occasionally a substantial residual thromboembolic burden remains. In this setting, the clot becomes organized and adherent and is not amenable to thrombolysis. If the obstruction becomes extensive, pulmonary hypertension develops. At least 50 percent of patients who develop chronic thromboembolic pulmonary hypertension have no documented history of DVT or PE. This feature may delay the diagnosis. Fatigue and dyspnea with exertion are the most common complaints. The $\dot{V}/\dot{Q}$ scan nearly always indicates a high probability of PE, but occasionally it is less impressive. Right heart catheterization and pulmonary arteriography are performed, both to establish the diagnosis with certainty and to determine operability. Pulmonary angioscopy has frequently proven complementary to arteriography in assessing these patients.

While anticoagulation should be instituted and IVC filter placement is recommended in patients with chronic thromboembolic pulmonary hypertension, the only was to alleviate symptoms and affect survival is with surgery. The group from the University of California at San Diego has had tremendous experience with evaluation and surgical therapy of these patients. Pulmonary thromboendarterectomy is performed via median sternotomy on cardiopulmonary bypass. The overall mortality, which has continued to improve, is now less than 5 percent. Lung transplantation can be performed in patients in whom thrombi are too distal to extract.

OTHER FORMS OF EMBOLISM

Fat embolism can cause a severe acute syndrome with sudden severe respiratory failure. This may be associated with confusion and petechiae. The entry of free fat globules into the lung most commonly occurs after long bone fractures of the lower extremities. Fat can also enter via direct trauma to subcutaneous fat. The exact pathophysiology of fat embolism syndrome is unknown and probably differs among patients. There is evidence that physiobiochemical alterations in circulating fat can result in the production of macroglobules of fat that may act as emboli. These fat droplets may obstruct small pulmonary arterial branches, including arterioles and capillaries. Other mechanisms include the release of thromboplastin from traumatized tissue, with resultant platelet aggregation; excess free fatty acidemia from the superimposition of fat on platelet aggregations, liberation of toxic free fatty acids in the lungs by enzymatic hydrolysis of embolic fat, with subsequent pulmonary capillary leak; and release of vasoactive and bronchoactive substances. Patients often develop acute respiratory distress syndrome (ARDS). Arterial hypoxemia is one of the earliest and most important laboratory findings. The chest radiograph usually shows extensive infiltrates. There is no specific therapy for fat embolism; the most important principle is maintenance of pulmonary oxygenation and function. High-dose glucocorticoids may decrease alveolar damage, although adequate clinical trials are lacking. Other forms of emboli include air embolism, amniotic fluid embolism; tumor embolism; embolism from heroin (talc), bullets, or shotgun shot, cardiac catheters, or indwelling venous catheters; embolism from bone marrow, parasites, and cardiac vegetations; and bile thromboembolism. The acuity and severity of these entities depend upon the specific embolic event and the clinical circumstances.

SUGGESTED READING

Ahearn G, Bounameaux H: The utility of D-dimer testing for acute venous thromboembolism. *Semin Respir Crit Care Med* 2001. In press.

Anderson FA, Wheeler HB: Venous thromboembolism: Risk factors and prophylaxis. *Clin Chest Med* 1995; 16:235–251.

Garg K, Sieler H, Welsh CH, et al: Clinical validity of helical CT being interpreted as negative for pulmonary embolism: Implications for patient treatment. *AJR* 1999; 172:1627–1631.

Goldhaber SZ, Haire WD, Feldstein ML, et al: Alteplase versus heparin in acute pulmonary embolism: Randomized trial assessing right ventricular function and pulmonary perfusion. *Lancet* 1993; 341:507–510.

Goldhaber SZ, Hennekens CH, Evans DA, et al: Factors associated with correct antemortem diagnosis of major pulmonary embolism. *Am J Med* 1982; 73:822–826.

Hyers TM, Agnelli G, Hull RD, et al: Antithrombotic therapy for venous thromboembolic disease: Fifth American College of Chest Physicians Consensus Conference on Antithrombotic Therapy. *Chest* 1998; 114:561S–578S.

Layish DT, Tapson VF: Pharmacologic hemodynamic support in massive pulmonary embolism. *Chest* 1997; 111:218–224.

Levine M, Gent M, Hirsh J, et al: A comparison of low molecular-weight-heparin administered primarily at home with unfractionated heparin administered in the hospital for proximal deep vein thrombosis. *N Engl J Med* 1996; 334:677–681.

Raschke RA, Reilly BM, Guidry JR, et al: The weight-based heparin dosing nomogram compared with a "standard care" nomogram. *Ann Intern Med* 1993; 119:874.

Tapson VF: Pulmonary embolism. In: Fuster V, Alexander RW, O'Rourke RA, et al (eds): *Hurst's The Heart,* 10th ed. New York: McGraw-Hill; 2001:1625–1643.

Tapson VF, Carroll BA, Davidson BA, et al: The diagnostic approach to venous thromboembolism. Clinical practice guideline. *Am J Respir Crit Care Med* 1999; 160:1043–1066.

Tapson VF, Witty LA: Massive pulmonary embolism: Diagnostic and therapeutic strategies. *Clin Chest Med* 1996; 16:329.

The PIOPED Investigators: Value of the ventilation/perfusion scan in acute pulmonary embolism. Results of the prospective investigation of pulmonary embolism diagnosis. *JAMA* 1990; 263:2753–2759.

DEFINITION

The term *cor pulmonale* describes the pathologic effects of lung dysfunction on the right side of the heart. Pulmonary hypertension is the link between lung dysfunction and the heart in cor pulmonale. Cor pulmonale can be an elusive clinical diagnosis because pulmonary hypertension can exist without clinical manifestations and because clinical signs, such as dyspnea, may be shared with the underlying disease. Acute pulmonary hypertension leads to acute dilatation of the right ventricle; chronic pulmonary hypertension leads to ventricular hypertrophy followed by dilatation. Right heart dysfunction secondary to left heart failure, valvular dysfunction, or congenital heart disease is excluded in the definition of cor pulmonale.

ETIOLOGIES (TABLE 21-1)

Chronic Obstructive Pulmonary Disease

Chronic obstructive pulmonary disease (COPD) causes cor pulmonale through several interrelated mechanisms, including hypoventilation, hypoxemia from ventilation/perfusion ($\dot{V}/\dot{Q}$) mismatch, and reduction of perfused surface area. Physical examination in advanced COPD shows an increase in the thoracic diameter, flattened diaphragms, hyperresonance to percussion, decreased breath sounds with expiratory wheezes, distant heart sounds, distended neck veins during expiration, and a palpable liver. The chest roentgenogram may show characteristic changes of emphysema, such as hyperlucent lungs, bullae, increased anteroposterior (AP) diameter, and flattened diaphragms. Pulmonary function tests show an increased residual volume and total lung capacity, decreased forced vital capacity (FVC), and markedly decreased expiratory flow rates (FEV_1, $FEF_{25-75\%}$). Arterial blood studies at rest can be normal when disease is mild, but in severe disease show decreased PO_2, increased PCO_2, and decreased pH. With cor pulmonale, PO_2 is likely to be below 55 mmHg. The

---

TABLE 21-1

ETIOLOGIES OF CHRONIC COR PULMONALE BY MECHANISM OF PULMONARY HYPERTENSION

I. Hypoxic vasoconstriction
  A. Chronic bronchitis and emphysema, cystic fibrosis
  B. Chronic hypoventilation
    1. Obesity
    2. Sleep apnea
    3. Neuromuscular disease
    4. Chest wall dysfunction
  C. High-altitude dwelling and chronic mountain sickness (Monge's disease)

II. Occlusion of the pulmonary vascular bed
  A. Pulmonary thromboembolism, parasitic ova, tumor emboli
  B. Primary pulmonary hypertension
  C. Pulmonary venoocclusive disease/pulmonary capillary hemangioma
  D. Sickle cell disease/sickle crisis/marrow embolism
  E. Fibrosing mediastinitis, mediastinal tumor
  F. Pulmonary angiitis from systemic disease
    1. Collagen-vascular diseases
    2. Drug-induced lung disease
    3. Necrotizing and granulomatous arteritis

III. Parenchymal disease with loss of vascular surface area
  A. Bullous emphysema, alpha$_1$ antiproteinase deficiency, hyperinflation
  B. Diffuse bronchiectasis, cystic fibrosis
  C. Diffuse interstitial disease
    1. Pneumoconiosis
    2. Sarcoid, idiopathic pulmonary fibrosis, histiocytosis X
    3. Tuberculosis, chronic fungal infection
    4. Adult respiratory distress syndrome
    5. Collagen-vascular disease (autoimmune lung disease)
    6. Hypersensitivity pneumonitis

$\dot{V}/\dot{Q}$ inequality and alveolar hypoventilation both contribute to the hypoxemia. A P_{CO_2} above 45 mmHg at rest defines net alveolar hypoventilation. Asthma rarely if ever leads to chronic cor pulmonale.

Diffuse Interstitial Lung Disease

These patients have dyspnea, tachypnea, exercise intolerance, and occasionally clubbing of the digits. Basilar crackles are heard frequently on auscultation of the chest and may persist throughout inspiration. The chest roentgenogram shows diffuse reticular, reticulonodular, or fibrotic lesions, but the appearance does not always correlate well with physiologic impairment. A lung biopsy frequently is required to identify the basic pathologic process. Transbronchial biopsy can be diagnostic in some interstitial diseases such as sarcoidosis, and bronchoalveolar ravage may point to a diagnosis in many cases. Pulmonary function tests show a restrictive process with reduced lung volumes and decreased diffusing capacity without airway obstruction. The forced expiratory volume in 1 s (FEV_1) as a percentage of FVC is usually at least 80 percent.

The presence of cor pulmonale in interstitial lung disease implies extensive lung dysfunction, and cor pulmonale may not occur even in end-stage disease. Treatment of idiopathic pulmonary fibrosis frequently is unsatisfactory despite the use of high-dose corticosteroids and either cyclophosphamide or azathioprine. Recent trials using interferon-alpha with corticosteroids show promise of improved efficacy.

Hypoventilation Syndromes

Some disorders (i.e., kyphoscoliosis, postpolio syndrome) may impair or restrict mechanisms of ventilation, causing general alveolar hypoventilation and alveolar hypoxia. Extreme obesity may be associated with hypoventilation, cyanosis, polycythemia, and somnolence (without intrinsic lung disease), often called the Pickwickian syndrome. Patients with daytime somnolence, morning headaches, and personality disturbances have been found to have periodic apnea during sleep associated with sleep deprivation. Diagnosis of hypoventilation is confirmed by blood gas analysis, a depressed ventilatory response to inhaled CO_2, or sleep studies. Noninvasive assisted nocturnal ventilation with continuous positive airway pressure (CPAP) with or without added O_2 is the most efficacious therapy in most patients with nocturnal hypoventilation.

Pulmonary Vascular Disease

Chronic cor pulmonale is a consequence of several diseases that involve the pulmonary vessels, including primary pulmonary hypertension and recurrent (or unresolved) pulmonary emboli, and sickle cell disease (SS or SC hemoglobinopathy). Pulmonary veno-occlusive disease is a rare disease of the pulmonary veins that presents with pulmonary hypertension and variable pulmonary infiltrates. Cirrhosis of the liver and HIV infection are associated with a disorder clinically and pathologically identical to primary pulmonary hypertension. Collagen-vascular disease can cause cor pulmonale by primary vasculitis as well as by diffuse interstitial fibrosis. Systemic sclerosis, systemic lupus erythematosus (SLE), and rheumatoid arthritis (RA) are the collagen-vascular diseases that most commonly cause pulmonary hypertension. Patients with SLE and RA occasionally present with cor pulmonale without interstitial disease but with primary pulmonary arteritis alone. The anorectic drug dexfenfluramine has been banned in the United States by the U.S. Food and Drug Administration (FDA) because of its association with primary pulmonary hypertension and perhaps valvular dysfunction.

PATHOPHYSIOLOGY

Physiologic variables determining pulmonary arterial pressure are shown in Table 21-2. These variables can be described in part by Poiseuille's law. Fortunately, most pulmonary diseases and disorders do not produce enough pulmonary hypertension to cause cor pulmonale. The effective cross-sectional area of the pulmonary vascular bed must be reduced by 25 to 50 percent before any change in PAP can be detected at rest. Exercise will dramatically raise PAP if the vascular bed is reduced. It is now well established, however, that arteriolar constriction resulting from alveolar hypoxia is the predominant cause of pulmonary hypertension in chronic airways diseases. The degree of hypoxic vasoconstriction depends primarily on the alveolar Po_2, and when alveolar Po_2 is less than 55 mmHg, PAP rises sharply. Hypoxic vasoconstriction is enhanced by acidosis and blunted by alkalosis.

Increases in cardiac output and blood volume contribute to pulmonary hypertension. Sustained or repetitive severe hypoxemia causes secondary erythrocytosis. Blood viscosity increases rapidly after the hematocrit exceeds about 55 percent, raising pulmonary vascular resistance (PVR) and also decreasing cerebral function. If left ventricular failure (LVF) is superimposed on an already reduced pulmonary vascular bed, pulmonary hypertension will be worsened by elevated downstream left atrial pressure. Once established, pulmonary hypertension may be self-perpetuating. Chronic hypoxia alone results in muscularization of pulmonary arterioles and exaggerated increases in PAP with stimuli.

TABLE 21-2

GENESIS OF PULMONARY VASCULAR PRESSURE: POISEUILLE'S LAW

$$Ppa = CO \left(\frac{8}{\pi} \times n \times \frac{1}{N} \times \frac{1}{r^4} \right) + Pla$$

Flow = cardiac output (usually ↑ elevated in COPD; if PRV is fixed, ↑ CO will ↑ PAP).

$\frac{8}{\pi}$ = numerical constant related to tubular structure of vessels.

n = blood viscosity (increased in polycythemia vera, secondary erythrocytosis, and cryoglobulinemia).

N = number of perfused vessels of a particular radius. N is decreased in any occlusive or destructive disease (see Table 61-1). N for pulmonary capillaries is >200 million.

$\frac{1}{r^4}$ = radius of a vessel is a critical determinant of flow (r is decreased by vasoconstriction, luminal obstruction, or hyperinflation. A change in r from 1 to 2 units changes resistance 16-fold).

Pla = left atrial pressure. Passive pulmonary hypertension can result from left atrial pressure elevation due to either LV or valvular disease.

Right Ventricular Response to Pulmonary Hypertension

Response of the right ventricle to pulmonary hypertension depends on the acuteness and severity of the pressure load. Acute cor pulmonale occurs after a sudden and severe stimulus (i.e., massive pulmonary emboli) with ventricular dilatation and failure but without hypertrophy. Acute cor pulmonale may develop within minutes to hours. Chronic cor pulmonale, however, is associated with a more slowly evolving and slowly progressive hypertension, and the response involves increased protein synthesis and right ventricular hypertrophy (RVH). At some stage, the myocardium is unable to function at the high pressure load; it therefore dilates and fails. Extreme pulmonary hypertension and RVH can occur in normal persons living at high altitude (>10,000 ft, or 3033 m) with no evidence of heart failure.

Left Ventricular Function and Edema Formation

Dysfunction of the left ventricle occurs in some patients with cor pulmonale, but the usual cause is coronary arteriosclerosis or hypertensive left ventricular disease. The dilated hypertensive right ventricle in cor pulmonale can reduce left ventricular compliance and impair left ventricular filling through effects on the shared ventricular septum. Despite these effects, most patients with chronic cor pulmonale demonstrate normal resting cardiac output, normal pulmonary artery wedge pressure, and normal resting left ventricular ejection fraction.

Peripheral edema occurs in some cases of chronic cor pulmonale. The mechanism of edema formation is poorly understood but is probably related to increased systemic venous pressure, hypercarbia, and hypoxemia. Hypercarbia stimulates plasma renin activity, and hypercarbic, edematous patients with COPD have increased plasma levels of aldosterone and antidiuretic hormone. Severe hypoxemia is associated with reduced renal blood flow and glomerular filtration rate and a decrease in urine sodium excretion of arginine vasopressin. Pulmonary edema and pleural effusion are not seen as a consequence of chronic cor pulmonale.

CLINICAL MANIFESTATIONS OF COR PULMONALE

Symptoms and Physical Examination

Shortness of breath is a nearly universal symptom in cor pulmonale. Episodes of leg edema, atypical chest pain, dyspnea on exertion, exercise-induced peripheral cyanosis, prior respiratory failure, and excessive daytime somnolence are all historical clues suggesting the presence of cor pulmonale. Chest pain may be related to right ventricular ischemia. Cough and complaints of easy fatigability are common. Some patients with nocturnal hypoventilation and sleep apnea may present with personality changes, mild systemic hypertension, and headache. Abdominal pain may be present if bowel edema results from venous hypertension.

The most sensitive sign of pulmonary hypertension is an accentuated pulmonic component of S_2 (see Chap. 1). With very high PAP, a characteristic systolic murmur of tricuspid valvular regurgitation may be heard with a systolic ejection click and right ventricular S_3 gallop. In overt right ventricular failure (RVF), cardiac enlargement, distended neck veins, hepatomegaly, and peripheral edema are present. In emphysema, the heart sounds may be best heard in the subxiphoid area. Extremities may be warm due to peripheral vasodilatation caused by hypercapnia, or there may be cyanosis due to low flow or hypoxemia.

Electrocardiogram

Absence of changes indicating right ventricular disease does not rule out cor pulmonale. The standard criteria for right ventricular enlargement were absent in two-thirds of patients with COPD who had RVH on postmortem examination. Diagnosis can be suspected on the combination of rS in V_5 to V_6, RAD, qR in aV_R, and P pulmonale. Tall peaked P waves in leads II and aV_F may reflect positional changes rather than right atrial enlargement. Right bundle branch block occurs in about 15 percent of patients. A pattern of S_1, Q_3, and T_3 carries reasonable sensitivity and specificity for cor pulmonale in COPD. Arrhythmias are infrequent in uncomplicated cor pulmonale; when present, they are usually supraventricular and may reflect blood gas abnormalities, hypokalemia, or excess of drugs such as digitalis, theophylline, and beta agonists.

Chest Roentgenogram

Radiographic manifestations are cardiomegaly, enlargement of the right ventricular shadow beyond the vertebral column, enlarged main PA, and dilated left and right descending pulmonary arteries. Right ventricular enlargement may be difficult to detect in the vertical heart of emphysema; comparison with previous films may be helpful. Pulmonary hypertension precedes right ventricular dilatation; thus a normal film does not exclude pulmonary hypertension. One indicator of pulmonary hypertension is measurement of the dimensions of the right and left PAs. Enlargement is considered to exist if the diameter of the right descending PA is greater than 16 mm and the left descending PA is greater than 18 mm. These findings occurred in 43 of 46 patients with known pulmonary hypertension, but the true sensitivity and specificity of these measurements are not known.

Echocardiogram

Echo-Doppler techniques have become the noninvasive standard to detect pulmonary hypertension and infer cardiac output. These techniques are relatively accurate when PAP is above 30 mmHg, but they may not detect milder yet pathologic pulmonary hypertension. Echo-Doppler is useful for longitudinal follow-up of pharmacologic treatment of pulmonary hypertension and cor pulmonale.

RIGHT-SIDED HEART CATHETERIZATION

Right-sided catheterization is the only technique available for the direct measurement of PAP, PA wedge pressure, and cardiac output. It is occasionally important in differentiating cor pulmonale from left ventricular dysfunction when the clinical presentation is confusing. Catheterization is important in patients with primary pulmonary hypertension (PPH) or unresolved pulmonary emboli, where airway function may appear normal, as well as with restrictive cardiomyopathy. In cor pulmonale, unlike LVF or mitral stenosis, PA diastolic pressure is usually significantly higher than wedge pressure. Mean PAP can be very high in obliterative vascular diseases but only moderately high in interstitial lung diseases. In COPD, PAP is not usually as severely increased as in PPH. About 50 percent of patients with severe COPD have pulmonary hypertension at rest.

USUAL STRATEGY OF WORKUP

No single strategy of workup exists. Spirometry, lung volumes (functional residual capacity), DL_{CO}, and an arterial blood sample for pH, P_{O_2}, and P_{CO_2} should be obtained. Transbronchial biopsy via a fiberoptic bronchoscope, bronchoalveolar lavage, and open lung biopsy are diagnostic options in patients with interstitial lung disease. Hematocrit above 50 percent gives a clue to the presence of chronic hypoxemia or nocturnal hypoventilation. Patients with cryptogenic pulmonary hypertension should receive a perfusion radionuclide lung scan to detect pulmonary emboli or other causes of obstruction of the pulmonary arteries, such as fibrosing mediastinitis. If pulmonary vasculopathy is suspected, serum can be screened for the presence of antinuclear antibody, antiphospholipid antibody, hepatitis B surface antigen, rheumatoid factor, and cryoglobulins. Factor V Leiden is likely to be a frequent abnormality in thrombotic pulmonary hypertension.

Polysomnography should be performed in patients with any signs or symptoms of sleep apnea. Exercise tests may reveal cardiac or ventilatory limitation not appreciated on examination at rest. Echo-Doppler is an important addition to the noninvasive workup of a patient suspected to have pulmonary hypertension.

TREATMENT

Relief of hypoxia is of prime importance in reducing pulmonary hypertension. All hypoxemic patients should be treated with oxygen to restore arterial O_2 tension to greater than 60 mmHg.

In COPD, oxygenation may be improved by bronchodilators for bronchospasm and antibiotics for acute exacerbations of bronchitis. Nocturnal aspiration of gastric fluid is now known to be a common cause of exacerbation of chronic lung disease and proton pump inhibitors are useful in patients with nocturnal aspiration.

Tranquilizers, sedatives, and narcotics should be avoided in unstable patients and patients with hypoventilation. Short-term ventilatory stimulants may be useful in some cases of decreased ventilatory drives, although nasal CPAP has become the first choice in most cases of sleep apnea.

Oxygen therapy is usually well tolerated in patients with stable lung disease but not in patients with acute acidosis or respiratory muscle fatigue. When low-flow nasal O_2 causes significant increases in P_{CO_2}, mechanical ventilation may be required to relieve hypoxia. Studies have shown conclusively that home oxygen therapy, nocturnal or continuous, is effective in treating cor pulmonale or in postponing its onset. Continuous 24-h/day oxygen therapy is the desired goal in most patients, because desaturation occurs during both sleep and physical activity.

Treatment of Heart Failure

General principles of management of heart failure apply. Diuretics are the mainstay therapy for treatment of RVF. Pulmonary vasodilators are efficacious in some patients with primary pulmonary hypertension but are of unproven value in cor pulmonale from COPD. Vasodilator use has not become widespread because of small observed reductions in pulmonary hypertension and occasional worsening of gas exchange. Diuretics are effective in the treatment of RVF, and indications for their use are the same as in other forms of heart disease. The effects of diuretics should be monitored carefully by measurement of electrolytes as well as arterial P_{O_2}, P_{CO_2}, and pH, because acid-base abnormalities are often present in cor pulmonale. Contraction alkalosis can be a problem in hypercarbic patients with a large buffer base who have had vigorous diuresis. When the hematocrit is above 55 to 60 percent, phlebotomy may reduce PAP and PVR and possibly improve right ventricular function. The phlebotomy should be in small volumes (200 to 300 mL) and done cautiously.

SURGICAL TREATMENT

There is no surgical treatment for most diseases that cause chronic cor pulmonale. Pulmonary embolectomy is efficacious for unresolved pulmonary emboli causing chronic thrombotic pulmonary hypertension. Adenoidectomy in children with chronic airways obstruction and uvulopalatopharyngioplasty in selected patients with sleep apnea can relieve cor pulmonale related to hypoventilation. Single-lung, double-lung, and heart-lung transplantations are all used for salvage in the terminal phase of several diseases complicated by cor pulmonale. The diseases most commonly treated by lung transplantation are primary pulmonary hypertension, emphysema, idiopathic pulmonary fibrosis, and cystic fibrosis. Two-year survival for single- and double-lung transplant has risen to 66 percent, still lower than the approximately 80 percent for heart transplant alone. One interesting finding is that the right ventricle can recover function after lung transplant even after the chronic stress of severe pulmonary hypertension. Volume-reduction surgery for selected patients with emphysema improves ventilatory function and gas exchange, and the long-term benefit of this approach is under study.

SUGGESTED READING

Cooper JD, Trulock EP, Triantafillon AN, et al: Bilateral pneumectomy (volume reduction) for chronic obstructive pulmonary disease. *J Thorac Cardiovasc Surg* 1995; 109:106–116.

Kawakami Y, Kishi F, Yamamoto H, et al: Relation of oxygen delivery, mixed venous oxygenation and pulmonary hemodynamics to prognosis in COPD. *N Engl J Med* 1983; 308:1045–1049.

Lange PA, Stoller JK: The hepatopulmonary syndrome. *Ann Intern Med* 1995; 122:521–529.

MacNee W: Pathophysiology of cor pulmonale in chronic obstructive pulmonary disease. State of the art. *Am J Pulm Crit Care Med* 1994; 150(4):833–892, 1158–1163.

Newman JH: Chronic cor pulmonale. In: Fuster V, Alexander RW, O'Rourke RA, et al (eds): *Hurst's The Heart,* 10th ed. New York: McGraw-Hill; 2001:1645–1654.

Palevsky Hl, Fishman AP: Chronic cor pulmonale. *JAMA* 1990; 263:2347–2354.

Schiller N: Pulmonary artery pressure estimation by Doppler and two-dimensional echocardiography. *Cardiol Clin* 1990: 8:277–287.

Standards for the diagnosis and care of patients with chronic obstructive pulmonary disease: ATS statement. *Am J Respir Crir Care Med* 1995; 152(55):S77–S120.

Strohl KP, Rogers RM: Obstructive sleep apnea. *N Engl J Med* 1996; 334:99–104.

CHAPTER

22

AORTIC VALVE DISEASE

Aly Rahimtoola
Shahbudin H. Rahimtoola

AORTIC STENOSIS

Definitions, Etiology, and Pathology

Aortic stenosis (AS) is obstruction to outflow of blood flow from the left ventricle to the aorta. The obstruction may be at the valve, above the valve (supravalvular), or below the valve (membranous; subvalvular).

The most common causes of valvular AS are congenital, rheumatic, and calcific ("degenerative"). Calcific AS is seen in patients 35 years of age or older and is the result of calcification of a congenital or rheumatic valve or of a normal valve that has undergone degenerative changes. Degenerative/calcific AS may represent an immune reaction to antigens present in the valve and is related to atherosclerosis. Rare causes of AS include obstructive infective vegetations, homozygous type II hyperlipoproteinemia, Paget's disease of the bone, systemic lupus erythematosus, rheumatoid involvement, ochronosis, and irradiation.

At the present time, calcific AS in the older patient is the most common valve lesion requiring valve replacement. Among patients under the age of 70, congenital bicuspid valve have accounted for one-half of the surgical cases; degenerative changes were the cause in 18 percent. In contrast, in those aged 70 or older, degenerative changes accounted for almost one-half of the surgical cases and a congenital bicuspid valve for approximately one-quarter of the cases.

Supravalvular and membranous subvalvular AS is usually congenital. Congenital bicuspid valves can produce severe obstruction to left ventricular (LV) outflow after the first few years of life. The valvular abnormality produces turbulent flow, which traumatizes the leaflets and eventually leads to fibrosis, rigidity, and calcification of the valve. In a congenitally abnormal tricuspid aortic valve, the cusps are of unequal size and have some degree of commissural fusion; the third cusp may be diminutive. Eventually, the abnormal structure leads to changes similar to those seen in a bicuspid valve, and significant LV outflow obstruction often results. In calcific (so-called degenerative) AS, early changes show chronic inflammatory cell infiltrate (macrophages and T lymphocytes), lipid within the lesion and in adjacent fibrosa, and thickening of fibrosa with collagen and elastin. These patients also have a higher incidence of risk factors for coronary atherosclerosis.

Rheumatic AS results from adhesions and fusion of the commissures and cusps. The leaflets and the valve ring become vascularized, which leads to retraction and stiffening of the cusps. Calcification occurs.

Rheumatoid AS is extremely rare and results from nodular thickening of the valve leaflets and the involvement of the proximal part of the aorta. In severe forms of hypercholesterolemia, lipid deposits occur not only in the aortic wall but also in the aortic valve, and occasionally producing AS.

The LV is concentrically hypertrophied. The hypertrophied cardiac muscle cells are increased in size. There is an increase of connective tissue and a variable amount of fibrous tissue in the interstitium. Myocardial ultrastructural changes may account for the LV systolic dysfunction that occurs late in the disease. Subclinical calcific emboli are commonly found in calcific AS if diligently sought at autopsy.

Pathophysiology

The aortic valve must be reduced to one-fourth of its natural size before significant changes occur in the circulation. The normal aortic valve is 3.0 to 4.0 cm^2; an area exceeding 0.7 to 1.0 cm^2 is not usually considered to indicate severe AS. In average-sized individuals, a valve area of greater than 1.0 cm^2 and in smaller people greater 0.75 cm^2 may be adequate.

Based on natural history and hemodynamic studies, AS is graded as mild when the valve area is >1.5 cm^2, moderate when the valve area is >1.0 to 1.5 cm^2, and severe when valve area is ≤1.0 cm^2. With reduction in the aortic valve area (AVA), energy is dissipated during the transport of blood from the LV to the aorta. The AVA must be reduced by about 50 percent of normal before a measurable gradient can be demonstrated in humans.

The outflow obstruction imposes a pressure overload on the LV, which compensates by an increase in wall thickness and mass. The concentric hypertrophy normalizes systolic wall stress and preserves normal systolic function; however, diastolic function may be abnormal. Eventually, there is impaired contractility of the LV and LV dilatation.

Left atrial contraction is of considerable benefit to these patients. Loss of effective atrial contraction—either due to atrial fibrillation or because of an inappropriately timed atrial contraction—results in elevation of mean left atrial pressure, reduction of cardiac output, or both. This may precipitate clinical heart failure with pulmonary congestion.

In most patients with AS, cardiac output is in the normal range and initially increases normally with exercise. Later, as the severity of AS increases progressively, the cardiac output remains within the normal range at rest. On exercise, however, it no longer increases in proportion to the amount of exercise undertaken or does not increase at all.

In severe AS, myocardial oxygen needs are increased because of an increased muscle mass, elevations in LV pressures, and prolongation of the systolic ejection time. As a result, patients may have classic angina pectoris even in the absence of coronary artery disease.

Clinical Findings

HISTORY

Patients with congenital valvular stenosis may give a history of a murmur since childhood or infancy; those with rheumatic stenosis may have a history of rheumatic fever. Most patients with valvular AS, including some with severe valvular stenosis, are asymptomatic.

The classic triad of symptoms of AS is angina pectoris, syncope, and heart failure. Sudden cardiac death is said to occur in 5 percent of patients with AS. It occurs only in those with severe valvular stenosis, most of whom have had some cardiac symptoms before the fatal episode.

Angina pectoris may be the initial clinical manifestation. Syncope is the result of reduced cerebral perfusion. Syncope occurring on effort is caused by systemic vasodilatation in the presence of a fixed or inadequate cardiac output, an arrhythmia, or both. Syncope at rest is usually due to a transient tachyarrhythmia from which the patient recovers spontaneously.

Dyspnea on exertion, orthopnea, paroxysmal nocturnal dyspnea, and pulmonary edema result from varying degrees of pulmonary venous hypertension.

There is an increased incidence of gastrointestinal arteriovenous malformations. As a result, these patients are susceptible to gastrointestinal hemorrhage and anemia. Calcific systemic embolism may occur.

PHYSICAL FINDINGS

There is a spectrum of physical findings in patients with AS, depending on the severity of the stenosis, stroke volume, LV function, and the rigidity and calcification of the valve. The arterial pulse rises slowly, taking longer than normal to reach peak pressure, the peak is reduced (parvus et tardus), and the pulse pressure may be narrowed. A systolic thrill may be felt in the carotid arteries (see Chap. 1). The cardiac impulse is heaving and sustained in character, and there may be a palpable fourth heart sound. (S_4). An aortic systolic thrill is often present at the base of the heart. In 80 to 90 percent of adult patients with severe AS, there is an S_4 gallop sound, a midsystolic ejection murmur that peaks late in systole, and a single second heart sound (S_2) because A_2 and P_2 are superimposed or A_2 is absent or soft. There is often a faint early diastolic murmur of minimal aortic regurgitation. The S_2 may be paradoxically split due to late A_2, and there may be no early diastolic murmur. In many patients, particularly the elderly, the systolic ejection murmur is atypical and may be heard only at the apex of the heart.

In many of these patients who are 60 years of age or older, the clinical features tend to be somewhat different from those typical of younger patients. Systemic hypertension is common, being present in about 20 percent of the patients, half of whom have moderate or severe systolic and diastolic hypertension. A fifth of the patients first present in congestive heart failure. The male : female ratio is 2 : 1. Because of thickening of the arterial wall and its associated lack of distensibility, the arterial pulse rises normally or even rapidly, and the pulse pressure is wide.

CHEST X-RAY

The characteristic finding is a normal-sized heart with a dilated proximal ascending aorta (poststenotic dilation). Calcium in the aortic valve can be seen on the lateral film but is better appreciated by fluoroscopy with image intensification. In the current era, calcification is most easily recognized on two-dimensional echocardiography. Calcium in the aortic valve is the hallmark of AS in adults 40 to 45 years of age. In patients aged 45 years or above, the diagnosis of severe AS is doubtful if there is no calcium in the aortic valve. The presence of calcium, however, does not necessarily mean that the valve is stenotic or that the AS is severe. The cardiac silhouette on chest x-ray shows mild to moderate enlargement if any. In patients with heart failure, the cardiac size is increased because of dilatation of the left ventricle and left atrium; the lung fields show pulmonary edema and pulmonary venous congestion and the right ventricle and atrium may be dilated.

ELECTROCARDIOGRAM

The electrocardiogram (ECG) in severe AS shows LV hypertrophy with or without secondary ST-T-wave changes. Conduction abnormalities are common and range from bundle branch block to first-degree block; higher grades of block occur but are uncommon. The patients are usually in sinus rhythm.

Atrial fibrillation indicates the presence of either associated mitral valve disease, coronary artery disease (CAD), or heart failure.

Laboratory Investigations

ECHOCARDIOGRAPHY/DOPPLER ULTRASOUND

Echocardiography/Doppler (echo/Doppler) ultrasound is an extremely important and useful noninvasive test. On the echocardiogram, the aortic valve leaflets normally are barely visible in systole, and the normal range of aortic valve opening is 1.6 to 2.6 cm. In the presence of a bicuspid aortic valve, eccentric valve leaflets may be seen. The aortic valve leaflets may appear to be thickened as a result of calcification and/or fibrosis; however, the older patient without valve stenosis may also have thickened cusps. The aortic valve may have a reduced opening, but this also occurs in other conditions in which the cardiac output is reduced. The LV hypertrophy often results in thickening of both the interventricular septum and the posterior LV wall. The cavity size is normal. When LV systolic function is impaired, the left ventricle and left atrium are dilated and the percentage of dimensional shortening is reduced. When properly applied, Doppler echocardio- graphy is extremely useful for estimating the valve gradient and aortic valve area (AVA) non-invasively. The calculated mean gradient from continuous-waveform Doppler interrogation correlates reasonably closely with that obtained at cardiac catheterization. The AVA can be calculated from the velocity of the jet across the aortic valve and from the velocity and character of the LV out flow tract.

Transesophageal echo/Doppler ultrasound is very useful in defining aortic valve abnormality and in assessing its severity when an adequate examination cannot be obtained with the transthoracic technique.

CARDIAC CATHETERIZATION/ ANGIOGRAPHY

Cardiac catheterization remains the standard technique to assess the severity of AS "accurately." This is done by measuring simultaneous LV and ascending aortic pressures and the cardiac output by either the Fick principle or the indicator dilution technique. The AVA can be calculated. The state of LV systolic pump function can be quantitated by measuring LV end-diastolic and end-systolic volumes and ejection fraction. *It must be recognized that ejection fraction may underestimate myocardiac function in the presence of the increased afterload of severe AS.*

The presence of CAD and its site and severity can be estimated only by selective coronary angiography, which should be performed in all patients 35 years of age or older being considered for valve surgery and in those <35 years if they have LV systolic dysfunction, symptoms or signs suggesting CAD, or two or more risk factors for premature CAD (excluding gender).

OTHER LABORATORY STUDIES

Gated blood pool radionuclide scans provide information on ventricular function similar to that provided by two-dimensional echocardiography and LV cineangiography.

Exercise tests of any kind should not be undertaken in patients with severe AS unless there is a specific reason for such studies. Ambulatory ECG recordings may be needed in an occasional patient suspected of having an arrhythmia or painless ischemia.

Natural History and Prognosis

Valvular AS is frequently a progressive disease, the severity increasing over time. The factors that control this progression and the time it takes for severe outflow obstruction to develop are unknown. In one study, patients with "mild" stenosis (catheterization-proven AVA > 1.5 cm^2), the rate of progression to severe stenosis was 8 percent in 10 years and 22 percent in 20 years. The duration of the asymptomatic period after the development of severe AS is also unknown; some recent data suggest that it may be less than 2 years. In patients aged 63 ± 16 years, the actuarial probability of death or aortic valve surgery was 7 ± 5 percent at 1 year, 38 ± 8 percent at 3 years, and 74 ± 10 percent at 5 years.

Severe disease in adults is lethal, particularly if the patient is symptomatic, with a prognosis that is worse than for many forms of neoplastic disease. The 3-year mortality is approximately 36 to 52 percent, the 5-year mortality is about 52 to 80 percent, and the 10-year mortality is 80 to 90 percent; the average life expectancy is 2 to 3 years. Almost all patients with heart failure are dead in 1 to 2 years.

Medical Therapy

All patients with AS need antibiotic prophylaxis against infective endocarditis (see Chap. 36). Those in whom the valve lesion is of rheumatic origin need additional prophylaxis against recurrence of rheumatic fever. Patients with mild or moderate stenosis rarely have symptoms or complications and do not need any specific medical therapy. In mild stenosis, the patient should be encouraged to lead a normal life. Those with moderate AS should avoid moderate to severe physical exertion and competitive sports. If atrial fibrillation should occur, it should be reverted rapidly to sinus rhythm. In severe AS, reversion to sinus rhythm often becomes a matter of some urgency.

Surgical Therapy

Operation should be advised for the symptomatic patient who has severe AS. In young patients, if the valve is pliable and mobile, simple commissurotomy or valve repair may be feasible; the operative mortality is <1 percent. Such a procedure will relieve outflow obstruction to a major degree. In these patients, catheter balloon valvuloplasty is the procedure of choice in experienced and skilled centers. Both of these are palliative procedures that postpone valve replacement. Catheter balloon valvuloplasty is a temporary palliative procedure for high-risk elderly patients with advanced symptoms and for emergency situations.

The natural history of symptomatic patients with severe AS is dismal—i.e., a 10-year mortality of 80 to 90 percent—but there is good outcome after surgery, particularly in patients without any comorbid cardiac and noncardiac conditions. Given the unknown natural history of the asymptomatic patient with severe AS, which may not be benign, it is reasonable to recommend surgery even to the asymptomatic patient. Some recommend valve replacement in all asymptomatic patients with severe AS, while others would recommend it in those with AVA ≤ 0.7 cm^2 and in selected patients with AVA of 0.76 to 1.0 cm^2.

The operative mortality of valve replacement is about 5 percent or less. In patients without associated CAD, heart failure, or other comorbid factors, it may be 1 to 2 percent in centers with experienced and skilled staff. Patients with associated CAD should have coronary bypass surgery at the same time as valve surgery because it results in a lower operative and late mortality. Patients with severe AS who need coronary bypass surgery should have aortic valve replacement at the same time.

In severe AS, valve replacement results in an improvement of survival, even in those with normal preoperative LV function. Aortic valve replacement is not recommended for asymptomatic patients with severe AS to prevent sudden death (Table 22-1).

For choice(s) of prosthetic valve, see Chap. 26.

AORTIC REGURGITATION

Definition; Etiology, and Pathology

Aortic regurgitation (AR) is a flow of blood in diastole from the aorta into the LV due to incompetence of the aortic valve. The two most common causes of acute AR are infective endocarditis and prosthetic valve dysfunction. Other common causes include dissection of the aorta, systemic hypertension, and trauma.

TABLE 22-1

RECOMMENDATIONS FOR AORTIC VALVE REPLACEMENT
IN AORTIC STENOSIS

Indication	Class
1. Symptomatic patients with severe AS	I
2. Patients with severe AS undergoing coronary artery bypass surgery	I
3. Patients with severe AS undergoing surgery on the aorta or other heart valves	I
4. Patients with moderate AS undergoing coronary artery bypass surgery or surgery on the aorta or other heart valves (see sections III.F.6, III.F.7, and VIII.D of the ACC/AHA Guidelines)	IIa
5. Asymptomatic patients with severe AS and	
LV systolic dysfunction	IIa
Abnormal response to exercise (e.g., hypotension)	IIa
Ventricular tachycardia	IIb
Marked or excessive LV hypertrophy (≥ 15 mm)	IIb
Valve area <0.6 cm^2	IIb
6. Prevention of sudden death in asymptomatic patients with none of the findings listed under indication 5	III

SOURCE: Bonow RO et al: ACC/AHA Guidelines. *J Am Coll Cardiol* 1998;
32:1486–1588, with permission.

In North America, the most common cause of chronic, isolated severe AR is aortic root/annular dilatation that is presumably the result of medial disease. Common causes include a congenital (bicuspid) valve, previous infective endocarditis, and rheumatic disease. Chronic AR also occurs in association with a variety of other diseases, particularly those that result in dilatation of the aortic root. Between 40 and 60 percent of the surgically removed valves from patients with isolated severe AR are classified as idiopathic; half show histologic criteria of myxomatous degeneration. Incompetence of the aortic valve can result from changes in the aortic valve or from the aortic wall.

In AR, volume overload of the LV is the basic hemodynamic abnormality. The extent of overload depends on the volume of the regurgitant blood flow, which is determined by the area of the regurgitant orifice, the diastolic pressure gradient between the aorta and LV, and the duration of diastole.

Pathophysiology

The LV diastolic pressure-volume relationship plays a very important role in the pathophysiology of acute valve regurgitation. The ability of the left ventricle to dilate acutely is limited; as a result, the volume overload of acute AR produces a rapid increase of LV diastolic pressure. If the left ventricle is already stiff or less compliant than normal from an associated lesion (e.g., AS or systemic hypertension), the LV diastolic pressure will rise more precipitously as a result of the volume overload of acute AR than if the LV were normal. On the other hand, if the left ventricle is somewhat dilated from a previous lesion—for example, mild AR—the LV pressure will initially rise more gradually with acute AR but may subsequently rise to the same high levels as seen with a normal or stiff LV. Acute AR that is mild produces little or no hemodynamic abnormality—for example, when associated with systemic hypertension. Increasing severity of regurgitation produces greater degrees of hemodynamic abnormalities, and severe AR often produces the clinical picture of "heart failure."

Acute AR that is severe results in a large volume of regurgitant blood; the increased LV diastolic pressure results in increases in mean left atrial and pulmonary venous pressures and produces varying degrees of pulmonary edema. Two compensatory mechanisms are utilized: an increase of myocardial contractility and tachycardia to maintain an adequate forward cardiac output.

In chronic AR, the AR becomes severe over a period of time; therefore the LV diastolic pressure-volume relationships are different from those seen in acute AR. If the AR is mild to moderate, the LV end-diastolic volume is increased moderately, the LV diastolic pressure-volume curve is moved to the right of normal, and the LV diastolic pressure is usually normal. In severe AR, the LV diastolic pressure-volume curves are moved further to the right. If the LV systolic pump function is normal, the LV end-diastolic volume can be quite large without significant elevation of LV end-diastolic pressure. If the LV diastolic volume increases further, however, the LV diastolic pressures will be increased. If LV systolic pump dysfunction supervenes, the LV diastolic pressure-volume curve relationships are moved even further to the right, with quite marked LV dilatation and increases in LV diastolic pressure.

In severe chronic AR, the increase of LV end-diastolic volume is a result of the regurgitant volume (and is proportional to the amount of regurgitation) and LV systolic dysfunction. The subsequent large

LV stroke volume produces LV systolic hypertension. Both of these increase LV wall stress (afterload), which can result in an impairment of LV function. The heart responds by becoming hypertrophied, and function remains normal. In time, the hemodynamic burden of the volume overload will result in depressed myocardial contractility and decreased LV compliance. Total coronary blood flow is increased but coronary flow reserve is reduced and some patients with severe AR may complain of angina pectoris.

Clinical Features

HISTORY

Patients with mild to moderate AR usually do not have symptoms that can be attributed to the heart. Even patients with severe AR may be asymptomatic for many years. The earliest symptom may be an awareness of the increased force of contraction of the dilated heart that undergoes a large volume change in systole; patients complain of pounding of the head or palpitations. The main symptoms of severe AR result from elevated pulmonary venous pressures and include dyspnea on exertion, orthopnea, and paroxysmal nocturnal dyspnea. Heart failure occurs in 20 percent of such patients and may be present even in the absence of CAD.

PHYSICAL FINDINGS

The arterial pulse is very characteristic and consists of an abrupt distention with a rapid rise and a quick collapse (Corrigan's pulse). The arterial pulse may be bisferiens, a double impulse during systole. The systolic arterial pressure is increased, the diastolic pressure is reduced, and Korotkoff's sounds persist down to 0 mmHg. The absence of a wide pulse pressure (greater than 50 percent of peak systolic pressure) or diastolic pressure greater than 70 mmHg in a patient without heart failure makes severe, chronic aortic regurgitation unlikely. The LV dilatation with severe AR displaces the apical impulse inferiorly and laterally. The AR murmur is a high-pitched, blowing, early diastolic murmur along the left sternal border. A third heart sound (S_3 gallop) and low-pitched diastolic and/or presystolic murmurs (Austin-Flint) may be heard at the apex. The wide pulse pressure, significant LV dilatation, and Austin-Flint murmur are not features of acute AR.

CHEST X-RAY

The LV is increased in size, and this can be appreciated by an increase in the cardiothoracic ratio. A better noninvasive quantification of LV size can be obtained by echocardiography. The ascending aorta is dilated, and there may be calcium in the aortic valve. With increased filling pressures in the later stages, there might be evidence of an enlarged left atrium and an increased left atrial and pulmonary venous pressure, which are manifest in the pulmonary vascular shadows by a redistribution of blood flow, pulmonary congestion, and pulmonary edema. In the presence of heart failure, enlargement of the right atrium and superior vena cava may be appreciated. Calcification that is limited to the ascending aorta is strongly suggestive of luetic aortitis.

ELECTROCARDIOGRAM

The ECG shows LV hypertrophy with or without associated ST-T-wave changes. In some patients, ECG evidence of LV hypertrophy is absent in spite of severe AR. Conduction abnormalities, such as atrioventricular block or left or right bundle branch block with or without axis deviation, may be present. The PR interval may be prolonged, particularly in patients with ankylosing spondylitis. The rhythm is usually sinus. The presence of atrial fibrillation should make one suspect the presence of associated mitral valve disease or heart failure.

ECHOCARDIOGRAPHY/DOPPLER

The echocardiogram can provide information about the etiology of AR as well as LV size and function and severity of AR. Diastolic fluttering of the anterior leaflet of the mitral valve is often present on M-mode and two-dimensional echo. Echocardiography is of particular value for excluding the presence of associated mitral stenosis in patients with an Austin Flint diastolic murmur. Two-dimensional echocardiography is much superior to the M-mode technique for assessing LV volumes and systolic function. A dilated ascending aorta can be detected on echocardiography, as can an enlarged left atrium. Aortic valve vegetations suggest infective endocarditis. Some other conditions can easily be detected by echocardiography—for example, prolapse of the aortic leaflet into the left ventricle in diastole. Doppler ultrasound is useful for diagnosing and assessing the severity of AR. There is a significant incidence of false-positive mild regurgitation. There is also an overlap between the various grades of severity of assessment of AR by Doppler as compared with angiography. Transesophageal echocardiography is a useful technique when transthoracic echocardiogram is unsatisfactory and in certain instances for identifying the anatomy of the valve leaflets and aortic root/annulus; it is essential to evaluate if the valve is suitable for repair. Echo/Doppler ultrasound is also very useful for assessing disease of other valves.

CARDIAC CATHETERIZATION/ ANGIOGRAPHY

Cardiac catheterization permits the measurement of intracardiac and intravascular pressures and cardiac output, both at rest and during exercise. In addition, other valvular disease—for example, mitral stenosis, aortic stenosis, and mitral regurgitation—can be excluded. LV angiography demonstrates enlarged LV and allows the calculation of LV volumes and LV ejection fraction. Angiography performed with injection of contrast medium in the ascending aorta demonstrates AR and allows a semiquantitative assessment of the degree of AR. In addition, the angiogram demonstrates the dimensions of the aortic root and the state of the ascending aorta. The indications for selective coronary angiography are the same for aortic stenosis.

OTHER LABORATORY TESTS

Gated blood pool radionuclide scans also allow the measurement of LV volumes and ejection fraction. In addition, with this technique, it is possible to quantify the amount of AR. These scans, however, assess regurgitation present at both the aortic and mitral valves. This technique also allows measurement of LV ejection fraction on exercise and on serial studies.

A treadmill exercise test provides an objective assessment of the degree of functional impairment and documentation of arrhythmias related to exertion. In some patients, however, the exercise test may remain normal despite deterioration of LV function.

Ambulatory ECG recording may be needed in an occasional patient suspected of having an arrhythmia.

MRI can demonstrate AR but is rarely needed clinically.

Natural History and Prognosis

Patients with mild AR that does not progress should have a normal life expectancy. Their major risk is the development of infective endocarditis and further valve destruction. Patients with moderate AR, if their disease does not progress, would be expected to have a life expectancy that is reasonably close to the normal range. The disease does progress, however, and mortality at the end of 10 years appears to be about 15 percent.

Patients with severe AR are known to have a long asymptomatic period before the condition is discovered. In asymptomatic patients with normal LV function at rest, symptoms and/or LV dysfunction (and/or sudden death) develop at the rate of about 3 to 6 percent per year. The predictor of development of symptoms is LV systolic dysfunction and/or an increased LV size (LV dimension at end-diastole of ≥ 70 mm and at end-systole of ≥ 50 mm). Sudden death in asymptomatic patients appears to occur only in those with a massively dilated left ventricle (LV end-diastolic dimension of ≥ 80 mm).

Medical Therapy

All patients with AR need antibiotic prophylaxis to prevent infective endocarditis. Patients with AR of a rheumatic origin need antibiotic prophylaxis to prevent recurrences of rheumatic carditis. Patients with syphilitic AR need a course of antibiotics to treat syphilis.

Patients with mild AR need no specific therapy. They do not need to restrict their activities and can lead a normal life. Patients with moderate AR also usually need no specific therapy. These patients, however, should avoid heavy physical exertion, competitive sports, and isometric exercise. Asymptomatic patients with severe AR and normal LV systolic function should be treated with a vasodilator (a calcium antagonist such as long-acting nifedipine) unless there is a contraindication to its use.

Surgical Therapy

Patients with severe chronic AR need valve surgery. The correct timing of surgical therapy is now better defined but is not fully clarified. Valve replacement should be performed before irreversible LV dysfunction occurs.

Decisions about surgery in AR should be based on the clinical functional class and on the LV ejection fraction. Patients with chronic severe AR who are symptomatic [New York Heart Association (NYHA) functional classes II to IV] need valve replacement. The benefit from valve replacement has been demonstrated even when the LV ejection fraction is 0.25 or less. Recent data indicate that patients with severe AR, LV end-diastolic dimension on echocardiography of ≥ 80 mm, and mild to moderate reduction of LV ejection fraction can obtain benefit from valve replacement. Postoperatively, they are symptomatically improved, LV ejection fraction increases, and LV size is reduced; the 5- and 10-year survivals are 87 and 71 percent, respectively.

Although the issue is controversial, most authorities recommend that patients who are asymptomatic and have a reduced ejection fraction at rest should be offered aortic valve replacement. If the ejection fraction is normal at rest, one should consider valve replacement in NYHA functional class I patients if they have severe obstructive CAD and/or need surgery for other valve disease. Patients with associated significant CAD should have coronary bypass surgery performed at the time of valvular surgery.

TABLE 22-2

RECOMMENDATIONS FOR AORTIC VALVE REPLACEMENT IN CHRONIC SEVERE AORTIC REGURGITATION

Indication	Class
1. Patients with NYHA functional class III or IV symptoms and preserved LV systolic function, defined as normal ejection fraction at rest (ejection fraction ≥ 0.50)	I
2. Patients with NYHA functional class II symptoms and preserved LV systolic functional (ejection fraction ≥ 0.50 at rest) but with progressive LV dilatation or declining ejection fraction at rest on serial studies or declining effort tolerance on exercise testing	I
3. Patients with Canadian Heart Association functional class II or greater angina with or without coronary artery disease	I
4. Asymptomatic or symptomatic patients with mild to moderate LV dysfunction at rest (ejection fraction 0.25 to 0.49)	I
5. Patients undergoing coronary artery bypass surgery or surgery on the aorta or other heart valves	I
6. Patients with NYHA functional class II symptoms and preserved LV systolic function (ejection fraction ≥ 0.50 at rest) with stable LV size and systolic function on serial studies and stable exercise tolerance	IIa
7. Asymptomatic patients with normal LV systolic function (ejection fraction >0.50) but with severe LV dilatation (end-diastolic dimension >75 mm or end-systolic dimension >55 mm)	IIa
8. Patients with severe LV dysfunction (ejection fraction <0.25)	IIb

(*continued*)

<table>

TABLE 22-2

(Continued)

9. Asymptomatic patients with normal systolic function at rest (ejection fraction >0.50) and progressive LV dilatation when the degree of dilatation is moderately severe (end-diastolic dimension 70 to 75 mm, end-systolic dimension 50 to 55 mm)	IIb
10. Asymptomatic patients with normal systolic function at rest (ejection fraction >0.50) but with decline in ejection fraction during	
Exercise radionuclide angiography	IIb
Stress echocardiography	III
11. Asymptomatic patients with normal systolic function at rest (ejection fraction >0.50) and LV dilatation when degree of dilatation is not severe (end-diastolic dimension <70 mm, end-systolic dimension <50 mm)	III

</table>

*Lower threshold values should be considered for patients of small stature of either gender. Clinical judgment is required.

SOURCE: Bonow RO et al: ACC/AHA Guidelines. *J Am Coll Cardiol* 1998; 32:1486–1588, with permission.

Aortic valve replacement, with or without associated coronary bypass surgery for obstructive CAD, can be performed at many surgical centers with an operative mortality of 5 percent or less (see Chap. 26). In those without associated CAD or reduced LV systolic function, the operative mortality may be in the range of 1 to 2 percent. If aortic valve replacement is successful and uncomplicated, LV volume and hypertrophy regress but do not return to normal. Impaired LV systolic pump function improves postoperatively in 50 percent or more of patients. The 5-year survival of patients with LV ejection fraction ≥ 0.45 is 87 percent, versus 54 percent in patients with an ejection fraction <0.45.

New techniques of aortic valve repair are being developed and evaluated, and early results are encouraging in selected subgroups. It is possible that selected patients may eventually need to have valve repair rather than valve replacement for AR.

The recommendations of the American College of Cardiology/ American Heart Association (ACC/AHA) Practice Guidelines are shown in Table 22-2.

SUGGESTED READING

Bonow RO, Carabello B, de Leon AC Jr, et al: ACC/AHA guidelines for the management of patients with valvular heart disease: A report for the American College of Cardiology/American Heart Association Task Force on Practice Guidelines (Committee on Management of Patients with Valvular Heart Disease). *J Am Coll Cardiol* 1998; 32:1486–1588.

Currie PJ, Seward JB, Reeder GS, et al: Continuous-wave Doppler echocardiographic assessment of severity of calcific aortic stenosis: A simultaneous Doppler-catheter correlative study in 100 adult patients. *Circulation* 1985; 71:1162–1169.

Hammermeister KL, Sethi GK, Henderson WG, et al: A comparison of outcomes in men 15 years after heart-valve replacement with a mechanical valve or bioprosthesis. *J Am Coll Cardiol* 2000; 36:1152–1158.

Horstkotte D, Loogen F: The natural history of aortic valve stenosis. *Eur Heart J* 1988; 9(suppl E):57–64.

Mullany CJ, Elveback ER, Frye RL, et al: Coronary artery disease and its management: Influence on survival in patients undergoing aortic valve replacement. *J Am Coll Cardiol* 1987; 10:66–72.

Murphy ES, Lawson RM, Starr A, Rahimtoola SH: Severe aortic stenosis in the elderly: State of left ventricular function and result of valve replacement on ten-year survival. *Circulation* 1981; 64(suppl II):184–188.

Otto CM, Knusisto J, Reichenbach D, et al: Characterization of the early lesion of "degenerative" valvular aortic stenosis: Historical and immunohistochemical studies. *Circulation* 1994; 90:844–853.

Pantely G, Morton MJ, Rahimtoola SH: Effects of successful, uncomplicated valve replacement on ventricular hypertrophy, volume, and performance in aortic stenosis and aortic incompetence. *J Thorac Cardiovasc Surg* 1978; 75:383–391.

Rahimtoola SH: Aortic valve disease. In: Fuster V, Alexander RW, O'Rourke RA, et al (eds): *Hurst's The Heart,* 10th ed. New York: McGraw-Hill; 2001:1667–1695.

Rahimtoola SH: Recognition and management of acute aortic regurgitation. *Heart Dis Stroke* 1993; 2:217–221.

Ross J Jr: Afterload mismatch and preload reserve: A conceptual framework for the analysis of ventricular function. *Prog Cardiovasc Dis* 1976; 18:255–264.

Ross J Jr, Braunwald E: Aortic stenosis. *Circulation* 1968; 36 (suppl IV):61–67.

Smith N, McAnulty JH, Rahimtoola SH: Severe aortic stenosis with impaired left ventricular function and clinical heart failure: Results of valve replacement. *Circulation* 1978; 58:255–264.

CHAPTER

23

MITRAL VALVE DISEASE

Shahbudin H. Rahimtoola
Maurice Enriquez-Sarano
Hartzell V. Schaff
Robert L. Frye

MITRAL STENOSIS

Definition, Etiology, and Pathology

Mitral stenosis (MS), an obstruction to blood flow between the left atrium (LA) and the left ventricle (LV), is caused by abnormal mitral valve function. In virtually all adult patients, the cause of MS is previous rheumatic carditis. About 60 percent of patients with rheumatic mitral valve disease do not give a history of rheumatic fever or chorea, and about 50 percent of patients with acute rheumatic carditis do not eventually have clinical valvular heart disease. Other causes of MS are uncommon, but obstruction to LV inflow can be congenital or due to active infective endocarditis, neoplasm, massive annular calcification, systemic lupus erythermatosus, carcinoid, methysergide therapy, Hunter-Hurler syndromes, Fabry's disease, Whipple's disease, rheumatoid arthritis, left atrial myxoma, massive left atrial ball thrombus, and cortriatum.

Acute rheumatic carditis is a pancarditis involving the pericardium, myocardium, and endocardium. In temperate climates and developed countries, there is usually a long interval (10 to 20 years) between an episode of rheumatic carditis and the clinical presentation of symptomatic MS. In tropical and subtropical climates and in less developed countries, the latent period is often shorter, and MS may occur during childhood or adolescence.

The pathologic hallmark of rheumatic carditis is an Aschoff's nodule. Rheumatic valvulitis results in scarring and fusion. The combination of commissural fusion, valve leaflet contracture, and fusion of the chordae tendineae results in a narrow, funnel-shaped orifice.*

Pathophysiology

The pathophysiologic features of MS all result from obstruction of the flow of blood between the LA and the LV. With reduction in valve area, energy is lost to friction during the transport of blood from the LA to the LV. Accordingly, a pressure gradient is present across the stenotic valve.

The pressure gradient between the LA and the LV increases markedly with increased heart rate or cardiac output (CO); this is responsible for LA hypertension. The LA gradually enlarges and hypertrophies. Pulmonary venous pressure rises with LA pressure increase and is passively associated with an increase in pulmonary arterial (PA) pressure. In up to 20 percent of patients, the pulmonary vascular resistance is also elevated, which further increases PA pressure. PA hypertension results in right ventricular (RV) hypertrophy and RV enlargement. The changes in RV function eventually result in right atrial (RA) hypertension and enlargement and systemic venous congestion; frequently, tricuspid regurgitation also occurs.

Pulmonary venous hypertension alters lung function in several ways. Distribution of blood flow in the lung is altered, with a relative increase in flow to the upper lobes and therefore in physiologic dead space. Pulmonary compliance generally decreases with increasing pulmonary capillary pressure, increasing the work of breathing, particularly during exercise. Chronic changes in the pulmonary capillaries and pulmonary arteries include fibrosis and thickening. These changes protect the lungs from the transudation of fluid into the alveoli (alveolar pulmonary edema).

Long-standing MS with severe PA hypertension and resultant RV dysfunction may be accompanied by chronic systemic venous hypertension. Tricuspid regurgitation is frequently present, even in the absence of intrinsic disease of this valve.

Clinical Manifestations

HISTORY

An asymptomatic interval is usually present between the initiating event of acute rheumatic fever and the presentation of symptomatic MS. Initially, there is little or no gradient at rest, but with increased cardiac output, LA pressure rises and exertional dyspnea develops. As mitral valve obstruction increases, dyspnea occurs at lower work levels. The progression of disability is so subtle and protracted that patients may adapt by circumscribing their lifestyles. It becomes

---

*Mitral stenosis section written by Dr. Rahimtoola. Mitral regurgitation section written by Drs. Enriquez-Sarano, Schaff, and Frye.

imperative, then, to document what activities the patient can perform without symptoms and at what activity level symptoms begin.

As obstruction progresses, the patients note orthopnea and paroxysmal nocturnal dyspnea, apparently resulting from redistribution of blood to the thorax on assuming the supine position. With severe MS and elevated pulmonary vascular resistance, fatigue rather than dyspnea may be the predominant symptom. Dependent edema, nausea, anorexia, and right-upper-quadrant pain reflect systemic venous congestion resulting from elevated systemic venous pressure and salt and water retention. Symptoms of RV failure (hepatomegaly, edema, and ascites) may predominate in patients with severe pulmonary hypertension.

Palpitations are a frequent complaint in patients with MS and may represent frequent premature atrial contractions or paroxysmal atrial fibrillation/flutter. Of patients with severe symptomatic MS, 50 percent or more have chronic atrial fibrillation.

Systemic embolism, a frequent complication of MS, may result in stroke, occlusion of extremity arterial supply, occlusion of the aortic bifurcation, and visceral or myocardial infarction. Hemoptysis, hoarseness, and exertional chest pain are infrequent manifestations of MS.

Progression of symptoms in MS is generally slow but relentless. Thus, a sudden change in symptoms rarely reflects a change in valve obstruction. Rather, there is usually a noncardiac precipitating event or paroxysmal atrial fibrillation.

PHYSICAL FINDINGS

During the latent, presymptomatic interval, incidental physical findings may be normal or may provide evidence of mild MS. Frequently, the only characteristic finding noted at rest will be a loud S_1 and a presystolic murmur. A short diastolic decrescendo rumble may be heard only with exercise. In patients with symptomatic stenosis, the findings are more obvious, and careful physical examination usually leads to the correct diagnosis (see also Chap. 1).

The jugular venous pressure may be normal or may show evidence of elevated RA pressure. A prominent a wave is a result of RV hypertension/hypertrophy or of associated tricuspid stenosis. A prominent v wave is caused by tricuspid regurgitation. Atrial fibrillation produces an irregular venous pulse with absent a waves. The chest findings may be normal or may reveal signs of pulmonary congestion with rales or pleural fluid (dullness and absent breath sounds). Marked LA enlargement may produce egophony at the tip of the left scapula.

The precordium is usually unremarkable on inspection. On palpation, the apical impulse should feel normal or be tapping. An abnormal LV impulse suggests disease other than isolated MS. A diastolic thrill is usually appreciated only when the patient is examined in the left lateral decubitus position. When PA hypertension is present, a sustained RV lift along the left sternal border and pulmonic valve closure may be palpable.

On auscultation in the supine position, the only abnormality appreciated may be the accentuated S_1, which is caused by flexible valve leaflets and the wide closing excursion of the valve leaflets. Failure to examine the patient in the left lateral decubitus position accounts for most of the missed diagnoses of symptomatic MS. The diastolic rumble is heard best with the bell of the stethoscope applied at the apical impulse. Nevertheless, the murmur may be localized, and the region around the apical impulse also should be auscultated. The *opening snap* (OS) occurs when the movement of the domed mitral valve into the LV is suddenly stopped. It is heard best with the diaphragm and is often most easily appreciated midway between the apex and the left sternal border. In this intermediate region, the S_1, P_2, and the OS can be identified.

The OS occurs after the LV pressure falls below LA pressure in early diastole. When LA pressure is high, as in severe MS, the snap occurs earlier in diastole. Although the OS is present in most cases of MS, it is absent in patients with stiff, fibrotic, or calcified leaflets. Thus, absence of the OS in severe MS suggests that mitral valve replacement rather than commissurotomy may be necessary.

The low-pitched diastolic rumble follows the OS and is best heard with the bell of the stethoscope. In some patients with low cardiac output or mild MS, brief exercise, such as sit-ups or walking, is adequate to increase flow and bring out the murmur. The murmur is low-pitched, rumbling, and decrescendo. In general, the more severe the MS, the longer the murmur. Presystolic accentuation of the murmur occurs in sinus rhythm and has been reported even in atrial fibrillation.

The two most important auscultatory signs of severe MS are a short A_2-OS interval and a full-length diastolic rumble. The diastolic murmur may not be full-length in severe MS if the stroke volume is low and there is no tachycardia.

Systolic murmurs also may be heard in association with the murmur of MS. A blowing murmur at the apex suggests associated mitral regurgitation, whereas a systolic blowing murmur heard best at the lower left sternal border that increases with inspiration usually signifies tricuspid regurgitation. The Graham Steell murmur is a high-pitched diastolic decrescendo murmur of pulmonic regurgitation caused by severe PA hypertension. In most patients with MS, such a murmur usually indicates aortic regurgitation. In general, a left-sided S_3 is not compatible with severe MS, with the possible exception of concomitant severe AR and/or significant LV systolic dysfunction. If an S_3 and a rumble are present, mitral regurgitation is usually the predominant lesion.

CHEST ROENTGENOGRAM

The posteroanterior and lateral chest films are often so typical that experienced clinicians can make the tentative diagnosis from them. The thoracic cage is normal. The lung fields show evidence of elevated pulmonary venous pressure. Blood flow is more evenly redistributed to the upper lobes, resulting in apparent prominence of upper-lobe vascularity. Increased pulmonary venous pressure results in transudation of fluid into the interstitium. Accumulation of fluid in the interlobular septa produces linear streaks in the bases, which extend to the pleura (Kerley B lines). Interstitial fluid may also be seen as perivascular or peribronchial cuffing (Kerley A lines). With transudation of fluid into the alveolar spaces, alveolar pulmonary edema is seen. These changes represent long-standing elevated LA pressure. PA hypertension results in enlargement of the main PA and right and left main pulmonary arteries.

The cardiac silhouette usually does not show generalized cardiomegaly, but the LA is invariably enlarged. In the posteroanterior chest film, LA enlargement is recognized by a density behind the RA border (double atrial shadow), prominence of the LA appendage on the left heart border between the main PA and LV apex, and elevation of the left main bronchus. The lateral film shows the LA bulging posteriorly. The combination of a normal-sized LV, enlarged LA, and pulmonary venous congestion should immediately raise the possibility of MS. Mitral valve calcification is occasionally seen on the plain chest x-ray.

ELECTROCARDIOGRAM

Patients in sinus rhythm may have a widened P wave caused by interatrial conduction delay and/or prolonged LA depolarization. Classically, the P wave is broad and notched in lead II and biphasic in lead V_1; it measures 0.12 s or more. Atrial fibrillation is common. LV hypertrophy is not present unless there are associated lesions. RV hypertrophy may be present if PA hypertension is marked.

CLINICAL INDICATIONS OF SEVERE MITRAL STENOSIS

Some clinical features make it virtually certain that MS is severe. These include (1) moderate to severe PA hypertension, as indicated by clinical and ECG evidence of RV hypertrophy or PA hypertension or both, and/or (2) moderate to severe elevation of LA pressure as indicated by orthopnea, a short P_2-OS interval, a diastolic rumble that occupies the whole length of a long diastolic interval in patients with atrial fibrillation, and pulmonary edema on the chest x-ray. In both these clinical circumstances, one must be certain that there is no other cause for elevated LA pressure and that LA hypertension is not caused mainly by a correctable transient elevation of LV diastolic pressure.

Laboratory Tests

ECHOCARDIOGRAPHY/DOPPLER ULTRASOUND

Echocardiography/Doppler ultrasound has proved to be both sensitive and specific for MS when adequate studies are done. The characteristic M-mode echocardiographic features are a decreased EF slope of the anterior mitral leaflet. Two-dimensional (2D) echocardiography will demonstrate the valve orifice and allow calculation of mitral valve area. Doppler echocardiography will provide estimates of the gradient across the valve and of pulmonary artery pressure.

Transesophageal echocardiography (TEE) is a useful technique to assess LA thrombus, the anatomy of the mitral valve and subvalvular apparatus, and the suitability of the patient for catheter balloon commissurotomy or surgical valve repair.

Echocardiography/Doppler ultrasound is a most useful test in MS and should be performed in all patients. It is essential to determine suitability of the valve for commissurotomy and/or repair and to determine the likely result.

CARDIAC CATHETERIZATION/ANGIOGRAPHY

In most patients with disabling symptoms from presumed MS, right and left heart catheterization should be performed as part of a preoperative assessment. Simultaneous measurement of cardiac output and the gradient between the LA and the LV and calculation of valve area remain the "gold standard" for assessing the severity of MS. LV angiography assesses the competence of the mitral valve, an important determinant of operability for mitral commissurotomy. Quantification of LV function provides a useful prognostic indicator of operative and late survival and of the expected functional result. Aortic valve function should be evaluated in all patients. Selective supraventricular aortography should be performed in all patients unless there is a contraindication. Tricuspid valve function can be assessed when there is a question of coexisting lesions. In certain circumstances, dynamic exercise in the catheterization laboratory with measurement of mitral valve gradient, CO, and LA and PA pressures can be extremely useful. Selective coronary arteriography establishes the site, severity, and extent of coronary artery disease and should be performed in patients with angina, LV dysfunction, and/or risk factors for coronary artery disease and in those 35 years of age or older who are being considered for interventional therapy.

OTHER LABORATORY STUDIES

In most clinical situations, other investigations are not needed. Occasionally, a treadmill exercise test to evaluate functional capacity may be very useful clinically—for example, when a patient denies symptoms in spite of severe hemodynamic abnormalities.

Natural History and Prognosis

The population presenting with MS is changing because of the sharp decline in the incidence of acute rheumatic fever in the past 40 years. Native-born American citizens with symptomatic MS are presenting at an older age. Young adults in the third and fourth decades with symptomatic MS are more likely to come from low socioeconomic backgrounds and from the inner city or to be immigrants, particularly from Latin America, the Middle East, Africa, or Asia. The mechanism for the progression from no symptoms to mild to severe symptoms is progressive stenosis of the mitral valve. Approximately 50 percent of patients develop symptoms gradually. Sudden deterioration is usually the result of atrial fibrillation, systemic embolization, and other conditions that result in tachycardia and/or increased cardiac output.

The 10-year survival of patients with MS who are asymptomatic is approximately 84 percent, and that of those who are mildly symptomatic is 34 to 42 percent. Patients in the New York Heart Association functional class IV have a very poor survival without treatment: 42 percent at 1 year and 10 percent or less at 5 years. All are dead by 10 years.

Medical Treatment

All streptococcal infections should be diagnosed rapidly and correctly treated. All patients with known previous acute rheumatic fever/rheumatic carditis with or without obvious valve disease should receive appropriate antibiotic prophylaxis against recurrent streptococcal infection (Table 23-1). Prophylaxis against infective endocarditis is a lifelong requirement. If atrial fibrillation is present, however, digitalis plays a critical role in controlling ventricular rate. In selected patients, beta-adrenergic blocking agents, diltiazem, or amiodarone may be added if digoxin alone is not satisfactory in controlling ventricular rate at rest or on exercise. Diuretics reduce pulmonary congestion and peripheral edema and allow most patients freedom from severe salt restriction. For the patient with mild symptoms, maintenance of sinus rhythm is desirable. Cardioversion of atrial fibrillation and maintenance of sinus rhythm using antiarrhythmic therapy with either digitalis and quinidine or digitalis and amiodarone should be offered to these patients. In patients who need interventional therapy, cardioversion is usually performed after

TABLE 23-1

SECONDARY PREVENTION OF RHEUMATIC FEVER

Agent	Dose	Mode
Benzathine Penicillin G	1,200,000 U every 4 weeks (every 3 weeks for high-risk* patients such as those with residual carditis)	Intramuscular
Penicillin V	250 mg twice daily	Oral
	or	
Sulfadiazine	0.5 g once daily for patients ≤27 kg (60 lb)	Oral
	1.0 g once daily for patients >27 kg (60 lb)	
For individuals allergic to penicillin and sulfadiazine:		
Erythromycin	250 mg twice daily	Oral

*High-risk patients include those with residual rheumatic carditis as well as patients from economically disadvantaged populations.

SOURCE: Bonow RA et al: ACC/AHA guidelines. *J Am Coll Cardiol* 1998; 32:1486–1588, with permission.

completion of the procedure. Anticoagulation with warfarin is usually begun about 3 weeks in advance of cardioversion and for 4 weeks after the procedure. Alternatively, if left atrial thrombus is excluded by TEE, 2 to 3 days of intravenous heparin should be instituted, the patient cardioverted to sinus rhythm, and warfarin therapy continued for at least 4 weeks. Patients with chronic atrial fibrillation and those with a previous history of embolism should receive anticoagulation with warfarin [International Normalized Ratio (INR) of 2 to 3] unless there is a specific contraindication. Systemic embolization necessitates permanent anticoagulation. A single systemic embolic episode is not an absolute indication for mitral valve surgery; emboli can and do occur in patients with mild mitral stenosis.

INTERVENTIONAL THERAPY

Unless there is a contraindication, surgery or catheter balloon commissurotomy (CBC) should be recommended to an MS patient with functional class III or IV symptoms. For younger patients with a pliable, non-calcified valve and without important mitral regurgitation, this means valve repair or CBC. The hemodynamic results of surgical commissurotomy or CBC are excellent. Because of the low morbidity and mortality of CBC/valve repair, surgery is also offered to those patients when functional class II symptoms are present. The results of successful commissurotomy are excellent; in experienced and skilled centers, surgical mortality is less than 1 percent. Late mortality at 10 years is less than 5 percent, the thromboembolism rate is 2 percent per year or less, and the reoperation rate ranges from 0.5 to 4.5 percent per year (Table 23-2).

For the older patient with a stiff or calcified valve or when moderate mitral regurgitation is present, mitral valve replacement is usually performed. Valve replacement carries a higher operative mortality than does commissurotomy (up to 5 percent) and the morbidity associated with prostheses. Hemodynamic results of mitral valve replacement are often not ideal (see also Chap. 26). Survival at 10 years after mitral valve replacement for functional class III and IV patients is better than 60 percent (Table 23-3).

Use of the double balloon technique or the Inoue balloon produces immediate and 3-month hemodynamic and clinical results comparable to those obtained by surgical commissurotomy. The mitral valve area increases from a mean of 1.0 to 2.0 cm^2. There are reductions of LA and PA pressures at rest and on exercise and an increase of exercise capacity. The immediate results of CBC are greatly influenced by the characteristics of the valve and its supporting apparatus, which are best determined by 2D echocardiography (transthoracic and/or transesophageal) (Table 23-4). Echocardiographic scores of ≤8 or of 0-1 determined by the two different methods provide a clue to the best immediate results. Repeat CBC or mitral valve replacement is needed in 20 percent of patients within 5 to 7 years. Late survival is poorer in those in whom functional class IV, higher echocardiographic score, higher LV end-diastolic pressure, or higher PA systolic pressure is present prior to the CBC.

MITRAL REGURGITATION

Definition, Etiology, and Pathology

Mitral regurgitation (MR) is characterized by an abnormal reversed blood flow from the left ventricle (LV) to the left atrium (LA) due to abnormalities in the mitral apparatus.

TABLE 23-2

RECOMMENDATIONS FOR MITRAL VALVE REPAIR
FOR MITRAL STENOSIS

Indication	Class
1. Patients with NYHA functional class III to IV symptoms, moderate or severe MS (mitral valve area ≤ 1.5 cm^2),* and valve morphology favorable for repair if percutaneous mitral balloon valvotomy is not available	I
2. Patients with NYHA functional class III to IV symptoms, moderate or severe MS (mitral valve area ≤ 1.5 cm^2),* and valve morphology favorable for repair if a left atrial thrombus is present despite anticoagulation	I
3. Patients with NYHA functional class III to IV symptoms, moderate or severe MS (mitral valve area ≤ 1.5 cm^2),* and a nonpliable or calcified valve with the decision to proceed with either repair or replacement made at the time of the operation	I
4. Patients in NYHA functional class I, moderate or severe MS (mitral valve area ≤ 1.5 cm^2), and valve morphology favorable for repair who have had recurrent episodes of embolic events on adequate anticoagulation	IIb
5. Patients with NYHA functional classes I to IV symptoms and mild MS	III

*The committee recognizes that there may be variability in the measurement of mitral valve area and that the mean transmitral gradient, pulmonary artery wedge pressure, and pulmonary artery pressure at rest or during exercise should also be taken into consideration.

SOURCE: Bonow RA et al: ACC/AHA guidelines. *J Am Coll Cardiol* 1998; 32:1486–1588, with permission.

Mitral valve prolapse (Chap. 24) is now the most common cause of MR, followed by that due to coronary artery disease. MR due to rheumatic valvulitis remains an important cause. Additional causes include infective endocarditis, mitral annular calcification, hypertrophic cardiomyopathy, trauma, connective tissue disorders, and congenital deformities. The competence of the mitral valve depends

TABLE 23-3

RECOMMENDATIONS FOR MITRAL VALVE REPLACEMENT FOR MITRAL STENOSIS

Indication	Class
1. Patients with moderate or severe MS (mitral valve area ≤1.5 cm²)* and NYHA functional class III to IV symptoms who are not considered candidates for percutaneous balloon valvotomy or mitral valve repair 2. Patients with severe MS (mitral valve area ≤1 cm²)* and severe pulmonary hypertension (pulmonary artery systolic pressure > 60 to 80 mmHg) with NYHA functional class I to II symptoms who are not considered candidates for percutaneous balloon valvotomy or mitral valve repair	I IIa

*The committee recognizes that there may be variability in the measurement of mitral valve area and that the mean transmitral gradient, pulmonary artery wedge pressure, and pulmonary artery pressure at rest or during exercise should also be taken into consideration.
SOURCE: Bonow RA et al: ACC/AHA guidelines. *J Am Coll Cardiol* 1998; 32:1486–1588, with permission.

on the normal structure and function of every part of the mitral apparatus—that is, the leaflets, chordae tendineae, annulus, left atrium, papillary muscles, and LV myocardium surrounding the papillary muscles. There is a report of MR and AR with use of anorectic drugs.

Pathophysiology

The abnormal coaptation of the mitral leaflets creates a *regurgitant orifice* during systole. The systolic pressure gradient between the LV and LA is the driving force of the regurgitant flow, which results in a *regurgitant volume*. This regurgitant volume represents a percentage of the total ejection of the LV and may be expressed as the *regurgitant fraction*. The regurgitant volume creates a volume overload by entering the LA in systole and the LV in diastole, modifying LV loading and function because it is additive to the systolic output of the right ventricle.

TABLE 23-4

RECOMMENDATIONS FOR PERCUTANEOUS MITRAL
BALLOON VALVOTOMY

Indication	Class
1. Symptomatic patients (NYHA functional class II, III, or IV), moderate or severe MS (mitral valve area ≤1.5 cm^2),* and valve morphology favorable for percutaneous balloon valvotomy in the absence of left atrial thrombus or moderate to severe MR	I
2. Asymptomatic patients with moderate or severe MS (mitral valve area ≤1.5 cm^2)* and valve morphology favorable for percutaneous balloon valvotomy who have pulmonary hypertension (pulmonary artery systolic pressure >50 mmHg at rest or 60 mmHg with exercise) in the absence of left atrial thrombus or moderate to severe MR	IIa
3. Patients with NYHA functional class III to IV symptoms, moderate or severe MS (mitral valve area ≤1.5 cm^2),* and a nonpliable calcified valve who are at high risk for surgery in the absence of left atrial thrombus or moderate to severe MR	IIa
4. Asymptomatic patients, moderate or severe MS (mitral valve area ≤1.5 cm^2)^a and valve morphology favorable for percutaneous balloon valvotomy who have new onset of atrial fibrillation in the absence of left atrial thrombus or moderate to severe MR	IIb
5. Patients in NYHA functional class III to IV, moderate or severe MS (MVA ≤1.5 cm^2), and a nonpliable calcified valve who are low-risk candidates for surgery	IIb
6. Patients with mild MS	III

*The committee recognizes that there may be variability in the measurement of mitral valve area and that the mean transmitral gradient, pulmonary artery wedge pressure, and pulmonary artery pressure at rest or during exercise should also be taken into consideration.

SOURCE: Bonow RA et al: ACC/AHA guidelines. *J Am Coll Cardiol* 1998; 32:1486–1588, with permission.

In acute MR, the hemodynamic burden is different. The sudden burden of the MR on normal chambers does not allow compensatory dilatation of the LA and LV. Consequently, marked elevations of the LA and pulmonary venous pressures are produced, which leads to acute pulmonary edema.

LV dysfunction is a frequent and dismal complication of MR; its exact mechanism is unknown. The changes in myofiber contractility parallel changes in global LV function and are associated with reduced myofiber content. During diastole, LV relaxation is frequently abnormal, but chamber stiffness is usually reduced. Age and decreased systolic function are associated with increased chamber stiffness.

Clinical Manifestations

HISTORY

Patients with MR usually have no symptoms. Severe MR may be associated with no or minimal symptoms. Fatigue and mild dyspnea on exertion are the most usual symptoms and are rapidly improved by rest, and these progress to orthopnea, paroxysmal nocturnal dyspnea, and peripheral edema. Often, the history provides clues to the etiology—for example, history of angina/myocardial infarction, rheumatic carditis, infective endocarditis, chronic heart failure (HF) with a markedly dilated heart, or sudden onset of severe symptoms with a normal-sized heart.

With severe MR of *acute onset,* symptoms are usually more dramatic—pulmonary edema or congestive heart failure—but may progressively subside with administration of diuretic and increased LA compliance.

PHYSICAL FINDINGS

Blood pressure is usually normal. The arterial upstroke is brisk, especially when ejection time is reduced in MR.

On palpation, the cardiac impulse (enlarged LV) is often laterally displaced, diffuse, and brief. An apical thrill is characteristic of very severe MR. The left sternal border lift is observed with right ventricular dilatation and may be difficult to distinguish from the LA lift in later systole due to the dilated, expansive LA, which is more substernal and lower (see also Chap. 1).

The first heart sound is included in the murmur and is usually normal but may be increased in rheumatic disease. The second heart sound is usually normal but may be paradoxically split if the LV ejection time is markedly shortened. The presence of a third heart sound (S_3) is directly related to the volume of the regurgitation in patients with organic MR. MR is often associated with an early diastolic rumble due to the increased mitral flow in diastole even without mitral stenosis. The S_3 and diastolic rumble are low-pitched sounds and may be difficult to detect without careful auscultation in the left lateral decubitus position. The S_3 increases with expiration. In ischemic and/or functional MR, S_3 corresponds more often to restrictive LV filling. An atrial gallop (S_4) is heard mainly in MR of recent onset and in ischemic and/or functional MR in sinus rhythm. Midsystolic clicks are markers of valve prolapse and are due to sudden tension of the chordae (discussed later).

The hallmark of MR is the systolic murmur, most often holosystolic, including first and second heart sounds. If an opening snap or S_3 is mistakenly interpreted as S_2, the murmur may appear midsystolic. The murmur is of a high-pitched and blowing type but may be harsh, especially in valve prolapse. The maximum intensity is usually at the apex, and it may radiate to the axilla when the anterior leaflet results in greater regurgitation and to the left sternal border when the posterior leaflet results in greater regurgitation. In posterior leaflet prolapse, the jet is usually superiorly and medially directed and the murmur radiates toward the base of the heart. In anterior leaflet prolapse, the murmur may be heard in the back, in the neck, and sometimes on the skull. In the cases where the murmur radiates to the base, it may be difficult to distinguish from the murmur of aortic stenosis or obstructive cardiomyopathy; pharmacologic maneuvers show that the murmur decreases with reduction of afterload or LV size and increases with increase of afterload or LV size. Murmur intensity does not increase with postextrasystolic beats because the degree of MR is not increased (see Chap. 1).

Murmurs of shorter duration usually correspond to mild MR; they may be mid- or late systolic in mitral valve prolapse or early systolic in functional MR.

ELECTROCARDIOGRAM

Chronic MR produces LA or LV enlargement typically manifest by increased amplitude of the P waves and QRS complex. If atrial fibrillation is present, the LA enlargement is associated with coarse fibrillatory waves. RV hypertrophy is uncommon. The electrocardiogram, especially in acute MR, may be entirely normal. When papillary muscle ischemia or infarction is the cause of MR, evidence of inferior or posterior infarction (old or new) may be present.

CHEST ROENTGENOGRAM

In chronic severe MR, the chest x-ray shows LA and LV enlargement. In rheumatic disease, the valve leaflets may be calcified; with degenerative disease, a calcified mitral annulus is often present. Acute severe MR is usually associated with normal cardiac size and pulmonary edema.

Laboratory Tests

ECHOCARIOGRAPHY/DOPPLER

The echocardiogram is usually helpful in defining the etiology of the MR (e.g., flail leaflets, severe prolapse, mitral annulus calcification, systolic anterior motion of the anterior leaflet, and endocarditis vegetation) and determining its consequences. The echo/Doppler technique provides an estimate of the severity of the regurgitation by assessing the velocity, width, and length of the regurgitant jet. Color-flow imaging demonstrates the origin and direction of the jet. Accordingly, the jet length, the ratio of the jet area to the left atrial area, or more simply size of the jet area have been suggested as good indices of the severity of MR. Small jets, such as those seen in normal subjects, consistently correspond to mild regurgitations. Color-flow imaging for defining regurgitant lesions has significant limitations that are intrinsically related to the nature of regurgitant jets. The extent of a jet is determined by its momentum and thus as much by regurgitant velocity as by regurgitant flow. Also, jets are constrained by the LA and expand more in large atria. The eccentric jets of valvular prolapse depend on the left atrial wall and tend to underestimate regurgitation. In contrast, the central jets of ischemic and functional MR expand markedly in a large atrium and tend to overestimate regurgitation. Transesophageal echocardiography usually shows larger jets but does not eliminate these limitations of color-flow imaging. The pulmonary venous velocity profile is useful to assess the degree of regurgitation. Systolic reversal of flow in the pulmonary veins is a strong argument for severe MR. Several quantitative methods have been used to measure parameters that reflect the degree of MR; however, the reliability of these techniques for the quantitative assessment of MR remains to be demonstrated.

CARDIAC CATHETERIZATION AND ANGIOGRAPHY

Cardiac catheterization is utilized to assess hemodynamic status, the severity of MR, LV function, and coronary artery anatomy. It confirms the diagnosis of MR as well. A large v wave in the pulmonary capillary wedge pressure tracings suggests MR but its absence does not exclude MR. A balloon flotation catheter, inserted at the bedside to determine oxygen saturation in the right heart chambers and the presence or absence of the v wave in the pulmonary capillary pressures, is helpful in establishing the cause of a new systolic murmur that develops in a patient after acute myocardial infarction. The assessment of the degree of regurgitation can be obtained by LV contrast angiography and can be qualitatively graded in three or four grades on the basis of the degree and persistence of opacification of the LA. The assessment of LV function can be performed using quantitative angiography. LV volumes are determined by the regurgitant volume, duration of regurgitation, etiology of regurgitation, and LV function. The most frequently utilized indices of LV function are the end-systolic volume and the LV ventricular ejection fraction. Both have been shown to be useful prognostically. The hemodynamic response to exercise (e.g., cardiac output, pulmonary artery pressure) often help to determine the need for valve replacement in borderline circumstances.

Regional wall motion abnormalities have been observed in patients with MR even in the absence of coronary lesions. Selected coronary angiography is at present the only technique for defining the coronary artery anatomy. It is usually performed in patients above 35 years of age or in those with angina or multiple risk factors for coronary artery disease.

OTHER LABORATORY STUDIES

Radionuclide angiography can be used to estimate the LV end-diastolic and end-systolic volumes as well as the RV and LV ejection fractions. The detection of exercise-induced LV dysfunction is frequent; however, the significance of such measurements on the long-term prognosis has not been analyzed in large series of patients. The comparison of the counts measured over the RV and LV allows the calculation of the mitral valve regurgitant fraction. Exercise testing is often useful for determining the patient's exercise capacity, particularly in those who appear relatively asymptomatic despite severe MR.

Natural History and Prognosis

Because of the qualitative and imprecise assessment of the degree of regurgitation, the natural history of MR is poorly defined. Patients with mild rheumatic MR appear to have a good prognosis. The prognosis of patients with mitral valve prolapse and no or mild regurgitation is usually excellent. Some deaths may occur in patients with murmurs of MR and more often when LV function is markedly decreased.

The predictors of poor outcome in patients with MR who are treated medically include severe symptoms (classes III to IV) even if the symptoms are transient, pulmonary hypertension, markedly increased LV end-diastolic volume, decreased cardiac output, and reduced LV ejection fraction. A comparison of the outcome of medically and surgically treated patients shows a trend in favor of the surgical treatment, especially early surgery, with a definite improvement of outcome with surgery in patients who have decreased systolic LV function.

Medical Treatment

Prevention of infective endocarditis with use of antibiotics is necessary in patients with MR. Young patients with rheumatic MR should receive rheumatic fever prophylaxis. In patients with AF, rate control is achieved using digoxin and/or beta blockers, diltiazem, and amiodarone. Long-term maintenance of sinus rhythm after cardioversion in patients with severe MR or enlarged LA is usually not possible in those who are treated medically. Oral anticoagulation should be used inpatients with atrial fibrillation (INR 2.0 to 3.0).

Afterload reduction decreases the amount of regurgitation not only by reducing the LV systolic pressure but also by decreasing the effective regurgitant orifice area. The acute utilization of sodium nitroprusside in unstable patients with severe MR, especially in the context of myocardial infarction, may be lifesaving in patients being prepared for mitral valve surgery. Chronic afterload reduction is more controversial. Diuretic treatment is extremely useful for the control of heart failure and for the chronic control of symptoms, especially dyspnea.

Surgical Treatment

Mitral valve reconstruction for MR is often possible. The frequency with which valve repair can be used in patients with MR varies with the experience of the operating team and the spectrum of underlying valve disease; repair is more often feasible in patients with degenerative valve disease than in those with regurgitation caused by rheumatic valvulitis or endocarditis. LV systolic function and late survival in general are better with mitral valve repair than with mitral valve replacement because of the lesser decline or maintenance of normal LV function when the chordae are preserved at the time of surgery. In patients whose mitral valves cannot be repaired, mitral valve replacement with chordal preservation is less likely to depress LV function than mitral valve replacement without preservation of the chordae tendineae. Patients with severe symptoms due to MR should be treated surgically even if symptoms are markedly improved by medical treatment (Table 23-5). Patients who are functional class I or II but with signs of overt LV dysfunction (LV ejection fraction <60 percent, end-systolic diameter >45 mm) should be treated surgically, particularly if they are candidates for valve repair or valve replacement with chordal preservation. In patients with *severe* MR who have no or minimal symptoms and no signs of LV dysfunction, surgery is a reasonable option when it is likely that the mitral valve can be repaired with chordal preservation. This pertains to patients with a low operative risk of 1 to 2 percent and valvular lesions that can be repaired as indicated by echocardiography. Intraoperative TEE

TABLE 23-5

RECOMMENDATIONS FOR MITRAL VALVE SURGERY IN NONISCHEMIC SEVERE MITRAL REGURGITATION

Indication	Class
1. Acute symptomatic MR in which repair is likely	I
2. Patients with NYHA functional class II, III, or IV symptoms with normal LV function defined as ejection fraction > 0.60 and end-systolic dimension <45 mm	I
3. Symptomatic or asymptomatic patients with mild LV dysfunction, ejection fraction 0.50 to 0.60, and end-systolic dimension 45 to 50 mm	I
4. Symptomatic or asymptomatic patients with moderate LV dysfunction, ejection fraction 0.30 to 0.50, and/or end-systolic dimension 50 to 55 mm	I
5. Asymptomatic patients with preserved LV function and atrial fibrillation	IIa
6. Asymptomatic patients with preserved LV function and pulmonary hypertension (pulmonary artery systolic pressure >50 mmHg at rest or > 60 mmHg with exercise	IIa
7. Asymptomatic patients with ejection fraction 0.50 to 0.60 and end-systolic dimension <45 mm and asymptomatic patients with ejection fraction > 0.60 and end-systolic dimension 45 to 55 mm	IIa
8. Patients with severe LV dysfunction (ejection fraction <0.30 and/or end-systolic dimension >55 mm) in whom chordal preservation is highly likely	IIa
9. Asymptomatic patients with chronic MR with preserved LV function in whom mitral valve repair is highly likely	IIb
10. Patients with MVP and preserved LV function who have recurrent ventricular arrhythmias despite medical therapy	IIb
11. Asymptomatic patients with preserved LV function in whom significant doubt about the feasibility of repair exists	III

*The committee recognizes that there may be variability in the measurement of mitral valve area and that the mean transmitral gradient, pulmonary artery wedge pressure, and pulmonary artery pressure at rest or during exercise should also be taken into consideration.

SOURCE: Bonow RA et al: ACC/AHA guidelines. *J Am Coll Cardiol* 1998; 32:1486–1588, with permission.

should be performed by physicians to monitor the repair procedure and help with decisions warranted by an imperfect result.

Patients who have no symptoms due to severe MR and normal LV systolic function who are candidates for mitral valve repair and have severe pulmonary hypertension at rest or with exercise, atrial fibrillation, or recurrent thromboemboli despite anticoagulation therapy are commonly recommended for early surgery if mitral valve repair with preservation of the chordae is the likely procedure.

SUGGESTED READING

Bonow RO, Carabello B, De Leon AC Jr, et al: ACC/AHA guidelines for valvular heart disease. *J Am Coll Cardiol* 1998; 32:1486–1588.

Committee on Rheumatic Fever, Endocarditis, and Kawasaki Disease of the Council on Cardiovascular Disease in the Young of the American Heart Association: Treatment of streptococcal pharyngitis and prevention of rheumatic fever: A statement for health professionals. *Pediatrics* 1995; 96:758–764.

Crawford MH, Souchek J, Oprian CA, et al: Determinants of survival and left ventricular performance after mitral valve replacement. Department of Veterans Affairs Cooperative Study on Valvular Heart Disease. *Circulation* 1990; 81:1173–1181.

Currie PJ, Seward JB, Chan KL, et al: Continuous wave Doppler determination of right ventricular pressure: A simultaneous Doppler-catheterization study in 127 patients. *J Am Coll Cardiol* 1985; 6:750–756.

Hatle L, Angelsen B, Tromsdal A: Noninvasive assessment of atrioventricular pressure half-time by Doppler ultrasound. *Circulation* 1979; 60:1096–1104.

Manning WJ, Silverman DI, Keighley CS, et al: Transesophageal echocardiographically facilitated early cardioversion from atrial fibrillation using short-term anticoagulation: Final results of a prospective 4.5 year study. *J Am Coll Cardiol* 1995; 256:1354–1361.

Nishimura RA, Rihal CS, Tajik AJ, Holmes DR Jr: Accurate measurement of the transmitral gradient in patients with mitral stenosis: A simultaneous catheterization and Doppler echocardiographic study. *J Am Coll Cardiol* 1994; 2:152–158.

Palacios IF, Tuzcu ME, Weyman AE: Clinical follow-up of patients undergoing percutaneous mitral balloon valvotomy. *Circulation* 1995; 91:671–676.

Rahimtoola SH, Enriquez-Sarano M, Schaff HV, Frye RL: Mitral valve disease. In: Fuster V, Alexander RW, O'Rourke RA, et al (eds): *Hurst's The Heart,* 10th ed. New York: McGraw-Hill; 2001: 1697–1727.

Reid CL, McKay CR, Chandraratna PA, et al: Mechanisms of increase in mitral valve area and influence of anatomic features in double-balloon, catheter balloon valvuloplasty in adults with rheumatic mitral stenosis: A Doppler and two-dimensional echocardiographic study. *Circulation* 1987; 76:628–636.

Tuzcu EM, Block PC, Griffin BP, et al: Immediate and long-term outcome of percutaneous mitral valvotomy in patients 65 years and older. *Circulation* 1992; 85:963–971.

Wisenbaugh T, Skudicky D, Sareli P: Prediction of outcome after valve replacement for rheumatic mitral regurgitation in the era of chordal preservation. *Circulation* 1994; 89:191–197.

CHAPTER

24

MITRAL VALVE PROLAPSE SYNDROME

Raja Naidu
Robert A. O'Rourke

DEFINITION, ETIOLOGY, AND TIMING

Mitral valve prolapse (MVP) refers to the systolic billowing of one or both mitral leaflets into the left atrium, with or without mitral regurgitation. MVP often occurs as a clinical entity with no or only mild mitral regurgitation, and it is frequently associated with unique clinical characteristics when compared with the other causes of mitral regurgitation (MR). Nevertheless, MVP is the most common cause of significant MR and the most frequent substrate for mitral valve endocarditis in the United States. The mitral valve apparatus is a complex structure composed of the mitral annulus, valve leaflets, chordae tendineae, papillary muscles, and supporting left ventricular, left atrial, and aortic walls. Disease processes involving any one or more of these components may result in dysfunction of the valvular apparatus and prolapse of the mitral leaflets toward the left atrium during systole, when left ventricular pressure exceeds left atrial pressure.

In primary MVP (Table 24-1), there is interchordal hooding due to leaflet redundancy involving both the rough and clear zones of the involved leaflets. The basic microscopic feature of primary MVP is marked proliferation of the spongiosa, the delicate myxomatous connective tissue between the atrialis (a thick layer of collagen and elastic tissue forming the atrial aspect of the leaflet) and the fibrosa or ventricularis, which is composed of dense layers of collagen and forms the basic support of the leaflet. In primary MVP, myxomatous proliferation of the mucopolysaccharide-containing spongiosa tissue causes focal interruption of the fibrosa. Secondary effects of the primary MVP syndrome include fibrosis of the surface of the mitral valve leaflets, thinning and/or elongation of the chordae tendineae, and ventricular friction lesions. Fibrin deposits often form at the

451

TABLE 24-1

CLASSIFICATION OF MITRAL VALVE PROLAPSE

Primary mitral valve prolapse
   Familial
   Nonfamilial
   Marfan's syndrome
   Other connective tissue diseases
   Cardiomyopathies
   "Flail" mitral valve leaflet(s)
Secondary mitral valve prolapse
   Coronary artery disease
   Rheumatic heart disease
Normal variant
   Inaccurate auscultation
   "Echocardiographic" heart disease

mitral valve–left atrial angle. The primary form of MVP may occur in families, where it appears to be inherited as an autosomal dominant trait with varying penetrance. Primary MVP has also been found with increasing frequency in patients with Marfan's syndrome and in other heritable connective tissue diseases.

In secondary forms of MVP (Table 24-1), myxomatous proliferation of the spongiosa portion of the mitral valve leaflet is absent. Echocardiographic evidence of MVP, often with MR, can be produced in closed-chest dogs undergoing transient coronary artery occlusion. Serial studies in patients with known ischemic heart disease have occasionally documented unequivocal MVP following an acute coronary syndrome that was previously absent; however, in most patients with coronary artery disease (CAD) and MVP, the two entities are coincident but unrelated.

Recently, several studies have indicated that valvular regurgitation caused by MVP may result from postinflammatory changes, including those following rheumatic fever. Mitral valve prolapse has also been observed in patients with hypertrophic cardiomyopathy, in whom posterior MVP may result from a disproportionally small left ventricular cavity, altered papillary muscle alignment, or a combination of factors. Patients with primary and secondary MVP must be distinguished from those with normal variations on cardiac auscultation or echocardiography that are misinterpreted to represent the MVP syndrome.

PATHOPHYSIOLOGY

In patients with MVP, there is frequently left atrial (LA) and left ventricular (LV) enlargement, depending upon the presence and severity of mitral regurgitation. In patients with connective tissue syndromes, the mitral annulus is usually dilated and sometimes calcified; it does not decrease its circumference by the usual 30 percent during left ventricular systole. The hemodynamic effects of mild to moderate MR are similar to those from other causes of MR.

CLINICAL MANIFESTATIONS

Symptoms

The diagnosis of MVP is most commonly made by cardiac auscultation in asymptomatic patients or by echocardiography performed for some other purpose. The patient may be evaluated because of a family history of cardiac disease or occasionally may be referred because of an abnormal resting electrocardiogram. The most common presenting complaint is palpitations, which are usually due to premature ventricular beats. Supraventricular arrhythmias are also frequent; the most common sustained tachycardia is paroxysmal reentry supraventricular tachycardia.

Chest pain is a frequent complaint in patients with MVP. It is atypical in most patients without coexistent ischemic heart disease and rarely resembles classic angina pectoris. Dyspnea and fatigue are also frequent symptoms in patients with MVP, including many without severe MR. Objective exercise testing often fails to show an impairment in exercise tolerance, and some patients exhibit distinct episodes of hyperventilation. Neuropsychiatric complaints are not uncommon in patients with MVP. Some have panic attacks and others frank manic-depressive syndromes. Transient cerebral ischemic episodes occur with increased incidence in patients with MVP, and some develop stroke syndromes. Reports of amaurosis fugax, homonymous field loss, and retinal artery occlusion have been described; occasionally the visual loss persists. These signs likely are due to embolization of platelets and fibrin deposits occurring on the atrial side of the mitral valve leaflets. It is important to note that both MVP and panic attacks occur relatively frequently. Accordingly, the occurrence of both syndromes in the same individual would be expected to occur frequently by chance, so that the panic attacks are not necessarily part of the primary MVP syndrome.

Physical Examination

The presence of thoracic skeletal abnormalities—the most common being scoliosis, pectus excavatum, straightened thoracic spine, and narrowed anteroposterior diameter of the chest—may suggest the diagnosis of MVP. The principal cardiac auscultatory feature of this syndrome is the midsystolic click, a high-pitched sound of short duration. The click may vary considerably in intensity and location in systole according to LV loading conditions and contractility. It results from the sudden tension of the mitral valve apparatus as the leaflets prolapse into the left atrium during systole. Multiple systolic clicks may be generated as different portions of the mitral leaflets prolapse at various times during systole. The major differentiating feature of the midsystolic click of MVP from that due to other causes is that its timing during systole may be altered by maneuvers that change hemodynamic conditions.

Dynamic auscultation is often useful for establishing the clinical diagnosis of the MVP syndrome. Changes in the LV end-diastolic volume lead to changes in the timing of the midsystolic click and murmur. When end-diastolic volume is decreased, the critical volume is achieved earlier in systole and the click-murmur complex occurs shortly after the first heart sound. In general, any maneuver that decreases the end-diastolic LV volume, increases the rate of ventricular contraction, or decreases the resistance to LV ejection of blood causes the MVP to occur early in systole and the systolic click and murmur to move toward the first heart sound. This occurs when the patient suddenly stands from the supine position, does submaximal hand-grip exercise, or performs the Valsalva maneuver (see Table 24-2).

DIAGNOSTIC STUDIES

Electrocardiogram

The electrocardiogram (ECG) is usually normal in patients with MVP. The most common abnormality in the MVP syndrome is the presence of ST-T wave depression or T-wave inversion in the inferior leads. MVP is associated with an increased incidence of false-positive exercise ECG results in patients with normal coronary arteries, especially females. Myocardial perfusion imaging with thallium or technetium sestamibi has been useful for differentiating false from true abnormal exercise ECG findings in patients with MVP.

Although arrhythmias may be observed on the resting ECG or during treadmill or bicycle exercise, they are detected more frequently by continuous ambulatory ECG recordings. The reported incidence of documented arrhythmias is higher in patients with MVP;

TABLE 24-2

RESPONSE OF THE MURMUR OF MITRAL VALVE PROLAPSE
TO INTERVENTIONS

Intervention	Timing	Intensity
Standing upright	←	↑
Recumbent	→	↓ or 0
Squatting	→	↓ or 0
Hand grip	←	±
Valsalva	←	±
Amyl nitrite	±	↑

NOTE: ↑ = increase; ↓ = decrease; 0 = no change; ± = variable; ← =
earlier; → = later.

however most are not life-threatening and often do not correlate with
the patient's symptoms.

Chest Roentgenogram

Posteroanterior and lateral chest x-ray films usually show normal cardiopulmonary findings. The skeletal abnormalities described above
can be seen. When severe MR is present, both LA and LV enlargement often result. Various degrees of pulmonary venous congestion
are evident when left heart failure results. Acute chordal rupture with
a sudden increase in the amount of mitral regurgitation may present
as pulmonary edema without obvious LV or LA dilatation. Calcification of the mitral annulus may be seen, particularly in adults with
Marfan's syndrome.

Echocardiography

Echocardiography is the most useful noninvasive test for defining
MVP. The M-mode echocardiographic definition of MVP includes
≥2-mm posterior displacement of one or both leaflets or holosystolic
posterior "hammocking" >3 mm. On two-dimensional (2D) echocardiography, systolic displacement of one or both mitral leaflets, particularly when they coapt on the left atrial side of the annular plane in
the parasternal long-axis view, indicates a high likelihood of MVP.
There is disagreement concerning the reliability of an echocardiographic diagnosis of MVP when these signs are observed only in
the apical four-chamber view. The diagnosis of MVP is even more

certain when the leaflet thickness is >5 mm during ventricular diastole. Leaflet redundancy is often associated with an elongated mitral annulus and elongated chordae tendineae. On Doppler velocity recordings, the presence or absence of MR is an important consideration, and MVP is more likely when the MR is detected as a high-velocity jet in late systole, midway or more posterior in the left atrium.

At present, there is no consensus on 2D echocardiographic criteria for MVP. Since echocardiography is a tomographic cross-sectional technique, no single view should be considered diagnostic. The parasternal long-axis view permits visualization of the medial aspect of the anterior mitral leaflet and middle scallop of the posterior leaflet. If the findings of prolapse are localized to the lateral scallop in the posterior leaflet, they would best be visualized by the apical four-chamber view. All available echocardiographic views should be utilized, with the provision that anterior leaflet billowing alone in the four-chamber apical view is not evidence of prolapse; however, a displacement of the posterior leaflet or the coaptation point in any view including the apical views suggests the diagnosis of prolapse. The echocardiographic criteria for MVP should include structural changes such as leaflet thickening, redundancy, annular dilatation, and chordal elongation.

Patients with echocardiographic criteria for MVP but without evidence of thickened/redundant leaflets or definite MR are more difficult to classify. If such patients have auscultatory findings typical of MVP, the echocardiogram usually confirms the diagnosis. 2D/Doppler echocardiography is also useful for defining LA size as well as LV size and function and for the detection and semiquantitation of MR. Recommendations for echocardiography in MVP are listed in Table 24-3.

Cardiac Catheterization

Cardiac catheterization is rarely used as a diagnostic technique for MVP. Also, contrast ventriculography is unnecessary for determining LV function, since it can usually be quantitated by 2D echocardiography or radionuclide ventriculography. While contrast cineventriculography is often useful for assessing the severity of mitral regurgitation, cardiac catheterization and angiography are most commonly used in patients with MVP to exclude the possibility of CAD.

Intracardiac pressures and cardiac output are usually normal in uncomplicated MVP; however, these measurements become progressively more abnormal as MR becomes more severe. LV angiography usually confirms the presence of MVP. LV wall motion is usually normal in patients with primary MVP, but some patients show abnormal contraction patterns in the absence of CAD.

TABLE 24-3

RECOMMENDATIONS FOR ECHOCARDIOGRAPHY IN MITRAL VALVE PROLAPSE

Indication	Class
1. Diagnosis, assessment of hemodynamic severity of MR, leaflet morphology, ventricular compensation in patients with physical signs of MVP	I
2. To exclude MVP in patients who have been given the diagnosis where there is no clinical evidence to support the diagnosis	
3. To exclude MVP in patients with first-degree relatives with known myxomatous valve disease	IIa
4. Risk stratification in patients with physical signs of MVP with no or mild regurgitation	IIa
5. To exclude MVP in patients in the absence of physical findings suggestive of MVP positive family history	III
6. Routine repetition of echocardiography in patients with MVP with no or mild regurgitation and no changes in clinical signs or symptoms	III

Class I: Conditions for which there is evidence and/or general agreement that a given procedure or treatment is useful and effective

Class II: Conditions for which there is conflicting evidence and/or a divergence of opinion about the usefulness/efficacy of a procedure or treatment

    Class IIa: Weight of evidence/opinion is in favor of usefulness/efficacy

    Class IIb: Usefulness efficacy is less well established by evidence/opinion

Class III: Conditions for which there is evidence and/or general agreement that the procedure/treatment is not useful/effective and in some cases may be harmful

KEY: MR = mitral regurgitation; MVP = mitral valve prolapse.
SOURCE: Bonow et al, with permission.

Other Diagnostic Tests

Exercise myocardial perfusion imaging with thallium or technetium sestamibi has been recommended as an adjunct to exercise ECG for determining the presence or absence of coexistent myocardial ischemia in patients with MVP. Most MVP patients with clinical evidence of CAD have an abnormal exercise scintigram. The indications for electrophysiologic testing in a patient with MVP are similar to those in general practice. The upright tilt test with monitoring of blood pressure and rhythm may be valuable in patients with light-headedness or syncope and in diagnosing autonomic dysfunction.

NATURAL HISTORY, PROGNOSIS, AND COMPLICATIONS

In most patient studies, the MVP syndrome is associated with a benign prognosis. The age-adjusted survival rate for both males and females with MVP is similar to that in patients without this common clinical entity. The gradual progression of mitral regurgitation in patients with mitral prolapse, however, may result in progressive dilatation of the LA and LV. LA dilatation often results in atrial fibrillation, and moderate to severe MR eventually results in left ventricular dysfunction and the development of congestive heart failure in certain patients. Several long-term prognostic studies suggest that complications occur most commonly in patients with a mitral systolic murmur, thickened redundant mitral valve leaflets, or increased LV or LA size. Sudden death is uncommon but obviously the most severe complication of mitral valve prolapse. Although sudden death is infrequent, its highest incidence has been reported in the familial form of MVP. Infective endocarditis is a serious complication of MVP, and MVP is the leading predisposing cardiovascular lesion in most series of patients reported with endocarditis. Recommendations for antibiotic endocarditis prophylaxis for patients with MVP undergoing procedures associated with bacteremia are listed in Table 24-4. Fibrin emboli are responsible in some patients for visual problems consistent with involvement of the ophthalmic or posterior cerebral circulation. Therefore, it has been recommended that antiplatelet drugs such as aspirin be administered to patients who have MVP and suspected cerebral emboli. Warfarin therapy is usually reserved for patients with MVP who have atrial fibrillation or poststroke patients with prolapse, particularly when symptoms occur on aspirin therapy. However, neither antiplatelet drugs nor anticoagulants should be prescribed routinely for patients with MVP, because the incidence of embolic phenomena is very low.

TABLE 24-4

RECOMMENDATIONS FOR ANTIBIOTIC ENDOCARDITIS
PROPHYLAXIS FOR PATIENTS WITH MITRAL VALVE PROLAPSE
UNDERGOING PROCEDURES ASSOCIATED
WITH BACTEREMIA

Indication	Class
1. Patients with characteristic systolic click-murmur complex	I
2. Patients with isolated systolic click and echo evidence of MVP and MR	I
3. Patients with isolated systolic click, echo evidence of high-risk MVP	IIa
4. Patients with isolated systolic click and no or equivocal evidence of MVP	III

KEY: MR = mitral regurgitation; MVP = mitral valve prolapse.
SOURCE: ACC/AHA guidelines for the clinical application of echocardiography. *Circulation* 1997; 95:1686–1744, with permission.

TREATMENT

The majority of patients with MVP are asymptomatic and lack the high-risk profile described earlier. These patients—with mild or no symptoms and findings of milder forms of prolapse—should be assured of a benign prognosis. A normal lifestyle and regular exercise are encouraged. Patients with MVP and palpitations associated with sinus tachycardia or mild tachyarrhythmias and those with chest pain, anxiety, or fatigue often respond to therapy with beta blockers. Symptoms of orthostatic hypotension are best treated with volume expansion, preferably by liberalizing fluid and salt intake. In survivors of sudden cardiac death and patients with symptomatic complex arrhythmias, specific antiarrhythmic therapy should be guided by monitoring techniques, including electrophysiologic testing when indicated. Restriction from competitive sports is recommended when moderate LV enlargement, LV dysfunction, uncontrolled tachyarrhythmias, long-QT interval, unexplained syncope, prior sudden death, or aortic root enlargement is present, individually or in combination. Asymptomatic patients with MVP and no significant MR can be evaluated clinically every 2 to 3 years. Patients with MVP who have high-risk characteristics, including those with moderate to severe regurgitation, should be followed more frequently even if no symptoms are present.

Surgical Considerations

Certain patients with MVP may require valve surgery, particularly those who develop a flail mitral leaflet due to rupture of chordae tendineae or their marked elongation. Most such valves can be repaired successfully by surgeons experienced with mitral valve repair, especially when the posterior leaflet valve is predominantly affected. Symptoms of heart failure, the severity of MR, the presence or absence of atrial fibrillation, LV systolic function, LV end-diastolic and end-systolic volumes, and pulmonary artery pressure (rest and exercise) all influence the decision to recommend mitral valve surgery. Recommendations for surgery in patients with MVP and MR are the same as for those with other forms of nonischemic severe MR and include class III to IV symptoms, LVEF ≤ 60 percent, and/or marked increases in LV end-diastolic and end-systolic volumes.

SUGGESTED READING

Bonow RO, Carabello B, De Leon AC Jr, et al: ACC/AHA guidelines for the management of patients with valvular heart disease. *J Am Coll Cardiol* 1998; 32:1486–1588.

Freed LA, Levy D, Levine RA, et al: Prevalence and clinical outcomes of mitral valve prolapse. *N Engl J Med* 1999; 341: 1–7.

Gilon D, Buonanno FS, Jaffee MM, et al: Lack of evidence of an association between mitral valve prolapse and stroke in young patients. *N Engl J Med* 1999; 341:8–13.

Ling LH, Enriquez-Sarano M, Seward JB, et al: Clinical outcome of mitral regurgitation due to flail leaflet. *N Engl J Med* 1996; 335;1417.

Nishimura R, McGoon MD: Perspectives on mitral valve prolapse. *N Engl J Med* 1999; 341:48–58.

O'Rourke RA: Mitral valve prolapse syndrome. In: Fuster V, Alexander RW, O'Rourke RA, et al (eds): *Hurst's The Heart*, 10th ed. New York: McGraw-Hill; 2001:1729–1740.

O'Rourke RA: The mitral valve prolapse syndrome. In: Chizner MA (ed): *Classic Teachings in Clinical Cardiology*. Cedar Grove, NJ: Laennec; 1996:1049–1070.

O'Rourke RA: The syndrome of mitral valve prolapse. In: Albert JA (ed): *Valvular Heart Disease*. New York: Lippincott-Raven; 1999:157–182. In press.

Shah PM: Echocardiographic diagnosis of mitral valve prolapse. *J Am Soc Echocardiogr* 1994; 7(3 pt 1):286–293.

Zuppiroli A, Rinaldi M, Kramer-Fox R, et al: Natural history of mitral valve prolapse. *Am J Cardiol* 1995; 75:1028–1032.

25

TRICUSPID VALVE AND PULMONIC VALVE DISEASE

Nilesh J. Goswami
Robert A. O'Rourke

DEFINITION, ETIOLOGY, AND PATHOLOGY

TRICUSPID VALVE DISEASE

Tricuspid regurgitation occurs when the tricuspid valve allows blood to enter the right atrium (RA) during a right ventricular (RV) contraction. *Tricuspid stenosis* results from obstruction to diastolic flow across the valve during diastolic filling of the RV.

Diseases causing tricuspid regurgitation are more numerous than those causing tricuspid stenosis (Fig. 25-1). Importantly, the normal tricuspid valve commonly does not completely coapt in systole, as is shown by the frequent occurrence of tricuspid regurgitation jets on Doppler ultrasound. Usually the volume of regurgitant blood is so small that the tricuspid regurgitation is silent; this finding occurs in 24 to 96 percent of normal individuals and thus must be considered a variant of normal by Doppler ultrasound.

Primary diseases of the tricuspid valve apparatus—which includes the tricuspid annulus, the leaflets, the chordae, the papillary muscle, and the RV wall—also cause tricuspid regurgitation. The most common etiology of isolated tricuspid regurgitation is infective endocarditis in drug addicts. Less common causes include myocardial infarction, trauma, carcinoid, leaflet prolapse, and congenital abnormalities such as atrial septal defect and Ebstein's anomaly. Tricuspid valve regurgitation has been reported to occur in patients with rheumatoid arthritis or Marfan's syndrome and those who have undergone radiation therapy. Primary involvement of the tricuspid valve due to rheumatic fever results in tricuspid stenosis, usually associated with tricuspid regurgitation.

The most common cause of tricuspid stenosis is rheumatic fever. This is usually associated with concomitant mitral stenosis. Isolated

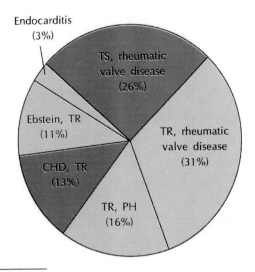

FIGURE 25-1

Pathologic findings in tricuspid valve (TV).

KEY: TR = tricuspid regurgitation; TS = tricuspid stenosis. [From Virmani R et al. Pathology of valvular heart diseases. In: Rahimtoola SH (ed). Philadelphia: Mosby (Current Medicine, Inc.), 1997:116, with permission.]

stenosis of the tricuspid valve can be seen with the carcinoid syndrome, infective endocarditis, endocardial fibroelastosis, endomyocardial fibrosis, and systemic lupus erythematosus. It has also been reported to occur in patients with Fabry's disease, Whipple's disease, and those receiving methysergide therapy. Mechanical obstruction of the valve can occur with a myxoma of the RA, tumor metastases, and thrombi in the RA, each resulting in the hemodynamic abnormalities of tricuspid stenosis. Additionally, RV inflow tract obstruction can be due to thrombosis, endocarditis, degeneration, or calcification affecting a prosthetic tricuspid valve.

Carcinoid heart disease is seen in up to 53 percent of patients with a malignant carcinoid tumor (usually originating in the ileum) with extensive metastases. Carcinoid usually causes tricuspid regurgitation and stenosis and, less often, pulmonic stenosis and regurgitation. Although tricuspid stenosis may result, the major functional abnormality is usually tricuspid regurgitation. The most common type of tricuspid regurgitation is the secondary type and results from the enlargement of the orifice and annulus secondary to congestive heart failure with RV dilation due to left ventricular (LV) disease. Tricuspid regurgitation may diminish when the heart failure is treated successfully, but it can be permanent with long-standing dilatation of the RV.

In infective endocarditis, the tricuspid regurgitation results from improper coaptation of the leaflets because of interposed vegetations. Major degrees of regurgitation may be due to rupture of chordae tendineae of the RV or perforation of the valve leaflets.

Until recently, myocardial infarction was not considered a common cause of tricuspid regurgitation except when secondary to chronic congestive heart failure. Currently, RV infarction is being recognized more often and is frequently associated with tricuspid regurgitation.

Various degrees of prolapse of the tricuspid valve are commonly present in the general population and may occur in 3 to 54 percent in patients with mitral valve prolapse, although incidents of *severe* tricuspid regurgitation from prolapse have been relatively uncommon.

External blunt trauma, most commonly occurring in automobile accidents, is a classic cause of tricuspid regurgitation. Primary congenital lesions of the tricuspid valve that cause regurgitation are Ebstein's malformation and valvular dysplasia.

PULMOMIC VALVE DISEASE

Acquired lesions of the pulmonic valve generally lead to *pulmonic regurgitation* (Table 25-1). On rare occasions, an inflammatory process can create stenosis and regurgitation of the valve. Pulmonary hypertension from any cause—such as mitral stenosis, chronic lung disease, or pulmonary emboli—can produce pulmonic regurgitation. Inflammatory diseases such as endocarditis, rheumatic fever, and, on rare occasions, tuberculosis can result in pulmonic regurgitation.

Pulmonic stenosis is created by obstruction to systolic flow across the valve and is most commonly congenital. Sarcomas and myxomas can sometimes extend to the pulmonic valve, causing pulmonic stenosis. Previous cardiac surgery on a congenital pulmonic valve lesion can result in pulmonic regurgitation. The carcinoid syndrome with cardiac involvement can create mild pulmonic stenosis and associated regurgitation.

CLINICAL MANIFESTATIONS

Symptoms

TRICUSPID VALVE DISEASE

Since tricuspid regurgitation generally accompanies LV failure or mitral stenosis, presenting symptoms include dyspnea, orthopnea,

TABLE 25-1

ACQUIRED LESIONS OF THE PULMONIC VALVE

Pulmonary hypertension with pulmonic regurgitation
   Mitral stenosis
   Chronic lung disease
   Pulmonary emboli
Inflammatory lesions
   Endocarditis
   Rheumatic fever
   Tuberculosis
Tumors
   Sarcoma
   Myxoma
Previous surgery or angioplasty for congenital lesions
Mediastinal lesions
   Tumor
   Aneurysm
   Constrictive pericarditis
Miscellaneous
   Carcinoid syndrome

and peripheral edema. Even though LV failure is usually present, paroxysmal nocturnal dyspnea is often absent. Tricuspid regurgitation under these conditions may occasionally ameliorate the pulmonary symptoms and provide a physiologic basis for the alleviation of left-sided heart failure by the development of right-sided heart failure. Some patients also have less pulmonary edema due to the development of pulmonary arteriolar disease. If the tricuspid regurgitation is produced by infective endocarditis, symptoms of febrile illness may be accompanied by fatigue and peripheral edema.

The most frequent symptoms in tricuspid stenosis are dyspnea and fatigue. When mitral stenosis coexists, the development of significant tricuspid stenosis can diminish the paroxysmal symptoms of dyspnea, pulmonary congestion, and pulmonary hypertension. Occasionally, patients with tricuspid stenosis complain of prominent pulsations in the neck veins, which may precede the development of peripheral edema.

PULMONIC VALVE DISEASE

Isolated pulmonic regurgitation can be tolerated without symptoms. Severe pulmonary hypertension may cause syncope in addition to shortness of breath and fatigue. With inflammatory lesions of the pulmonic valve, febrile manifestations and pulmonary infection may be present. The carcinoid syndrome is characterized by episodes of facial flushing, increased intestinal activity, diarrhea, and bronchospasm. Tumors involving the pulmonic valve may exert pressure from expansion and metastases that affect the heart and lungs.

Physical Examination

TRICUSPID VALVE DISEASE

In patients with primary tricuspid regurgitation not due to pulmonary hypertension, there are large v waves in the jugular venous pulse (see Chap. 1). There is a dilated RV with a precordial lift and right-sided third or fourth heart sounds. There is usually a long systolic murmur in the third and fourth intercostal spaces at the left sternal border that increases with inspiration. When a large amount of blood returns to the RV in diastole, a short diastolic rumble along the left sternal border may be heard. All of these findings are increased with inspiration (Rivero Carvallo's sign). When RV failure occurs, the mean central venous pressure becomes elevated and the jugular veins are pulsatile and engorged. When tricuspid regurgitation is due to pulmonary hypertension, there is an accentuated pulmonic component of the second heart sound, and a high-pitched decrescendo diastolic murmur of pulmonic valve regurgitation is often heard with a greater intensity during inspiration. In patients with tricuspid regurgitation and atrial fibrillation, there is a prominent cv wave in the internal jugular veins, produced by the regurgitant flow into the RV. The characteristic physical finding of tricuspid regurgitation due to pulmonary hypertension is a holosystolic murmur at the left sternal border that increases during inspiration.

In tricuspid stenosis, the internal jugular veins will display the prominent a wave indicative of impaired RV diastolic filling with atrial systole. The cv wave is small, and the y descent is slow and insignificant.

PULMONIC VALVE DISEASE

The murmur of acquired pulmonic regurgitation is a high-pitched diastolic blow along the left sternal border. This murmur may be difficult to differentiate from the murmur of aortic regurgitation, but the absence of peripheral findings of aortic regurgitation is useful in identifying regurgitation of the pulmonic valve as the source of the diastolic blow. Congenital pulmonic regurgitation characteristically is associated with a low-pitched, decrescendo murmur along the left sternal border, the peak of the murmur occurring shortly after the pulmonic component of the second heart sound. (see also Chap. 1).

Electrocardiogram

TRICUSPID VALVE DISEASE

Atrial fibrillation is frequent in patients with tricuspid regurgitation. When tricuspid regurgitation results from myocardial infarction, acute or chronic electrocardiographic (ECG) changes will be seen in the inferior ECG leads, and ST-segment elevation indicating RV infarction may be present in the right-sided precordial leads. The characteristic ECG finding in tricuspid stenosis is a large P wave of RA enlargement in the absence of RV hypertrophy.

PULMONIC VALVE DISEASE

Although there are no characteristic changes with pulmonic valvular lesions, preexisting pulmonary hypertension will produce RV hypertrophy, right axis deviation, and changes in the P wave, suggesting RA enlargement. If pulmonary hypertension is secondary to mitral stenosis, P mitrale with characteristic notches will be presented in lead II.

Chest Roentgenogram

TRICUSPID VALVE DISEASE

Tricuspid regurgitation may produce some degree of RA enlargement, but there will usually be accompanying RV enlargement. In tricuspid stenosis, the most characteristic radiographic finding is prominence of the RA without significant pulmonary arterial enlargement or changes due to pulmonary hypertension.

PULMONIC VALVE DISEASE

Patients with pulmonic valve regurgitation have pulmonary artery prominence along with an increase in RV dimensions. If stenosis of the pulmonary valve is acquired, there may be poststenotic dilatation or prominence of the main pulmonary artery.

Echocardiogram

TRICUSPID VALVE DISEASE

With tricuspid regurgitation, there may be echocardiographic evidence of systolic prolapse, rupture of the chordae or papillary muscle, or vegetative lesions on the valve. Increased RV dimensions indicate impaired RV function and the likelihood of secondary tricuspid regurgitation. Contrast echocardiography with peripheral venous injection can identify the back-and-forth flow across the valve. The echo/Doppler technique can estimate the severity of the regurgitation and the systolic pressure in the RV. Color-flow Doppler imaging can delineate the patterns and sites of regurgitation across the valve apparatus.

A characteristic pattern of stenosis of the tricuspid valve can often be recorded with the echocardiogram. Fibrosis and calcification of the valve can be identified. Obstructive lesions such as myxoma, thrombus, or other tumors can be recognized echocardiographically. The echo/Doppler technique can be used to estimate the diastolic gradient across the valve with generally good accuracy.

PULMONIC VALVE DISEASE

Echocardiography can delineate the anatomy of the pulmonic valve as well as intrinsic or extrinsic lesions impinging on the valve apparatus. Sometimes a vegetative lesion or tumor can be detected in the pulmonary valve area. The echo/Doppler technique can estimate both the severity of the regurgitation and the stenosis of the valve, and analysis of echo/Doppler recordings can provide estimates of pulmonary artery pressure. Color-flow imaging can further confirm the patterns of regurgitation in the RV outflow tract.

Cardiac Catheterization

TRICUSPID VALVE DISEASE

If tricuspid stenosis is clinically suspected, simultaneous pressures should be recorded in the RA and in the RV in order to measure the gradient across the valve accurately. Since the normal gradient across the tricuspid valve is less than 1 mmHg, small gradients may not be detected if pullback pressure is recorded from the RV to the RA. The area of the tricuspid valve in significant stenosis is usually less than 1.5 cm^2; in severe stenosis it is less than 1 cm^2.

PULMONIC VALVE DISEASE

Pulmonic regurgitation is not readily demonstrated angiographically, but a right-sided injection can outline the pulmonary valve as well as poststenotic dilatation. An aortic root injection can be helpful in the elimination of aortic regurgitation as the etiology of a diastolic murmur along the left sternal border. Nevertheless, this distinction is usually best made by echo/Doppler studies.

NATURAL HISTORY AND PROGNOSIS

TRICUSPID VALVE DISEASE

With tricuspid regurgitation due to RV hypertension, the symptoms and clinical course are primarily related to the left-sided heart conditions that produce a pressure-volume overload on the RV. Tricuspid regurgitation virtually always develops with severe RV failure. In infective endocarditis of the tricuspid valve, the type of organism may significantly influence the course and the response to antibiotics.

With tricuspid stenosis, the symptoms are usually those of mitral stenosis; the absence of pulmonary congestion in the presence of peripheral edema should raise the possibility of underlying stenosis of the tricuspid valve. Significant tricuspid stenosis may slow the development of characteristic symptoms of mitral stenosis and result in an underestimation of the severity of mitral valve obstruction.

PULMONIC VALVE DISEASE

The clinical history is important in delineating the causes of left-sided heart failure that can lead to pulmonary hypertension and regurgitation of the pulmonic valve. Mild to moderate pulmonary regurgitation can be relatively well tolerated, and the natural history in patients with pulmonic regurgitation really depends upon the severity of left heart failure or of the other syndromes involving the pulmonic valve. The natural history and prognosis of congenital valvular stenosis are discussed in Chap. 29.

MEDICAL MANAGEMENT

TRICUSPID VALVE DISEASE

With tricuspid regurgitation, treatment of RV failure requires digitalis and diuretics; vasodilating agents are also required in cases of LV failure. If failure of the right side of the heart is caused by mitral stenosis, early intervention to enlarge or replace the mitral valve is appropriate.

In tricuspid stenosis, the usual precautionary measures of antibiotic coverage and prevention of endocarditis apply. Peripheral edema may not respond well to administration of digitalis, diuretics, and vasodilator therapy, thus emphasizing the clinical importance of detecting underlying tricuspid stenosis. Tricuspid balloon valvuloplasty has been used successfully in patients with predominant tricuspid stenosis.

PULMONIC VALVE DISEASE

Patients with congenital pulmonic valve stenosis are usually best treated by catheter balloon valvotomy. Antibiotic prophylaxis is appropriate for patients with pulmonic valve regurgitation. Therapy for pulmonary hypertension may include management of left-sided failure, correction of mitral stenosis, or use of vasodilating agents.

Anticoagulation should be considered in pulmonary hypertension, particularly if emboli are a contributing source.

If rheumatic fever is the likely etiology of combined aortic and mitral valve disease, prophylactic penicillin should usually be continued until age 35 years. Dental prophylaxis with antibiotic coverage, using either amoxicillin or erythromycin, should be provided in all patient groups prior to dental procedures. For genitourinary or other abdominal procedures, gram-negative antibiotic coverage should be provided.

SURGICAL MANAGEMENT

TRICUSPID VALVE DISEASE

The decision to proceed with valvular heart surgery is usually based on the severity of the aortic and mitral valve disease rather than on the severity of the disease of the tricuspid valve. The usual decisions to be made regarding the tricuspid valve are (1) whether or not a procedure should be added to the mitral and/or aortic valve procedures, and, if so, (2) which procedure—annuloplasty or valve replacement—should be performed.

Indications for Surgery

TRICUSPID VALVE DISEASE

The severity of the symptoms and clinical signs of tricuspid valve disease are used to determine whether or not to perform tricuspid valve surgery. If there are signs of tricuspid stenosis and particularly if stenosis is demonstrated by cardiac catheterization and two dimensional echocardiography, the tricuspid valve is directly visualized at operation with the anticipation of performing commissurotomy or valve replacement.

When there are signs of severe tricuspid regurgitation secondary to mitral stenosis, it is important to document the duration of the regurgitation and the severity and duration of pulmonary artery hypertension. If the tricuspid regurgitation is severe and long-standing and if there is chronic pulmonary artery hypertension, it is unlikely that the tricuspid regurgitation will resolve in the early postoperative period after mitral valve surgery alone. In this circumstance, tricuspid valve surgery is usually indicated. In contrast, if the tricuspid regurgitation and pulmonary artery hypertension are of short duration, mitral valve replacement will usually reduce pulmonary artery pressure in the early postoperative period; this will result in a decrease in the tricuspid valve regurgitation. In this situation, the surgeon usually

TABLE 25-2

RECOMMENDATIONS FOR SURGERY FOR
TRICUSPID REGURGITATION

Indication	Class
Annuloplasty for severe TR and pulmonary hypertension in patients with mitral valve disease requiring mitral valve surgery	I
Valve replacement for severe TR secondary to diseased or abnormal tricuspid valve leaflets not amenable to annuloplasty or repair	IIa
Valve replacement of annuloplasty for severe TR with mean pulmonary artery pressure <60 mmHg when symptomatic	IIa
Annuloplasty for mild TR in patients with pulmonary hypertension secondary to mitral valve disease requiring mitral valve surgery	IIb
Valve replacement or annuloplasty for TR with pulmonary artery systolic pressure <60 mmHg in presence of a normal mitral valve in asymptomatic patients or in symptomatic patients who have not received a trial of diuretic therapy	III

waits until discontinuation of bypass after mitral valve surgery to decide whether or not a procedure to reduce tricuspid regurgitation is indicated. The ACC/AHA guidelines recommending surgery for TR are listed in Table 25-2.

Tricuspid stenosis may be treated successfully by commissurotomy, which is usually performed under direct vision. The procedure may be combined with annuloplasty to correct valve regurgitation. Valve replacement is occasionally necessary if the changes in the leaflets and subvalvular structures are advanced or if severe regurgitation cannot be relieved by annuloplasty.

When the leaflets and subvalvular apparatus are severely deformed as a result of rheumatic fever, reconstruction may not be feasible. In such cases, replacement is performed with either a mechanical or tissue valve. Anticoagulation with warfarin is generally advisable in patients with tricuspid valve replacement, and therefore the major advantage of a bioprosthetic valve is negated. Nevertheless, the bioprosthetic valve has been the prosthesis of first choice of many surgeons.

In general, the early and late results of tricuspid annuloplasty have been superior to those of valve replacement, and valve replacement should be avoided when possible. Valvulectomy is often the best option for patients with tricuspid valve endocarditis and is usually well tolerated.

PULMONIC VALVE DISEASE

Pulmonic valve surgery for acquired disease is performed infrequently. Pulmonic valve stenosis on an acquired basis is rare. Although there are a variety of causes of pulmonic valve regurgitation, this hemodynamic condition is relatively well tolerated if pulmonary vascular resistance is normal. Pulmonic valve replacement may be performed for acquired conditions such as carcinoid heart disease and infective endocarditis, but it usually is limited to cases where RV dysfunction has become severe after congenital heart disease surgery.

Although pulmonic regurgitation is generally well tolerated for several years after correction of malformations such as tetralogy of Fallot, the regurgitation may become hemodynamically significant, especially if pulmonary artery hypertension is present or develops. In such a case, the placement of a pulmonic valve prosthesis may significantly improve the patient's functional status. In general, bioprosthetic valves have been preferred because of the tendency for mechanical valve thrombosis in this position. Valvulectomy in combination with antibiotic therapy is often the most effective treatment patients with pulmonic valve endocarditis.

MULTIVALVULAR HEART DISEASE

For surgical options of mutivalvular heart disease please refer to Chap. 59 in the full text (see Suggested Reading, under O'Rourke, on page 474).

SUGGESTED READING

Bonow RO, Carabello B, De Leon AC Jr, et al: ACC/AHA guidelines for valvular heart disease. *J Am Coll Cardiol* 1998; 32:1486–1588.

Cheitlin MD, Alpert JS, Armstrong WF, et al: ACC/AHA guidelines for the clinical application of echocardiography. *Circulation* 1997; 95:1696–1744.

Kern MJ, Aguirre F, Donohue T, Bach R: Interpretation of cardiac pathophysiology from pressure waveform analysis:

Multivalvular regurgitant lesions. *Cathet Cardiovasc Diagn* 1993; 28:167–172.

O'Rourke RA: Tricuspid valve, pulmonic valve, and multivalvular disease. In: Fuster V, Alexander RW, O'Rourke RA, et al. (eds): *Hurst's The Heart,* 10th ed. New York: McGraw-Hill; 2001: 1741–1758.

Waller BF, Howard J, Fess S: Pathology of tricuspid valve stenosis and pure tricuspid regurgitation—Parts I–III. *Clin Cardiol* 1995; 18:97–102; 167–174; 225–230.

26

CLINICAL PERFORMANCE OF PROSTHETIC HEART VALVES

Gary L. Grunkemeier
Albert Starr
Shahbudin H. Rahimtoola

A heart valve prostheses consist of an orifice through which blood flows and an occluding mechanism that closes and opens the orifice. There are two classes of heart valves: *mechanical prostheses,* with rigid, manufactured occluders, and *biological* or *tissue valves,* with flexible leaflet occluders of animal or human origin. Among the mechanical valves there are three basic types, depending on whether the occluding mechanism is a reciprocating ball, a tilting disk, or two semicircular hinged leaflets. The biological valves include those whose origin is from the patient, another human, or another species.

PROSTHETIC HEART VALVES

Mechanical Valves

Ball valves appeared in the early 1960s, disk valves in the early 1970s, and bileaflet valves predominantly during the 1980s.

BALL VALVES

The first successful valve replacement devices, which led to long-term survivors and a design that has endured until today, used a ball-in-cage design. Several modifications of this design have been used, but only the *Starr-Edwards* valve has endured; it has been used about 200,000 times.

DISK VALVES

The first successful low-profile design was the *Bjork-Shiley* tilting-disk valve, introduced in 1969. It evolved through several design refinements, and about 360,000 valves have been used. These refinements also introduced a structural failure mode cause by strut fracture in the Convexo-Concave model; it is no longer used.

BILEAFLET VALVES

Current development in mechanical valves is based on the bileaflet design, introduced by St. Jude Medical in 1977. The two semicircular leaflets of a bileaflet valve are connected to the orifice housing by a hinge mechanism. The leaflets swing apart during opening, creating three flow areas, one central and two peripheral. The *St. Jude* bileaflet valve has been used over 900,000 times and the *Carbomedics* valve has been used about 300,000 times since its clinical introduction in 1986.

Biological Valves

Biological valves include an equally wide variety of models, as do mechanical valves.

AUTOGRAFT

The pulmonary autograft procedure consists of an autotransplant of the pulmonary valve to the aortic position; the pulmonary valve is then replaced by an aortic or pulmonary homograft. This operation was first described in 1967 and is called the Ross procedure.

HOMOGRAFT

The homograft or allograft valve may be a preferred substitute for aortic valve replacement in younger patients. There is transplantation from a donor of the same species—from the donor's aortic or pulmonic valve into the recipient's aortic or pulmonic valve. Several methods of procurement, sterilization, and preservation have been used.

PORCINE HETEROGRAFT

This utilizes transplantation of a valve from another species, the pig. Glutaraldehyde sterilizes valve tissue, renders it bioacceptable by destroying antigenicity, and stabilizes the collagen cross links for durability. The two major porcine valves are the Hancock and Carpentier-Edwards.

Most porcine valves are mounted on rigid or flexible stents, to which the leaflets and the sewing ring are attached. Unstented versions have also been devised by several manufacturers. The St. Jude Medical Toronto SPV and the Medtronic Freestyle stentless porcine valves are available.

BOVINE PERICARDIAL HETEROGRAFT

Pericardial valves are tailored and sewn into a valvular configuration using bovine pericardium as a fabric and results in a valve that opens more completely than a porcine valve, providing better hemodynamics. The Carpentier-Edwards Perimount pericardial bioprosthesis is available for use in the aortic and mitral positions.

GUIDELINES FOR CLINICAL REPORTING (AMERICAN ASSOCIATION FOR THORACIC SURGEONS/ SOCIETY OF THORACIC SURGEONS)

The complications that were determined to be of critical importance by these guidelines, developed in 1988 and revised in 1996, include *structural valvular deteriorations and nonstructural dysfunction,* including *prosthesis-patient mismatch, valve thrombosis, embolism, bleeding event, and operated valvular endocarditis.*

The *consequences* of these morbid events include reoperation, valve-related mortality, sudden unexpected unexplained death, cardiac death, total deaths, and permanent valve related impairment.

VALVE SELECTION CRITERIA

Because of the wide variation in results among and between various valve models, it is impossible to rank valves within valve types on the basis of complication rates. Some general recommendations, however, can be made with regard to valve selection.

A biological valve should be used when the patient cannot or will not take anticoagulants or has a short life expectancy. Its use in relation to subsequent pregnancy is controversial. A mechanical valve should be used if the patient needs anticoagulant therapy (e.g., because of atrial fibrillation), has a mechanical valve in another position, previously had a stroke, requires double valve replacement, or has a long life expectancy. Mechanical valves should be considered for double valve replacement because the risk of structural deterioration for two porcine valves is additive, whereas the thromboembolic risk of two mechanical valves is not additive. The American College of Cardiology/American Heart Association recommendations are shown in Tables 26-1 and 26-2.

MANAGEMENT

All patients with prosthetic valves need appropriate antibiotics for prophylaxis against infective endocarditis (Chap. 26). Patients with rheumatic heart disease continue to need antibiotics as prophylaxis against the recurrence of rheumatic carditis. Adequate antithrombotic therapy is needed for appropriate patients (Chap. 36).

TABLE 26-1

RECOMMENDATIONS FOR VALVE REPLACEMENT
WITH A MECHANICAL PROSTHESIS

Indication	Class
1. Patients with expected long life spans	I
2. Patients with a mechanical prosthetic valve already in place in a different position than the valve to be replaced	I
3. Patients in renal failure, on hemodialysis, or with hypercalcemia	II
4. Patients requiring warfarin therapy because of risk factors[a] for thromboembolism	IIa
5. Patients ≤65 years for AVR and ≤70 years for MVR[b]	IIa
6. Valve rereplacement for thrombosed biological valve	IIb
7. Patients who cannot or will not take warfarin therapy	III

[a] Risk factors: atrial fibrillation, severe LV dysfunction, previous thromboembolism and hypercoagulable condition.

[b] The age at which patients may be considered for bioprosthetic valves is based on the major reduction in rate of structural valve deterioration after age 65 and the increased risk of bleeding in this age group.

KEY: AVR = aortic valve replacement; LV = left ventricle; MVR = mitral valve replacement.

SOURCE: Bonow et al: ACC/AHA guidelines for the management of patients with valvular heart disease. *J Am Coll Cardiol* 1998; 32:1486–1588, with permission.

During the 4 to 6 weeks after surgery, the physician and surgeon jointly manage the patient, directing their attention toward relieving postoperative discomfort, readjusting cardiac medications, and instituting anticoagulation if not contraindicated. A graduated plan of activity is started that, in most cases, enables the patient to return to full activity in 4 to 6 weeks.

The *4- to 6-week postoperative visit* is critical, because by this time the patient's physical capabilities and expected improvement in functional capacity can usually be assessed. The recommendations for follow-up strategy are shown in Table 26-3.

TABLE 26-2

RECOMMENDATIONS FOR VALVE REPLACEMENT WITH BIOPROSTHESES

Indication	Class
1. Patients who cannot or will not take warfarin therapy	I
2. Patients ≤65 years[a] needing AVR who do not have risk factors for thromboembolism[b]	I
3. Patients considered to have possible compliance problems with warfarin therapy	IIa
4. Patients >70 years[a] needing MVR who do not have risk factors for thromboembolism[b]	IIa
5. Valve replacement for thrombosed mechanical valve	IIb
6. Patients <65 years[a]	IIb
7. Patients in renal failure, on hemodialysis, or with hypercalcemia	III
8. Adolescent patients who are still growing	III

[a]The age at which patients should be considered for bioprosthetic valves is based on the major reduction in rate of structural valve deterioration after age 65 and increased risk of bleeding in this age group.

[b]Risk factors: atrial fibrillation, severe LV dysfunction, previous thromboembolism, and hypercoagulable condition.

KEY: AVR = aortic valve replacement; LV = left ventricle; MVR = mitral valve replacement.

SOURCE: Bonow et al: ACC/AHA guidelines for the management of patients with valvular heart disease. *J Am Coll Cardiol* 1998; 32:1486–1588, with permission.

Echocardiography/Doppler ultrasound is the most useful noninvasive test. It provides information about prosthesis stenosis/regurgitation, valve area, other valve disease(s), pulmonary hypertension, atrial size, left ventricular hypertrophy, left ventricular size and function, and pericardial effusion/thickening. It is essential at the first postoperative visit because it allows an assessment of the effects and results of surgery and serves as a baseline for comparison should complications and/or deterioration occur later. Subsequently, it is performed as is needed in both symptomatic and asymptomatic patients at 1- to 2-year intervals. In patients with a bioprosthesis in

TABLE 26-3

RECOMMENDATIONS FOR FOLLOW-UP STRATEGY OF PATIENT WITH PROSTHETIC HEART VALVES

Indication	Class
1. History, physical exam, ECG, chest x-ray, echocardiogram, complete blood count, serum chemistries, and INR (if indicated) at first postoperative outpatient evaluation[a]	I
2. Radionuclide angiography or magnetic resonance imaging to assess LV function if result of echo-cardiography is unsatisfactory	I
3. Routine follow-up visits at yearly intervals with earlier reevaluations for change in clinical status	I
4. Routine serial echocardiograms at time of annual follow-up visit in absence of change in clinical status	IIb
5. Routine serial fluroscopy	III

[a]This evaluation should be performed 3 to 4 weeks after hospital discharge. In some settings, the outpatient echocardiogram may be difficult to obtain: if so, an inpatient echocardiogram may be obtained before hospital discharge.
Key: INR = International Normalized Ratio; LV = left ventricle.
Source: Bonow et al: ACC/AHA guidelines for the management of patients with valvular heart disease. *J Am Coll Cardiol* 1998; 32:1486–1588, with permission.

the mitral position, echocardiography/Doppler ultrasound should be performed annually after 5 years and in the aortic position annually after 8 years because of the increasing incidence of bioprosthetic structural valve deterioration.

ANTITHROMBOTIC THERAPY

All patients with mechanical valves require warfarin therapy. With use of warfarin, the risk of thromboemboli in these patients is reduced but is still 1 to 2 percent per year; the risks are higher in the mitral than in the aortic position. Therefore, the International Normalized Ratio (INR) of the patient with aortic mechanical valve should be about 2.5 (range 2 to 3) and the INR of the patient with mitral mechanical valve should be about 3.0 (range 2.5 to 3.5). Many authorities recommend the addition of low-dose aspirin (81 mg) to warfarin unless there is a contraindication to its use. Importantly, the risk of thromboemboli is increased early after insertion of a prosthetic valve (mechanical and biological); this is a reason to start heparin within 24 to 48 h of surgery, as soon as it is safe to do so with maintenance of the a PPT between 60 and 80 s until the recommended INR level is achieved. Patients with biological valves can have the warfarin discontinued after 2 to 3 months. However, even patients with biological valves need continued warfarin therapy (INR 2.5; range 2 to 3) if they have atrial fibrillation, severe left ventricular dysfunction, previous thromboembolism, and/or a hypercoagulable condition.

SUGGESTED READING

Barratt-Boyes BG: Homograft aortic valve replacement in aortic incompetence and stenosis. *Thorax* 1964; 19:131–135.

Bonow RO, Carabello B, de Leon AC Jr, et al: ACC/AHA guidelines for the management of patients with valvular heart disease: A report of the American College of Cardiology/American Heart Association Task Force on Practical Guidelines (Committee on Management of Patients with Valvular Heart Disease). *J Am Coll Cardiol* 1998; 32:1486–1588.

Carpentier A, Dubost C: From xenograft to bioprosthesis. In: Ionescu MI, Ross DN, Wooler GH (eds): *Biological Tissue in Heart Valve Replacement.* London: Butterworth; 1971:515–541.

Edmunds LH Jr, Clark RE, Cohn LH, et al: Guidelines for reporting morbidity and mortality after cardiac valvular operations. *J Thorac Cardiovasc Surg* 1996; 112:708–711.

Grunkemeier GL, Li H-H, Starr A, Rahimtoola SH: Long-term performance of heart valve prostheses. *Curr Probl Cardiol* 2000; 25:75–154.

Grunkemeier GL, Starr A, Rahimtoola SH: Clinical performance of prosthetic heart valves. In: Fuster V, Alexander RW, O'Rourke RA, et al (eds): *Hurst's The Heart,* 10th ed. New York: McGraw-Hill; 2001:1759–1773.

Grunkemeier GL, Starr A, Rahimtoola SH: Replacement of heart valves. In: O'Rourke RA, (ed): *The Heart: Update I.* New York: McGraw-Hill; 1996:98–123.

Grunkemeier GL, Starr A, Rahimtoola SH: Prosthetic heart valve performance: A long-term follow-up. *Curr Probl Cardiol* 1992; 26:355–406.

Hammermeister K, Sethi GK, Henderson WG, et al: Outcomes 15 years after valve replacement with a mechanical vs bioprosthetic valve: Final report of the VA randomized trial. *J Am Coll Cardiol* 2000; 36:1152–1158.

McAnulty JH, Rahimtoola SH: Antithrombotic therapy for valvular heart disease. In: Fuster V, Alexander RW, O'Rourke RA, et al (eds): *Hurst's The Heart,* 10th ed. New York: McGraw-Hill; 2001:1775–1782.

Ross DN: Replacement of aortic and mitral valves with a pulmonary autograft. *Lancet* 1967; 2:956–958.

Starr A, Edwards M: Mitral replacement: Clinical experience with a ball valve prosthesis. *Ann Surg* 1961; 154:726–740.

Turpie AG, Gent M, Laupacis A, et al: A double blind randomized trial of acetylsalicylic acid (100 mg) versus placebo in patients treated with oval anticoagulants following heart valve replacement. *N Engl J Med* 1991; 329:1365–1369.

ANTITHROMBOTIC THERAPY FOR VALVULAR HEART DISEASE

John H. McAnulty
Shahbudin H. Rahimtoola

A stroke. It is the most important reason to address the issue of protection against thromboemboli in every patient with valve disease. In addition, the consequences of valve thrombosis and of emboli to other organs make the risk of antithrombotic therapy reasonable or essential in many patients with valve disease. Treatment must be individualized, but some issues and principles are widely applicable (Table 27-1). Although some recommendations are appropriate for affluent American communities, the risk, benefit, and cost ratio may not be applicable in poorer areas, where the resources are simply not available. Thromboemboli are not ignored, but alternative therapy—for example, a greater use of antiplatelet agents, in particular aspirin—may, on balance, be more appropriate.

Intracardiac thrombosis most often presents as an embolic event; in over 80 percent of cases this is a cerebrovascular event. Less commonly, thrombosis becomes manifest by causing valve dysfunction. The physical examination should include careful attention to the peripheral pulses and to the skin, fundi, and soft tissues (mouth, conjunctiva), looking for clues to an embolus. A detailed neurologic assessment for focal deficits is essential. Although thrombosis most often occurs without any change in the cardiac examination, auscultation to assess for a change in a murmur or quality of heart sounds is important.

Thrombus is the most common but not the exclusive cause of an embolus. Infective endocarditis must be considered and excluded as a cause, particularly in individuals with valve disease. Disruption of a vascular plaque in the ascending aorta, arch, or descending aorta and in the cerebral vessels may be a common cause of peripheral and cerebral emboli in patients with atherosclerotic disease. Intracardiac tumors and calcified emboli from the heart or aorta are other rare causes.

TABLE 27-1

VALVE DISEASE AND ANTITHROMBOTIC THERAPY[a,b]

1. Prevention of thromboemboli should be addressed each time a patient with valve disease is seen.
2. Lifelong antithrombotic therapy is required in patients with artial fibrillation (paroxysmal or persistent) (Table 27-2).
3. Warfarin therapy is required in all patients with a mechanical prothesis (Table 27-3).
4. Antithrombotic therapy should be started early after valve surgery.
5. Warfarin should be avoided in the first trimester of pregnancy.
6. Antithrombotic therapy should be individualized during noncardiac surgery and cardiovascular procedures.

[a] See text for discussion.

[b] In general, whenever warfarin/aspirin therapy is recommended, it is assumed that there is no specific contraindication to its use.

NATIVE VALVE DISEASE

The risk of thromboembolism in patients with native valve disease is most directly related to associated risk factors; atrial fibrillation, a history of thromboembolism, left ventricular (LV) dysfunction, and known hypercoagulability. Antithrombotic therapy is not required in the patient with native valve disease unless it is associated with one of these factors (Fig. 27-1).

Risk of Thromboemboli with Native Valve Disease

The risk factors and treatment recommendations are as outlined in Table 27-1.

ATRIAL FIBRILLATION

Most is known about the stroke risk with atrial fibrillation. Six recent large, prospective randomized trials have demonstrated a 60 to 70 percent decrease in the incidence of stroke with warfarin–reducing it from 3 to 8 percent down to 0.5 to 2 percent yearly. Some

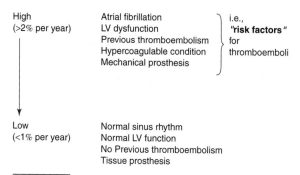

FIGURE 27-1

Risk of thromboembolism. Clinical variables define valve disease patients as being at high or low risk of thromboembolic events.

patients in the studies had valve disease. If a patient is a reasonable candidate for warfarin therapy, its use [maintaining an International Normalized Ratio (INR) of 2 to 3] is appropriate when atrial fibrillation (constant or paroxysmal) occurs in combination with reduced LV function (heart failure or an LV ejection fraction ≤0.30), with associated severe hypertension, or if there is a history of thromboemboli. The risk of emboli with atrial fibrillation increases with age, but the increased risk of warfarin must be balanced against its benefit. If a patient with atrial fibrillation has reasonable LV function, has not had a previous thromboembolism, and does not have other risk factors, aspirin (325 mg/day) is just as likely as warfarin to be protective against thromboemboli, without the associated expense and risk of warfarin therapy.

LEFT VENTRICULAR DYSFUNCTION

Systemic or pulmonary thromboemboli occur at a rate of over 5 percent per year in patients with LV dysfunction. While antithrombotic therapy is of unproven value, the risk of an embolic event is sufficient that, with or without valve disease, consideration should be given to treatment. One approach (including the authors') is to use warfarin if the LV ejection fraction (EF) is ≤0.30 and the patient is a reasonable candidate for this treatment.

PREVIOUS THROMBOEMBOLI

In other clinical situations (e.g., in patients with atrial fibrillation or with a prosthetic valve), a thromboembolic event defines patients at high risk for having an embolic event—i.e., a recurrent event. It is unclear whether this is true in patients with native valve disease, but we recommend lifelong warfarin.

HYPERCOAGULABLE CONDITIONS

Reasons to consider anticoagulant therapy are the presence of protein C, protein S, or antithrombin III deficiencies; the anticardiolipin antibody syndrome; resistance to activated protein C; or an associated malignancy. This is also true in patients with native valve disease.

Screening for Patients at High Risk for Thromboemboli

The risk factors described above define patients requiring antithrombotic therapy. Transthoracic and transesophageal echocardiography (TTE and TEE) are often performed in patients with valvular heart disease and in those who have had a systemic embolic episode. The use of these procedures in determining which patients are at risk of thromboemboli is not yet well defined. Until more is known, it is not appropriate to screen patients with native valve disease who do not have one of the obvious clinical risk factors listed above.

PROSTHETIC HEART VALVES

All patients with mechanical valves require warfarin therapy. Even with the use of warfarin, the risk of thromboemboli in these patients is 1 to 2 percent per year. The risk of an embolus in patients with biological valves in sinus rhythm was approximately 0.6 to 0.7 percent per year.

Antithrombotic Treatment for Prosthetic Valves (Table 27-2)

MECHANICAL VALVES

All patients with mechanical valves require warfarin. In patients with an aortic prosthesis without risk factors for emboli, the INR should be between 2.0 and 3.0; in those with risk factors and those with a mitral prosthesis, the INR should be between 2.5 and 3.5. The addition of low-dose aspirin (50 to 100 mg/day) to warfarin therapy further decreases the risk of thromboembolism and is recommended unless there is a contraindication.

BIOLOGICAL (TISSUE) VALVES

Because of an increased risk of thromboemboli during the first 3 months after implantation of a biological prosthetic valve,

TABLE 27-2

ANTITHROMBOTIC THERAPY—NATIVE VALVE DISEASE

I. *No therapy* if no thrombosis risk factor
II. *Therapy* if thrombosis risk factor present
   A. *Atrial fibrillation*
     1. Warfarin (INR 2–3) if congestive heart failure, hypertension, or previous thromboembolism
     2. Warfarin (INR 2–3) if valve lesion is mitral stenosis
     3. Aspirin (325 mg/day) or warfarin (INR 2–3) if valve lesion other than mitral stenosis
   B. *Previous thromboembolism*—warfarin (INR 2–3)
   C. *LV dysfunction* (ejection fraction ≤0.30)—warfarin (INR 2–3)
   D. *Hypercoagulable state*—warfarin (INR 2–3)

KEY: INR = international normalized ratio.

anticoagulation with warfarin is indicated. After that time, the tissue valve can be treated in the same way as native valve disease (see Table 27-2), and warfarin can be discontinued in approximately two-thirds of patients with biological valves. Associated atrial fibrillation or an LV ejection fraction ≤0.30 are reasons for lifelong warfarin therapy.

SPECIAL CLINICAL SITUATIONS

Altered Native Valves

Valve disease is increasingly being treated by interventional catheter techniques or surgical valve repair. It is difficult to give firm recommendations about antithrombotic therapy in these patients, but the recommendations given for treatment of native valve disease would seem most applicable in patients who have had surgical valve repair or catheter valve procedures (see Table 27-2).

Pregnancy

Pregnancy makes decisions regarding antithrombotic therapy for valve disease more difficult. Warfarin should be avoided in the first trimester of pregnancy, particularly in weeks 6 through 12. It crosses the placental barrier and has a 5 to 20 percent chance of causing an embryopathy manifest in the live born as mental impairment, ocular atrophy, and facial and digital abnormalities. Therefore warfarin should be discontinued immediately when pregnancy is recognized, and heparin therapy should be initiated. The value of switching from warfarin to heparin *before* conception is uncertain. We suggest this when pregnancies are planned, since little is known about the consequences of warfarin taken in the first 6 weeks of pregnancy; however, this is often not clinically practical or feasible. While a return to warfarin during the second and third trimesters is recommended by some, there is concern that this drug may continue to endanger the fetus.

Heparin does not cross the placenta. While not devoid of problems (maternal bleeding, heparin-initiated thrombocytopenia, an increased risk of osteoporosis when used for longer than 1 month), successful pregnancies have occurred when adequate doses of the drug are administered subcutaneously at home throughout gestation. Thromboembolic complications have occurred with heparin use during pregnancy in women with a mechanical prosthesis. To minimize this, it is important to give a dose that will result in high "therapeutic effect" heparin levels prior to the next dose (this usually requires 15,000 to 30,000 U every 12 h). Activated PTT measurements do not accurately reflect heparin levels during pregnancy.

Low-molecular-weight heparin (LMWH) is currently approved only for treatment of venous thrombosis. There are no data about its use in patients with native valve disease or with prosthetic heart valves. Therefore, LMWH cannot be recommended in such patients at this time.

Surgery and Dental Care

Although antithrombotic therapy must be individualized, some generalizations apply. For procedures where bleeding is unlikely or would be inconsequential if it occurred, antithrombotic therapy should not be stopped. This can apply to surgery on the skin, dental prophylaxis, or simple treatment for dental caries. When bleeding is likely or its potential consequences are severe, antithrombotic treatment should be altered. If a patient is on aspirin, it should be discontinued 1 week before the procedure and restarted as soon as it is considered safe by the surgeon or dentist.

For most patients on warfarin, the drug should be stopped 48 to 72 h before surgery to ensure the INR is ≤1.5 and restarted within 24 h after a procedure; admission to the hospital or a delay in discharge to give heparin is usually unnecessary. Deciding who is at very high risk of thrombosis and thus should require heparin until warfarin can be reinstated may be difficult; clinical judgment is required. Heparin can usually be reserved for those who have had a recent thrombosis or embolus (arbitrarily within 1 year), those with demonstrated thrombotic problems when previously off therapy, and those with three or more risk factors. When used, unfractionated heparin should be started 24 h after warfarin is stopped (i.e., 48 h before surgery) and stopped 4 to 6 h before the procedure. The heparin should be restarted as early after surgery as bleeding stability allows, and the activated partial thromboplastin time (aPTT) maintained at a "therapeutic level" (Table 27-2) until warfarin is restarted and the desired INR can be achieved. Home administration and management of heparin (and warfarin) can be arranged to minimize time in the hospital. LMWH is even more easily utilized outside of the hospital; however, there are no data with its use in patients with valve disease.

Cardiac Catheterization and Angiography

Antiplatelet therapy or heparin does not have to be stopped for these procedures. Protamine can be given to the patient on heparin if bleeding occurs. In an emergent or semiemergent situation, cardiac catheterization can be performed with a patient on warfarin, but preferably the drug should be stopped 72 h before the procedure and restarted the day of the procedure. If a patient is at very high risk of thromboembolism, heparin should be started 48 h before the procedure and continued until warfarin is restarted and the desired INR is achieved.

Therapy at the Time of an Active Thromboembolic Event

VALVE THROMBOSIS
Thrombosis of a valve, usually a prosthetic valve, can result in severe hemodynamic compromise. If recognized (TEE can be diagnostic), this complication may be treated with thrombolytic therapy. We recommend emergency surgery rather than thrombolytic therapy in the patient with severe hemodynamic compromise (see Chap. 26). If a patient is a nonsurgical candidate, thrombolysis should be attempted. Streptokinase or urokinase should be initiated but stopped at 24 h if there is no improvement by Doppler echocardiography and at 72 h even if hemodynamic recovery is incomplete. This should be followed by heparin until high INR levels are achieved with concommitant warfarin therapy (INR 3 to 4 for aortic prostheses or 3.5 to 4.5 with mitral prostheses).

THROMBOEMBOLIC EVENT
An embolic event often indicates inadequate therapy for that patient's circumstances. Data and opinions about optimal timing for initiating

or continuing anticoagulants in patients in whom an embolus is the presumed cause of a stroke are conflicting. Ideally, treatment would be started early to prevent recurrent emboli, but the early use of heparin (within 72 h) is associated with a 15 to 25 percent chance of converting a nonhemorrhagic into a hemorrhagic stroke. While a case can still be made for immediate use of heparin, the early recurrence of an embolus in patients with valve disease while off anticoagulants has not been clearly documented.

ACUTE MANAGEMENT OF AN EMBOLIC EVENT

Antithrombotic therapy should be withheld or stopped for 72 h. If a computed tomography (CT) scan at that time reveals little or no hemorrhage, heparin should be administered to maintain an aPTT at the lower end of the "therapeutic level" until warfarin, started at the same time, results in the desired INR (see Table 27-2). If the CT scan demonstrates significant hemorrhage, antithrombotic therapy should be withheld until the bleed is treated or has stabilized (7 to 14 days). Anticoagulation can then be started as just described.

LONG-TERM MANAGEMENT

If the embolic event occurs when a patient is *off* antithrombotic therapy, long-term warfarin therapy is required (see Tables 27-2 and 27-3). If the embolic event occurs while the patient is *on* antithrombotic treatment, therapy should be individualized. Those who are on warfarin, but in whom the INR was low at the time of the embolus should have the dose increased into the high end of the desired range (see Table 27-2). If the embolus occurs in a patient despite an INR in the desirable range, aspirin (50 to 100 mg/day) should be added to the warfarin. Embolism recurring with this combination should lead to consideration of possible valve surgery if the valve is the likely source of the thrombus.

At the Time of a Bleed

With significant bleeding, antithrombotic therapy should be stopped and, if the patient is at risk, drug effects should be reversed. If possible, the site of bleeding should be corrected and antithrombotic therapy restarted as soon as possible. If this is not possible, treatment decisions are difficult. In patients with a mechanical prosthesis or multiple risk factors for thromboemboli, acceptance of intermittent bleeding with acute management for the bleeds may be necessary. In valve patients who are at lower risk of emboli or in whom the role of antithrombotic treatment is less clear (e.g., LV dysfunction), it may be optimal to withhold chronic therapy or, if a patient is on warfarin, to switch to aspirin. In some patients with mechanical valves,

TABLE 27-3
ANTITHROMBOTIC THERAPY[a]—PROSTHETIC HEART VALVES

	Mechanical Prosthetic Valves			Biological Prosthetic Valves		
	Warfarin, INR 2–3	Warfarin, INR 2.5–3.5	Aspirin, 50–100 mg	Warfarin, INR 2–3	Warfarin, INR 2.5–3.5	Aspirin, 50–100 mg
First 3 months after valve replacement		+			+	+
After first 3 months						
Aortic valve	+					+
Aortic valve + risk factor[b]		+	+	+		+
Mitral valve		+	+			+
Mitral valve + risk factor		+	+		+	

[a]Depending on the clinical status of patient, antithrombotic therapy must be individualized (see special situations in text).
[b]Risk factors—atrial fibrillation, previous thromboembolus, LV dysfunction, hypercoagulable state.

491

consideration should be given to replacing the mechanical valve with a biological valve—for example, in those who have had multiple large life- or organ-threatening bleeds.

Infective Endocarditis

If a patient with valve disease develops endocarditis, antithrombotic therapy should be continued. If the patient presents with or develops an embolic event involving the central nervous system, therapy should be as described above for acute embolic events.

SUGGESTED READING

Bloomfield P, Wheatley DJ, Prescott RJ, Miller HC:. Twelve-year comparison of a Bjork-Shiley mechanical heart valve with porcine bioprostheses. *N Engl J Med* 1991; 324:573–579.

Bonow RJ, Carabello B, De Leon AC Jr, et al: ACC/AHA guidelines for the management of patients with valvular heart disease: A report of the American College of Cardiology/American Heart Association Task Force on Practice Guidelines (Committee on Management of Patients With Valvular Heart Disease). *J Am Coll Cardiol* 1998; 32:1486–1588.

Hammermeister K, Sethi GK, Henderson WG, et al: Outcomes 15 years after valve replacement with a mechanical versus a bioprosthetic valve: Final report of the veterans affairs randomized trial. *J Am Coll Cardiol* 2000; 36(4):1152–1158.

Levin HJ, Pauler SG, Eckman MH: Antithrombotic therapy in valve disease. Fourth ACCP conference on antithrombotic therapy. *Chest* 1995; 108(suppl):360S–370S.

McAnulty JH, Rahimtoola SH: Antithrombotic therapy for valvular heart disease. In: Fuster V, Alexander RW, O'Rourke RA, et al (eds): *Hurst's The Heart,* 10th ed. New York: McGraw-Hill; 2001: 1775–1782.

North RA, Sadler L, Stewart AW, et al: Long-term survival and valve-related complications in young women with cardiac valve replacements. *Circulation* 1999; 99:2669–2676.

28

CARDIOVASCULAR DISEASES DUE TO GENETIC ABNORMALITIES

Jeffrey A. Towbin
Robert Roberts

Genetic factors play a significant role in the pathogenesis of many if not all cardiovascular disorders. Malformations of the heart and blood vessels account for the largest number of human birth defects, occurring in about 1 percent of all live births; among stillbirths, the prevalence is estimated to be tenfold higher. Inherited forms of cardiovascular disease have become increasingly recognized over the past decade and the genetic basis of several diseases is now known. In addition, cardiac diseases are common in patients with dysmorphic syndromes. In this chapter, a wide spectrum of cardiovascular diseases due to genetic abnormalities is discussed.

GENOTYPE—PHENOTYPE

Important definitions: *Genome* refers to all of the genes of an individual. *Genotype* refers to the gene or genes inherited. *Phenotype* refers to the physical, physiologic, or biochemical features that are manifest. Even in single-gene disorders, the phenotype is a result not just of the primary genetic defect but also of its interaction with other genes and, in turn, their interaction with environmental factors. *Penetrance* refers to what percentage of individuals inheriting a mutation develop one or more features of the expected phenotype. Penetrance is an all-or-none phenomenon. *Expressivity* refers to variability of the features manifest for a particular phenotype.

CARDIOVASCULAR DISEASE DUE TO SINGLE-GENE MUTATIONS

Familial Hypertrophic Cardiomyopathy

GENETIC BASIS

Familial HCM is an autosomal dominant disorder characterized by myocardial hypertrophy with a wide spectrum of symptoms, including dyspnea, chest pain, and syncope. The annual mortality rate, initially reported as 2 to 4 percent (but now thought to be 0.1 percent), is primarily due to sudden death, which often occurs in asymptomatic individuals. This disorder is the leading cause of sudden death in the young and in athletes in the United States. The annual incidence of sudden death is higher in younger patients with familial HCM than in the elderly. The diagnosis is based on typical clinical features and the demonstration of unexplained left ventricular (LV), right ventricular (RV), or biventricular hypertrophy on two-dimensional echocardiography. The LV hypertrophy is commonly asymmetrical, localized to the septum, but it may involve the entire ventricle in a concentric pattern. Isolated RV hypertrophy occurs in fewer than 5 percent of cases. Isolated apical hypertrophy is rare except in Japan, where it is claimed to account for 20 to 30 percent of the cases. Dynamic outflow tract obstruction occurs in about 30 percent. Histologically, the myocardial hypertrophy consists of myocyte hypertrophy, cellular and myofibrillar disarray, and myocardial fibrosis. The hallmark of familial HCM is myocyte and myofibrillar disarray. The disorder exhibits marked variability of expressivity, even in the same family.

Familial HCM was the first primary cardiomyopathy to yield to molecular genetics. Genetic linkage of the disease to the chromosomal locus of 14q1 was identified in 1989. The β-myosin heavy chain (βMHC) gene was identified as the responsible gene and is now known to be the most common mutated gene in HCM. A total of nine genes have now been found to be responsible for familial HCM; a brief description of the loci, the proteins they encode, and their function is presented in Table 28-1. All genes indentified to date involve the sarcomere.

The hypertrophy of familial HCM is markedly variable in its degree, distribution, and age at onset as well as in the type and severity of its associated clinical manifestations. The natural course of familial HCM in certain families is riddled with sudden cardiac death, whereas sudden cardiac death is almost absent in others and the life span is essentially normal. None of the clinical features is a reliable predictor of sudden death. Hypertrophy, while present in all individuals, since it is required for the clinical diagnosis, does not correlate

TABLE 28-1
HYPERTROPHIC CARDIOMYOPATHY GENES, mRNA, AND PROTEINS

Gene	Chromosomal Locus	Frequency	Function and Location
β-MyHC	14q1	35–50%	Contractile molecule that forms a thick filament of the sarcomere
MyBP-C	11q11	15–20%	Binds to myosin and titin
Cardiac troponin T (cTnT)	1q3	15–20%	Regulation of contraction via calcium binding
α-Tropomyosin	15q2	<5%	Binds the troponin complex to actin
Cardiac troponin I	19q13	<1%	Inhibits contractility
MLC-1	3p	<1%	Unknown
MLC-2	12q	<1%	Unknown
α-Cardiac actin	15q11	<1%	Forms the actin thin filament of the sarcomere
Titin	2q31	<1%	Binds MyBP-C
Unknown	7q3	?	Unknown
Unknown	11q	?	Unknown

495

with the incidence of sudden death. Familial HCM due to mutations in the troponin T gene is associated with a high incidence of sudden death, yet there is often minimal hypertrophy. The occurrence of palpitations, arrhythmias, and/or syncope is a poor predictor of sudden death. A family history of sudden death usually indicates that the presenting individual is affected. While most individuals affected with familial HCM due to the βMHC mutation manifest the disease in the second or third decade of life, those with familial HCM due to mutations in myosin binding protein C frequently do not develop any evidence of the disease until the fourth or fifth decade. However, once the disease develops, the particular mutation is highly predictive of risk for sudden death.

Dilated Cardiomyopathy

IDIOPATHIC DILATED CARDIOMYOPATHY

Idiopathic DCM is a disease of unknown etiology characterized by increased ventricular chamber size, decreased wall thickness, and impaired systolic ventricular function. The prevalence of idiopathic DCM has been estimated to be approximately 40 cases per 100,000. The diagnosis of DCM is typically made by echocardiography, and symptoms usually are those of sudden death and heart failure. Familial DCM is estimated to account for 30 percent of patients with idiopathic DCM. Autosomal dominant inheritance is the most common form of transmission. However, X-linked autosomal recessive and mitochondrial inheritance is also seen. In most cases of DCM, symptoms of congestive heart failure (CHF) predominate; ventricular tachyarrhythmias are also common. In a relatively uncommon subgroup of patients, conduction disease predates the development of DCM by years. Transient arrhythmias, which present in the second or third decade, become sustained and commonplace by the third or fourth decade. The abnormal rhythms include second- or third-degree AV block, atrial fibrillation, or marked bradycardia, commonly requiring a pacemaker. DCM usually develops in the fourth or fifth decade. Sudden death commonly occurs in the late stages of the disease. On autopsy, marked right and left ventricular dilatation, interstitial fibrosis, myocyte degeneration characterized by cytoplasmic vacuolization, and AV nodal cell replacement by fibrous tissue are typical. The genetic basis of DCM is now unraveling. Multiple genetic loci have been identified for families with pure DCM. Three genes have now been identified as being responsible for autosomal dominant familial DCM: those governing actin, desmin, and δ-sarcoglycan. Actin, in addition to forming the thin filaments of the sarcomere, essential to the generation of force, is also an important cytoskeletal protein involved in structural integrity and the transmission of force. Desmin is the specific intermediate filament for muscle and an essential cytoskeletal protein for maintaining cardiac structure and for the transmission of force and other signals to the cytoplasm and the nucleus of the cell. Desmin stretches from its attachment to the sarcomere Z-band to the nuclear membrane and other organelles. The δ-sarcoglycan gene encodes a dystrophin-associated glycoprotein which is an integral membrane cytoskeletal protein. It is of note that all of these genes have been also associated with musculoskeletal disorders such as nemaline myopathy (actin), desmin myopathy (desmin), and limb-girdle muscular dystrophy (δ-sarcoglycan). There is thus the strong suggestion that familial DCM may be a disease of cytoskeletal proteins analogous to HCM, being a disease of the sarcomere, and the genes involved also cause muscular disease in some patients.

A gene for DCM associated with conduction system disease was recently identified in families linked to chromosome 1p1-q21. The gene, lamin A/C, is a nuclear lamina protein and has also been shown to cause autosomal dominant Emery-Dreifuss muscular dystrophy, further supporting the concept that cardiac and skeletal muscle diseases are interrelated.

X-LINKED CARDIOSKELETAL MYOPATHY (BARTH SYNDROME)

This X-linked recessive disease is characterized by the triad of dilated cardiomyopathy with endocardial fibroelastosis, neutropenia, and skeletal myopathy. All affected males were initially reported to die in infancy or early childhood from cardiac decompensation or septicemia. However, it is now known that long-term survival is possible. No affected females have been reported. Ultrastructural abnormalities are detected in mitochondria from cardiac and skeletal muscle as well as in neutrophil bone marrow cells. Furthermore, respiratory chain abnormalities are commonly observed and isolated skeletal muscle mitochondria demonstrate diminished cytochrome concentrations. Lactic acidemia not provoked by prolonged fasting, increased plasma and muscle carnitine concentrations, growth retardation, and increased levels of urinary 3-methylglutaconic acid and 2-ethyl-hydracrylic acid have also been seen. The gene causing Barth syndrome is G4.5, which codes for a novel protein known as taffazin, whose function is unclear. Mutations in G4.5 have also been shown to cause other infantile cardiomyopathies, including isolated left ventricular noncompaction and dilated hypertrophic cardiomyopathy.

FAMILIAL ARRHYTHMOGENIC RIGHT VENTRICULAR DYSPLASIA

Arrhythmogenic right ventricular dysplasia (ARVD) is characterized by fatty infiltration of the right ventricle, fibrosis, and ultimately thinning of the wall with chamber dilatation. It is the most common cause of sudden cardiac death in the young in Italy and is said to account for about 17 percent of sudden death in the young in the United States. This is a very devastating disease, since the first symptom is often sudden death. ECG abnormalities include inverted T waves in the right precordial leads, late potentials, and right ventricular arrhythmias with left bundle branch block (LBBB). There is still great difficulty in making the diagnosis even when this condition occurs in a family with the disease history. Since the disease affects only the RV in most cases, it is difficult to detect. There is no diagnostic definitive standard. RV biopsy is definitive when positive but often gives a false-negative result, since the disease initiates in the epicardium and spreads to the endocardium of the RV free wall, making it inaccessible to biopsy. A consensus diagnostic criterion was developed which includes findings on right ventricular biopsy, magnetic resonance imaging (MRI), echocardiography, and ECG. Identification of the gene will have tremendous diagnostic impact and hopefully will provide an explanation as to why ARVD is typically restricted to the right ventricle. The disorder is inherited as an autosomal dominant trait, and multiple genetic loci have been identified. No gene has been found thus far. A large Greek family with arrhythmogenic right ventricular dysplasia associated with diffuse nonepidermolytic palmoplantar keratoderma and woolly hair (Naxos disease) has been reported, and autosomal recessive inheritance was noted in this family. The gene for Naxos disease has been identified. The gene was identified to be plakoglobin, which encodes a cell-cell adhesion protein.

MUCOPOLYSACCHARIDOSES

The mucopolysaccharidoses (MPS) are a group of diseases caused by deficiency of lysosomal enzymes involved in the degradation of glycosaminoglycans. Undegraded glycosaminoglycans accumulate in lysosomes and affect tissue function. MPS have been divided into seven major types. The classification (types I to VII) is based on the deficient enzyme responsible for the disorder. These disorders carry such eponyms as *Hurler, Scheie, Hurler-Scheie, Hunter, Sanfilippo, Morquio, Maroteaux-Lamy, and Sly*. They share many clinical features, including multiple system involvement, organomegaly, dysostosis multiplex, facial abnormalities, hearing and vision loss, joint involvement, cardiac involvement, and central nervous system (CNS) involvement. Cardiac disease includes myocardial hypertrophy, pulmonary and systemic hypertension, valvular disease, coronary occlusion, and myocardial infarction. Congestive heart failure and sudden death are relatively frequent. The most common mucopolysaccharidosis with cardiac involvement is MPS I (Hurler syndrome). Valvular disease is prominent in the Scheie's syndrome (late-onset form). Less commonly, heart disease has been noted in Sanfilippo A syndrome with aortic regurgitation, as well as in severe Maroteaux-Lamy syndrome with valvular heart disease. The diagnosis for either of these disorders is made by assaying the enzyme activity in cultured skin fibroblasts or leukocytes.

Duchenne Muscular Dystrophy

Duchenne muscular dystrophy (DMD) is an X-linked disorder characterized by the early onset of progressive, generalized muscle weakness and "pseudohypertrophy" of certain muscle groups. The incidence of DMD is estimated to be 1 in 3300 live male births with little ethnic variation, and the calculated mutation rate of 10^4 is an order of magnitude higher than that for most other genetic diseases. About one-third of cases arise by spontaneous mutation, with the remaining two-thirds occurring by inheritance of the disease-causing gene from the carrier mother. Female carriers of DMD are usually asymptomatic but occasionally have a slowly progressive myopathy of moderate severity. This "manifesting female carrier" state occurs in approximately 8 percent of carriers and is thought to occur due to random X-inactivation. The disease may also be expressed in females with Turner syndrome having a single X chromosome and in females with X-autosome translocations that disrupt the DMD gene. In the latter case, the translocation not only disrupts the DMD gene but also causes the nonrandom inactivation of the normal allele on the other X chromosome, resulting in the expression of the disease phenotype.

The heart is commonly involved in DMD, with ECG abnormalities and dilated cardiomyopathy being most typical. However, cardiac symptoms are unusual before the terminal stages of the disease. Congestive heart failure tends to occur. A midsystolic click and late systolic murmur associated with mitral valve prolapse is also common. In addition, an S_3 or S_4 gallop, sinus tachycardia, and a mitral regurgitation murmur are usually heard along with cardiomegaly and increased pulmonary vascular markings. At this stage, bilateral diaphragmatic elevations may be seen due to diaphragmatic dystrophy. Unlike the late-onset findings of dilated cardiomyopathy, the ECG is abnormal early in the course of DMD, with a tall R wave, an abnormally increased R/S ratio in the right precordial chest leads, and a deep, narrow Q wave in leads I, aV_L, V_5, and V_6. These abnormalities progress over time and are attributed to the finding of the greatest dystrophic myocardial changes in the posterobasal and contiguous lateral left ventricular myocardium. In addition, P waves with negative terminal deflections in V_1 exceeding 20 ms and 0.1 mV appear in 20 to 45 percent of patients; in the absence of left atrial enlargement on the echocardiogram, this is attributed to an intrinsic disorder of left atrial or intraatrial conduction. A short PR interval may be seen in up to 50 percent of patients but is not thought to be due to a bypass tract, as seen in Wolff-Parkinson-White syndrome. However, infranodal conduction abnormalities may be seen in patients with

DMD; these include complete or incomplete bundle branch block and left anterior or posterior fascicular block. Atrial and ventricular premature beats and atrial flutter are seen in some patients.

Echocardiography reveals LV dilatation and dysfunction, with significantly reduced shortening fraction or ejection fraction and LV hypokinesis of the posterobasal ventricular wall identified. Doppler and color Doppler commonly demonstrate mitral regurgitation, either secondary to the dilated cardiomyopathy or to the associated mitral valve prolapse, which occurs secondary to papillary muscle dysfunction. In some patients systolic function appears normal but diastolic dysfunction is present.

Emery-Dreifuss Muscular Dystrophy

Emery-Dreifuss muscular dystrophy (EDMD) is a relatively rare disorder characterized by weakness in the humeroperoneal distribution, early joint contractures, and dilated cardiomyopathy, with X-linked or autosomal dominant inheritance. The onset of disease in these patients occurs between 2 and 10 years of age, with weakness initially noted in the shoulder girdles and upper extremities. Contractures of the elbows and posterior cervical muscles appear early. The disease is slowly progressive, with involvement of the distal leg musculature following that of the upper extremities; contractures of the knees and ankles follow contractures of the elbows. Unlike the case in DMD and Becker's muscular dystrophy (BMD), muscle pseudohypertrophy does not occur. The disease evolves slowly and usually stabilizes in the third decade, with most patients remaining ambulatory. Dilated cardiomyopathy is a common occurrence, but the severity of disease varies from family to family. Varying degrees of atrioventricular block are common, and atrial standstill may occur. These electrical abnormalities may lead to episodes of syncope, transient ischemic attacks, stroke, and sudden death. A pacemaker is commonly required. Atrial fibrillation has also been observed. As in DMD and BMD, muscle enzyme activity is elevated, albeit to a lesser extent. The gene responsible for X-linked EDMD, on Xq28, is called emerin, a nuclear lamina protein. The autosomal dominant form of EDMD was initially mapped to chromosome 1 and the gene was identified as lamin A/C. The encoded protein is also thought to be a nuclear lamina–associated protein.

Myotonic Dystrophy (Steinert's Disease)

Myotonic dystrophy (DM) is the most common form of inherited muscular dystrophy in adults, with an incidence of 1 in 8000 to 10,000 persons. This autosomal dominant disorder affects multiple organ systems; its name is derived from the combined myopathy, dystrophy, and myotonia of skeletal muscle. Myotonia, an abnormality in relaxation after muscle contraction, is the primary feature of this disease. DM is variably expressed and individuals may present with signs and symptoms involving many different organ systems. Penetrance varies with age and the disease may affect different tissues at different periods of life; a severe form of DM exists, with symptoms at birth.

Serious complications of DM involve the heart. Cardiac conduction abnormalities are common and may be progressive, particularly in younger patients. These are identified by periodic ECG monitoring and usually occur without obvious cardiac complaints. Sudden cardiac death in athletically inclined adolescents is relatively frequent. In studies of families with DM, cardiac findings may be the initial clinical manifestation of the disease, with bradycardia and first-degree heart block being common. Progression to complete heart block may occur over time and is not well tolerated, potentially ending in death and frequently requiring pacing. In some cases, ventricular tachycardia or dilated cardiomyopathy may also occur. Typically, however, systolic function is preserved but diastolic dysfunction occurs.

Defects of Metabolism Causing Cardiomyopathy

CARNITINE DEFICIENCY

L-carnitine, a small, water-soluble molecule containing seven carbon atoms, is important in the shuttling of long-chain fatty acids and activated acetate across the intermitochondrial membrane. A specific translocase facilitates this exchange of long-chain acylcarnitine and acetylcarnitine. Carnitine also serves as the shuttle for the end products of peroxisomal fatty acid oxidation and for α-keto acids derived from branched-chain amino acids. These metabolites are transferred into the mitochondrial matrix for terminal oxidation.

Primary carnitine deficiency syndrome is characterized by a profound decrease in carnitine in affected tissues. The mechanism underlying the primary disorder is defective transport of carnitine from the serum into the affected cells. End-stage disease of many different organs including the heart may induce depletion of carnitine stores and must be differentiated from the chronic inherited type. Based on carnitine levels, carnitine deficiency is usually divided into two forms: a myopathic form and a systemic form. In the myopathic form, carnitine levels are decreased only in muscle tissue, while in the systemic form multiple tissues are affected, including muscle, liver, and plasma. The systemic form presents in infancy or early childhood with episodes of hypoglycemia, ammonemia, acidemia, hepatomegaly, and endocardial fibroelastosis (EFE). Therapy includes oral carnitine, occasionally reversing the cardiomyopathy. Additional therapy includes bicarbonate to reverse the acidemia, intravenous glucose, and anticongestive measures. Intercurrent illness commonly causes acute decompensation and death.

Homocystinuria

Homocystinuria, inherited as an autosomal recessive defect, occurs with a frequency of 1 in 75,000 individuals. There is a deficiency of cystathionine β-synthase (CBS), which leads to elevated methionine in the blood and homocystine and methionine in the urine. In the homozygous individuals, major clinical features include a marfanoid habitus with a thin, tall body build and arachnodactyly, pectus excavatum, kyphoscoliosis, and osteoporosis. Subluxation of the lens, usually in a downward position, is frequently seen by 10 years of age, and myopia is common. Approximately 60 percent of affected individuals are mentally retarded to some degree. Schizophrenic behavior has also been noted in some patients. Cardiovascular abnormalities consist primarily of arterial and venous thrombosis, with medial degeneration of the aorta and large arteries as well as intimal hyperplasia and fibrosis. It is estimated that about one-third of patients with familial homocystinuria will experience arterial or venous thrombosis. It is interesting that even within the same family with the same mutation, there is marked variability among affected siblings. The thrombotic episodes usually occur before the age of 30 and include deep venous thrombosis, pulmonary embolism, and arterial thrombosis in the cerebral, peripheral, and coronary arteries. However, when this disease occurs in individuals with other thrombogenic risk factors, such as factor V Leiden, the incidence of thrombosis, both arterial and venous, is significantly increased. An increased risk of cardiovascular disease has also been observed in carriers of the gene for homocystinuria. The latter disease, although rare, has received increased attention because of several studies indicating that homocysteine is an important and independent risk factor for atherosclerosis and thrombosis. The disorder can be treated in some cases by pyridoxine supplementation. The percentage of pyridoxine responders ranges between 13 and 47 percent. Betaine, low-methionine diet, and aspirin treatments have also been tried with varying success.

Mitochondrial Cardiomyopathies

The human mitochondrial genome is a small, circular DNA molecule that is maternally inherited. Mitochondrial DNA (mtDNA) encodes

13 of the 69 proteins required for oxidative metabolism, 22 transfer RNAs (tRNAs), and 2 ribosomal RNAs (rRNAs) required for their translation. Mitochondria are dependent on nucleocytoplasmic mechanisms for most structural components but also contribute vital peptides that are central to cellular respiration. The electron transport chain, which generates cellular adenosine triphosphate (ATP), is organized into complexes I to IV and the ATP synthase (complex V). The 13 mtDNA genes that encode enzymes in the respiratory chain include seven complex I subunits (ND1, 2, 3, 4L, 4, 5, and 6); one complex III subunit (cytochrome b); three complex IV subunits (COI, II, and III); and two complex V subunits (ATPase 6 and 8). Each cell contains numerous mitochondria and each mitochondrion contains multiple copies of mtDNA. In most mitochondrial disorders, patients carry a mix of mutant and normal mitochondria—a condition known as *heteroplasmy,* with the proportions varying from tissue-to-tissue and individual-to-individual within a pedigree in a manner correlating with severity of phenotype.

Mitochondrial diseases often produce disturbances of brain and muscle function and are usually evident during infancy or early childhood. Cardiac disease is most commonly seen with respiratory chain defects. Ragged red fibers are almost invariably present in muscle biopsy specimens when the molecular defect involves mtDNA. These defects represent the genetics of ATP production. The diverse clinical syndromes associated with various respiratory chain complexes are thought to result from involvement of tissue-specific isoforms in some cases, involvement of tissue-nonspecific (generalized) subunits in other cases, and the residual enzyme activity in affected tissues. The cardiac diseases seen associated with mitochondrial defects include both hypertrophic cardiomyopathy and dilated cardiomyopathy.

Therapy for these disorders is generally symptom-based. Conduction disturbance generally requires placement of a permanent pacemaker, and heart failure is treated with the usual therapy. In some patients, beta blockers may be useful. Hypertrophic heart disease is usually treated much the same as other forms of HCM. Mitochondrial-based therapy may include coenzyme Q_{10}, carnitine, or vitamins, but these therapeutic approaches typically do not alter the clinical course.

Connective Tissue Disorders

MARFAN SYNDROME

Marfan syndrome is a heritable disorder of connective tissue caused by a defect in the fibrillin protein encoded by the fibrillin-1 gene on chromosome 15 at 15q15-q20. The Marfan syndrome occurs in approximately 1 in 10,000 individuals and is equally common in males and females. There is marked variation in clinical expression, and the diagnosis can be made at any age from the newborn period through adulthood. Because of the variability in expression, overlap with nonpathologic features (such as tall stature) can be observed in the general population. Since fibrillin is diffuse, Marfan syndrome affects the skeletal, ocular, cardiovascular, skin, pulmonary, and central nervous systems. The skeletal manifestations of Marfan syndrome include tall stature, thin body build, long arms and legs (dolichostenomelia), long fingers and toes (arachnodactyly), hyperextensibility, pectus deformity, scoliosis, joint contractures, and narrow, high-arched palate. Cardiovascular abnormalities, particularly affecting the mitral apparatus and aorta, are also common. There may also be overlap with other disorders that share some of the same phenotypic features, such as the condition termed *congenital contractual arachnodactyly* (CCA). Clinical manifestations of CCA include dolichostenomelia and arachnodactyly, contractures of large joints, and abnormal pinna formation. The gene for Marfan syndrome is fibrillin-1 (FBN1), a component of microfibrils that are ubiquitous in the connective tissue space. Defects in this gene cause not only Marfan syndrome but also severe neonatal Marfan syndrome, which is also due to fibrillin-1 mutations. Furthermore, fibrillin defects have been found in patients with atypical phenotypes, including autosomal dominant ectopia lentis with skeletal features and milder forms such as the MASS phenotype (mitral valve, aorta, skeleton, and skin) or isolated ascending aortic aneurysm with dissection. Mutations in FBN1 also have been associated with the marfanoid-craniosynostosis (Shprintzen-Goldberg) syndrome.

The majority of cardiac abnormalities associated with Marfan syndrome affect the ascending aorta, the aortic valve, and the mitral valve. Physical examination alone is insufficient to detect subtle changes in the heart and in the aorta. The dilation of the ascending aorta may occur gradually before physical findings occur. Echocardiograms are recommended annually and beta-blocker therapy should be considered. If the diameter of the aorta corrected for body surface area exceeds the upper limits of normal by 50 percent, the frequency of evaluations should be increased to at least every 6 months. Prophylactic repair with composite graft, including aortic valve, should be performed when ascending aortic dilation reaches a diameter of 6 cm. Repair of a severe pectus excavatum may be indicated at an earlier stage, not only for cosmetic reasons but also to allow easier and safer aortic surgery should it be indicated. After surgery, the use of beta blockers and anticoagulants should be maintained and individuals should avoid contact sports and marked physical exertion. Surveillance of the aorta should continue after surgery. Prophylactic antibiotics should be administered to all patients to decrease the risk of bacterial endocarditis. In general, contact sports (e.g., football, basketball) should be avoided—along with isometric exercises, weight lifting, and extreme physical activity—and replaced with noncompetitive sports such as swimming and bicycling. Other abnormalities include mitral valve prolapse, mitral regurgitation, and aortic regurgitation. The cardiovascular abnormalities in neonatal Marfan syndrome differs somewhat from those seen in older patients, demonstrating significant mitral regurgitation as well as tricuspid and pulmonary valve regurgitation. In addition, these children have significant heart failure, as previously noted.

Primary Disorders of Rhythm and Conduction

Virtually all rhythm and conduction abnormalities have been reported to be familial. However, many families have been small, so that the mode of inheritance (or even whether the inheritance is Mendelian) is uncertain. In many cases, these rhythm and conduction defects have been associated with other cardiac and systemic disorders. However, the genetics of several disorders has recently been unraveled (Table 28-2).

Romano-Ward Long-QT syndrome

The association of stress-induced syncope, sudden death, and ventricular arrhythmias in families has long been noted, including a distinct syndrome having prolongation of the QT interval and abnormal T waves on ECG. Multiple families with long-QT syndrome (LQTS) have demonstrated autosomal dominant inheritance, with torsades de pointes polymorphic ventricular tachycardia, bradycardia, and T-wave alternans. The diagnosis is made when the QT interval corrected for heart rate (QTc) is greater than 480 ms using Bazzett's formula; T-wave abnormalities are usually seen. In symptomatic patients (i.e., patients with syncope or "seizures"), the diagnosis may be made with a shorter QTc (i.e., 470 ms).

Six genetic loci and five genes, all encode ion channels (LQT1, KVLQT1 potassium channel; LQT2, HERG potassium channel; LQT3, SCN5A sodium channel; LQT5, minK potassium channel subunit; LQT6, MiRP1 potassium channel subunit). Heterozygous mutations lead to this disorder.

Phenotype-genotype studies have been reported in LQTS. Distinct ECG differences between patients have been demonstrated, with mutations of different genes (LQT1-LQT3). Important prognostic differences appear to occur with various mutations of the different genes. Mutations in LQT1 and LQT2 were shown to result in earlier onset of syncope than LQT3 (usually by age 15 years) and more

TABLE 28-2
FAMILIAL PRIMARY DISORDERS OF RHYTHM AND CONDUCTION

Disease	Rhythm Abnormality	Inheritance	Chromosome	Gene Location
Ventricular arrhythmias				
Romano–Ward syndrome	TdP, VF	AD	11p15.5, 7q35, 3p21, 4q25, 21q22[b]	KVLQT1 (11p15.5); HERG (7q35); SCN5A (3p21); minK (21q22); MiRP1 (21q22)
Jervell and Lange-Nielsen syndrome[a]	TdP, VF	AD/AR[b]	11p15.5, 21q22	KVLQT1 (11p15.5); minK (21q22)
Brugada syndrome	VT, VF	AD	3p21	SCN5A
Sudden unexpected death syndrome	VT/VF	AD	?	?
Familial VT	VT	AD	?	?
Familial bidirectional VT	VT	AD	?	?
Familial polymorphic VT	VT	AD	1q42[b]	?

506

Supraventricular arrhythmias				
Familial atrial fibrillation	AF	AD	10q22	?
Familial total atrial standstill	SND, AF	AD	?	?
Familial absence of sinus rhythm	SND, AF	AD	?	?
Wolff-Parkinson-White syndrome	AVRT, AF, VF	AD	7q3	?
Familial PJRT	AVRT	AD	?	?
Conduction abnormalities				
Familial AV block	AVB, AF, SND, VT, SD	AD	19q13	?
Lev-Lenègre syndrome	AVB, AF, SND, VT, SD	AD	3p21	SCN5A
Familial bundle branch block	RBBB	?	?	?

KEY: AF = atrial fibrillation; AVB = atrioventricular block; AVRT = atrioventricular reciprocating tachycardia; RBBB = right bundle branch block; SD = sudden death; SND = sinus node dysfunction; TdP = torsade de pointes; VT = ventricular tachycardia; VF = ventricular fibrillation; AD = autosomal dominant; AR = autosomal recessive; PJRT = permanent form of junctional reciprocating tachycardia.

[a] Jervell and Lange-Nielsen syndrome: autosomal dominant rhythm abnormality and autosomal recessive sensorineural deafness.

[b] At least one other unknown.

frequent episodes of syncope. However, LQT3 patients appear to be at higher risk of death than either LQT1 or LQT2. The mode of symptoms and death also appears to be gene-specific to some extent. LQT1 mutations have been associated with episodes of syncope, seizures, or sudden death during diving/swimming or emotional upset. LQT2 also appears to be triggered by emotions, but auditory triggers (i.e., phone or alarm clock ringing) are also important. LQT3, on the other hand, is associated with a high incidence of events during sleep. LQT3 patients appear to shorten their QT intervals with exercise, while exercise seems to trigger events in LQT1 and LQT2 patients.

Recently, sudden infant death syndrome (SIDS) has been speculated to be due to QT prolongation. Mutation of SCN5A has been reported in at least one baby.

Gene-based therapy has been reported to improve the ECG features of LQTS, including QTc shortening and T-wave normalization. Patients with LQT2 and LQT3 have been treated with the sodium channel blocker mexiletine, and significant QTc shortening was found only in the LQT3 patients. Exogenous potassium has been used to increase the serum potassium in LQT2 patients, with QTc shortening noted; potassium channel openers appear to achieve similar results. However, no long-term results or outcomes have been reported with any of these therapies.

Jervell and Lange-Nielsen Long-QT Syndrome

This syndrome, described in 1957, is characterized by autosomal recessive congenital deafness, syncope, autosomal dominant prolonged QT interval, sudden death, and autosomal recessive inheritance. Affected individuals are usually diagnosed in childhood with congenital, severe high-tone-perceptive bilateral deafness; fainting spells precipitated by exertion, rage, or fright; and ECG evidence of QT-interval prolongation and T-wave abnormalities. As would be expected for rare autosomal recessive traits, the parents of affected individuals are more likely than usual to be consanguineous. Homozygous mutations or compound heterozygous mutations in either KVLQT1 or *minK* (i.e., I_{Ks}) have been shown to result in Jervell and Lange-Nielsen syndrome.

BRUGADA SYNDROME (IDIOPATHIC VENTRICULAR FIBRILLATION)

First described in detail in 1992, the Brugada syndrome is characterized by ST-segment elevation in leads V_1 to V_3 with or without RBBB. Clinical symptoms occur due to ventricular fibrillation. Brugada syndrome appears to be due to mutations in ion channels as well. Mutations in SCN5A, the cardiac sodium channel gene previously shown to cause LQT3, have been identified. This disorder appears to be relatively common in Europe and Southeast Asia and often is familial, usually with autosomal dominant inheritance.

FAMILIAL ATRIAL FIBRILLATION

Familial atrial fibrillation appears to be rare, but autosomal dominant inheritance occurs. A gene responsible for the disease has been mapped to 10q22. The signs and symptoms are those related to atrial fibrillation, which include palpitations, syncope, and dyspnea.

Autosomal Dominant Atrioventricular Block When it is familial, this disorder presents with adult onset (age 20 to 50 years) and has an autosomal dominant inheritance pattern. Approximately 50 families have been identified with it, and in each, transmission is consistent with autosomal dominant inheritance with full penetrance and variable expression. Whether all of these conditions represent a single disorder is not known. The common presentation of this disease includes one of the following: (1) RBBB alone; (2) left axis deviation (LAD) alone; (3) RBBB plus LAD; or (4) complete heart block. In addition, atrioventricular block has been associated with DCM and skeletal myopathy. In progressive conduction system disease (Lev-Lenègre syndrome), mutations in SCN5A have been identified.

Congenital Heart Disease with or without Genetic Syndromes

FAMILIAL ATRIAL SEPTAL DEFECT

Two Mendelian forms of atrial septal defect (ASD) exist as autosomal dominant traits. One form has no other associated abnormalities and is due to mutations in the transcription factor Nkx2.5 in families and sporadic cases of ASD. The more common form of familial secundum ASD is associated with atrioventricular conduction delay, which rarely progresses to heart block. In these patients, attention should be directed to the upper limbs, particularly the thumbs, to rule out the Holt-Oram syndrome, which is described below.

HOLT-ORAM SYNDROME

The cardinal manifestations of this autosomal dominant condition include upper limb dysplasia, ASD, and marked variability within families. The abnormalities of the arm demonstrate a wide spectrum in heterozygous individuals, ranging from undetectable to distally placed thumbs and hypoplastic thenar eminences, triphalangeal thumbs, anomalies of the carpus, and radial aplasia to phocomelia and hypoplasia of the clavicles and shoulders. The deformity of the upper extremity is typically bilateral, but the left side is commonly more severe than the right. In addition to the ASD, other cardiac malformations are occasionally found, the most frequent of which is a ventricular septal defect (VSD). Cardiac conduction disturbances, usually involving the atrioventricular node in patients with septal defects and hypoplastic peripheral arteries, are also found. Other noncardiac manifestations include dermatoglyphic abnormalities and pectus excavatum. Since the noncardiac abnormalities have a very wide spectrum, all patients with ASD should be evaluated closely for upper limb deformities.

A gene for HOS, *TBX5* [a member of the Brachyury (T) gene family], located at 12q24.1, has been identified.

SUPRAVALVULAR AORTIC STENOSIS AND WILLIAMS SYNDROME

Supravalvular aortic stenosis (SVAS) occurs in three different situations, with an estimated incidence of 1 in 20,000 births. The most common type is associated with the Williams syndrome, which is usually sporadic but may be a highly variable autosomal dominant condition. The full spectrum of Williams syndrome includes dysmorphic facies—often called "elfin" facies—infantile hypercalcemia, mental retardation, short stature, SVAS, and multiple peripheral pulmonic stenoses. Many of these individuals have robust ("cocktail party") personalities. Late-onset problems may include progressive joint contractures, gastrointestinal dysfunction, and genitourinary dysfunction.

Cardiovascular features of Williams syndrome are present in about 75 percent of patients, the most characteristic being supravalvular aortic stenosis. Other findings include peripheral pulmonic arterial stenosis and pulmonic valvular stenosis. Occasionally, VSD or ASD may be present. Peripheral vascular anomalies—including renal arterial stenosis, diffuse narrowing of the aorta, and coarctation of the aorta—may be present and may be associated with systemic hypertension. Sudden death has occurred in children with Williams syndrome, especially after cardiac catheterization. Coronary arterial stenosis may occur and lead to myocardial infarction. Histopathology in these patients suggests the possibility of abnormal elastic fibers.

A second setting for SVAS is the autosomal dominant entity, which is distinct from that of Williams syndrome (WS). Mental retardation and abnormal facies are not found, and these individuals present with SVAS and/or peripheral pulmonary artery stenoses. In some cases, family members present with moderate pulmonic valve and branch pulmonary artery stenoses but without SVAS. Later, the valvular and branch pulmonary stenoses may disappear while SVAS becomes evident. The stenotic aortic lesion requires surgery in less than one-half of these patients. The diagnosis relies on echocardiography, but cardiac catheterization is sometimes required. Finally,

SVAS may present as sporadic cases. Many investigators have long believed that the sporadic SVAS, WS, and autosomal dominant SVAS are all interrelated. SVAS and the cardiovascular features of WS are due to a WS submicroscopic deletion involving elastin on chromosome 7q11.23.

DOWN'S SYNDROME (TRISOMY 21)

Chromosome 21 is the smallest of all human chromosomes, containing less than 2 percent of the genomic DNA. Down's syndrome, however, is the most common phenotype caused by a human chromosome abnormality, occurring approximately once in every 500 to 600 births. This disorder is usually due to the presence of an extra chromosome 21 (i.e., trisomy 21), but in some cases is caused by the presence of only the distal one-half of chromosome 21, band q22 (i.e., 21q22)—the "Down's syndrome critical region"—so called owing to the presence of a subset of major phenotypic features of Down's syndrome, including mental retardation, congenital heart disease, characteristic facial appearance, and hand and dermatoglyphic changes. In order to produce this syndrome, the region of 21q22 must be triplicated. The gene(s) responsible for manifesting Down's syndrome is unknown, but the severity of the disease is believed to depend on the extent of the region q22 and beyond that is triplicated. Creation of a linkage map of chromosome 21 has allowed for consideration of potential candidate genes. Several genes have been implicated in some of the phenotypic features, but the cardiac features currently have no known cause.

TURNER'S SYNDROME

This disorder, which is due to a single X chromosome in females (i.e., XO genotype), occurs in approximately 1 female in 2500. The frequency of nonmosaic XO karyotypes is significantly higher in spontaneous abortuses than in liveborns, with less than 2 percent of such conceptuses reaching term. Clinically, there is a variable and often mild phenotype, and the diagnosis may go unsuspected until a child's short stature is evaluated or a woman complains of amenorrhea. The clinical findings of patients with Turner's syndrome include lymphedema of the hands and feet, inguinal hernias, short stature, primary amenorrhea, facial features including a slightly triangular face with down-slanted palpebral fissures, epicanthal folds, and ptosis. Ears are frequently low-set and posteriorly rotated, and the mandible is commonly micrognathic. The neck is typically short, with marked webbing, and the posterior hairline may be low, extending to the upper shoulders. A broad thorax with widely spaced nipples is common, as is cubitus valgus and shortening of the fourth and fifth metacarpals. Abnormalities of sexual development are usually associated, including hypogonadotropic hypogonadism with ovarian dysgenesis. Intelligence is normal. Many cases are mosaic for cell lines with the normal 46XX or 46XY makeup. The frequency of congenital cardiac disease varies from 20 to 50 percent, with at least one-half of these having CoA. A variety of other cardiac defects may also occur either singly or in combination with CoA. The majority of these are other left heart abnormalities, including bicuspid aortic valve, aortic stenosis, dilated ascending aorta, and hypoplastic left heart syndrome (HLHS). ASD and VSD, as well as partial anomalous pulmonary venous return, have also been reported.

DIGEORGE ANOMALY

First described in 1965, the combination of thymic hypoplasia, parathyroid hypoplasia, and cardiac defects has been termed DiGeorge syndrome or DiGeorge anomaly. Eighty percent of affected infants present with congenital heart defects within the first 48 h of life. The two types of defects associated with DiGeorge anomaly are conotruncal defects and branchial arch mesenchymal tissue defects. Among conotruncal defects, truncus arteriosus is the most common type. Among the branchial arch mesenchymal tissue defects, interrupted aortic arch type b and right aortic arch are the most common.

The second key feature is persistent hypocalcemia, occurring either as the initial presenting feature or in combination with the cardiac defect. Parathyroid glands may be absent or reduced in size and number, and serum parathyroid hormone levels are decreased. Hypocalcemia may require continuous calcium infusions and/or frequent calcium supplementation. In cases of partial defect, the hypocalcemia may improve over time.

There are multiple etiologies for DiGeorge anomaly, which include chromosomal abnormalities, single-gene defects, teratogenic exposures, and association with other defects. Approximately 5 to 10 percent of infants with features of DiGeorge anomaly will have an obvious abnormality of chromosome 22, with monosomy of the proximal portion of the long arm. However, approximately 70 percent of patients will have submicroscopic deletions of 22q11 detectable only by FISH. In addition, many of these patients have features of the Shprintzen velocardiofacial (VCF) syndrome and the Takao conotruncal face syndrome. These syndromes are currently referred to as a group by the mnemonic CATCH-22 for the associated defects: cardiac, abnormal facies, thymic hypoplasia, cleft palate, hypocalcemia, 22q11 deletions.

SUGGESTED READING

Cox GF, Kunkel LM: Dystrophies and heart disease. *Curr Opin Cardiol* 1997; 12:329–343.

Marian AJ, Roberts R: Molecular pathophysiology of cardiomyopathies. In: Sperelakis N (ed): *Cardiac Physiology.* San Diego, CA: Academic Press; 1999.

Srivastava D: Developmental and genetic aspects of congenital heart disease. *Curr Opin Cardiol* 1999; 14:263–268.

Towbin JA: Pediatric myocardial disease. *Pediatr Clin North Am* 1999; 46:289–312.

Towbin JA, Casey B, Belmont J: The molecular basis of vascular disorders. *Am J Hum Genet* 1999; 64: 678–684.

Towbin JA, Greenberg F: Genetic syndromes and clinical molecular genetics. In: Bricker JT, Garson A Jr, Fisher DJ, Neish SR (eds): *The Science and Practice of Pediatric Cardiology.* Baltimore: Williams & Wilkins, 1998: 2627–2700.

Towbin JA, Roberts R: Cardiovascular disease due to genetic abnormalities. In: Fuster V, Alexander RW, O'Rourke RA, et al (eds): *Hurst's The Heart*, 10th ed. New York: McGraw-Hill; 2001: 1785–1835.

CHAPTER

29

CONGENITAL HEART DISEASE IN ADULTS

Carole A. Warnes
Luc M. Beauchesne

The adult with congenital heart disease usually presents in one of three ways: (1) with a prior history of surgical intervention in childhood (either palliated or repaired), (2) known heart lesion without prior intervention (asymptomatic with mild lesion or severe defect deemed unrepairable), or (3) unrecognized defect, which is diagnosed in adulthood. The patient with cyanotic heart disease requires special care. Cyanosis usually occurs because of right-to-left shunting through an atrial septal defect, ventricular septal defect, or patent ductus arteriosus, which may be associated with pulmonary stenosis or acquired pulmonary vascular disease (Eisenmenger syndrome). Common to all are certain medical and surgical considerations that must be addressed in these patients (see Tables 29-1, 29-2, and 29-3).

SELECTED LESIONS

Atrial Septal Defect

- Seventy-five percent of atrial septal defects (ASDs) are ostium secundum defects and are among the most common anomalies in adulthood. Twenty percent are ostium primum defects, and 5 percent are sinus venosus defects.
- Associated lesions must be ruled out (cleft mitral valve in primum defect, anomalous pulmonary venous return in venosus defect).
- Patients are frequently asymptomatic in early adulthood; presenting as murmur or abnormal electrocardiogram (ECG) or chest x-ray (CXR). Most will eventually develop symptoms later in life related to chronic right ventricular (RV) volume overload,

TABLE 29-1

ISSUES IN THE CARE OF THE PATIENT WITH CYANOTIC HEART DISEASE

Erythrocytosis	This is a physiologic response to chronic hypoxia. At a certain level [usually a hemoglobin (Hgb) greater than 20 g/dL] may cause hyperviscosity symptoms (headache, dizziness, fatigue).
Phlebotomy	Perform only if Hgb greater than 20 g/dL and there are symptoms of hyperviscosity. Remove 500 mL of whole blood at a time and always replace with an equal amount of dextrose or saline.
Iron deficiency	Common and frequently secondary to injudicious phlebotomies. Microcytes increase blood viscosity, and this not only causes symptoms but increases the risk of stroke.
Bleeding	Secondary to coagulation factor deficiency, platelet dysfunction, and increased vascular permeability. As a rule, avoid anticoagulation and antiplatelet agents unless absolutely necessary.
Cardiovascular	Supraventricular arrhythmias are common. Ventricular arrhythmias also occur and are more common with ventricular dysfunction. Right heart failure develops with end-stage disease.
Other	Gout, renal dysfunction, paradoxical embolization (use filters in all IV lines), cerebral abscesses, hemoptysis, kyphoscoliosis.

pulmonary hypertension, atrial arrhythmias, and rarely paradoxical embolization.
- Typical ECG findings in secundum ASD: right axis deviation, incomplete right bundle branch block (RBBB).
- Rarely (<5 percent) patients may develop Eisenmenger physiology.

TABLE 29-2

CARE OF THE ADULT WITH CONGENITAL HEART DISEASE

Ventricular function	Defects with single-ventricle physiology or when the morphologic right ventricle (RV) functions as the systemic pump are at increased risk of dysfunction and may benefit from ACE inhibitors or beta blockers.
Arrhythmias	Arrhythmias are common. Underlying hemodynamic problems should always be sought. Atrial arrhythmias are frequently not well tolerated and need to be aggressively treated. VT may be secondary to fibrosis, ventricular dilation, or reentry adjacent to a surgical scar.
Conduction disease	Intrinsic or postoperative sinus node disease and AV node dysfunction common. Pacing may require epicardial lead placement in certain situations.
Endocarditis	Both operated and unoperated patients are at risk. Patients need meticulous dental, skin, and nail care. Antibiotic prophylaxis is important, and American Heart Association guidelines must be followed.
Pregnancy	As a rule stenotic lesions and right-to-left shunts are tolerated poorly, whereas regurgitant lesions and left-to-right shunts do better. Patients need very close follow-up and should deliver in centers with appropriate expertise.
Contraception	Low-dose estrogen is usually safe provided there is no cyanosis or pulmonary hypertension.
Exercise	Exercise testing is a useful tool to assess fitness level, rule out exertion-induced tachy-arrhythmias, and provide an exercise prescription. As a rule, isometric exercise is to be avoided.

KEY: RV = right ventricular; ACE = angiotensin-converting enzyme; VT = ventricular tachycardia; AV = atrioventricular.

TABLE 29-3

SURGICAL CONSIDERATIONS IN THE CARE OF THE ADULT
WITH CONGENITAL HEART DISEASE

Type of procedure	May be palliative (e.g., systemic-to-pulmonary artery shunt) or reparative.
Sternal reentry	Reoperation poses a higher risk than first operations. They are more risky when an extracardiac conduit or high-pressure ventricular chamber lies beneath the sternum.
RV to pulmonary artery conduit	Need close follow-up and frequently require multiple replacements throughout life, since valve replacements degenerate.
Transplantation	May be used in selected subjects with end-stage disease. Donor supply, however, is limited.
Noncardiac surgery	Frequent cause of morbidity and mortality in the adult with congenital heart disease. High-risk patients benefit from special expertise, particularly with cardiac anesthesia.

KEY: RV = right ventricular.

MANAGEMENT
- Routine catheterization is unnecessary unless coexistent coronary disease or pulmonary vascular disease is suspected.
- Closure should be performed in any patient with a shunt of any significance ($Qp/Qs \geq 1.5$)* or right ventricular (RV) volume overload on echocardiogram—certainly if symptomatic. Symptoms improve in the majority. Surgical closure carries a low risk (<1 percent mortality) provided that pulmonary vascular resistance is not significantly elevated. The management of

---

*KEY: Qp = pulmonary blood flow; Qs = systemic blood flow; PVR = pulmonary vascular resistance; SVR = systemic vascular resistance.

asymptomatic patients is less clear, but closure halts progression of RV volume overload, pulmonary hypertension, and tricuspid regurgitation.

- Benefit of repair is debatable when irreversible pulmonary vascular disease (PVR/SVR greater than two-thirds).
- Device closure is increasingly used for secundum ASD and is attractive, since it avoids sternotomy or thoracotomy. The long-term data are limited, however.
- Closure of the ASD in adult life does not prevent atrial fibrillation.

Ventricular Septal Defect

- There are four types of ventricular septal defects (VSDs): perimembranous (most common), muscular, inlet, and outlet.
- Associated lesions are common: bicuspid aortic valve and aortic coarctation.

CLINICAL PRESENTATION

- Different modes of presentation in the adult: (1) the patient with prior surgical repair or spontaneous closure, (2) the patient with a small VSD with left-to-right shunt who is asymptomatic, (3) the patient with a large VSD and Eisenmenger physiology.
- Spontaneous closure may still occur in adult life.
- Perimembranous or outlet defects may be associated with aortic insufficiency due to cusp prolapse.

MANAGEMENT

- A small restrictive defect does not require surgical repair unless it is causing hemodynamically significant aortic insufficiency.
- Patients have a significant risk of endocarditis: antibiotic prophylaxis and diligent dental care is crucial.

Atrioventricular Septal Defect

Atrioventricular septal defects (AVSDs) are also known as AV canal defects or endocardial cushion defects and form a spectrum of lesions secondary to a deficiency of the normal AV septum. The partial form consists of a defect in the lower part of the atrial septum (primum ASD), usually with a cleft mitral valve, which may or may not be regurgitant. The diagnosis may be missed until adulthood, and patients have a presentation similar to that of secundum ASD, often with coexistent mitral regurgitation.

- Typical ECG: left axis deviation and incomplete RBBB.
- The complete form comprises a common AV valve with the atrial defect above and a ventricular defect below.
  —This is the most common cardiac lesion seen in Down's syndrome.
  —If not repaired early in childhood, it presents with Eisenmenger physiology in adults.

MANAGEMENT

- The complete form requires early surgical repair (age < 6 months) to prevent pulmonary hypertension and pulmonary vascular disease.
- Residual mitral regurgitation is common and frequently must be addressed surgically.
- In the partial form, the need and timing of repair are dictated by the hemodynamic severity of the dominant lesion. Surgical closure of the defect is usually indicated, with repair of the mitral cleft if necessary.

Tetralogy of Fallot

- The tetrad consists of RV outflow tract obstruction, which occurs at the infundibular and often valvular levels. In addition, there is a nonrestrictive subaortic VSD, aortic override, and compensatory RV hypertrophy. Pentalogy includes an associated ASD.

CLINICAL PRESENTATION

- Most patients will have had intracardiac repair during childhood. Rarely they can present in adulthood without prior surgery (these patients usually have mild pulmonary outflow tract obstruction and are said to have acyanotic or pink tetralogy of Fallot).
- Details of the surgical intervention are important, as they predict long-term complications. If repair involved a pulmonary valvectomy or the use of a transannular patch, resultant severe pulmonary regurgitation is the rule—which, though well tolerated for many years, ultimately leads to progressive RV enlargement, dysfunction, and secondary tricuspid regurgitation. Pulmonary valve replacement should be performed before irreversible RV dysfunction occurs. While the timing is controversial, decreasing exercise tolerance and the new onset of arrhythmia also warrant consideration of pulmonary valve replacement.
- Other important issues after repair include recurrent RV outflow tract obstruction, residual VSD, peripheral pulmonary stenosis, and the development of RV outflow tract aneurysm after patch outflow repair. Aortic regurgitation results from prolapse of the

aortic cusps into the VSD prior to repair with aortic dilatation. The late functional outcome is excellent in the majority of patients, but atrial and ventricular arrhythmias also occur.

MANAGEMENT
Reoperation should be considered for a large residual VSD (Qp/Qs ≥ 1.5), significant residual RV outflow tract obstruction, large RV outflow tract aneurysm, or hemodynamically significant aortic regurgitation.

Isolated Pulmonary Stenosis

In the adult, this is usually due to a trileaflet pulmonary valve with fused commissures. A dysplastic valve is seen in Noonan's syndrome (webbed neck, hypertelorism, low-set ears, small chin, and deformed auricles). Coexistent subvalvular stenosis due to infundibular hypertrophy also occurs. Survival to adulthood is common.

MANAGEMENT
Moderate stenosis is usually well tolerated. Balloon valvuloplasty should be considered if the peak gradient is ≥40 mmHg.

Left Ventricular Outflow Tract Obstruction

CLINICAL PRESENTATION
Obstruction may be valvular (usually bicuspid valve), subvalvular (discrete membrane or more diffuse tunnel), or supravalvular. Multilevel obstruction is common. Common associations include VSD and aortic coarctation. Abnormal chordal attachments of the mitral valve may contribute to the obstruction. Aortic regurgitation is commonly associated with valvular and subvalvular forms. A bicuspid aortic valve may be associated with aortopathy and the propensity for dilatation and dissection.

MANAGEMENT
The development of symptoms (angina, dyspnea, or syncope) mandates intervention in aortic valve stenosis. In asymptomatic patients, intervention may be considered if the stenosis is severe. Surgical valvotomy may be appropriate for young adults without valvular calcification but should be considered palliative. Catheter balloon valvotomy is also palliative. Valve replacement may be necessary for valves unsuitable for valvotomy, and various prostheses are available (mechanical, bioprosthesis, and Ross procedure). For subvalvular obstruction, surgical intervention may consist of membrane

excision together with myotomy and myectomy. Multilevel obstruction may require a Konno procedure (aortic annulus enlargement, aortic valve replacement, and ventricular septal myotomy with patch enlargement).

Coarctation of the Aorta

CLINICAL PRESENTATION

In > 95 percent of cases the lesion consists of a discrete narrowing in the descending aorta just distal to the origin of the left subclavian artery. In adults it is often discovered in asymptomatic patients who are found to have upper limb hypertension. A bicuspid valve occurs in 25 to 50 percent of patients, and aortic stenosis may be the presenting condition. An associated aortopathy makes the aorta more vulnerable to aneurysm formation and dissection. Death occurs from complications of hypertension, such as stroke or aortic dissection but also endarteritis, congestive heart failure, and premature coronary disease.

MANAGEMENT

- Assessment of severity includes a combination of measuring upper limb versus lower limb gradient with bedside sphygmomanometry, blood pressure response to exercise, echocardiogram, magnetic resonance imaging, and sometimes angiography.
- Intervention should be considered if the peak gradient across the coarctation is ≥20 mmHg.
- Surgical repair is well established, with a low complication rate. Techniques include end-to-end anastomosis, patch grafting, and the use of a subclavian flap. The role of percutaneous intervention is not entirely clear. Currently this is used mostly for recoarctation with a balloon angioplasty with or without stent placement. Many adults remain hypertensive, however, even after successful repair, and all require lifelong follow-up.

Transposition of The Great Arteries

In complete transposition of the great arteries, or d-TGA, the aorta arises from the right ventricle (RV), and the pulmonary artery arises from the LV (ventriculoarterial discordance). This causes deoxygenated systemic venous flow to be directed to the aorta and pulmonary venous flow directed to the lungs. Survival to adulthood without intervention is rare. Frequent associations include VSD, left ventricular outflow tract obstruction, and coronary anomalies.

The earlier surgical approach consisted of atrial switch, which redirected atrial flow through the creation of a baffle, so that systemic venous blood was diverted to the LV and pulmonary venous flow to the RV (Mustard and Senning operations). Long-term survivals of 80 percent at 28 years have been reported. Since the early 1980s, the surgical approach has consisted of anatomic repair by reconnecting the aorta to the LV, the pulmonary artery to the RV, and coronary artery reimplantation (arterial switch).

LATE RESULTS

- Mustard and Senning patients need close follow-up. Complications include: sinus node dysfunction, supraventricular arrhythmias, obstruction or leak of the atrial baffle, failure of the RV (which still functions as a systemic pump), and secondary tricuspid regurgitation. The last may necessitate cardiac transplantation.
- Long-term results in adults with arterial switch are not known but appear promising.

Congenitally Corrected Transposition of the Great Arteries

In this anomaly (1-TGA), the aorta arises from the RV and the pulmonary artery arises from LV (ventriculoarterial discordance). In addition, the left atrium enters the RV and the right atrium enters the LV (atrioventricular discordance). This "double discordance" permits blood to flow in the appropriate direction, hence the term *congenitally corrected transposition.* The morphologic RV, however, still functions as a systemic ventricle.

- The majority of patients (about 90 percent) have associated anomalies: pulmonary stenosis, VSD, and an abnormal systemic (tricuspid) atrioventricular valve are the most common.
- Patients are frequently diagnosed in adulthood, when they present with heart block or exercise intolerance secondary to systemic AV valve regurgitation.

MANAGEMENT

- The conduction system is intrinsically abnormal in this condition. Patients frequently require pacing.
- Significant systemic AV valve regurgitation requires replacement with a prosthesis before ventricular dysfunction becomes established.
- Since the RV is a systemic ventricle and frequently abnormal, patients may benefit from angiotensin-converting enzyme (ACE) inhibitor therapy.

Ebstein's Anomaly of the Tricuspid Valve

CLINICAL PRESENTATION

This lesion consists of an apically displaced and dysplastic tricuspid valve, which divides the RV into an "atrialized" portion above and a "ventricularized" portion below. Fifty percent of patients have an associated ASD or patent foramen ovale and may develop progressive cyanosis from right-to-left shunting. The anomaly embraces a wide spectrum of disease from asymptomatic to severe tricuspid regurgitation (TR) and cyanosis. Twenty-five percent of patients have one or more accessory pathways with ventricular preexcitation (usually right-sided). Patients often present in adulthood with arrhythmias or exercise intolerance.

MANAGEMENT

- If functionally mild, TR may not require intervention.
- Progressive RV dysfunction, impaired functional capacity, right-to-left shunting, and/or paradoxical embolization require surgical intervention.
- If a large, mobile anterior leaflet is present, the tricuspid valve may be repaired in surgical centers with expertise. Otherwise, a biological prosthesis is usually inserted. The ASD will also be closed, and any accessory pathway can be interrupted at the time of surgical repair.

Marfan's Syndrome

This autosomal dominant defect occurs because of an abnormal fibrillin protein on chromosome 15. It may occur secondary to spontaneous genetic mutation. Cardiovascular manifestations occur in 30 to 60 percent of patients and consist of aortic root dilatation with the potential for dissection or rupture or severe aortic valve regurgitation. Mitral valve prolapse is the most common finding in the pediatric population. The diagnosis at the present time remains clinical and based on the presence of phenotypical features, cardiovascular abnormalities, and family history.

MANAGEMENT

- The aorta should be electively replaced when its diameter is greater than 5.5 cm and probably earlier if there is rapid progression or a family history of aortic dissection or rupture.
- Beta blockers have been shown to decrease the rate of aortic dilatation in some patients.

SUGGESTED READING

Ammash N, Connolly H, Abel M, et al: Noncardiac surgery in Eisenmenger syndrome. *J Am Coll Cardiol* 1999; 33:222–227.

Brickner ME, Hillis LD, Lange RA: Congenital heart disease in adults. First of two parts. *N Engl J Med* 2000; 342:256–263.

Brickner ME, Hillis LD, Lange RA: Congenital heart disease in adults. Second of two parts. *N Engl J Med* 2000; 342:334–342.

1996 Consensus Conference on Adult Congenital Heart Disease. Montreal: Canadian Cardiovascular Society; 1996.

Somerville J: How to manage the Eisenmenger syndrome. *Int J Cardiol* 1997; 63:1–8.

Warnes CA: Congenital heart disease and pregnancy. In: Elkayam U, Gleicher N (eds): *Cardiac Problems in Pregnancy.* New York: Wiley; 1998.

Warnes CA, Deanfield JE: Congenital heart disease in adults. In: Fuster V, Alexander RW, O'Rourke RA, et al (eds): *Hurst's The Heart,* 10th ed. New York: McGraw-Hill; 2001: 1907–1938.

CHAPTER

30

DILATED CARDIOMYOPATHIES

Michael R. Bristow
Luisa Mestroni
Teresa J. Bohlmeyer
Edward M. Gilbert

INTRODUCTION

This chapter describes characteristics of the primary and secondary dilated cardiomyopathies, the most common causes of the clinical syndrome of chronic heart failure. Heart failure is an important clinical problem that threatens to overwhelm health care resources. As discussed in Chap. 4, the clinical syndrome of heart failure is a complex process where the primary pathophysiology is quickly obscured by a variety of superimposed secondary adaptive, maladaptive, and counterregulatory processes. Heart failure is best understood and approached from the vantage point of *myocardial failure,* most commonly associated with a dilated cardiomyopathy phenotype.

The vast majority of the cases of heart failure are caused by heart muscle disease (cardiomyopathy). Within the World Health Organization (WHO) categorization (Table 30-1) of cardiomyopathy, the most common cause of the clinical syndrome of heart failure is a secondary (ischemic, valvular, hypertensive, etc.) or primary dilated cardiomyopathy, defined as a ventricular chamber exhibiting increased diastolic and systolic volumes and a low (<40) left ventricular (LV) ejection fraction. The natural history of the clinical syndrome of heart failure is dependent on the course of myocardial failure.

THE WHO/ISFC CLASSIFICATION OF CARDIOMYOPATHIES

The WHO/International Society and Federation of Cardiology (ISFC) classification of cardiomyopathies was recently revised to

TABLE 30-1

THE WORLD HEALTH ORGANIZATION/INTERNATIONAL SOCIETY AND FEDERATION OF CARDIOLOGY CLASSIFICATION OF THE CARDIOMYOPATHIES

Category	Definition
I. Dilated (DCM) 1. Primary 2. Secondary	↑ EDV, ↑ ESV; low EF
II. Restrictive (RCM) 1. Primary 2. Secondary	↓ EDV, ↔ ESV; ↑ FP, ↔EF
III. Hypertrophic (HCM)	↑↑ septal and ↑ posterior wall thickness, myofibrillar disarray Mutation in sarcomeric protein, autosomal dominant inheritance
IV. Arrhythmogenic right ventricular (ARVC)	Fibrofatty replacement of RV myocardium Autosomal dominant (most) and recessive inheritance
V. Unclassified 1. Primary 2. Secondary	Not meeting criteria for other categories Features of > one category

KEY: EDV = end-diastolic volume; ESV = end-systolic volume; EF = LV ejection fraction; FP = LV filling pressure.
SOURCE: Richardson et al, 1996.

accommodate our greater understanding of the pathophysiology of these conditions. Since the molecular genetic basis of previously unknown types of heart muscle disease is rapidly being elucidated, it has become unnecessary to reserve the classification for "unknown etiologies" of cardiomyopathy. The mechanisms responsible for progression of myocardial dysfunction and the response to treatment are qualitatively similar in both primary and secondary dilated cardiomyopathies. Because of this, it is no longer justified to exclude secondary or "known cause" cardiomyopathies from inclusion in the classification of dilated cardiomyopathy. This change allows all cardiomyopathies to be classified under one scheme.

As shown in Table 30-1, the WHO/ISFC classification of cardiomyopathy utilizes two separate methods to define the individual categories. The first is based on the global anatomic description of chamber dimensions in systole and diastole. Thus the dilated and restrictive categories have definitions based on LV dimensions and function. The justification for this is that these two groups have distinct natural histories and respond differently to medical treatment. The second method of creating individual categories within the WHO/ISFC classification is genetically based. These categories include cardiomyopathies associated with an individual gene mutation that results in a unique myocardial phenotypic feature without extracardiac manifestations. Examples of such individual categories include hypertrophic cardiomyopathy and arrhythmogenic right ventricular dysplasia. On the other hand, genetic cardiomyopathies without unique phenotypes, such as the dilated cardiomyopathy of Becker-Duchenne, are included as one form of dilated cardiomyopathy (category I).

The WHO/ISFC classification includes another assignment of nomenclature in "secondary" cardiomyopathies, i.e., those associated with known cardiac or systemic processes. These are referred to as *specific cardiomyopathies,* named for the disease processes with which they are associated. Thus an ischemic cardiomyopathy would be a specific cardiomyopathy related to previous myocardial infarction and the subsequent remodeling process, which would usually fall within the dilated class. On the other hand, a hypertensive cardiomyopathy might be classified as either dilated or restrictive depending on the chamber dimensions. Therefore the correct terms for these cardiomyopathies would be *ischemic dilated cardiomyopathy* and *hypertensive dilated (or restrictive) cardiomyopathy.*

COMPENSATORY MECHANISMS AND THE PROGRESSION OF MYOCARDIAL FAILURE

There is now a large body of information supporting the idea that activation of the adrenergic and renin-angiotensin compensatory mechanisms contributes to, or is responsible for, the progressive nature of both myocardial failure and the natural history of the heart failure clinical syndrome. This evidence includes the observations that activation of both these systems is associated with progression of myocardial dysfunction and the heart failure syndrome and clinical trial data consistently demonstrating that inhibition of these systems can prevent deterioration in or improve myocardial function as well as reduce mortality. While we know that chronic activation of the adrenergic and renin-angiotensin systems contributes to the progressive

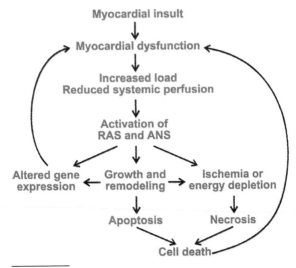

FIGURE 30-1

Relationship of neurohormonal activation and production of cardiac myocyte loss due to apoptosis and necrosis and altered gene expression. Cell loss and altered gene expression result in more myocardial dysfunction, and a vicious cycle is established. RAS = renin-angiotensin system; ANS = autonomic nervous system.

nature of myocardial dysfunction in human heart failure, we know virtually nothing about how these systems adversely affect the biology of the cardiac myocyte. Change in contractile proteins; E-C coupling mechanisms; bioenergetics; cytoskeleton, sarcomere, and cell remodeling; receptor–G protein–adenyl cyclase pathways; and receptor–G protein–phospholipase pathways are all likely contributors to this process.

Regardless of the type or cause of dilated cardiomyopathy, an initial myocardial insult resulting in this phenotype exhibits common pathophysiologic features (Fig. 30-1). Any myocardial insult that produces systolic dysfunction will be followed by the initiation of processes designed to temporarily stabilize pump function. These changes, in chronological order of onset, are (1) increase in heart rate and contractility mediated by an increase in cardiac beta-adrenergic signaling (produced within seconds of the onset of pump dysfunction); (2) volume expansion in order to utilize the

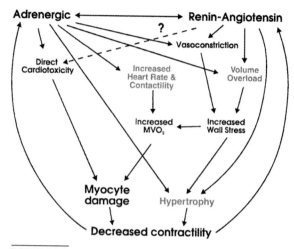

FIGURE 30-2
Heart failure compensatory mechanisms activated to support the failing heart. Lighter-colored type areas indicate physiologic mechanisms that stabilize pump function.

Frank-Starling mechanism to increase stroke volume (evident within hours of the onset of pump dysfunction); and (3) cardiac myocyte hypertrophy to increase the number of contractile elements (evident within days or weeks of the onset of pump dysfunction). As shown in Fig. 30-2, these compensatory adjustments are largely accomplished by activation of the renin-angiotensin system (RAS) and adrenergic nervous (ANS) system. However, despite the short-term (days to months) stability achieved via these mechanisms, they ultimately prove harmful.

Much current work is focused on the precise pathophysiologic mechanisms by which activation of the RAS and ANS produces remodeling and adverse effects on myocardial function. Some of the possibilities are given in Fig. 30-1. They include an exacerbation of ischemia and/or energy depletion leading to cell loss via necrosis, cell loss by programmed cell death, direct promotion of hypertrophy and remodeling through stimulation of cell growth, and alterations in cardiac myocyte gene expression. A key feature of the schema shown in Fig. 30-1 is the process of *remodeling*. Virtually all dilated cardiomyopathies undergo this process, which is characterized by progressive dilatation, progressive myocardial systolic dysfunction in viable segments, and a change in chamber shape whereby the ventricle becomes less elliptical and more spherical. This places the ventricle at an energetic disadvantage, which likely contributes to further myocardial dysfunction, which then contributes to progressive remodeling.

SCOPE OF DILATED CARDIOMYOPATHIES

The number of cardiac or systemic processes that produce or are associated with a dilated cardiomyopathy are plentiful and remarkably varied, as shown in Table 30-2. The dilated phenotype is by far the most common form of cardiomyopathy, comprising over 90 percent of subjects referred to specialized centers. The most common dilated cardiomyopathy in the United States is ischemic dilated cardiomyopathy, or the cardiomyopathy that follows myocardial infarction. Other common secondary dilated cardiomyopathies are hypertensive and valvular dilated cardiomyopathies, both produced in part by chronically increased wall stress. The primary cardiomyopathy, idiopathic dilated cardiomyopathy, is another relatively common dilated phenotype.

SELECTED COMMON TYPES OF DILATED CARDIOMYOPATHIES

Ischemic Cardiomyopathy

Ischemic cardiomyopathy is defined as a dilated cardiomyopathy in a subject with a history of myocardial infarction or evidence of clinically significant (i.e., ≥70 percent narrowing of a major epicardial artery) coronary artery disease, in whom the degree of myocardial dysfunction and ventricular dilatation is not explained solely by the extent of previous infarction or the degree of ongoing ischemia. Dilatation of the left ventricle and a decrease in ejection fraction occurs in 15 to 40 percent of subjects within 12 to 24 months following an anterior myocardial infarction and in a smaller percentage of subjects following an inferior infarction. Although the remodeling process undoubtedly is effective in increasing ventricular performance for the short term, it correlates with an adverse outcome in the long term. Several studies have concluded that patients with ischemic cardiomyopathy have a worse prognosis than subjects with a "nonischemic" dilated cardiomyopathy, probably because the risk of ischemic events is added to the risk of having a dilated cardiomyopathy.

The gross pathology of ischemic cardiomyopathy includes transmural or subendocardial scarring, representing old myocardial

TABLE 30-2

TYPES OF DILATED CARDIOMYOPATHIES

Ischemic insult (ischemic cardiomyopathy)
Valvular disease (mitral regurgitation, aortic
 regurgitation, aortic stenosis); (valvular
 cardiomyopathy)
Chronic hypertension (hypertensive cardiomyopathy)
Tachyarrhythmias (supraventricular, ventricular, atrial
 flutter)
Familial (autosomal dominant, X-linked)
Idiopathic
Toxins
　Ethanol
　Chemotherapeutic agents (anthracyclines such as
　　doxorubicin and daunorubicin)
　Cobalt
　Antiretroviral agents (zidovudine, didanosine,
　　zalcitabine)
　Phenothiazines
　Carbon monoxide
　Lithium
　Lead
　Cocaine
　Mercury
Metabolic abnormalities
　Nutritional deficiencies (thiamine, selenium, carnitine,
　　protein)
　Endocrinologic disorders (hypothyroidism, acromegaly,
　　thyrotoxicosis, Cushing's disease, pheochromocytoma,
　　catecholamines, diabetes mellitus)
　Electrolyte disturbances (hypocalcemia,
　　hypophosphatemia)
Infectious
　Viral (coxsackie virus, cytomegalovirus, HIV)
　Rickettsial
　Bacterial
　Mycobacterial
　Spirochetal
　Fungal
　Parasitic (toxoplasmosis, trichinosis, Chagas' disease)

(*continued*)

TABLE 30-2

(Continued)

Systemic disorders
    Systemic lupus erythematosus
    Juvenile rheumatoid arthritis
    Polyarteritis nodosa
    Kawasaki disease
    Collagen vascular disorders (scleroderma,
       lupus erythematosus, dermatomyositis)
    Hemochromatosis
    Amyloidosis
    Sarcoidosis
    Pseudoxanthoma elasticum
    Hypereosinophilic syndrome
Hypersensitivity myocarditis
Peri-/postpartum dysfunction
Arrhythmogenic right ventricular
    dysplasia or cardiomyopathy
Infantile histiocytoid
Neuromuscular dystrophies
    Becker's or Duchenne's muscular dystrophy,
       X-linked cardioskeletal myopathy
Facioscapulohumoral muscular dystrophy
Erb's limb-girdle dystrophy
Myotonic dystrophy
Fridreich's ataxia
Emery-Dreifuss muscular dystrophy
Inborn errors of metabolism
Mitochondrial cardiomyopathies
Keshan cardiomyopathy

infarction(s), which may comprise up to 50 percent of the ventricular chamber. The histopathology of the noninfarcted regions is similar to changes occurring in idiopathic dilated cardiomyopathy, as discussed below.

The treatment of all dilated cardiomyopathies includes the treatment of chronic heart failure (see Chap. 4). Patients with ischemic cardiomyopathy should also be assessed for the presence of viable but ischemic myocardium. If documented, ischemia should be treated aggressively, including antianginal therapy, control of the heart failure state, and revascularization.

Hypertensive Cardiomyopathy

Hypertensive dilated cardiomyopathy is diagnosed when myocardial systolic function is depressed out of proportion to the increase in wall stress associated with hypertension. In addition to producing a "pure" form of hypertensive cardiomyopathy, hypertension is a major risk factor for heart failure from any cause. Within the WHO/ISFC classification, hypertensive heart disease may present in the dilated, restrictive, or unclassified categories.

In the absence of comorbid conditions, the prognosis of patients with hypertensive cardiomyopathy is usually better than that of patients with other dilated cardiomyopathies as long as hypertension is controlled. Therefore, therapy includes vigorous control of afterload, including the addition or pure antihypertensive vasodilators such as third-generation calcium channel blockers or alpha-blocking agents to standard heart failure therapy.

Valvular Cardiomyopathy

A valvular cardiomyopathy occurs when a valvular abnormality is present and myocardial systolic function is depressed out of proportion to the increase in wall stress. This most commonly occurs with left-sided regurgitant lesions (mitral regurgitation and aortic regurgitation), less commonly with aortic stenosis, and never as a consequence of pure mitral stenosis. The pattern of eccentric hypertrophy derives from increased diastolic wall stress. Thus, long-standing mitral regurgitation most commonly results in compensated eccentric hypertrophy, which can progress to a dilated failing phenotype. Aortic regurgitation is a particularly poorly tolerated hemodynamic insult because wall stress is increased in both systole and diastole. Aortic stenosis classically results in compensated concentric hypertrophy; but when decompensation occurs, a variety of phenotypes can be observed that are similar to hypertensive cardiomyopathies.

The most important prognostic variable is the severity of the cardiomyopathy at the time of surgical correction of the valvular abnormality. In general, severely depressed myocardial function will not improve much with surgical repair of aortic regurgitation or mitral regurgitation (MR). Replacement of the mitral valve should not be attempted in the majority of subjects with severe MR and LV ejection fraction below 25 percent because of prohibitively high operative/perioperative mortality rates. On the other hand, there is no impairment of LV systolic function severe enough to preclude valve replacement of severe aortic stenosis, as function will invariably improve on relief of the hemodynamic insult and the prognosis is relatively good.

Idiopathic Dilated Cardiomyopathy, Including Familial Forms

Idiopathic dilated cardiomyopathy (IDC) is diagnosed by excluding significant coronary artery disease, valvular abnormalities, and other causes. IDC is a relatively common cause of heart failure, with an estimated prevalence rate of 0.04 percent and incidence rates of 0.005 percent. Although the diagnosis is not difficult, problems arise when an apparent IDC presents in someone with a history of hypertension or excessive alcohol intake. In such cases it is best to reassign the etiology to alcohol only when the intake has exceeded 80 g/day for men and 40 g/day for women for more than 5 years and to hypertensive heart disease when blood pressure has been uncontrolled and high (>160/100 mmHg) as well as sustained (for years). All subjects with an unexplained dilated cardiomyopathy need a TSH level done to exclude hypo- or hyperthyroidism. IDC may be familial in as many as 30 to 50 percent of the cases when first-degree relatives are carefully screened. However, analysis of the IDC phenotype identifies a wide range of clinical and pathologic forms, indicating genetic heterogeneity.

The major morphologic feature of IDC on postmortem examination is dilatation of the cardiac chambers. Although there is an increase in muscle mass and myocyte cell volume in IDC, LV wall thickness is usually not increased because of the marked dilatation of the ventricular cavities. Grossly visible scars may be present in either ventricle, and while most scars are small, some may be large and transmural. Scarring occurs in the absence of significant narrowing of the epicardial coronary arteries. In most cases, the degree of fibrosis does not appear to be extensive enough to cause changes in systolic or diastolic function.

The characteristic findings of IDC on microscopy are marked myocyte hypertrophy, very large, bizarrely shaped nuclei, increased interstitial fibrosis, myocyte atrophy, and myofilament loss. In isolated cardiac myocytes, the major cellular phenotypic change is marked increase in cell length without a concomitant increase in diameter. As described earlier, this cellular lengthening contributes to the chamber remodeling that characterizes IDC and other cardiomyopathies. These morphologic changes in IDC are not specific and are generally found in secondary cardiomyopathies, as in the noninfarcted regions of ischemic dilated cardiomyopathy.

A number of immune-regulatory abnormalities have been identified in IDC, including humoral and cellular autoimmune reactivity against myocytes, decreased natural killer cell activity, and abnormal suppressor cell activity. These abnormalities suggest that immune defects may be important etiologic factors in the development of IDC. These findings, however, are not universally present in patients with

IDC, and some abnormalities are also present in other types of heart muscle disease. Thus, while the autoimmune hypothesis is an attractive one for the etiology of some cases of IDC, it remains unproved.

SELECTED, SPECIFIC DILATED CARDIOMYOPATHIES WITH UNIQUE MANAGEMENT ISSUES

Anthracycline Cardiomyopathy

The commonly used and highly efficacious anthracycline antibiotic anticancer agents doxorubicin and daunorubicin produce a cardiomyopathy that depends on the total cumulative dose. For doxorubicin (Adriamycin), the incidence of heart failure due to cardiomyopathy dramatically increases above total cumulative doses of 450 mg/m^2 in subjects without underlying cardiac problems or other risk factors. Mediastinal radiation involving the heart, regardless of timing, is a powerful risk factor for anthracycline cardiomyopathy. In subjects with risk factors, anthracycline cardiomyopathy can present at cumulative doses lower than 450 mg/m^2.

Although the diagnosis of anthracycline cardiomyopathy can be made clinically, the definitive diagnosis depends on the demonstration of a substantial number of cardiac myocytes exhibiting the characteristic anthracycline effect. Tissue sampling is best done by endomyocardial biopsy, which allows for "thin-section" electromyographic processing of the sample and more definitive resolution of the anthracyline effect with light microscopy. With increasing exposure to anthracyclines, there is cell vacuolization progressing to cell dropout. Myocardial dysfunction results when 16 to 25 percent of the total number of sampled cells exhibit this morphology.

Postpartum Cardiomyopathy

Post- or peripartum cardiomyopathy is defined as the presentation of systolic dysfunction and clinical heart failure during the last trimester of pregnancy or within 6 months of delivery. Postpartum cardiomyopathy is likely a heterogeneous group of disorders, consisting of the addition of the hemodynamic load of pregnancy to a variety of underlying myocardial processes including hypertensive heart disease, familial or idiopathic dilated cardiomyopathy, and myocarditis. Approximately half of subjects who develop postpartum cardiomyopathy will completely recover, and most of the rest will improve. Subjects who have developed a postpartum cardiomyopathy should never become pregnant again, even if myocardial function has fully recovered.

Chagas' Cardiomyopathy

Chagas' disease is a cause of myocarditis and is the most common cause of nonischemic cardiomyopathy in South and Central America, afflicting over 10 million people. It is caused by a parasite, the leishmanial or tissue form of the protozoan *Trypanosoma cruzi*. Chagas' disease may be transmitted by blood transfusions; as a result, it could become relatively more important in the United States. The natural history consists of an initial myocarditis—most commonly presenting in childhood—associated with acute myocardial infection, followed by recovery and in some individuals the development of a dilated cardiomyopathy 10 to 30 years later. The diagnosis of Chagas' cardiomyopathy is based on clinical criteria and a positive serologic test for *T. cruzi*. The histologic lesion of chronic Chagas' consists of mononuclear infiltrates, fibrosis, and foci of the leishmanial form of *T. cruzi* in myocardial fibers. The basis for the Chagas' cardiomyopathy is unknown but may be immunologic, whereby antibodies generated against *T. Cruzi* cross-react with cardiac myocyte antigens, including myosin.

There is no definitive treatment for Chagas' cardiomyopathy. Nonspecific treatment includes pacemaker implantation for heart block and heart failure treatment, as for idiopathic dilated cardiomyopathy. The one exception may be the more frequent use of amiodarone, which appears to be particularly effective in treating arrhythmias associated with Chagas' cardiomyopathy. The role of cardiac transplantation is still somewhat uncertain, but transplantation can be done at acceptable risk, especially when coupled with trypanocidal agents.

SUGGESTED READING

Bristow MR, Mestroni L, Bohlmeyer TJ, Gilbert EM: Dilated cardiomyopathies. In: Fuster V, Alexander RW, O'Rourke RA, et al (eds): *Hurst's The Heart,* 10th ed. New York: McGraw-Hill; 2001:1947–1966.

Codd MB, Sugrue DD, Gersh BJ, Melton LJ: Epidemiology of idiopathic dilated and hypertrophic cardiomyopathy: A population based study in Olmstead County, MN 1975–1984. *Circulation* 1989; 80:564–572.

Cohn JN: Structural basis for heart failure: Ventricular remodeling and its pharmacological inhibition. *Circulation* 1995; 91:2504–2507.

Cohn JN, Johnson GR, Shabetai R, et al, for the V-HeFT VA Cooperative Studies Group: Ejection fraction, peak exercise oxygen consumption, cardiothoracic ratio, ventricular arrhythmias, and plasma norepinephrine as determinants of prognosis in heart failure. *Circulation* 1993; 87(suppl VI):VI-5–VI-16.

Lowes BD, Minobe WA, Abraham WT, et al: Changes in gene expression in the intact human heart: Downregulation of alpha-myosin heavy chain in hypertrophied, failing ventricular myocardium. *J Clin Invest* 1997; 100:2315–2324.

Richardson P, McKenna W, Bristow MR, et al: Report of the 1995 World Health Organization/International Society and Federation of Cardiology Task Force on the definition and classification of cardiomyopathies. *Circulation* 1996; 93:841–842.

CHAPTER

31

HYPERTROPHIC CARDIOMYOPATHY

Barry J. Maron

DEFINITION

The cardinal feature of *hypertrophic cardiomyopathy* (HCM) is an unexplained increase in left ventricular wall thickness without ventricular chamber dilatation. Left ventricular systolic function is characteristically normal and often hypercontractile.

ETIOLOGY

HCM is usually familial and genetically transmitted as an autosomal dominant trait. A myriad of mutations in nine genes encoding proteins of the cardiac sarcomere have been identified as disease-causing.

PATHOLOGY

Characteristic abnormalities at necropsy include (1) an asymmetrical pattern of left ventricular hypertrophy in which the ventricular septum is thicker than portions of the left ventricular free wall; (2) a small or normal-sized left ventricular cavity; (3) a fibrous mural endocardial plaque on the ventricular septum in the outflow tract in apposition to the anterior mitral leaflet; (4) mitral valve enlargement and elongation with or without secondary thickening; (5) atrial dilatation; (6) abnormal intramural coronary arteries with thickened walls and narrowed lumina; (7) areas of replacement scarring; (8) increased interstitial (matrix) collagen; and (9) disorganized left ventricular architecture with myocardial cell (myocyte) disarray.

The abnormal intramural coronary arteries are regarded as a form of "small vessel disease" and are probably responsible for myocardial ischemia and replacement fibrosis. Areas of myocyte disorganization, often diffusely distributed throughout the myocardium, are thought to potentially represent the arrhythmogenic substrate in this disease, possibly serving as a nidus for ventricular tachyarrhythmias.

CLINICAL MANIFESTATIONS

History

Exertional dyspnea and chest pain are the most common symptoms. Patients also frequently experience impaired consciousness (syncope, near-syncope, or dizziness), palpitations, or occasionally orthopnea or paroxysmal nocturnal dyspnea when more advanced stages of heart failure evolve. Dyspnea usually results from abnormal ventricular compliance and increased pulmonary venous pressure; it is accentuated by tachycardia. Chest pain may be characteristic of angina pectoris (in the absence of coronary artery disease) but often is atypical in character.

Physical Examination

In the presence of a left ventricular outflow tract pressure gradient (which occurs at rest in only 20 to 25 percent of patients), the characteristic physical findings include (1) systolic ejection murmur along the lower left sternal border and at the apex, decreasing with squatting and handgrip but intensified with standing, the Valsalva maneuver, or amyl nitrite inhalation; (2) abrupt upstroke to the arterial pulse, at times demonstrating bisferiens (bifid) configuration with initial brisk percussion wave and a subsequent tidal wave; (3) a bifid apical systolic impulse, often preceded by a prominent presystolic impulse giving a triple-beat character; and (4) an A wave in the jugular venous pulse associated with a prominent fourth heart sound at the cardiac apex. These findings are absent in patients with the much more common nonobstructive form of the disease in which there is no systolic ejection murmur or only a soft one.

DIAGNOSTIC TESTS

Electrocardiogram

The 12-lead ECG is abnormal in 90 to 95 percent of the patients with HCM, and a wide variety of patterns occur; however, none of these abnormalities is either diagnostic or specific. Patterns of left ventricular hypertrophy with increased QRS voltage and ST-T-wave abnormalities are common. Also frequent are left anterior hemiblock, deep inferior Q waves (which may simulate healed myocardial infarction), prominent T-wave inversion, left atrial enlargement, and "pseudoinfarction" patterns with diminished R-wave voltages in the precordial leads.

Chest X-ray

The cardiac silhouette is often enlarged, and left atrial enlargement and interstitial pulmonary edema may be present. The assessment of cardiac size on x-ray usually adds little to the clinical evaluation, since chamber dimensions are best assessed with echocardiography.

SPECIAL DIAGNOSTIC EVALUATION

Echocardiography

The two-dimensional echocardiogram is the most useful test for the clinical diagnosis of HCM. The echocardiographic diagnosis of HCM is based on the identification of a hypertrophied, nondilated left ventricle in the absence of another cardiac or systemic disease capable of producing the degree of wall thickening evident in a given patient. A wide variety of patterns of left ventricular wall thickening may be present in patients with HCM—i.e., not uncommonly involving diffuse hypertrophy of both septum and free wall but also frequently demonstrating only localized thickening of relatively small portions of the left ventricular wall. The mitral valve (which is often elongated) is displaced anteriorly, toward the septum within the small left ventricular outflow tract. Systolic anterior motion (SAM) of the mitral valve with ventricular septal contact is responsible for dynamic obstruction to left ventricular outflow. Doppler echocardiography can accurately assess the magnitude and dynamic characteristics of the outflow pressure gradient, the severity of mitral regurgitation (with color-flow imaging), and the diastolic filling and relaxation abnormalities commonly present in HCM.

Ambulatory Electrocardiography

The Holter ECG may be of value in identifying bursts of nonsustained ventricular tachycardia, which can represent markers for the risk of sudden cardiac death in some patients, particularly when multiple and repetitive.

Radionuclide Imaging Technique

Technetium-99m labeling of the blood pool and gated blood pool scanning can define cavity size and offer quantitation of the left ventricular ejection fraction and filling abnormalities. Myocardial perfusion imaging with thallium 201 may demonstrate reversible or fixed perfusion defects that suggest areas of myocardial ischemia or scarring.

Hemodynamics

Cardiac catheterization and angiography are usually performed only when surgery is contemplated in order to measure (1) intracardiac pressures and the presence of resting and/or provocable obstruction (with Valsalva maneuver, isoproterenol infusion, or amyl nitrite inhalation) and (2) the presence or absence of coronary artery disease. There is no generally accepted clinical indication for endomyocardial biopsy.

Left Ventricular Function

The predominant functional abnormality responsible for limiting symptoms in patients with HCM is impaired ventricular compliance with abnormal diastolic filling and relaxation, presumably due to the distorted myocardial architecture and resultant asynchronous myocardial contraction and relaxation. Of note, the heart failure that patients with HCM characteristically manifest occurs in the presence of a nondilated chamber and normal (or even hyperdynamic) left ventricular systolic function. Therefore the congestive symptoms so common in HCM are usually a consequence of impaired filling rather than pump failure. Only in the "end-stage" phase of the disease, associated with cavity enlargement and wall thinning, is left ventricular systolic dysfunction evident.

NATURAL HISTORY

HCM should be regarded as a highly complex disease process capable of leading to important clinical consequences and premature death in some patients; however, other patients experience little or no disability and may even achieve normal life expectancy, often without the aid of major therapeutic interventions. Nevertheless, the natural history of HCM is highly variable and unpredictable, reflecting the heterogeneity characteristic of this disease. The overall disease is associated with an annual mortality of 1 percent, but identification of higher- (and lower) risk subgroups is an important aim of the clinical evaluation. Premature sudden cardiac death may occur in young people (≤30 years old), and HCM is the most common cause of sudden death in young competitive athletes; however, sudden catastrophes may also occur in midlife and beyond. Both patients with and patients without outflow obstruction may die suddenly. Progressive symptoms of heart failure may dominate after age 35 to 40. While some patients may live their entire lives without incurring important functional limitation, some elderly patients with HCM may also experience severe heart failure after being free of symptoms for many decades.

Atrial fibrillation (present in 20 to 25 percent of HCM patients), with loss of the atrial contribution to ventricular filling, may result in acute clinical deterioration and long-term heart failure as well as peripheral embolization. Atrial fibrillation does not appear to be predictive of sudden and unexpected death. Infective endocarditis may occur occasionally in patients with outflow obstruction, the anterior mitral leaflet being the most common site. Pregnancy with vaginal delivery is usually well tolerated.

DIFFERENTIAL DIAGNOSIS

HCM has been regarded clinically as a "great masquerader." The murmur of obstructive HCM can mimic that of aortic valvular stenosis, ventricular septal defect, or mitral regurgitation. Some children with HCM have marked right ventricular outflow obstruction with a murmur similar to that in pulmonary valve stenosis. Chest pain in HCM may be typical of coronary artery disease (angina pectoris), and some ECG patterns suggest a prior healed myocardial infarction. In addition, other diseases (such as cardiac amyloidosis) may be characterized by a thickened left ventricular wall and in this way can mimic HCM.

TREATMENT

Therapeutic decisions in HCM (Table 31-1) also reflect the heterogeneity of the disease spectrum. Treatment is focused initially on *drug therapy* when cardiac symptoms and functional limitation are present.

Exertional dyspnea (and chest pain) often responds to a variety of beta-blocking agents. The calcium channel blocker verapamil has been shown to reduce symptoms and improve exercise capacity in a large proportion of patients who do not benefit from beta blockers, probably by improving ventricular filling. Some centers

TABLE 31-1

MANAGEMENT GUIDELINES FOR HYPERTROPHIC
CARDIOMYOPATHY

Congestive Symptoms	Treatment
Early	Beta blocker or verapamil
Progressive	Beta blocker or verapamil plus diuretic, or disopyramide (with or without a beta blocker)
Refractory	
Obstruction, at rest ($\geq$50-mmHg outflow gradient)	*Primary* → septal myotomy-myectomy *Alternative* → alcohol septal ablation or DDD pacing
Obstruction, provocable ($\geq$50 mmHg only with provocative maneuvers)	Septal myotomy-myectomy*
Nonobstructive (including "end stage")	Heart transplant
Asymptomatic	Reassurance and follow-up (if no identifiable risk factors or unfavorable prognostic indicators)
High risk for sudden death ($\geq$1 risk factors)	Implantable cardioverter/ defibrillator (ICD)

*If exertional symptoms can be shown to be related to development of marked outflow obstruction.

have utilized disopyramide (instead of verapamil) to relieve limiting symptoms.

In those patients judged to be at *high risk* for sudden cardiac death (due to risk factors including prior cardiac arrest, family history of premature HCM-related death, or massive left ventricular hypertrophy), the implantable cardioverter/defibrillator has proven effective.

Surgical treatment with muscular resection from the basal ventricular septum (septal myotomy-myectomy; Morrow procedure) is presently the "gold standard" reserved for severely symptomatic patients who become refractory to drug treatment, with a basal peak systolic left ventricular outflow tract gradient of at least 50 mmHg. As a result of this operation, the outflow gradient and mitral regurgitation are usually abolished, and symptoms are relieved or greatly reduced in the vast majority of patients. While operation can improve quality of life, it does not eliminate subsequent risk for disease progression or sudden cardiac death. In major centers, the operative risk is now acceptably low (≤ 1 to 2 percent).

Potential *alternatives to surgery* in selected patients to relieve symptoms or outflow obstruction include dual-chamber pacing and the experimental procedure of alcohol septal ablation, in which alcohol is injected into the first major septal perforator coronary artery and a myocardial infarction is produced.

Anticoagulation is indicated in those patients who have atrial fibrillation and should be continued indefinitely once this arrhythmia has been documented. Diuretics can be used judiciously in treating those patients with marked symptoms in conjunction with other cardioactive medications. Vasodilators and digitalis may increase the outflow gradient and therefore are contraindicated in patients with obstructive HCM. In patients with progressive congestive heart failure secondary to impaired systolic function (i.e., "end-stage" HCM), the therapeutic strategy is similar to that utilized for pump failure in other diseases, ultimately including the possibility of cardiac transplantation. Antibiotic prophylaxis is indicated to protect against infective endocarditis in patients with outflow obstruction.

SUGGESTED READING

Klues HG, Schiffers A, Maron BJ: Phenotypic spectrum and patterns of left ventricular hypertrophy in hypertrophic cardiomyopathy: Morphologic observations and significance as assessed by two-dimensional echocardiography in 600 patients. *J Am Coll Cardiol* 1995; 26:1699–1708.

Maron BJ: Hypertrophic cardiomyopathy. In: Fuster V, Alexander RW, O'Rourke RA, et al (eds): *Hurst's The Heart,* 10th ed. New York: McGraw-Hill; 2001:1967–1987.

Maron BJ: Hypertrophic cardiomyopathy. *Lancet* 1997; 350:127–133.

Maron BJ, Bonow RO, Cannon RO III, et al: Hypertrophic cardiomyopathy: Interrelations of clinical manifestations, pathophysiology, and therapy. *N Engl J Med* 1987; 316:780–789, 844–852.

Maron BJ, Shen W-K, Link MS, et al: Efficacy of implantable cardioverter-defibrillators for the prevention of sudden death in patients with hypertrophic cardiomyopathy. *N Engl J Med* 2000; 342:365–373.

Morrow AG, Reitz BA, Epstein SE, et al: Operative treatment in hypertrophic subaortic stenosis: Techniques and the results of pre- and postoperative assessments in 83 patients. *Circulation* 1975; 52:88–102.

Spirito P, Bellone P, Harris KM, et al: Magnitude of left ventricular hypertrophy predicts the risk of sudden death in hypertrophic cardiomyopathy. *N Engl J Med* 2000; 342:1778–1785.

Spirito P, Seidman CE, McKenna WJ, Maron BJ: The management of hypertrophic cardiomyopathy. *N Engl J Med* 1997; 336:775–785.

Wigle ED, Sasson Z, Henderson MA, et al: Hypertrophic cardiomyopathy: The importance of the site and extent of hypertrophy—A review. *Progr Cardiovasc Dis* 1985; 28:1–83.

CHAPTER

32

RESTRICTIVE, OBLITERATIVE, AND INFILTRATIVE CARDIOMYOPATHIES

Joseph M. Restivo
Brian D. Hoit

The World Health Organization and International Society and Federation of Cardiology (WHO/ISFC) define cardiomyopathies as heart muscle diseases of unknown etiology, and classify them according to hemodynamic and pathophysiologic criteria. Restrictive cardiomyopathy refers to either an idiopathic or systemic myocardial disorder characterized by restrictive filling, normal or reduced ventricular volmues, and normal or nearly normal systolic ventricular function (Table 32-1). Striking elevation of the jugular venous pulse and prominent X and especially Y descents are characteristic. A diastolic arterial pulse due to a reduced stroke volume and tachycardia may be seen in severe cases. The apical impulse is nondisplaced and systolic murmurs of atrioventricular regurgitation and filling sounds marking the abrupt cessation of rapid early diastolic filling may be present.

Electrocardiographic abnormalities such as abnormal voltage, atrial and ventricular arrhythmias, and conduction disturbances are frequent. Atrial enlargement and pericardial effusion may produce an enlarged cardiac silhouette on the chest radiogram, and pleural effusions and signs of pulmonary congestion may also be present. Echocardiographic findings are nonspecific but in many cases are useful to exclude other, more common causes of heart failure.

Several clinical, imaging, and hemodynamic features are helpful in distinguishing restrictive cardiomyopathy from constrictive pericarditis (Table 32-2). Although Doppler techniques have assumed an important role in characterizing the nature of transvalvular filling and helping to make this clinically crucial distinction, rigorous studies of the sensitivity and specificity of these Doppler findings are lacking, and relatively few patients have been examined. Thus, the diagnostic certainty is related to the number of "pathognomonic" findings

549

TABLE 32-1

CLASSIFICATION OF THE RESTRICTIVE CARDIOMYOPATHIES

Myocardial
   Noninfiltrative cardiomyopathies
      Idiopathic
      Familial
      Pseudoxanthoma elasticum
      Scleroderma
   Infiltrative cardiomyopathies
      Amyloidosis
      Sarcoidosis
      Gaucher's disease
   Storage disease
      Hemochromatosis
      Fabry's disease
      Glycogen storage diseases
Endomyocardial
   Obliterative
      Endomyocardial fibrosis
      Hypereosinophilc syndrome
   Nonobliterative
      Carcinoid
      Malignant infiltration
      Iatrogenic (radiation, drugs)

in concert with clinical information and additional imaging studies. Magnetic resonance imaging (MRI) and computed tomography (CT) are useful in that pericardial thickness can be accurately assessed.

Right- and left-sided heart catheterization is performed to document the diagnosis, assess the severity, and, in some patients, establish the etiology by means of endomyocardial biopsy. The venous pressure is elevated and the deep, precipitous nature of the right atrial Y descent is striking. The right ventricular systolic pressure is often elevated, and the early portion of diastole is characterized by a deep, sharp dip followed by a plateau (square root sign), during which no further increase in right ventricular pressure occurs. These hemodynamic features are similar to those of constrictive pericarditis and may create further diagnostic confusion; although it is not uncommon for the pulmonary wedge and the right atrial pressures to be identical, a higher left than right ventricular (RV) filling pressure strongly favors the diagnosis of restrictive cardiomyopathy.

TABLE 32-2

CLINICAL AND HEMODYNAMIC FEATURES THAT HELP TO DISTINGUISH RESTRICTIVE CARDIOMYOPATHY FROM CONSTRICTIVE PERICARDITIS

	Restrictive Cardiomyopathy	Constrictive Pericarditis
History	Systemic disease that involves the myocardium, multiple myeloma, amyloidosis, cardiac transplant	Acute pericarditis, cardiac surgery, radiation therapy, chest trauma, systemic disease involving the pericardium
Chest radiogram	Absence of calcification	Helpful when calcification persists
Electrocardiogram	Massive atrial enlargement Bundle branch blocks, AV block	Moderate atrial enlargement Abnormal repolarization
CT/MRI	Normal pericardium	Helpful if thickened (>4 mm) pericardium
Hemodynamics	Helpful if unequal diastolic pressures Concordant effect of respiration on diastolic pressures	Diastolic equilibration Dip and plateau
Biopsy	Fibrosis, hypertrophy, infiltration	Normal

KEY: AV = atrioventricular; CT = computed tomography; MRI = magnetic resonance imaging.

Treatment of restrictive cardiomyopathy is empiric and directed toward the treatment of diastolic heart failure. Judicious use of diuretics is warranted in view of the steep pressure-volume relation of the ventricles and the need to maintain a relatively high filling pressure. Vasodilators may also jeopardize ventricular filling and should be used cautiously.

NONINFILTRATIVE RESTRICTIVE CARDIOMYOPATHIES

Idiopathic restrictive cardiomyopathy may occur as an autosomal dominant disorder involving myocardium, conduction tissue, and skeletal muscle, with resultant restrictive ventricular filling and heart failure, atrioventricular (AV) block, and distal skeletal myopathy, respectively. Deposition of the intermediate filament desmin has been linked to this syndrome. Myocyte hypertrophy and fibrosis on endomyocardial biopsy are characteristic. Echocardiography reveals normal or reduced ventricular dimensions, variable systolic function, and increased atrial dimensions. A dominant early diastolic mitral "E" velocity (increased E/A ratio), an increased pulmonary venous atrial systolic "A" reversal velocity and duration, as well as shortened mitral deceleration time are typical features on Doppler.

Pseudoxanthoma elasticum is a rare disorder, characterized by fragmentation and calcification of elastic fibers, that uncommonly causes restrictive cardiomyopathy. Similarly, restrictive cardiomyopathy is a rare complication of scleroderma.

INFILTRATIVE RESTRICTIVE CARDIOMYOPATHIES

Amyloidosis

Amyloidosis is a systemic disorder characterized by interstitial deposition of amyloid protein fibrils in multiple organs. Cardiac involvement is most common in primary amyloidosis (AL type) and often occurs in association with multiple myeloma. Cardiac deposition of amyloid protein (protein A) may also occur in secondary amyloidosis due to chronic inflammation. Amyloidosis may also be familial; mutations of the protein transthyretin produce peripheral and autonomic neuropathy in addition to cardiac disease. Finally, senile amyloidosis is commonly seen in the elderly.

Amyloid deposits may be interstitial and widespread, resulting in restrictive cardiomyopathy, or localized to (1) conduction tissue, resulting in heart block and ventricular arrhythmias (especially in familial amyloidosis); (2) the cardiac valves, resulting in valvular regurgitation; (3) the pericardium, resulting in constriction; and (4) the coronary arteries, resulting in ischemia. In some cases, the clinical picture is dominated by autonomic neuropathy and nephropathy and cardiac involvement is unrecognized. Cardiac manifestations often progress from the asymptomatic to biventricular failure. The cardiac silhouette on the chest radiogram may be normal or moderately enlarged; decreased voltage, pseudoinfarction, and left axis deviation are typical. Arrhythmias and conduction disturbances may dominate the clinical course. The echocardiogram may reveal symmetrical wall thickness involving the right and left ventricles, a small or normal LV cavity with variably depressed systolic function, atrial and vena caval dilatation, thickening of the interatrial septum and valves, and a small pericardial effusion. Highly reflective echoes producing a granular or sparkling appearance and occurring in a patchy distribution are characteristic echocardiographic findings but are neither sensitive nor specific.

The earliest sign of amyloid cardiomyopathy is impaired LV relaxation, manifest by a mitral Doppler E/A ratio <1, and increased isovolumic relaxation and transmitral diastolic deceleration times. The restrictive pattern of LV filling—i.e., a transmitral E/A ratio ≥ 2 without respiratory variation, transmitral diastolic deceleration time <150 ms, and an isovolumic relaxation time ≤ 70 ms—are strong predictors of cardiac death.

The variable clinical, diagnostic, and prognostic features reflect the location, nature, and extent of amyloid deposition and the temporal course of the disease. Serum and urine protein electrophoresis is diagnostic in most cases of primary amyloidosis, but monoclonal protein may not be secreted. Endomyocardial biopsy of the right ventricle, which is most helpful if an abdominal fat aspirate is negative, provides the diagnosis and quantifies myocardial damage.

The treatment of amyloidosis is fraught with hazard; patients are sensitive to digoxin and calcium channel blockers, and hypotension with vasodilators and diuretics is a threat due to the steep LV pressure–volume relation. Immunosuppressive therapy with melphalan and prednisone is established—conventional therapy for primary amyloidosis. Orthotopic cardiac transplantation is generally not recommended, but liver transplantation may be lifesaving in patients with familial amyloidosis.

Other Infiltrative Cardiomyopathies

Noncaseating granulomas involve the heart in sarcoidosis in as many as 25 percent of patients but are frequently subclinical. The combination of extracardiac manifestations and cardiac abnormalities favors a presumptive diagnosis of sarcoidosis without biopsy. Interstitial granulomatous inflammation initially produces diastolic dysfunction and later may produce systolic abnormalities. Localized thinning and dilatation of the basilar left ventricle, resembling ischemic heart disease, are characteristic. Restrictive cardiomyopathy is uncommon; more often, sarcoid pulmonary involvement produces pulmonary hypertension and right heart failure. High-grade AV block and ventricular arrhythmias are principal manifestations and may result in syncope and sudden cardiac death. The electrocardiogram most commonly demonstrates T-wave and conduction abnormalities; with extensive myocardial involvement, pseudoinfarct patterns may appear. Thallium 201 and gallium 67 have been used to indicate areas of myocardial involvement and are used to predict the response to corticosteroids. MRI may detect sarcoid granulomata or scar. Endomyocardial biopsy is useful but, because of sampling error, may be falsely negative. Treatment with prednisone is warranted in highly suspicious or proven cases.

Gaucher's disease is due to an inherited deficiency of β-glucocerebroside, which results in accumulation of cerebroside in the reticuloendothelial system, brain, and heart. Diffuse interstitial infiltration of the left ventricle occurs, leading to reduced LV compliance and decreased cardiac output, but it is often subclinical. Ventricular and valvular thickening and pericardial effusion are seen on echocardiography.

STORAGE DISEASES

Myocardial iron deposition in hemochromatosis usually produces dilated cardiomyopathy, but it may cause restrictive cardiomyopathy. Congestive heart failure, arrhythmia, and conduction disturbances are common. Interstitial fibrosis is variable and unrelated to the extent of iron deposition, which is deposited within the myocyte; secondarily, myocardial fibrosis may develop. Findings consistent with either dilated or restrictive cardiomyopathy may be seen. Granular sparkling and atrial enlargement may be observed but are nonspecific signs. CT and MRI may demonstrate subclinical cardiac involvement, and tissue characterization may be possible with MRI. Endomyocardial biopsy is confirmatory. Repeated phlebotomy is recommended for primary hemochromatosis, and the chelating agent desferrioxamine is often beneficial in secondary hemochromatosis. Cardiac transplantation (with or without liver transplantation) may be considered in selected cases.

Fabry's disease is characterized by glycolipid accumulation in the myocardium as well as the vascular and valvular endothelium and may present with a restrictive, hypertrophic, or dilated cardiomyopathy, mitral regurgitation, ischemic heart disease, or aortic degeneration. Definitive diagnosis may require endomyocardial biopsy.

Pompe's disease is due to an autosomal recessive deficiency of acid maltase that causes glycogen deposition in the heart and skeletal muscles. The echocardiographic manifestations may be indistinguishable from hypertrophic obstructive cardiomyopathy. The diagnosis can be made by skeletal muscle biopsy.

ENDOMYOCARDIAL OBLITERATIVE DISEASES

Endomyocardial diseases that cause obliterative cardiomyopathy include endomyocardial fibrosis (EMF) and hypereosinophilic (Loeffler's) syndrome (Table 32-3). Endomyocardial disease is characterized by endocardial fibrosis of the apex and subvalvular regions of one or both ventricles, resulting in restriction to inflow to the affected ventricle. Although their clinical presentations differ, the pathology and therefore the cardiac imaging studies are generally similar in the endomyocardial diseases. Echocardiography reveals apical obliteration of the ventricles, apical thrombus, echodensities in the endocardium, and small ventricular and large atrial cavities. Involvement of the posterior mitral and tricuspid valve leaflets results in mitral and tricuspid regurgitation; less commonly, restricted motion may produce stenosis. Sparing of the outflow tracts is characteristic. Typical patterns of restriction, mitral and tricuspid regurgitation, and, less often, stenosis are seen on Doppler. Not surprisingly, the location, extent, and severity of involvement determine the clinical picture.

Medical therapy of Loeffler's is often ineffective and frustrating. Treatment consists of symptomatic relief, anticoagulants, corticosteroids, and hydroxyurea for myocarditis and palliative surgery in the late, fibrotic stage. Surgical excision of fibrotic endocardium and valve replacement may offer symptomatic improvement, but at the expense of high operative mortality. The prognosis of advanced disease is grim (50 percent 2-year mortality) but is considerably better in those with milder disease.

NONOBLITERATIVE ENDOMYOCARDIAL DISEASES

Carcinoid syndrome results from metastatic carcinoid tumors and consists of cutaneous flushing, diarrhea, and bronchoconstriction; involvement of the heart occurs as a late complication of carcinoid syndrome in approximately 50 percent of patients. Although tricuspid and pulmonic stenosis and regurgitation dominate the clinical picture, restrictive cardiomyopathy may occur.

Infiltrating tumors of the heart are generally metastatic and rarely produce restriction to ventricular filling unless the pericardium is

TABLE 32-3

ENDOMYOCARDIAL OBLITERATIVE DISEASE—ENDOMYOCARDIAL FIBROSIS (EMF) VERSUS HYPEREOSINOPHILIC (LOEFFLER'S) SYNDROME

	EMF	Loeffler's
Distribution	Worldwide; 10–20% of cardiac-related deaths in equatorial Africa	Temperate climates
Gender predilection	None; affects children and young adults	Primarily affects males
Etiology	Endemic form associated with high levels of cerium and low levels of magnesium	Parasitic infections, leukemia, and immunologic reactions
Onset	Insidious	Rapid
Course	Indolent	Aggressive and rapidly progressive; 50% two-year mortality in advanced cases
Cardiac involvement	Biventricular in only 50% of cases; atrial fibrillation common	Biventricular in majority of cases; Thromboembolic phenomena; >1500 eosinophils/mL

involved. Infiltration on echocardiography is suggested by a localized increase in wall thickness, often associated with abnormal wall motion and pericardial effusion.

Pericardial disease frequently complicates radiation therapy to the chest and may produce constrictive pericarditis; however, endo- and myocardial involvement may produce restrictive cardiomyopathy, at times presenting years after radiation therapy has been completed. Anthracyclines and methysergide can cause endomyocardial fibrosis. A restrictive pattern of LV filling is common soon after orthotopic cardiac transplantation and may persist for at least a year.

SUGGESTED READING

Arbustini E, Morbini P, Grasso M, et al: Restrictive cardiomyopathy, atrioventricular block and mild to subclinical myopathy in patients with desmin-immunoreactive material deposits. *J Am Coll Cardiol* 1998; 31(3):645–653.

Dabestani A, Child J, Henze E, et al: Primary hemochromatosis: Anatomic and physiologic characteristics of the cardiac ventricles and their response to phlebotomy. *Am J Cardiol* 1984; 54:153–159.

Hoit BD: Restrictive, obliterative, and infiltrative cardiomyopathies. In: Fuster V, Alexander RW, O'Rourke RA, et al (eds): *Hurst's The Heart,* 10th ed. New York: McGraw-Hill; 2001:1989–2000.

Kyle RA: Amyloidosis. *Circulation.* 1995; 91:1269–1271.

Olsen E, Spry C: Relation between eosinophilia and endomyocardial disease. *Prog Cardiovasc Dis* 1985; 27:241–254.

WHO/ISFC Task Force: Definition and classification of cardiomyopathies. *Br Heart J* 1980; 44:672–673.

33

INFLAMMATORY CARDIOMYOPATHIES— ENDOCRINE DISEASE AND ALCOHOL

Donna M. Mancini
Ainat Beniaminovitz

The diagnosis of cardiomyopathy encompasses a wide spectrum of diseases, with divergent pathogenic mechanisms; which have as their final common pathway the syndrome of congestive heart failure (CHF). These heart muscle diseases may be primary or secondary— i.e., resulting from specific cardiac or systemic disorders. Etiologies associated with the development of cardiomyopathy are listed in Table 33-1. (Hypertrophic cardiomyopathies and those due to coronary artery or valvular disease are not discussed.) Endomyocardial biopsy is generally a low-yield procedure; however, in this group of diseases, it can be diagnostic (Table 33-2).

MYOCARDITIS

Myocardial dysfunction from viral myocarditis may result from viral injury, immunologic responses initiated by the virus, or apoptotic cell death. Multiple infectious etiologies (Table 33-1) can cause myocarditis, the most common being viral, specifically, coxsackie B virus. The clinical manifestations of myocarditis are variable. The majority of patients are asymptomatic, as cardiac dysfunction is subclinical and self-limited. However, other patients present in cardiogenic shock. Antecedent flu-like symptoms occur in 60 percent of patients. Chest pain occurs in 35 percent of patients and may be typically anginal, atypical, or pericardial in character. Sudden death, syncope, and palpitations are other presentations. Complete atrioventricular (AV) block is common and generally transient; it rarely requires a permanent pacemaker. Sudden cardiac death can result from

TABLE 33-1
CAUSES OF MYOCARDITIS

Disease	Etiologies	Comment
Infectious myocarditis Viral	Viruses Coxsackie virus, echovirus, HIV, Epstein-Barr virus, influenza, cytomegalovirus, adenovirus, Hepatitis (A and B), mumps, poliovirus, rabies, respiratory synctyial virus, rubella, vaccinia, varicella zoster, arbovirus	The most common etiology of infectious myocarditis in North America is viral infection by coxsackie- or echoviruses. Most episodes are self-limited and asymptomatic. In patients with symptoms of congestive heart failure (CHF), acute and chronic viral titers are needed along with endomyocardial biopsy to confirm the diagnosis. In South America, the most common cause of myocarditis is Chagas' disease, caused by the bite of the reduviid bug carrying the parasite *Trypanosoma cruzi*
Bacterial	Bacteria *Corynebacterium diphtheriae, Streptococcus pyogenes, Staphylococcus aureus, Haemophilus pneumoniae, Salmonella* spp., *Neisseria gonorrhoeae*, leptospirosis, Lyme disease, syphilis, brucellosis, tuberculosis, actinomycosis, *Chlamydia* spp. *Coxiella burnetii, Mycoplasma pneumoniae, Rickettsia* spp.	

Fungal	Fungi	
		Candida spp. *Aspergillus* spp. histoplasmosis, blastomycosis, cryptococcosis, coccidioidomycosis
Parasitic	Parasites	
		Toxoplasmosis, schistosomiasis, trichinosis
Dilated cardiomyopathy	Unknown	May represent prior undiagnosed episode of myocarditis, untreated hypertension, or occult alcohol use.
Infiltrative	Amyloid	Myocardial inflammation may be present on biopsy. Routine and special stains are extremely valuable in confirming these diagnoses.
	Sarcoid	
	Hemochromatosis	
	Carcinoid syndrome	
	Hypereosinophilic (Loeffler's) heart disease	
	Glycogen storage disease	

(continued)

561

TABLE 33-1
(Continued)

Disease	Etiologies	Comment
Hypersensitivity/ Eosinophilic	*Antibiotics* Sulfonamides, penicillins, cefaclor, chloramphenicol, amphotericin B, tetracycline, streptomycin *Antituberculous drugs* Isoniazid, para-aminosalicylic acid *Anticonvulsants* Phenindione, phenytoin, carbamazepine, phenobarbital *Antidepressants* Amitriptyline, desipramine *Anti-inflammatories* Indomethcin, phenylbutazone, oxyphenylbutazone *Diuretics* Acetazolamide, chlorthalidone, hydrochlorothiazide, spironolactone *Others* Methyldopa, sulphonylureas, interleukin-2, interleukin-4, tetanus toxoid	Treatment is discontinuation of the offending agent with or without steroids. Potentially reversible.

Toxins	Cocaine, cyclophosphamide, emetine, lithium, methysergide, phenothiazines, interferon-alpha, interleukin-2, doxorubicin, cobalt, lead, chloroquine, hydrocarbons, carbon monoxide, anabolic steroids	Potentially reversible for some toxins.
Radiation	Past history of lymphoma	
Giant-cell myocarditis	Unknown	Generally a fulminant disease with a high mortality. May recur after transplant.
Postpartum cardiomyopathy	Unknown	CHF onset in last trimester or first 5 months after delivery in patient with no structural heart disease or known cause of CHF.
Genetic	Fabry disease, Kearns-Sayre syndrome, right ventricular dysplasia	Patients with right ventricular dysplasia present with ventricular arrhythmias.
Endocrine	Hypothyroidism, hyperthyroidism, pheochromocytoma, acromegaly, diabetes	
Metabolic	Hypocalcemia, hypophosphatemia, uremia, carnitine	

TABLE 33-2

DISEASES DIAGNOSED BY ENDOMYOCARDIAL BIOPSY

1. Myocarditis
   Giant-cell arteritis
   Cytomegalovirus infection
   Toxoplasmosis
   Chagas' disease
   Rheumatic fever
   Lyme disease
2. Infiltrative cardiomyopathy
   Amyloid
   Sarcoid
   Hemochromatosis
   Carcinoid
   Hypereosinophilic cardiomyopathy
   Glycogen storage disease
   Cardiac tumors
3. Toxins
   Doxorubicin
   Chloroquine
   Radiation injury
4. Genetic conditions
   Fabry disease
   Kearns-Sayre syndrome
   Right ventricular dysplasia

complete heart block or ventricular tachycardia. Systemic or pulmonary thromboembolic disease can also be seen.

Physical findings include fever, tachycardia, and signs of CHF. The first heart sound may be soft and a summation gallop may be present. An apical systolic murmur of functional mitral regurgitation may be auscultated. A pericardial friction rub can be heard. Laboratory findings are generally nondiagnostic. Some 60 percent of patients will have an elevated erythrocyte sedimentation rate (ESR) and 25 percent an elevated white blood cell (WBC) count. Elevated titers to cardiotropic viruses may be present. A fourfold rise in IgG titer over a 4- to 6-week period is required to document acute infection. Increase in the MB band of CPK is observed in 12 percent of patients and elevated troponin levels in 32 percent of patients. The electrocardiogram (ECG) frequently shows sinus tachycardia. Diffuse ST-T-wave changes, a prolonged QT interval, low voltage, an acute infarct pattern, and conduction delays also occur. Echocardiography can reveal left ventricular systolic dysfunction in patients with a normal-sized left ventricular cavity. Segmental wall motion abnormalities may be observed. Wall thickness may be increased early in the disease, when inflammation is fulminant. Ventricular thrombi are seen in 15 percent of those studied. Endomyocardial biopsy confirms the diagnosis. As myocarditis can be focal, four to six fragments are obtained to reduce sampling error to <5 percent. Active myocarditis is defined pathologically as an inflammatory infiltrate with myocyte necrosis. Endomyocardial biopsy must be applied quickly to maximize the diagnostic yield. Resolution of myocarditis can occur within 4 days of initial biopsy.

Approximately 40 percent of patients with acute myocarditis fully recover. The prognosis depends somewhat on the causative agent, but if clinical CHF develops, 5-year mortality rates are 50 to 60 percent. Predictors of recovery include the degree of left ventricular dysfunction at presentation, shorter duration of disease, and less intensive conventional drug therapy. A recent study suggests that patients with "fulminant" myocarditis—defined as rapid onset of symptoms, fever, and severe hemodynamic compromise—have a better survival than patients with acute nonfulminant myocarditis.

The Multicenter Myocarditis Treatment Trial randomized patients with biopsy-proven myocarditis between conventional medical therapy versus steroid/azathioprine or steroid/cyclosporine immunosuppression. The primary endpoint was change in ejection fraction. For all patients. the average increase in ejection fraction over baseline was 9 percent. Treatment assignment was not predictive of improvement in left ventricular ejection fraction, attenuation of clinical disease, or mortality. The IMAC trial (Intervention in Myocarditis and Acute Cardiomyopathy with Immune Globulin) used a single infusion of high-dose immunoglobulin (2 g/kg) to treat presumed inflammatory cardiomyopathies. Improvement in left ventricular ejection fraction and symptoms were similar in both groups. Thus no benefit of immunomodulation has been demonstrated in randomized trials. Standard CHF treatment remains the mainstay of therapy in acute myocarditis.

Human Immunodeficiency Virus

Human immunodeficiency virus (HIV) is increasingly recognized as a cause for dilated cardiomyopathy. This cardiomyopathy may result from infection of myocardial cells with HIV, coinfection with other viruses, post-viral autoimmune response, or cardiotoxicity from illicit drugs or therapy. Asymptomatic HIV-positive patients develop cardiomyopathy with an annualized incidence of 16 cases per 1000 patients. A CD4 count <400 cells per milliliter predisposes to the development of cardiomyopathy. As the symptoms of CHF and HIV can be similar (fatigue and wasting), careful follow-up is needed to detect left ventricular dysfunction in these patients.

Chagas' Disease

American trypanosomiasis, or Chagas' disease, is the most common cause of CHF in the world and is endemic to rural South and Central America. It results from the bite of the reduviid bug, leading to infection with *Trypanosoma cruzi*. In the acute phase, hematogenous spread of the parasite is accompanied by an intense inflammatory reaction. Patients experience fever, sweating, and myalgias. Most patients recover from the acute illness and enter an asymptomatic latent phase. Twenty to 30 percent of patients develop chronic disease up to 20 years after the initial infection. The gastrointestinal tract and the heart are the most commonly involved sites, with cardiac disease the primary cause of death. In the gut, destruction of the myenteric plexus leads to megaesophagus and megacolon. In the heart, fibrosis of the myofibrils and Purkinje fibers leads to cardiomegaly, CHF, heart block, and arrhythmia. Parasites are found in about a quarter of the patients on endomyocardial biopsy. The acute disease is diagnosed with the discovery of trypomastigotes in the blood. Xenodiagnosis and the complement-fixation test (Machado-Guerreiro test) are the most reliable diagnostic tests for chronic disease. Noninvasive assessment shows segmental wall motion abnormalities—specifically apical aneurysms. ECG findings include complete heart block, atrioventricular block, or right bundle branch block with or without fascicular block. The treatment of chronic Chagas' disease includes a pacemaker for complete heart block, an implantable cardioverter/defibrillator for recurrent ventricular arrhythmia, and standard therapy for CHF. Antiparasitic agents such as nifurtimox and benzimidazole eradicate parasitemia during the acute phase and are curative. They should be administered if the disease has not been treated and may be used as prophylaxis if there is a high likelihood of recurrence. Heart transplantation is effective for end-stage cardiac disease.

Lyme Carditis

Lyme disease may result from infection with the spirochete *Borrelia burgdorferi,* introduced by a tick bite. The initial presenting symptom in patients who progress to cardiac involvement is frequently complete heart block. Left ventricular dysfunction may be seen but is unusual. Endomyocardial biopsy may show active myocarditis and rarely spirochetes. Tetracycline and corticosteroid administration are the indicated treatments.

Rheumatic Carditis

The incidence of rheumatic myocarditis has declined dramatically in the United States but remains high in developing countries. Rheumatic fever follows a group A streptococcal pharyngitis. Clinical diagnosis is made using the Jones criteria. The major manifestations are carditis, polyarthritis, chorea, erythema marginatum, subcutaneous nodules, and evidence of preceding streptococcal infection. Minor criteria are nonspecific findings such as fever, arthralgia, previous rheumatic fever or rheumatic heart disease, elevated ESR or C-reactive protein, and prolonged PR interval. Two major criteria or one major and two minor criteria are needed for diagnosis. Sixty-seven percent of patients present with a pharyngitis followed by symptoms in 1 to 5 weeks (mean, 19 days). Severe carditis resulting in death is unusual. CHF is generally mild and is observed in 5 to 10 percent of cases. The physical examination is notable for fever and heart murmurs. The mitral valve is involved three times as often as the aortic valve; therefore mitral murmurs are more common. ECG findings include PR prolongation and nonspecific ST-T-wave changes. Endomyocardial biopsy demonstrates the pathognomonic Aschoff nodules. Laboratory tests suggestive of rheumatic fever include antibodies to antistreptolysin O and anti-DNAase B, an elevated ESR, and C-reactive protein. Aspirin and penicillin are the mainstays of therapy. Corticosteriods can provide symptomatic relief. Once the condition has been diagnosed, antibiotic prophylaxis using monthly injections of 1.2 million units of benzathine penicillin G is recommended until age 21.

NONINFECTIVE MYOCARDITIS

Hypersensitivity myocarditis due to an allergic reaction to drugs (Table 33-1) is characterized by peripheral eosinophilia and infiltration into the myocardium of eosinophils, multinucleated giant cells, and leukocytes. Resolution is reported with stopping of the offending agent and treatment with corticosteroids. Unfortunately, the presence of this condition often goes unnoticed, with the initial manifestation being sudden death.

Giant-Cell Myocarditis

Giant-cell myocarditis is a rare form of myocarditis. This disease is most prevalent in young adults with a mean age at onset of 42 years. Association with other autoimmune disorders occurs in 20 percent of cases. Diagnosis is made by endomyocardial biopsy. Widespread or multifocal necrosis with a mixed inflammatory infiltrate including lymphocytes and histiocytes is required for histologic diagnosis.

Eosinophils are often seen, as are multinucleated giant cells, in the absence of granuloma. The clinical course is characterized by progressive CHF and is often associated with refractory ventricular arrhythmia. It is almost uniformly and rapidly fatal. Rare reports of response to immunosuppressive regimens have been described. Cardiac transplant is the best treatment option, though most patients expire prior to identification of a donor. Giant-cell myocarditis may recur following transplant, but the frequency of recurrence is unknown.

Peripartum Cardiomyopathy

Peripartum cardiomyopathy has a reported incidence varying from 1 in 1300 to 1 in 15,000 pregnancies. Predisposing factors include black race, age >30 years, obesity, cesarean delivery, multiple gestations, preeclampsia, and chronic hypertension. Patients present with CHF in the last trimester of pregnancy or in the first 5 months postpartum. Absence of a demonstrable cause of CHF and structural heart disease is required to make the diagnosis. Proposed mechanisms include myocarditis due to a viral illness or autoimmune etiology, nutritional deficiencies, genetic disorders, hormonal imbalances, volume overload, alcohol, physiologic stress of pregnancy, or unmasking of latent idiopathic dilated cardiomyopathy. The presentation is that of CHF, syncope, sudden death, or thromboembolic phenomena. Physical findings include S_3, S_4, tricuspid, or mitral insufficiency murmurs, edema, rales, ascites, hepatomegaly, and jugular venous distention. The ECG frequently shows left ventricular hypertrophy. Echocardiographic findings can range from single- to four-chamber dilatation. In a small percentage of patients, endomyocardial biopsy may reveal myocarditis, but generally the findings are nonspecific. Serial echocardiograms have been used to predict prognosis. Patients with higher ejection fractions and smaller ventricular diastolic dimensions at the time of diagnosis have a better long-term prognosis. If the congestive cardiomyopathy persists for more than 6 months, it is likely to be irreversible and to be associated with a worse prognosis. Due to the high incidence of thromboembolism, anticoagulation is recommended. Patients referred for transplant have an excellent survival posttransplant. Patients with stable heart failure or those who have recovered are high risk for recurrence in subsequent pregnancies. Counsel on birth control and even sterilization is indicated.

INFILTRATIVE CARDIOMYOPATHIES

Amyloidosis

The most common infiltrative cardiomyopathy (see Table 33-1) is amyloidosis. Primary amyloidosis results from an overproduction of a monoclonal immunoglobulin protein, which deposits throughout the body. Secondary amyloidosis results from deposition of a protein other than immunoglobulin and is always associated with a chronic disease. The frequency of cardiac involvement varies with the different etiologies. With primary amyloidosis, 33 to 50 percent of patients have cardiac involvement and >25 percent have symptomatic CHF. Cardiac involvement in patients with secondary amyloidosis is less frequent. Familial amyloidosis occurs in 4 percent of cases; however, cardiomyopathy is present in 68 percent of those affected. Senile cardiac amyloidosis is common in the elderly but does not lead to CHF. The rigid amyloid fibrils lead to relaxation abnormalities and diastolic dysfunction; however, when myocardial replacement occurs, systolic dysfunction becomes prominent. The clinical presentation is predominately that of right-sided CHF. Sudden death and myocardial infarction may result from vascular involvement. Atrial arrhythmias are common. Diagnosis is made by characteristic echocardiographic features and endomyocardial biopsy. Echocardiography demonstrates symmetrical thickening of the left ventricular wall with a diffuse hyper-refractile, granular, sparkling appearance of the myocardium. The ECG typically demonstrates low voltage despite marked hypertrophy on echocardiography. A pseudoinfarct anterior wall pattern is often present. The majority of patients with CHF have a monoclonal protein spike in the serum or urine, reflecting the primary nature of the disease. Amyloid is detected on endomyocardial biopsy using Congo red staining. Prognosis is poor and treatment ineffective. Five-year survival is <5 percent. Cardiac transplant is not recommended due to recurrence in the transplanted heart.

Sarcoidosis

Sarcoidosis is a systemic granulomatous disease of unknown etiology characterized by enhanced cellular immune responses. The pathologic hallmark of this disease is the noncaseating granuloma. Less than 10 percent of patients with sarcoid have cardiac symptoms; however, cardiac involvement is more common than recognized. Frequently the initial presentation is sudden death. Because of the varied extent and location of the myocardial granulomas, presenting signs and symptoms range from first-degree heart block to fulminant CHF. Heart failure can present as a cardiomyopathy with restrictive hemodynamics or systolic dysfunction. Some 25 percent of the deaths due to cardiac sarcoid are from CHF and 33 to 50 percent from sudden cardiac death. In diagnosing cardiac sarcoid, evidence of other organ system involvement is sought. In cases where the heart is predominantly involved, little or no evidence of extracardiac sarcoidosis may be found. CXR, ECG, and echocardiography findings depend on the extent and location of involvement. Due to the scattered nature of the granulomas, endomyocardial biopsy lacks sensitivity and seldom makes the diagnosis despite high specificity. Magnetic resonance imaging is useful in diagnosing myocardial lesions due to sarcoid. While no controlled trials have been performed, high-dose corticosteroids are usually given. Corticosteroids can improve cardiac symptoms and reverse ECG changes in >50 percent of treated patients. Antiarrhythmic drugs are used as necessary, although drug therapy of ventricular tachycardia, even when guided with programmed ventricular stimulation, is associated with a high rate of arrhythmia recurrence or sudden death in these patients. Automatic internal cardioverter/defibrillators have been advocated. Prognosis after the diagnosis of cardiac sarcoid is poor, with survival of 41 percent at 5 years. Transplantation is a successful treatment, as the recurrence of sarcoid in the allograft is low.

Hemochromatosis

Primary hemochromatosis is an inborn error of metabolism leading to iron deposition in a variety of organs including the heart. Both restrictive and dilated presentations can occur. Treatment with phlebotomy is highly effective. In secondary forms of hemochromatosis due to multiple blood transfusions for blood dyscrasias, chelation therapy is highly effective. Diagnosis is made by symptom constellation in the presence of an elevated serum iron and ferritin. Endomyocardial biopsy is diagnostic.

Carcinoid

Carcinoid heart disease typically leads to a restrictive pattern and often has asymmetrical involvement due to the predilection of carcinoid for the tricuspid valve apparatus. Diagnosis is generally made with right-sided heart findings and systemic features of carcinoid syndrome. Cardiac involvement responds to control of the tumor with chemotherapy or catheter embolization. Tricuspid valve replacement and/or pulmonary valvulotomy and outflow tract enlargement have been recommended when hemodynamically indicated. Alternatively, balloon valvuloplasty for tricuspid or pulmonary stenoses has been used successfully.

Eosinophilic Heart Disease

Hypereosinophilic syndromes (Loeffler's disease) are characterized by peripheral eosinophilia and endocardial disease with eosinophilic infiltration, fibrosis, and eventual occlusion of the ventricular cavity by scar and thrombus. This leads to severe restrictive disease known as *obliterative myocardial disease*. It is an immunologic disorder caused by clones of abnormal eosinophils infiltrating the heart. It occurs primarily in men in their forties from temperate climates. Diffuse organ involvement may be observed (lungs, bone marrow, brain), with cardiac involvement in >75 percent of patients. Clinical presentation includes weight loss, fever, cough, skin rash, and CHF. Overt CHF occurs in 50 percent of patients and is the leading cause of death. Echocardiography demonstrates localized thickening of the left ventricle with valvular leaflet abnormalities and atrial enlargement. In advanced endomyocardial fibrosis, there may be apical obliteration by thrombus but normal systolic function. Diagnosis is by endomyocardial biopsy and echocardiogram. Early therapy with corticosteroids and cytotoxic drugs may substantially improve survival. Surgical therapy offers palliation once the later fibrotic stages have been reached.

CARDIOMYOPATHY DUE TO ENDOCRINE DISORDERS

Myocardial dysfunction can occur with several endocrine disorders. Cardiomyopathy can be caused by thyroid deficiency or excess. Thyroid hormone metabolism is frequently abnormal in patients with CHF. Low T3 levels may be an adaptive mechanism to decreased catabolism. Thyroid hormone replacement increases cardiac output, decreases peripheral vascular resistance, and improves exercise performance. Thyroid toxicity can lead to the development of both high- and low-output CHF. Prolonged tachycardia and the high-output state caused by thyrotoxicosis can produce left ventricular dilatation with a consequent decline in systolic function. This process can be reversed by reduction of excess hormone levels.

Hypertension and its sequelae are the major cardiovascular manifestations of pheochromocytoma. However, a specific catecholamine-induced myocarditis and/or cardiomyopathy has been reported. Although progression to cardiac involvement is unusual, pheochromocytoma patients typically die of cardiovascular causes, most commonly CHF or malignant ventricular arrhythmias. Hemodynamic stabilization is obtained with alpha and beta blockers and prompt adrenalectomy. Reversibility of the impaired cardiac function occurs with tumor resection.

Acromegalic cardiomyopathy may be a specific entity or simply secondary to the hypertension or atherosclerosis associated with this condition. Some 10 to 20 percent of patients with acromegaly develop CHF, which is difficult to treat due to the higher collagen content of the acromegalic heart. Surgery and irradiation are the mainstays of therapy, but often the cardiopathic manifestations persist despite a fall in growth hormone levels.

Analysis of the Framingham data showed that the risk of developing CHF was increased fivefold among diabetic patients. This increased incidence suggests that the metabolic abnormalities associated with diabetes may contribute to myocyte dysfunction and produce a diabetes-induced cardiomyopathy. Typically, interstitial fibrosis and arteriolar hyalinization are present. Both systolic and diastolic dysfunction can occur; the severity of the dysfunction is related to the degree of metabolic control.

TOXINS: ALCOHOLIC CARDIOMYOPATHY

Chronic alcohol abuse accounts for up to 45 percent of all dilated cardiomyopathies. Cardiac damage results from direct toxic effect of alcohol or its metabolites in addition to nutritional deficiencies, sympathetic stimulation, or coexistent hypertension. The disease occurs most frequently in males between 30 and 55 years of age with a >10-year history of heavy alcohol use. The disease is extremely rare in premenopausal women. Presenting symptoms include dyspnea on exertion, orthopnea, paroxysmal nocturnal dyspnea, fatigue, weakness, arrhythmias, and embolic phenomena. Atrial fibrillation is common. Sudden death can be the initial presentation. ECG findings include first-degree heart block, left ventricular hypertrophy, nonspecific interventricular conduction defects, bundle branch blocks, and prolongation of the QT interval. The echocardiogram frequently shows left ventricular hypertrophy, single- to four-chamber enlargement, and mural thrombi. Histologic changes observed on endomyocardial biopsies are not pathognomonic. The mainstay of treatment is abstinence from alcohol. In early stages of the disease, 91 percent of patients who become abstinent after diagnosis are alive at 42 months, versus 43 percent of those who continue to drink. Cessation of alcohol is no longer effective in reversing the disease in the later stages, when structural histologic abnormalities have occurred.

Cocaine

Myocardial ischemia, infarction, coronary spasm, cardiac arrhythmias, sudden death, myocarditis, and dilated cardiomyopathy are all reported cardiovascular complications of cocaine abuse. By blocking the reuptake of norepinephrine, cocaine induces tachycardia, vasoconstriction, hypertension, cardiomyopathy, and ventricular arrhythmias. Cardiomyopathy may then result from secondary changes in the heart due to tachycardia or sustained increased ventricular afterload or from a direct toxic effect. The risk and manifestations of toxicity in any given individual are unpredictable. The duration or amount of cocaine use does not predict disease. There are no clinical or histologic features specific for cocaine-induced myocardial damage. Treatment is nonspecific and focuses on abstinence and heart failure therapy.

Chemotherapeutic Agents

Several chemotherapeutic agents can cause cardiomyopathy. The anthracyclines (doxorubicin) and cyclophosphamide are the most common agents associated with CHF. Doxorubicin has been used for the treatment of many different tumors. Its cardiotoxicity may be due to increased oxidative stress from the generation of free radicals by this drug. Early or late cardiotoxicity can occur. Risk factors for the development of doxorubicin cardiomyopathy include age >70 years, combination chemotherapy, mediastinal irradiation, prior cardiac disease, hypertension, and liver disease. The early cardiotoxicity manifests as a pericarditis-myocarditis syndrome and is not dose-related. Left ventricular dysfunction is rarely seen, but arrhythmias, abnormalities of conduction, decreased QRS voltage, and nonspecific ST-segment and T-wave abnormalities are observed in 40 percent of patients. The prognosis is good with quick resolution with the discontinuation of therapy. In contrast, the late cardiotoxicity is due to a dose-dependent degenerative cardiomyopathy. This syndrome occurs at doses >550 mg/m^2. Serial assessment of ejection fractions is useful to monitor for toxicity. However, histopathologic grading delineates best the safety of continued doxorubicin administration. Cardiotoxicity may occur during therapy, within a year of the last dose or up to 10 years after cessation of chemotherapy. Therefore this chemotherapy commits patients to prolonged cardiac surveillance. Prognosis depends on the severity at time of presentation, but overall the mortality is high. The best management of anthracycline cardiotoxicity is prevention. Heart failure due to doxorubicin is typically refractory to conventional therapy. Diminished symptoms and improved left ventricular function have been described in patients on beta blockers.

In contrast to anthracyclines, cyclophosphamide leads to an acute cardiotoxicity that is not dose-related. Pericarditis, systolic dysfunction, arrhythmias, and myocardial edema can occur. Prior left ventricular dysfunction is a risk factor for the development of cardiomyopathy. Mortality is not trivial, but survivors regain normal cardiac function.

IDIOPATHIC CARDIOMYOPATHY

The term *idiopathic cardiomyopathy* describes a group of myocardial diseases of unknown cause. Idiopathic dilated cardiomyopathy probably represents the end result of a number of disease processes that lead to myocyte dysfunction, loss, hypertrophy, and fibrosis. It is a diagnosis of exclusion. Surreptitious alcohol use and undiagnosed and untreated hypertension represent other etiologies of cardiomyopathy in many of these cases. The incidence of IDC has been estimated at 0.005 to 0.006 percent, increasing with age and male gender. Mortality for untreated cardiomyopathy approaches 50 percent at 5 years.

SUGGESTED READING

Cooper LT, Berry GJ, Shabetai R: Idiopathic giant-cell myocarditis—Natural history and treatment. *N Engl J Med* 1997; 336:1860–1866.

Dec GW, Palacios IF, Fallon JT, et al: Active myocarditis in the spectrum of acute dilated cardiomyopathies: Clinical features, histologic correlates, and clinical outcomes. *N Engl J Med* 1985; 312:885–890.

Felker G, Thompson R, Hare J, et al: Underlying causes and long term survival in patients with initially unexplained cardiomyopathy. *N Engl J Med* 2000; 342:2001–2032.

Grogan M, Redfield M, Bailey K, et al: Long term outcome of patients with biopsy proved myocarditis: Comparison with idiopathic dilated cardiomyopathy. *J Am Coll Cardiol* 1995; 26:80–84.

Mancini DM, Beniaminovitz A: Myocarditis and specific cardiomyopathies—endocrine disease and alcohol. In: Fuster V, Alexander RW, O'Rourke RA, et al (eds): *Hurst's The Heart*, 10th ed. New York: McGraw-Hill; 2001: 2001–2032.

Mason JW, O'Connell JB, Herskowitz A, et al: A clinical trial of immunosuppressive therapy for myocarditis. *N Engl J Med* 1995; 333:269–275.

McCarthy R, Boehmer J, Hruban R, et al: Long-term outcome of fulminant myocarditis as compared with acute (nonfulminant) myocarditis. *N Engl J Med* 2000; 342:690–695.

THE HEART AND NONCARDIAC DRUGS, ELECTRICITY, POISONS, AND RADIATION

Andrew L. Smith

This chapter deals with the effects on the heart of a variety of non-cardiac drugs, electricity, poisons, and radiation.

NONCARDIAC DRUGS

Chemotherapeutic Agents

Chemotherapeutic agents may cause acute or chronic cardiovascular toxicity. Cardiomyopathy has generally been associated with the anthracyclines (doxorubicin, daunorubicin, epirubicin, idarubicin, mitoxantrone). Cyclophosphamide has been associated with reversible systolic dysfunction and occasionally hemorrhagic myocarditis. Interleukin-2 and interferon alpha may cause hypotension and rarely cardiomyopathy. 5-Fluorouracil has been associated with coronary vasospasm. Amsacrine and paclitaxel have been associated with cardiac arrhythmias. Herceptin, given in combination with doxorubicin, may cause systolic dysfunction.

ANTHRACYCLINES

Doxorubicin (Adriamycin) and daunorubicin (Cerubidine) cause dose-related cardiotoxicity possibly related to free-radical damage. The majority of cases of chemotherapy-related heart disease result from these agents. Acute cardiac toxicity may occur after the initial doses, and chronic cardiotoxicity occurs within months of therapy. Additionally, late cardiac toxicity with systolic dysfunction occurring years later is becoming increasingly recognized. Diffuse left ventricular dysfunction (cardiomyopathy) occurs in up to 7 percent of patients receiving 550 mg/m^2 of doxorubicin. Toxicity is less with newer dosing schedules, which incorporate prolonged infusions in order to avoid high peak concentrations. Once cardiomyopathy develops, treatment strategies are similar to those with other forms of systolic dysfunction. Further cardiac toxins are to be avoided. The clinical course varies from fulminant heart failure to gradually progressive deterioration. In some patients, systolic dysfunction is reversible. Serial echocardiography is of only moderate sensitivity and specificity in detecting cardiotoxicity during therapy. Endomyocardial biopsy provides more definitive detection, but it is not widely used clinically. Dexrazoxane, an iron-chelating agent, is approved as a preventive strategy in women with breast cancer after cumulative doses of doxorubicin of greater than 300 mg/m^2. Herceptin, a new treatment for metastatic breast cancer, when used in combination with doxorubicin and paclitaxel, is associated with heart failure in up to 30 percent of patients.

Psychotropic Agents

TRICYCLIC ANTIDEPRESSANTS

Tricyclic antidepressants have potentially serious cardiovascular effects, including tachycardia, orthostatic hypotension, ECG changes, and depression of ventricular function. These drugs have electrophysiologic properties similar to those of the type IA antiarrhythmics. These drugs are contraindicated in the recovery phase following myocardial infarction. While they may be indicated in the treatment of severely depressed patients, the threshold for use should rise as the severity of heart disease increases or when there is QT prolongation.

Tricyclic antidepressant overdose is lethal in approximately 2 percent of patients and is generally related to cardiac complications. Initial clinical status and initial serum drug levels are not predictive of prognosis. QRS prolongation is a sign of toxicity but is an insensitive finding. Gastric lavage, repeat dosing of activated charcoal, and sodium bicarbonate therapy are appropriate treatment strategies. Type I antiarrhythmics should not be used for cardiac rhythm disturbances. Sodium bicarbonate is the initial therapy for ventricular dysrhythmias. Hypotension refractory to volume loading and bicarbonate therapy should be treated with vasopressors such as norepinephrine, phenylephrine, or vasopressor doses of dopamine.

OTHER ANTIDEPRESSANTS

The selective serotonin reuptake inhibitors (SSRIs) have rarely been associated with orthostatic hypotension and bradycardia. These drugs may affect the cytochrome P450 system and interfere with other cardiovascular drugs. Case reports of cardiac toxicity are rare.

The monoamine oxidase (MAO) inhibitors have little effect on cardiac conduction or myocardial contractility. Orthostatic hypotension is common. The major concern with these agents is interaction with tyramine-containing substances, resulting in hypertensive crisis.

Lithium may suppress automaticity, particularly of the sinus node. Electrocardiographic changes may simulate hypokalemia, including T-wave inversion, prominent U waves, and QT prolongation. Overdose with lithium may result in severe bradycardia. A low anion gap suggests the presence of lithium toxicity. Phenothiazine antipsychotic agents, including chlorpromazine (Thorazine) and thioridazine (Mellaril), can produce tachycardia, postural hypotension, T-wave changes, QT prolongation, and bundle branch block. Sudden death, presumed to be due to cardiac arrhythmia, has occurred.

Noncardiac Drugs Causing Torsades de Pointes

Torsades de pointes has been associated with tricyclic antidepressants, tetracyclic antidepressants, phenothiazines, haloperidol, chloral hydrate, and probucol. Other implicated drugs include erythromycin, trimethoprim-sulfamethoxazole, terfenadine, astemizole, cisapride, and pentamidine.

Methylxanthines and Beta-Adrenergic Agonists

Caffeine, theophylline, and terbutaline may cause sinus tachycardia and thus exacerbate the tendency for cardiac arrhythmias. Controversy exists over the safety of long-term use of these agents in patients with cardiovascular disease.

Ergotamine, Methysergide, and Sumatriptan

These drugs are commonly used to treat migraine headaches. Ergotamine and methysergide have similar chemical structures. Valvular heart disease has been reported with both agents. Pericardial, pleural, or retroperitoneal fibrosis may occur. Methysergide is more strongly associated with regurgitant valvular lesions. Therapy should be discontinued if a new murmur is detected. Regression of valvular lesions may occur, although valve replacement is occasionally required. Ergotamine is a vasoconstrictor and may induce coronary artery spasm. Sumatriptan, a selective serotonin type I agonist, may cause coronary vasospasm and should not be taken with ergotamine-like medications. These medications are generally contraindicated in patients with obstructive coronary disease.

Chloroquine

Chloroquine and hydroxychloroquine can cause skeletal and rarely heart muscle disease. When cardiac involvement occurs, features of restrictive cardiomyopathy are most common. Acute chloroquine poisoning results in hypotension, tachycardia, and prolongation of the QRS; it is often fatal.

Weight-Loss Medications

Dexfenfluramine and the combination of fenfluramine and phentermine were in the past prescribed for weight loss in obese patients, but dexfenfluramine and fenfluramine were withdrawn from the market in 1997, when valvular regurgitation was noted. Recent reports suggest an incidence of valvular regurgitation in approximately 7 percent of dexfenfluramine-treated patients versus 2 to 5 percent of controls. Mild aortic regurgitation is the most common finding. Abnormalities often improve with cessation of therapy.

Oral Contraceptive Agents

The cardiovascular risk profile of newer-generation oral contraceptive agents is favorable. Thrombosis resulting in myocardial infarction or deep venous thrombosis may occur; the risk is significantly increased in smokers. Hypertension is rare. The risk of stroke in otherwise healthy women is only minimally increased. Women who use oral contraceptives should be advised to avoid smoking.

Anabolic Steroids

Illicit use of androgens is a problem in competitive athletes and body builders. Data on human toxicity is limited. Stanozolol and nandrolone have been associated with marked lipid abnormalities and an increase in coronary atherosclerosis. These agents may also cause left ventricular hypertrophy and hypertension.

Cocaine

The cardiovascular complications of cocaine use include sudden death, acute myocardial infarction, accelerated atherosclerosis, dilated cardiomyopathy, acute reversible myocarditis, acute severe hypertension, acute aortic dissection, and stroke. Endocarditis may result from intravenous drug use. Electrocardiographic abnormalities include sinus tachycardia, premature ventricular contractions (PVCs), ventricular tachycardia, torsades de pointes, prolongation of the QT interval, diffuse ST-segment changes, and ventricular fibrillation.

Chest pain is the most common reason for cocaine users to seek medical attention. The evaluation of cocaine-related chest pain is difficult. Approximately 6 percent of patients presenting to emergency departments with cocaine-related chest pain have myocardial infarction. These patients are often young men without other risk factors for coronary artery disease except tobacco smoking. The quality or duration of the chest discomfort is often not predictive of infarction. Because young patients often have early repolarization patterns on the electrocardiogram (ECG), ST-segment elevation in leads V_1 to V_3 may be confused with acute infarction. Patients may require cardiac monitoring for 6 to 12 h, until enzymes have excluded infarction.

Treatment strategies for cocaine-induced myocardial ischemia have been developed based on the known cardiac and nervous system toxicity of this agent. Patients presenting with anxiety, tachycardia, and/or hypertension may respond well to benzodiazepines. Nitroglycerin may reverse coronary vasoconstriction induced by cocaine. Aspirin may prevent thrombus formation. Patients not responding to these measures may benefit from phentolamine or from calcium channel blocker therapy with verapamil. Beta-adrenergic antagonists should generally be avoided due to unopposed alpha-mediated vasoconstriction. Combined alpha and beta blockade with labetalol has been used to treat tachyarrhythmias but is not an accepted therapy for myocardial ischemia. In documented cocaine-related myocardial infarction, thrombolytic therapy is highly effective. However, emergency coronary angiography may be necessary to distinguish patients with acute infarction from those with ST-segment elevation due to early repolarization. Cocaine-related cardiac rhythm disturbances are best managed initially with benzodiazepines. Intravenous sodium bicarbonate and magnesium may be beneficial. Lidocaine should be used cautiously because of concerns of lower seizure threshold. Beta blockade with propanolol or esmolol should be avoided.

ELECTRICITY

Environmental Accidents

The immediate cardiac effect of injury due to lightning or electrical equipment may be asystole or ventricular fibrillation. Cardiac arrest may also result from apnea and hypoxia. Atrial and ventricular arrhythmias, conduction abnormalities, and left ventricular dysfunction may occur. Cardiac abnormalities occur from direct myocardial injury or central nervous system injury, with intense catecholamine release. Hypertension and tachycardia may be managed with beta-blocking agents.

Cardiopulmonary resuscitation should be continued for a prolonged period after apparent death from lightning, since late recovery may occur. In lightning strikes involving multiple victims, attention should first be directed to those who are "apparently dead," since lightning victims with vital signs generally survive without immediate medical attention and those without vital signs may recover after prolonged resuscitation.

Electroconvulsive Therapy

Electroconvulsive therapy (ECT) may produce cardiac arrhythmias and ECG changes during the first few minutes after the shock. ECT produces brief, intense stimulation of the central nervous system. Cardiovascular complications may result from this stimulation or from the drugs used to modify the response. Patients with coronary artery disease should be pretreated with a beta blocker to blunt tachycardia and hypertension and to reduce the frequency of ventricular ectopic beats. Patients with cardiac pacemakers can safely undergo ECT.

POISONS

Plants

A variety of plants contain poisonous substances, some of which produce cardiac effects similar to those of digitalis. Others can produce myocardial depression, cardiac arrhythmias, hypotension, circulatory collapse, and death. Plants with cardiac glycoside effects include foxglove, oleander, lily-of-the-valley, Christmas rose, wallflower, and milkweed.

Herbal Therapies

The use of herbal and nonprescription remedies is common among cardiac patients. Aconite prolongs the QT interval. *Ephedra equisetina,* or Ma-huang, may cause hypertension, arrhythmias, and myocardial infarction. Garlic and ginger may potentiate warfarin. Gingko causes decreased platelet activity. Hawthorne may cause hypotension at high doses.

Snake and Scorpion Venoms

Snake venoms affect the coagulation system, cellular components of the blood, endothelium, nervous system, and heart. Cardiac arrhythmias, severe hypotension, and cardiac arrest may occur. Multiple pulmonary emboli may be seen in patients who survive 12 h or longer. Scorpion venom may cause hypertension, myocardial infarction, arrhythmias, conduction disturbances, and myocarditis.

Marine Toxins

Scorpion fish cause envenomation that may result in rhythm disturbances and heart failure. Ingestion of pufferfish may cause severe bradycardia and cardiovascular collapse. Stingray venom contains phosphodiesterases and rarely may cause cardiac rhythm disturbances.

Halogenated Hydrocarbons

These substances are used in fire extinguishers, solvents, refrigerants, pesticides, and plastics, paints, and glues. They can suppress myocardial contractility and produce arrhythmias and sudden death.

Carbon Monoxide

Carbon monoxide poisoning produces myocardial ischemia usually manifest by ST-segment and T-wave changes and atrial and ventricular arrhythmias. Extensive myocardial necrosis and cardiomyopathy can occur.

RADIATION

Radiation to the mediastinum can affect the pericardium, myocardium, endocardium, valves, and capillaries of the heart. Radiation may cause acute pericarditis, chronic pericarditis, and pericardial constriction. Pericardial involvement is most frequent 4 to 6 months after radiation therapy.

Clinically important myocardial dysfunction related to radiation generally occurs in combination with pericardial disease. Myocardial fibrosis may result in diastolic dysfunction and, less commonly, systolic dysfunction. Radiation-induced valvular heart disease is rare but usually involves the aortic or mitral valves. Premature coronary artery disease may occur years after radiation therapy.

Radiation may result in fibrosis of the nodal and infranodal pathways. Right bundle branch block is especially common; complete heart block is rare.

SUGGESTED READING

Arsenian MA: Cardiovascular sequelae of therapeutic thoracic radiation. *Prog Cardiovasc Dis* 1991; 33:299–311.

Carleton SC: Cardiac problems associated with electrical injury. *Cardiol Clin* 1995; 13:263–277.

Ernst E: Harmless herbs? A review of the recent literature. *Am J Med* 1998; 104:170–178.

Feenstra J, Grobbee DE, Remme WJ, Stricker BH: Drug induced heart failure. *J Am Coll Cardiol* 1999; 33:1152–1162.

Frishman WH, Sung HM, Yee HCM, et al: Cardiovascular toxicity with cancer chemotherapy. *Curr Probl Cardiol* 1996; 21:225–288.

Glassman AH, Roose SP, Bigger JT: The safety of tricyclic antidepressants in cardiac patients—risk benefit reconsidered. *JAMA* 1993; 269:2673–2675.

Jain S, Bandi V: Electrical and lightning injuries. *Crit Care Clin* 1999; 15:319–331.

Kloner RA, Hale S, Alker Rezkalla S: The effects of acute and chronic cocaine use on the heart. *Circulation* 1992; 85:407–419.

Rosenberg L, Begaud B, Bergan U, et al: What are the risks of third generation oral contraceptives? *Hum Reprod* 1996; 11:687–693.

Shan K, Lincoff AM, Young JB: Anthracycline-induced cardiomyopathy. *Ann Intern Med* 1996; 125:47–58.

Shively BK, Roldan CA, Gill EA, et al: Prevalence and determinants of valvulopathy in patients treated with dexfenfluramine. *Circulation* 1999; 100:2161–2167.

Smith AL, Book WM: Effect of noncardiac drugs, electricity, poisons, and radiation on the heart. In: Fuster V, Alexander RW, O'Rourke RA, et al (eds): *Hurst's The Heart,* 10th ed. New York: McGraw-Hill; 2001:2045–2058.

VanDenBrink AM, Reekers M, Bax W, et al: Coronary side-effect potential of current and prospective antimigraine drugs. *Circulation* 1998; 98:25–30.

35

DISEASES OF THE PERICARDIUM

Joseph M. Restivo
Brian D. Hoit

The pericardium consists of an inner visceral and an outer parietal layer, between which is a potential space, the pericardial cavity. Despite serving many important functions (Table 35-1), the pericardium is not essential for life and no adverse consequences follow either congenital absence or surgical removal of the pericardium. In view of its simple structure, clinicopathologic processes involving the pericardium are understandably few; indeed, pericardial heart disease comprises only pericarditis and its complications (tamponade and constriction) and congenital lesions. Nevertheless, the pericardium is affected by virtually every category of disease (Table 35-2).

ACUTE PERICARDITIS

Acute fibrinous or dry pericarditis is a syndrome characterized by typical chest pain, a pericardial friction rub, and specific electrocardiographic (ECG) changes. Findings on the history and physical examination are summarized in Fig. 35-1; it should be emphasized that the quality, severity, and location of pain vary greatly.

The ECG may either confirm the clinical suspicion of pericardial disease or first alert the clinician to the presence of pericarditis. Serial tracings may be needed to distinguish the ST-segment elevations caused by acute pericarditis from those caused by acute myocardial infarction (MI) or normal early repolarization. The ST-T-wave changes in acute pericarditis are diffuse and have characteristic evolutionary changes (Table 35-3).

The chest radiograph may reveal an enlarged cardiac silhouette because of a moderate or large pericardial effusion and may provide evidence of the underlying etiology. Echocardiography estimates the volume of pericardial fluid (however, the patient with purely fibrinous acute pericarditis often has a normal echocardiogram), identifies cardiac tamponade, suggests the basis of pericarditis, and

---

TABLE 35-1

FUNCTIONS OF THE PERICARDIUM

Mechanical
 Effects on chambers
  Limits short-term cardiac distention
  Facilitates cardiac chamber coupling and interaction
  Maintains pressure-volume relation of the cardiac
   chambers and output from them
  Maintains geometry of left ventricle
 Effects on whole heart
  Lubricates, minimizes friction
  Equalizes gravitation, inertial, hydrostatic forces
  Mechanical barrier to infection
Immunologic
Vasomotor
Fibrinolytic
Modulation of myocyte structure, function, and gene
 expression
Vehicle for drug delivery and gene therapy

documents associated acute myocarditis. Nonspecific blood markers of inflammation usually increase in cases of acute pericarditis, and serum cardiac isoenzymes may increase with extensive epicarditis.

Hospitalization is warranted for most patients who present with an initial episode of acute pericarditis in order to determine the etiology and to observe for the development of cardiac tamponade. Acute pericarditis usually responds to oral nonsteroidal antiinflammatory agents. Indomethacin reduces coronary blood flow and should be avoided. Addition of colchicine is effective for the acute episode and may prevent recurrences. The intensity of therapy is dictated by the distress of the patient; narcotics may be required for severe pain. Some cases necessitate high doses of steroids for a week to control pain, with the dosage tapered rapidly thereafter. Corticosteroids should be avoided unless there is a specific indication, as they enhance viral multiplication and may produce recurrences when the dosage is tapered. Nevertheless, corticosteroids are useful in acute pericarditis associated with uremic pericarditis and connective tissue diseases. Painful recurrences of pericarditis may respond to nonsteroidal anti-inflammatory agents but commonly require

TABLE 35-2

CAUSES OF PERICARDIAL HEART DISEASE

Idiopathic
Infectious
   Bacterial
   Viral
   Mycobacterial
   Fungal
   Protozoal
   AIDS-associated
Neoplastic
   Primary
   Secondary (breast, lung, melanoma, lymphoma, leukemia)
Immune/Inflammatory
   Connective tissue diseases (rheumatoid arthritis, systemic
      lupus erythematosus, scleroderma, acute rheumatic
      fever, dermatomyositis, mixed connective tissue
      disease, Wegener's granulomatosis)
   Arteritis (temporal arteritis, polyarteritis nodosa,
      Takayasu's arteritis)
   Acute myocardial infarction (MI) and post-MI (Dressler's
      syndrome)
   Postcardiotomy
   Posttraumatic
Metabolic
   Nephrogenic
   Aortic dissection
   Myxedema
   Amyloidosis
Iatrogenic
   Radiation injury
   Instrument/device trauma (implantable defibrillator,
      pacemakers, catheters)
   Drugs (hydralazine, procainamide, daunorubicin,
      isoniazid, anticoagulants, cyclosporine, methysergide,
      phenytoin, dantrolene, mesalazine)
   Cardiac resuscitation
Traumatic
   Blunt trauma
   Penetrating trauma
   Surgical trauma
Congenital
   Pericardial cysts
   Congenital absence of pericardium
   Mulibrey nanism

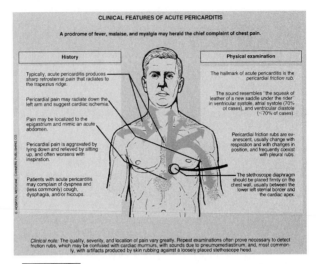

FIGURE 35-1
Clinical features of acute pericarditis: history and physical examination. (From Hoit BD: Acute pericarditis: Diagnosis and differential diagnosis. *Hosp Pract* 1991; 27:23–43, with permission.)

corticosteroids. Prednisone is begun at a high dose, but rapid tapering should be initiated within a few days of clinical resolution. Using the lowest possible dose, alternate-day therapy, combinations with non-steroidal drugs, or colchicine should minimize the risks of long-term steroids. Pericardiectomy should be considered only when repeated attempts at medical treatment have clearly failed, especially when there is evidence of steroid-induced complications.

PERICARDIAL EFFUSION

Accumulation of transudate, exudate, or blood in the pericardial sac is a frequent complication of pericardial disease and should be sought in all patients with acute pericarditis. Chronic effusive pericarditis may be associated with large, asymptomatic effusions. Transudative effusions (hydropericardium) occur in heart failure and other states associated with chronic salt and water retention, and exudative effusions occur in a large number of the infectious and inflammatory types of pericarditis. Although frank hemorrhagic

TABLE 35-3

ELECTROCARDIOGRAPHIC CHANGES IN ACUTE PERICARDITIS

Stage	Time Course	ECG Changes
1	ST-segment elevation occurs within hours of onset of chest pain and may persist for days	Upward concave ST-segment elevations usually not exceeding 5 mm; PR-segment depression (except aVR)
2	Hours to days following stage one	ST segments return to baseline; T waves normal or show loss of amplitude
3	T-wave inversions may persist indefinitely (especially when associated with TB, uremia, or neoplasm)	T-wave inversions
4	Usually completed within 2 weeks, but variability common	ECG normalizes

effusions suggest recent intrapericardial bleeding, sanguineous and serosanguineous effusions occur in many infectious and inflammatory disorders. Chylous pericarditis implies injury or obstruction to the thoracic duct, and cholesterol pericarditis is either idiopathic or associated with hypothyroidism, rheumatoid arthritis, or tuberculosis.

Echocardiography is the procedure of choice for the diagnosis of pericardial effusion. Computed tomography and magnetic resonance imaging may be useful to identify loculated or atypically loculated pericardial effusions and to characterize the nature of the effusion.

Drainage of a pericardial effusion is usually unnecessary unless either purulent pericarditis is suspected or cardiac tamponade supervenes, although on occasion pericardiocentesis is needed to establish the etiology of a hemodynamically insignificant pericardial effusion. Persistent or progressive effusion, particularly when the cause is uncertain, also warrants pericardiocentesis.

CARDIAC TAMPONADE

Cardiac tamponade is a hemodynamic condition characterized by equal elevation of atrial pericardial pressures, an exaggerated inspiratory decrease in arterial systolic pressure (pulsus paradoxus), and arterial hypotension. Although the absolute intracardiac pressures are elevated, the transmural pressures are practically zero or even negative. The greatly reduced preload is responsible for the fall in cardiac output, and when compensatory mechanisms are exhausted, arterial pressure decreases.

Cardiac tamponade may be acute or chronic and should be viewed hemodynamically as a continuum, ranging from mild (pericardial pressure less than 10 mmHg) to severe (pericardial pressure greater than 20 mmHg). Mild cardiac tamponade is frequently asymptomatic, whereas moderate and especially severe tamponade produces precordial discomfort and dyspnea. Both the severity of cardiac tamponade and the time course of its development dictate symptoms and physical findings. Careful inspection of the jugular venous pulse waveform is essential for the diagnosis; compression of the heart by pericardial fluid results in a characteristic loss of the venous Y descent. An inspiratory decline of systolic arterial pressure exceeding 10 mmHg defines pulsus paradoxus, a phenomenon with complex and multifactorial origins. However, in the presence of coexisting left ventricular disease, atrial septal defects, or aortic insufficiency, pulsus paradoxus may not develop. Nevertheless, in the appropriate clinical setting, pulsus paradoxus is a key finding signifying cardiac tamponade.

Low voltage on the ECG and/or electrical alternans should raise the suspicion of cardiac tamponade; unless even a brief delay might prove life threatening, an echocardiogram should be obtained. During inspiration, greater than normal increases in right ventricular dimensions and decreases in left ventricular dimensions occur in many cases of tamponade. These respiratory changes also accompany other conditions associated with pulsus paradoxus, such as chronic obstructive lung disease and pulmonary embolism. Diastolic collapse of the right ventricle and right atrium, which reflects negative transmural pressure, is useful but neither sensitive nor specific as a marker for tamponade. Exaggerated respiratory variation in transvalvular and venous velocities measured by Doppler echocardiography (flow velocity pulsus paradoxus) also helps diagnose cardiac tamponade.

The pericardial, right atrial, pulmonary capillary wedge, and pulmonary artery diastolic pressures are elevated and equal; the degree of elevation is related to both the severity of tamponade and the patient's intravascular volume status. The right atrial and wedge pressure tracings reveal an attenuated or absent Y descent. Cardiac output is reduced and systemic vascular resistance is elevated.

Removal of small amounts of pericardial fluid (~50 mL) produces considerable symptomatic and hemodynamic improvement because of the steep pericardial pressure-volume relation. Unless there is concomitant cardiac disease or coexisting constriction, removal of all of the pericardial fluid normalizes pericardial, atrial, ventricular diastolic and arterial pressures, and cardiac output. Although pericardiocentesis may provide effective relief and has relatively simple logistic and personnel requirements, *surgical drainage* offers several advantages. These include complete drainage, access to pericardial tissue for histopathologic and microbiological diagnoses, the ability to drain loculated effusions, and the avoidance of the risk of traumatic injury due to blind placement of a needle into the pericardial sac. The choice between needle pericardiocentesis and surgical drainage depends upon institutional resources and physician experience, the etiology of the effusion, the need for diagnostic tissue samples, and the patient's prognosis. Irrespective of the method of retrieval, pericardial fluid should be sent for smear, culture, and cytology. Repeat pericardiocentesis, sclerotherapy with tetracycline, surgical creation of a pericardial window, or pericardiectomy may treat recurrent effusions. A pericardial window is usually placed in patients with malignant effusions, and pericardiectomy may be required for recurrent effusions in dialysis patients. In critically ill patients, a pericardial window may be created percutaneously with a balloon catheter.

CONSTRICTIVE PERICARDITIS

Constrictive pericarditis is a condition in which a thickened, scarred, and often calcified pericardium limits diastolic filling of the ventricles. Although acute pericarditis from most causes may eventuate in constrictive pericarditis, the most common antecedents are idiopathic, cardiac trauma and surgery, tuberculosis and other infectious diseases, neoplasms, radiation therapy, renal failure, and connective tissue diseases.

Constrictive pericarditis resembles the congestive states due to myocardial disease and chronic liver disease. Patients generally complain of fatigue, dyspnea, weight gain, abdominal discomfort, nausea, and increased abdominal girth. Physical findings include ascites, hepatosplenomegaly, edema, and wasting; often these lead to an erroneous diagnosis of hepatic cirrhosis. Misdiagnosis is avoided by a careful examination of the neck veins—the venous pressure is elevated and displays deep Y and often deep X descents, and it fails to decrease with inspiration (Kussmaul's sign). Kussmaul's sign lacks specificity, as it is seen also in cases of restrictive cardiomyopathy, right ventricular failure and infarction, and tricuspid stenosis. A pericardial knock, similar in timing to the third heart sound, is pathognomonic but occurs infrequently. Pulsus paradoxus may occur with associated pericardial effusion (effusive-constrictive pericarditis).

Low QRS voltage and nonspecific P and T wave changes are common; atrial fibrillation is seen in approximately one-third of cases and atrial flutter less often. The cardiac silhouette may be normal or enlarged, and pericardial calcification is present in less than half of the cases. Pericardial thickening and calcification and abnormal ventricular filling produce characteristic but insensitive and nonspecific changes on the M-mode echocardiogram; these reflect abnormal filling of the ventricles. However, a normal study virtually rules out the diagnosis. Because of the close physiologic similarities of constrictive pericarditis and restrictive cardiomyopathy, increased pericardial thickness detected by computed tomography (CT) is the most reliable means of distinguishing between the two disorders. Accurate definition of pericardial thickness and its distribution is also possible with magnetic resonance imaging (MRI).

Cardiac catheterization is used to confirm the clinical suspicion of pericardial disease, uncover occult constriction, diagnose effusive-constrictive disease, and identify associated coronary, myocardial, and valvular disease. Endomyocardial biopsy is sometimes necessary to exclude restrictive cardiomyopathy.

Pericardiectomy is the definitive treatment for constrictive pericarditis but is unwarranted either in very early constriction or in severe, advanced disease, when the risk of surgery is excessive (30 to 40 percent mortality) and the benefits are diminished. Involvement of the visceral pericardium also increases the surgical risk. Symptomatic relief and normalization of cardiac pressures may take several months following pericardiectomy; it occurs sooner when the operation is carried out before the disease is too chronic and when the pericardiectomy is complete.

Evidence of transient (acute) constriction may occur in about 15 percent of patients with acute effusive pericarditis. Therefore, before proceeding with pericardiectomy, the possibility that pericardial constriction may be reversible and amenable to medical therapy should be considered. Constrictive pericarditis may resolve spontaneously or in response to various combinations of nonsteroidal anti-inflammatory agents, steroids, and antibiotics. Diuretics and digoxin are useful in patients who are not candidates for pericardiectomy because of their high surgical risk.

CONGENITAL PERICARDIAL HEART DISEASE

Congenital absence of the pericardium is an uncommon anomaly, usually involving a portion or the whole of the left parietal pericardium. Its presence is usually suspected from the chest radiogram and echocardiogram. Contrast-enhanced CT and MRI reliably establish the anatomy of the defect. Pericardial cysts are rare remnants of defective embryologic development and are benign; their importance lies in differentiation from neoplasm.

SUGGESTED READING

Appleton CP, Hatle LK, Popp RL: Relation of transmitral flow velocity patterns to left ventricular diastolic function: New insights from a combined hemodynamic and Doppler echocardiographic study. *J Am Coll Cardiol* 1988; 12:426–440.

Fowler NO: Constrictive pericarditis: Its history and current status. *Clin Cardiol* 1995; 18:341–350.

Fowler NO: *The Pericardium in Health and Disease.* Mt. Kisco, NY: Futura; 1985.

Hoit BD: Diseases of the pericardium. In: Fuster V, Alexander RW, O'Rourke RA, et al (eds): *Hurst's The Heart,* 10th ed. New York: McGraw-Hill; 2001:2061–2085.

Shabetai R: The pericardium: An essay on some recent developments. *Am J Cardiol* 1978; 42(6):1036–1043.

Spodick DH: *The Pericardium. A Comprehensive Textbook.* New York: Marcel Dekker; 1997.

36

Infective Endocarditis

Raja Naidu
Robert A. O'Rourke

Infective endocarditis is defined as an inflammation of the endocardium by invading microorganisms. Although the valvular surfaces are most commonly affected, other native or prosthetic cardiac structures may be involved. Before the antibiotic era, endocarditis was uniformly fatal. Previous classifications systems usually divided endocarditis according to the natural course of the disease when untreated. The clinical syndrome may be either acute or subacute in nature, depending on the causative organism, and this distinction may be useful in initiating empiric therapy. A timely diagnosis, proper identification of the etiologic agent, prompt bactericidal antibiotic treatment, recognition and management of potential complications, and appropriate surgical intervention are relevant to all cases of endocarditis.

EPIDEMIOLOGY

The spectrum of infective endocarditis continues to change. There are approximately 10,000 to 15,000 cases annually in the United States. While the incidence of endocarditis has remained relatively constant, several new features have developed. The median age of patients has increased from an average of 30 years in 1926 to over age 50. This is due to a different susceptible population. Degenerative valve disease and mitral valve prolapse have replaced rheumatic heart disease as the most common substrate for endocarditis. Moreover, the number of children with congenital heart disease surviving into adulthood has increased, owing to improved palliative and corrective surgical procedures. Common congenital lesions predisposing to endocarditis include ventricular septal defects, bicuspid aortic valves, patent ductus arteriosus, coarctation of the aorta, and tetralogy of Fallot.

The use of intravenous drugs is also associated with a high risk of endocarditis. Multiple bouts of transient bacteremia from poor sterile techniques and contaminated drug material commonly lead to right-sided valvular infections. New bioprosthetic material to correct congenital and acquired valvular disease has predisposed many patients with prosthetic heart valves to the risk of infective endocarditis. Despite differences in individual series, the risk appears similar in patients with mechanical or bioprosthetic valves. A prior history of endocarditis is an additional important risk factor.

A growing number of patients have no identifiable cardiac lesions. Most of these patients are older than 65 years of age and probably have degenerative changes that serve as a nidus for the initiation of endocarditis. Nosocomial infections due to intravenous devices and catheters as well as procedures involving the gastrointestinal and genitourinary tracts may facilitate development of the causal bacteremia in this group.

PATHOGENESIS

For endocarditis to develop, a complex interaction between the native endothelium, the host hemostatic system, and circulating microorganisms must occur (Fig. 36-1). The initial step in the development of the characteristic lesions of endocardial vegetations is injury to the endothelium. This is caused by immune complex deposition and/or turbulent blood flow due to pressure gradients or regurgitant lesions.

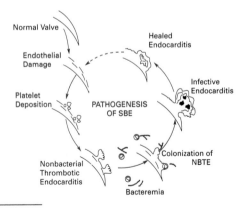

FIGURE 36-1

The main events in the pathogenesis of nonbacterial thrombotic endocarditis (NBTE) and subacute bacterial endocarditis (SBE).

Subendothelial connective tissue, composed of collagen, is exposed with endothelial damage, predisposing to a clot of platelets and fibrin. With stabilization and growth, the clot forms a vegetation of nonbacterial thrombotic endocarditis. Subsequently, this sterile vegetation becomes colonized by bacteria from a distant focal infection or from transient bacteremia. The microbes locally multiply, elude host defenses, recruit more fibrin and platelets, and a multilayered, mature infectious vegetation results.

The location and size of vegetations are important in understanding the pathogenesis of endocarditis. Endothelial damage occurs more commonly in high-pressure systems. Thus, left-sided valves are more commonly affected than right-sided ones and regurgitant lesions are more prone to infection than stenotic lesions. Vegetations also tend to occur just beyond the narrowed orifice through which high-velocity jets pass. The left ventricular surface of aortic regurgitant lesions, the left atrial chamber in mitral regurgitant lesions, and the pulmonary artery side of a patent ductus arteriosus are classic examples. Importantly, these generalizations are valid for subacute endocarditis but do not apply to most cases of acute endocarditis related to intravenous drug use (IVDU). In the latter case, the predilection for the tricuspid valve by *staphylococcus aureus* predominates. The actual size of a vegetation can vary greatly, from only several millimeters to several centimeters. Usually, right-sided lesions are larger than left-sided ones. Fungal species tend to produce larger lesions than bacteria. Rarely, vegetations may be large enough to cause valvular or vascular stenosis.

ETIOLOGY

The microbiology of infective endocarditis has undergone substantial changes in the last several decades (Table 36-1). Streptococci are the most common group of organisms causing endocarditis, accounting for more than 50 percent of cases. The *viridans* streptococci, normal inhabitants of the oropharynx and highly sensitive to penicillin, are the most common type. Although the *viridans* group are low-grade pathogens, their common association with endocarditis is secondary to their frequent presence in the bloodstream and unique adherence properties. Strains of enterococci are the next most frequent cause of endocarditis. They tend to cause a subacute infection in older men after genitourinary manipulation or in young women following an obstetric procedure. Moreover, today, they are a common cause of nosocomial endocarditis and sometimes associated with IVDU. *Streptococcus bovis* is an another common cause of endocarditis. It is particularly prevalent in elderly patients and has been associated with colonic polyps or colonic malignancy.

TABLE 36-1

FREQUENCY OF VARIOUS ORGANISMS CAUSING INFECTIVE ENDOCARDITIS[a]

Organism	NVE, %	IV Drug Abusers, %	Early PVE, %	Late PVE, %
Streptococci	60	15–25	5	35
Viridans, alpha-hemolytic	35	5–10	<5	25
Streptococcus bovis	10	<5	<5	<5
Enterococcus faecalis	10	10	<5	<5
Other streptococci	<5	<5	<5	<5
Staphylococci	25	50	50	30
Coagulase-positive	23	50	20	10
Coagulase-negative	<5	<5	30	20
Gram-negative aerobic bacilli	<5	5	20	10
Fungi	<5	<5	10	5
Miscellaneous bacteria	<5	5	5	5
Diphtheroids, propionibacteria	<1	<5	5	<5
Other anaerobes	<1	<1	<1	<1
Rickettsiae	<1	<1	<1	<1
Chlamydiae	<1	<1	<1	<1
Polymicrobial infection	<1	1–5	5	5
Culture-negative endocarditis	5–10	<5	<5	<5

[a]These are representative figures collated from the literature; wide local variations in frequency are to be expected.
KEY: NVE = native valve endocarditis; PVE = prosthetic valve endocarditis; IV = intravenous.

Staphylococcus infections are a frequent cause of endocarditis and now account for about 33 percent of cases. *Staph. aureus* is the predominant organism in cases of IVDU and prosthetic valve infection. The bacterium causes rapid local tissue destruction along with a high prevalence of local and distal complications. In left-sided lesions, the course is fulminant, with death from bacteremia after a few days and heart failure within 1 or 2 weeks. In contrast, right-sided lesions in IVDU follow a more indolent course and usually respond to intravenous antibiotics. *Staphylococcus epidermidis* rarely causes native valve endocarditis. However, it is a common cause of early prosthetic valve endocarditis (<60 days postoperatively).

Other bacteria responsible for endocarditis include gram-negative bacilli, which account for approximately 5 percent of all cases. These organisms are highly virulent and portend a poor prognosis. A subgroup of gram-negative bacilli that are slow-growing and fastidious are referred to as the HACEK group: *Haemophilus* species, *Actinobacillus, Cardiobacterium, Eikenella,* and *Kingella.* They are part of the oropharyngeal flora and produce endocarditis with subacute presentations and large vegetations. Fungal infections are a rare cause of native valve endocarditis in patients who do not use intravenous drugs. Large vegetations with frequent embolic events are characteristic of fungal endocarditis.

CLINICAL FEATURES

The presentation of infective endocarditis is quite variable (Table 36-2). Factors such as the virulence of the causative pathogen, the host immune response, and the underlying health of the patient all contribute to the clinical presentation. Certain cases may be subtle, with only nonspecific constitutional symptoms, while more acute cases present with sudden illness, heart failure, and overwhelming sepsis. Fever is present in almost all patients; the elderly and patients previously treated with antibiotics may be exceptions. Other common but nonspecific symptoms include malaise, fatigue, weight loss, anorexia, and myalgias.

In addition to the systemic features, patients with endocarditis exhibit a variety of striking physical findings related to embolic events or immunologic phenomena. Petechiae are a common physical finding and occur in the conjunctiva, buccal mucosa, and skin above the clavicle. Their presence is not a highly specific finding. Splinter hemorrhages (subungual dark, linear streaks) are caused by microembolization to small capillaries. Osler's nodes are painful, tender erythematous nodules on the pads of fingers and toes. Janeway lesions are erythematous, macular, nontender lesions on the fingers, palm, or sole. Ocular findings include Roth's spots, which are retinal

TABLE 36-2

SUMMARY OF THE MAJOR CLINICAL MANIFESTATIONS OF INFECTIVE ENDOCARDITIS

Manifestation	History	Examination	Investigations
Systemic infection	Fever, chills, rigors, sweats, malaise, weakness, lethargy, delirium, headache, anorexia, weight loss, backache, arthralgia, myalgia Portal of entry: oropharynx, skin, urinary tract, drug addiction nosocomial bacteremia	Fever, pallor, weight loss, asthenia, splenomegaly	Anemia, leukocytosis (variable), raised erythrocyte sedimentation rate, positive blood culture, abnormal cerebrospinal fluid
Intravascular lesion	Dyspnea, chest pain, focal weakness, stroke, abdominal pain, cold and painful extremities	Murmurs, signs of cardiac failure, petechiae (skin, eye, mucosae), Roth's spots, Osler's nodes, Janeway lesions, splinter hemorrhages, stroke, mycotic aneurysm, ischemia or infarction of viscera or extremities	Blood in urine, chest roentgenogram, echocardiography, arteriography, liver-spleen scan, lung scan, brain scan, CT scan, histology, culture of emboli
Immunologic reactions	Arthralgia, myalgia, tenosynovitis	Arthritis, signs of uremia, vascular phenomena, finger clubbing	Proteinuria, hematuria, casts, uremia, acidosis, polyclonal increases in gamma globulins, rheumatoid factor, decreased complement, immune complexes in serum, antistaphylococcal teichoic acid antibodies

hemorrhages with a white or yellow center. Although microembolic findings are helpful in the diagnosis of infective endocarditis, larger emboli may cause infarctions in the brain, lung, or gastrointestinal tract.

The localized intracardiac infection of endocarditis produces heart murmurs in more than 90 percent of patients. The triad of fever, bacteremia, and murmur should alert the physician to the possibility of infective endocarditis. Regurgitant murmurs from chordal rupture, valve perforation, or other valvular damage predominate. The most commonly associated murmurs are those of mitral, aortic, or tricuspid regurgitation.

LABORATORY FINDINGS

Diagnosis of infective endocarditis is dependent on isolation of an etiologic agent from blood cultures. Bacteria from vegetations are discharged at a relatively constant rate and thus produce a continuous bacteremia. A single blood culture is likely to demonstrate the organism. However, to maximize the diagnostic yield, it is generally recommended to draw three sets of blood cultures 1 h apart. Even with the most stringent collection and advanced culture techniques 5 to 10 percent of infective endocarditis cases will have negative blood cultures. While fastidious organisms must be considered as the cause, prior antibiotic treatment is a more common explanation. Serologic tests and environmental exposure may help identify rare cases of endocarditis caused by *Coxiella burnetii* (Q fever), *Brucella*, *Bartonella*, or *Chlamydia*.

Other laboratory findings common with endocarditis include a normochromic, normocytic anemia consistent with anemia of chronic disease. Leukocytosis with a leftward shift is seen in acute bacteria endocarditis, while a normal white blood cell count is characteristic of subacute bacterial endocarditis (SBE). Nonspecific inflammatory markers such as the erythrocyte sedimentation rate (ESR) or C-reactive protein are elevated in 90 percent of cases. Normalization of these markers may provide useful evidence of antibiotic success.

An electrocardiogram should be obtained at admission for all patients with suspected endocarditis and repeated according to the treatment response. Prolongation of the PR interval may indicate extension of the infection into the conduction system, focal myocarditis, or a ring abscess. Chest radiographs are important in the hemodyanmic assessment of endocarditis. They can provide early evidence of congestive heart failure and chamber enlargement. Moreover, in certain cases of tricuspid valve endocarditis, multiple small, patchy infiltrates often suggest septic pulmonary emboli.

ECHOCARDIOGRAPHY

Transthoracic two-dimensional images along with color-flow Doppler provide information concerning the presence and location of vegetations, the amount of regurgitation present, global left ventricular function, and the detection of complications such as valvular perforation or abscesses. Today, with meticulous examination, transthoracic echocardiography (TTE) has 60 to 75 percent sensitivity for the detection of valvular vegetations. Usually vegetations larger than 5 mm in diameter are reliably detected by TTE, while those smaller than 3 mm are often missed.

The transesophageal approach provides improved visualization of the cardiac valves, especially posterior cardiac structures such as the mitral valve. Transesophageal echocardiography (TEE) improves the rate of vegetation detection to 90 percent. Small vegetations of 1 to 1.5 mm can be readily detected by TEE. Transesophageal studies also improve the sensitivity for detecting prosthetic valve endocarditis, valvular perforation, and abscesses.

In general, most patients suspected of having endocarditis should have multiple blood cultures and a TTE. If the TTE is of

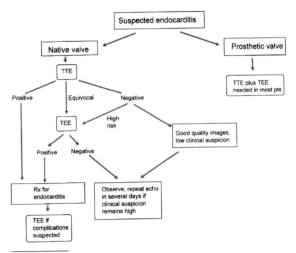

FIGURE 36-2

Flowchart for the role of echocardiography in the diagnosis of endocarditis. TEE, transesophageal echocardiography; TTE, transthoracic echocardiography. (From Otto CM: *Valvular Heart Disease*. Philadelphia: Saunders; 1999: 429, with permission.)

limited quality or equivocal, further study with a TEE is mandated (Fig. 36-2).

The role of cardiac catheterization in endocarditis is mainly limited to patients being considered for surgical intervention. It is important to delineate the coronary anatomy in all patients >35 years of age to rule out concomitant coronary artery disease. Catheterization can also be used to better clarify the hemodynamic severity of valvular lesions, detect any fistulous communications, and define the aortic root anatomy. Fluoroscopy is an excellent method to detect prosthetic valve dysfunction. A rocking motion of the valve may indicate valvular dehiscence, while a frozen leaflet may signal the presence of vegetation.

DIAGNOSTIC CRITERIA

The high variability and nonspecific clinical manifestations of endocarditis can make the diagnosis challenging. The application of strict diagnostic criteria can improve the sensitivity and specificity for the diagnosis of endocarditis. The Duke University Endocarditis Service recently developed clinical criteria that incorporated echocardiography with previously important diagnostic parameters such as persistent bacteremia, new regurgitant murmurs, and vascular complications (Tables 36-3 and 36-4).

TREATMENT

Once the diagnosis of infective endocarditis is suspected or diagnosed, appropriate treatment involves the proper selection of antimicrobial therapy along with prompt surgical intervention when needed. Antimicrobial therapy should be administered in doses assuring high bactericidal serum concentrations throughout the dosing interval. The cure of endocarditis requires complete sterilization of the vegetation; thus, bacteriostatic antibiotics should be avoided. Synergistic combinations are favored for certain pathogens. The duration of treatment required to sterilize the vegetation varies depending on the etiologic organism, the valve affected, and the antibiotic regimen. Most cases of endocarditis require 6 weeks of parental antibiotics. However, certain cases of endocarditis due to penicillin-susceptible *Strep. viridans* and right-sided endocarditis resulting from *Staph. aureus* can be cured in 2 to 4 weeks.

Acute bacterial endocarditis (ABE), because of its fulminant nature, usually requires treatment prior to the isolation of an organism. Delay of treatment until culture results are available can have deleterious consequences. Conversely, there is less clinical urgency for antimicrobial therapy in subacute forms of endocarditis. Prompt

TABLE 36-3

CRITERIA FOR DIAGNOSIS OF INFECTIVE ENDOCARDITIS

Definite Infective Endocarditis

PATHOLOGIC CRITERIA

Microorganisms: demonstrated by culture or histology in a vegetation, or in a vegetation that has embolized, or in an intracardiac abscess, *or*

Pathologic lesions: Vegetation or intracardiac abscess present, confirmed by histology showing active endocarditis

CLINICAL CRITERIA, USING SPECIFIC DEFINITIONS LISTED IN TABLE 36-8

Two major criteria, *or*
One major and three minor criteria, *or*
Five minor criteria

Possible Infective Endocarditis

Findings consistent with infective endocarditis that fall short of "definite," but not "rejected"

Rejected

Firm alternate diagnosis for manifestations of endocarditis, *or*

Resolution of manifestations of endocarditis, with antibiotic therapy for 4 days or less, *or*

No pathologic evidence of infective endocarditis at surgery or autopsy after antibiotic therapy for 4 days or less

SOURCE: From Durack et al., with permission.

treatment of SBE should be balanced against the benefit of isolating a specific organism. Common empiric treatment regimens are detailed in Table 36-5. Specific antimicrobial regimens are listed in Table 36-6.

COMPLICATIONS

Congestive heart failure (CHF) is the most important complication associated with infective endocarditis and has the greatest impact on prognosis. It tends to occur more frequently with aortic regurgitation

TABLE 36-4

DEFINITIONS OF TERMINOLOGY USED IN THE DIAGNOSTIC CRITERIA FOR ENDOCARDITIS

Major Criteria

POSITIVE BLOOD CULTURE FOR INFECTIVE ENDOCARDITIS

Typical microorganism for infective endocarditis from two separate blood cultures: viridans streptococci,[a] *Strep. bovis*, HACEK group, or community-acquired *Staph. aureus* or enterococci, in the absence of a primary focus, *or*

Persistently positive blood culture, defined as recovery of a microorganism consistent with infective endocarditis from

1. Blood cultures drawn more than 12 h apart *or*
2. All of three or a majority of four or more separate blood cultures, with first and last drawn at least 1 h apart

EVIDENCE OF ENDOCARDIAL INVOLVEMENT

Positive echocardiogram for infective endocarditis

1. Oscillating intracardiac mass, on valve or supporting structures, or in the path of regurgitant jet or on implanted material, in the absence of an alternative anatomic explanation, *or*
2. Abscess, *or*
3. New partial dehiscence of prosthetic valve, *or*
   New valvular regurgitation (increase or change in preexisting murmur not sufficient)

Minor Criteria

- Predisposition: predisposing heart condition *or* intravenous drug use
- Fever: $\geq 38.0°C$ (100.4°F)
- Vascular phenomena: major arterial emboli, septic pulmonary infarcts, mycotic aneurysm, intracranial hemorrhage, conjunctival hemorrhages, Janeway lesions
- Immunologic phenomena: glomerulonephritis, Osler's nodes, Roth's spots, rheumatoid factor
- Microbiologic evidence: positive blood culture but not meeting major criterion as previously defined[b] *or* serologic evidence of active infection with oganism consistent with infective endocarditis[c]
- Echocardiogram: consistent with infective endocarditis but not meeting major criterion as previously defined

[a] Including nutritional variant strains.

[b] Excluding single positive cultures for coagulase-negative staphylococci or organisms that do not cause endocarditis.

[c] Positive serologies for *Coxiella* or *Bartonella* may be considered major criteria.

KEY: HACEK = *Haemophilus* spp., *Actinobacillus actinomycetemcomitans*, *Cardiobacterium hominis*, *Eikenella* spp., and *Kingella kingae*.

SOURCE: Adapted from Durack et al., with permission.

TABLE 36-5
EMPIRIC TREATMENT REGIMENS

	Common Organisms	Antibiotics
Native valve endocarditis (NVE)	Viridans streptococci, enterococci, staphylococci	Nafcillin 2 gm IV q 4 h plus ampicillin 2 gm IV q 4 h plus gentamicin 1 mg/kg IV q 8 h
Right-sided endocarditis in IVDU	Staph. aureus	Nafcillin 2 gm IV q 4 h plus gentamicin 1 mg/kg IV q 8 h
Early prosthetic valve endocarditis (<60 d)	Staphylococci	Vancomycin 1 gm IV q 12 h plus gentamicin 1 mg/kg IV q 8 h
Late prosthetic valve endocarditis (>60 d)	Same as NVE	Similar to NVE

KEY: IVDU = intravenous drug use.

(30 percent) than in mitral valve disease (20 percent). The onset may be acute, due to a fulminant infection with valvular destruction, or it may take a more insidious form of progressively worsening valvular regurgitation and left ventricular dysfunction. Valvular perforations, rupture of infected chordae, or perivalvular abscess formation can all precipitate heart failure. Acute CHF mandates prompt surgical treatment. Delaying surgery to extend antibiotic treatment greatly increases perioperative mortality and the risk of permanent ventricular dysfunction.

Systemic embolization is another serious complication of endocarditis. It occurs in 25 to 50 percent of cases. Common sites of major emboli include the central nervous system, lungs, spleen, bowel, extremities, and coronary arteries. The highest rate of embolic complications is associated with *Staph. aureus* and *Candida* infections. Several studies have also shown that vegetations >1 cm in diameter have a higher embolic rate. The rate of embolization drops significantly after the first week of effective antibiotic therapy. However, failure of a vegetation to stabilize or diminish in size can predict future embolic events. Surgical therapy should be considered for recurrent major embolic events despite adequate antimicrobial therapy.

Extension of infective endocarditis beyond the valve annulus predicts a significantly higher risk of mortality and is an indication for surgical intervention. Perivalvular aortic abscess formation is more common than mitral annular abscess. It occurs in 10 percent of native valve endocarditis (NVE), but approximately 50 to 60 percent of prosthetic valves will be affected. The higher incidence of abscess formation with prosthetic valves is due to the fact that the annulus, rather than the leaflet, is the primary site of infection. Clinically, persistent bacteremia or fever, recurrent emboli, heart block, or CHF in a patient on appropriate antimicrobial therapy should alert the clinician to periannular extension of the infection. TEE is the best imaging modality for the diagnosis and evaluation of perivalvular complications. Two dimensional imaging with color-flow Doppler can help delineate possible perivalvular abscesses, fistulous communications, or the presence of a pseudoaneurysm.

Mycotic aneurysms are an unusual complication of infective endocarditis. They result from embolization of the valvular vegetation to the arterial vasa vasorum or the intraluminal space. Inflammatory response to the microbes causes vascular damage and weakens the arterial wall. The combined effects of intraarterial pressure and vascular damage will result in the formation of an aneurysm. Arterial branch points, which trap emboli, are the most common site for the formation of mycotic aneurysms. The most common locations include the proximal aorta, intracranial arteries, visceral arteries, and vessels of the extremities. Intracranial mycotic aneurysms, an extremely dangerous subset, usually present with severe localized

TABLE 36-6
TREATMENT REGIMENS FOR INFECTIVE ENDOCARDITIS[a,b]

Organism	Treatment Regimen: Dose and Route	Duration in Weeks	Comments
Fully penicillin-sensitive streptococci MIC ≤ 0.1 μg/mL viridans (α-hemolytic) streptococci; Strep. bovis; Strep. pneumoniae; Strep. pyogenes group A, C, etc.; Strep. agalactiae group B	1. Penicillin G 4 million units every 6 h IV alone (4 weeks) or	4	Suitable for hospitalized patients but less convenient for outpatient therapy
	2. Penicillin G 4 million units every 6 h IV with gentamicin (2 weeks)		
	3. Ceftriaxone 2 g IV or 1 M once daily alone (2 weeks) or	4	For patients allergic to penicillins but not cephalosporins or for out-patient therapy in selected patients
	4. Ceftriaxone 2 g IV or 1 M once daily or with gentamicin 1 mg/kg twice a day or 3 mg/kg 4 times a day (2 weeks)	4	For patients allergic to penicillins and cephalosporins
	5. Vancomycin 15 mg/kg IV every 12 h (4 weeks)[a,b]		

Relatively penicillin-resistant streptococci: MIC > 0.1 < 1.0 μg/mL, some viridans (α-hemolytic) streptococci; some *Strep. pneumoniae* etc.	1. Penicillin G 4 million units IV every 4 h *plus* gentamicin 1.0 mg/kg every 12 h IV or IM (for first 2 weeks only)[a] *or*	4(2)	For outpatient therapy in selected patients, ceftriaxone 2 g IV once daily may be substituted for penicillin if ceftriaxone MIC ≤ 4 μg/mL, *plus* gentamicin 2.0 mg/kg given once daily
	2. Vancomycin 15 mg/kg IV every 12 h[b]	4	For patients allergic to penicillins
Penicillin-resistant streptococci: MIC ≥ 1.0 μg/mL, *E. faecalis*, *E. faecium*, other enterococci; some other streptococci	1. Penicillin G 18–30 million units/day IV continuously or in divided doses *plus* gentamicin 1 mg/kg IV or IM every 8 h *or*	4–6	Susceptibility testing needed do not use penicillin- or ampicillin-containing regimen if strain produces β-lactamase.
	2. Ampicillin 12 g/day IV continuously or in divided doses *plus* gentamicin 1.0 mg/kg IV every 8 h, *or*	4–6	4-week regimen recommended for most cases with symptoms for <3 months, otherwise 6 weeks
	3. Vancomycin 15 mg/kg IV every 12 h *plus* gentamicin 1.0 mg/kg IV every 8 h[a,b]	4–6	For patients allergic to penicillin; 4 weeks should be adequate for most cases; serum levels should be monitored

(continued)

607

TABLE 36-6
(Continued)

Organism	Treatment Regimen: Dose and Route	Duration in Weeks	Comments
Staphylococci (in the absence of prosthetic material)	Methicillin-susceptible staphylococci:		β-lactam-containing regimens preferred over vancomycin unless patient is definitely hypersensitive to penicillins and cephalosporins; for patients with severe disseminated staphylococcal infection, antimicrobial synergy may be advantageous during early stages of treatment; therefore, gentamicin 1.0 mg/kg IV every 8 h for first 3–5 days only may be added to any of these regimens
	1. Nafcillin 2 g IV every 4 h IV 4–6 wks *or*	4–6	
	2. Nafcillin 2 g IV every 4 h IV × 4–6 wks plus gentamicin 1.0 mg/kg IV every 8 h IV × 3–5 days	4–6	
	3. Vancomycin 15 mg/kg IV every 12 h 4–6 wks[b]	4–6	
In right sided uncomplicated tricuspid endocarditis	Nafcillin 2 g IV every 4 h and gentamicin 1 mg/kg twice a day or 3 mg/kg 4 times a day	2	
	Methicillin-resistant staphylococci: Vancomycin 15 mg/kg IV every 12 h[b]	4–6	

Staphylococci (associated with prosthetic valve or other prosthetic material)	Methicillin-susceptible staphylococci: Nafcillin 2 g IV every 4 h *plus* gentamicin 1.0 mg/kg IV every 8 h[a] plus rifampin 600 mg orally 4 times a day	≥6	Cefazolin or vancomycin may be substituted for nafcillin if necessary due to drug hypersensitivity
	Methicillin-resistant staphylococci: Vancomycin 15 mg/kg IV every 12 h *plus* gentamicin 1.0 mg/kg IV or IM every 8 h *plus* rifampin 300 mg orally every 8 h[a,b]	≥6	
HACEK group organisms: *Haemophilus* species *Actinobacillus actinomycetemcomitans* *Cardiobacterium hominis* *Eikenella* species *Kingella kingae*	1. Ceftriaxone 2 g IV or IM once daily *or*	4	Other third-generation cephalosporins may be substituted, using appropriate dose adjustment
	2. Ampicillin 12 g/day IV continuously or in divided doses *plus* gentamicin 1.0 mg/kg every 12 h IV or IM[a]	4	Less convenient for outpatient therapy

(continued)

TABLE 36-6
(Continued)

Organism	Treatment Regimen: Dose and Route	Duration in Weeks	Comments
Pseudomonas aeruginosa, other gram-negative bacilli	Extended-spectrum penicillin *or* third-generation cephalosporin *or* imipenem *plus* aminoglycoside	4–6	Combination therapy recommended; final choice of antibiotic regimen to be made after sensitivity results available
Neisseria species	1. Penicillin G 2 million units IV every 6 h *or*	3–4	Organisms often highly sensitive to penicillin, but must be tested for β-lactamase production; 3 weeks should be adequate for most patients without complications
	2. Ceftriaxone 1 g IV or IM once daily	3–4	

[a] All gentamicin- and vancomycin-containing regimens require monitoring for potential toxicity; monitoring of serum concentrations usually will be required.

[b] Vancomycin dose not to exceed 2.0 g per 24 h.

TABLE 36-7

ESTIMATE OF MICROBIOLOGIC CURE RATES FOR VARIOUS FORMS OF ENDOCARDITIS[a]

Native Valve Endocarditis	Antimicrobial Therapy Alone	Antimicrobial Therapy Plus Surgery
Viridans streptococci, group A streptococci, Strep. bovis, pneumococci, gonococci	98	98
Enterococcus faecalis	90	>90
Staph. aureus (in young intravenous drug users)	90	>90
Staph. aureus (in elderly patients with chronic underlying diseases)	50	70
Gram-negative aerobic bacilli[b]	40	65
Fungi	<5	50

Prosthetic Valve Endocarditis	Antimicrobial Therapy Alone		Antimicrobial Therapy Plus Surgery	
	Early PVE	Late PVE	Early PVE	Late PVE
Viridans streptococci, group A streptococci, Strep. bovis, pneumococci, gonococci	c	80	c	90
Enterococcus faecalis	c	60	c	75
Staph. aureus	25	40	50	60
Staph. epidermidis	20	40	60	70
Gram-negative aerobic bacilli[b]	<10	20	40	50
Fungi	<1	<1	30	40

[a] Morbidity and mortality are significantly greater than these figures for microbiologic cure indicate.

[b] Excluding HACEK species.

[c] Insufficient data to estimate rates.

TABLE 36-8

RECOMMENDATIONS FOR SURGERY
IN INFECTIVE ENDOCARDITIS

Definite
    Acute aortic or mitral regurgitation with heart failure
    Evidence of periannular abscess or perivalvular extension
    Fungal endocarditis
    Suppurative pericarditis
    Prosthetic valve dehiscence or dysfunction
    Early prosthetic valve endocarditis (within 60 days after
        surgery)
Probable
    Recurrent emboli after appropriate antibiotic therapy
    Persistent bacteremia despite appropriate antibiotic
        therapy
    Enlarging vegetations
    Repeated relapses
    Infection with gram-negative organism
    Staphylococcus aureus infection of left-sided valve
        (esp. aortic)
Controversial
    Mobile vegetations >10 mm

headache or focal neurologic deficits. Appropriate diagnostic testing includes a contrast-enhanced computed tomography and/or magnetic resonance imaging.

Despite the availability of potent antimicrobial therapy, surgical intervention is needed for approximately one-third of all cases of infective endocarditis. Prosthetic valve endocarditis and fungal infections are difficult to eradicate with antibiotics alone (Table 36-7). Moreover, when infective endocarditis is complicated by valvular regurgitation and congestive heart failure, surgical therapy should be undertaken regardless of the duration of antibiotic therapy. If the patient is hemodyanmically stable, the indications for and timing of surgery are not as clear (Table 36-8). When feasible, several days of optimal antimicrobial therapy to eradicate or reduce the bacteremia is recommended prior to surgical intervention.

PREVENTION

Although no clinical trials have definitely proven the efficacy of antibiotic prophylaxis in preventing bacterial endocarditis, the substantial morbidity and mortality associated with this infection justifies

TABLE 36-9

SUGGESTED REGIMENS FOR PROPHYLAXIS OF INFECTIVE ENDOCARDITIS[a]

	Standard Regimen	
For dental procedures and oral or upper respiratory tract surgery		Amoxicillin 2.0 g orally 1 h before procedure[b]
	Special Regimens	
Parenteral regimen for high-risk patients; also for gastrointestinal (GI) or genitourinary (GU) tract procedures		Ampicillin 2.0 g IM or IV *plus* gentamicin 1.5 mg/kg IM or IV, 0.5 h before procedure,[b] 6 h later, ampicillin 1 g IM or IV or amoxicillin 1 g orally
Parenteral regimen for penicillin-allergic patients		Vancomycin 1.0 g IV *slowly* over 1–2 h; *plus* gentamicin 1.5 mg/kg IM or IV[b]; complete within 30 min of starting the procedure
Oral regimen for penicillin-allergic patients (oral and respiratory tract only)		Clindamycin 600 mg orally 1 h before procedure[b]
Oral regimen for minor GI or GU tract procedures		Amoxicillin 2.0 g orally 1 h before procedure[b]

(*continued*)

TABLE 36-9
(Continued)

Parenteral regimen for cardiac surgery including valve replacement	Cefazolin 2.0 g IV on induction of anesthesia, repeated 8 and 16 h later *or*
	Vancomycin 1.0 g IV *slowly* over 1 h starting on induction of anesthesia, then 0.5 g IV 8 and 16 h later[c]

[a]Note that (1) these regimens are empiric suggestions, no regimen has been proved effective for prevention of endocarditis, and prevention failures may occur with any regimen; (2) these regimens are not intended to cover all clinical situations, and the practitioner should use his or her own judgement on safety and cost-benefit issues in each individual case; (3) one or two additional doses may be given if the period of risk for bacteremia is prolonged.

[b]Pediatric dosages: ampicillin 50 mg/kg; gentamicin 1.5 mg/kg; amoxicillin: for children who weigh more than 60 lb, use same as for adults, for children less than 60 lb, use one-half the adult dose; vancomycin 20 mg/kg; clindamycin 20 mg/kg; cefazolin 30 mg/kg. Do not exceed 2.0 g ampicillin, 120 mg gentamycin.

[c]Vancomycin is preferred if *Staph. epidermidis* is an important cause of postoperative infection in that hospital. Gentamicin 1.5 mg/kg IV or IM may be added to each dose, only if postoperative gram-negative infections have occurred with significant frequency.

SOURCE: Durack DT. Nine controversies in the management of infective endocarditis. In: Petersdorf RG, et al., eds. *Update V: Harrison's Principles of Internal Medicine.* New York: McGraw-Hill; 1984:35; and Dajani, et al. (*JAMA* 1997; 277:1794–1801). Adapted and reproduced with permission of the publisher and author.

appropriate treatment. The rationale for therapy centers on the notion that certain medical procedures cause transient bacteremia and may cause predisposing organisms to lodge at sites of cardiac abnormality. Table 36-9 summarizes suggested regimens for endocarditis prophylaxis.

SUGGESTED READING

Chambers HF, Miller RT, Newman MD: Right-sided *Staphylococcus aureus* endocarditis in intravenous drug abusers: Two-week combination therapy. *Ann Intern Med* 1988; 109:619–624.

Dajani AS, Taubert KA, Wilson WR, et al: Prevention of bacterial endocarditis: Recommendations by the American Heart Association. *Circulation* 1997; 96:358–366; *JAMA* 1997; 227:1794–1801.

Durack DT, Bright DK, Lukes AS: Duke Endocarditis Service. New criteria for the diagnosis of infective endocarditis: Utilization of specific echocardiographic findings. *Am J Med* 1994; 96:200–209.

Linder JR, Case RA, Dent JM, et al: Diagnostic value of echocardiography in suspected endocarditis: An evaluation based on pretest probability of disease. *Circulation* 1996; 93:730–736.

Naidu RB, O'Rourke RA: Infective endocarditis. In: Rakel RE, Bope ET (eds): *Conn's Current Therapy.* Philadelphia: Saunders; 2001:314–325.

Sande MA, Kartalija M, Anderson JL: Infective endocarditis. In: Fuster V, Alexander RW, O'Rourke RA (eds): *Hurst's The Heart,* 10th ed. New York: McGraw-Hill; 2001:2087–2125.

Scheld WM, Sande MA: Endocarditis and intravascular infections. In: Mandel GL, Douglas RG Jr, Dolin R (eds): *Principles and Practice of Infectious Diseases,* 4th ed. New York: Churchill Livingstone; 1995:740–783.

Vlessis AA, Hoviguimian H, Jaggers J, et al: Infective endocarditis: Ten year review of medical and surgical therapy. *Ann Thorac Surg* 1996, 61:1217–1222.

Wilson WR, Karchmer A, Dajani A, et al: Antibiotic treatment of adults with infective endocarditis due to *viridans* streptococci, enterococci, staphylococci, and HACEK microorganisms. *JAMA* 1995; 274:1706–1713.

37

PERIOPERATIVE EVALUATION AND MANAGEMENT OF PATIENTS WITH KNOWN OR SUSPECTED CARDIOVASCULAR DISEASE WHO UNDERGO NONCARDIAC SURGERY

Michael J. Lim
Kim A. Eagle

Each year in the United States, approximately 25 million patients undergo noncardiac surgery; among these, 50,000 suffer perioperative myocardial infarction, and more than half of the 40,000 perioperative deaths are caused by cardiac events. Most perioperative cardiac morbidity and mortality is related to myocardial ischemia, congestive heart failure, or arrhythmia. The goals of perioperative evaluation are twofold: first, to identify patients at increased risk of an adverse perioperative cardiac event and second, to identify patients with a poor long-term prognosis due to cardiovascular disease who come to medical attention only because another noncardiac problem leads to noncardiac surgery.

This chapter summarizes available data and recommendations for the preoperative evaluation and perioperative management of patients with known or suspected cardiovascular disease undergoing noncardiac surgery. However, the nature of preoperative evaluation and perioperative management should be individualized to the patient and the clinical scenario surrounding surgery.

CLINICAL DETERMINANTS OF PERIOPERATIVE CARDIOVASCULAR RISK

The majority of patients at increased risk of adverse perioperative cardiac events can be identified using simple, clinically assessable features. Specifically, a careful history, physical examination, and review of the resting 12-lead electrocardiogram (ECG) are usually sufficient to allow stratification of most patients into low, intermediate, or high risk for an adverse perioperative cardiac event. Current recommendations of the American College of Cardiology (ACC) and the American Heart Association (AHA) designate risk factors as belonging to three groups: major, intermediate, and minor (Table 37-1).

History

Risk factors recognized as predictive of increased perioperative risk include advanced age, poor functional capacity, and prior history of coronary artery disease, congestive heart failure, arrhythmia, valvular heart disease, diabetes mellitus, uncontrolled systemic hypertension, and stroke. Coronary artery disease is a major risk factor in the setting of recent myocardial infarction or unstable angina pectoris and an intermediate risk factor in the setting of mild stable angina pectoris or remote myocardial infarction. Similarly, congestive heart failure is a major risk factor if decompensated and an intermediate risk factor if compensated. A history of arrhythmia may be a major, intermediate, or minor risk factor, depending on the nature and severity of the arrhythmia as well as the presence of the underlying heart disease.

A patient's preoperative functional capacity significantly influences the assessment of perioperative cardiac risk. Because most symptoms of cardiac disease are either associated exclusively with or exacerbated by increased physical activity, significant noncardiac limitations in physical capacity are associated with inherent problems in the ability to detect symptoms of underlying cardiac disease and thereby to diagnose it. Impaired conditioning, poor cardiac reserve, poor respiratory reserve, or a combination of these disorders result in a poor functional capacity. Whatever the cause, it results in a reduced ability to accommodate the cardiovascular stresses that may accompany noncardiac surgery.

Physical Exam

Several features of the physical exam may be useful in the assessment of perioperative risk. Systemic hypertension, elevated jugular venous pressure, pulmonary rales, the presence of a third heart sound, murmurs suggestive of significant valvular heart disease, and vascular bruits all may identify a patient to have a higher perioperative risk.

Comorbid Diseases

Many associated medical conditions can exacerbate risk or complicate perioperative cardiac management. Patients with diabetes

TABLE 37-1

CLINICAL PREDICTORS OF INCREASED PERIOPERATIVE
CARDIOVASCULAR RISK (MYOCARDIAL INFARCTION,
CONGESTIVE HEART FAILURE, DEATH)

MAJOR

→ Unstable coronary syndromes
  √ Recent myocardial infarction[a] with evidence
    of important ischemic risk by
    clinical symptoms or noninvasive study
  √ Unstable or severe[b] angina (Canadian class III or IV)
→ Decompensated congestive heart failure
→ Significant arrhythmias
  √ High-grade atrioventricular block
  √ Symptomatic ventricular arrhythmias in the
    presence of underlying heart disease
  √ Supraventricular arrhythmias with uncontrolled
    ventricular rate
→ Severe valvular disease

INTERMEDIATE

→ Mild angina pectoris (Canadian class I or II)
→ Prior myocardial infarction by history or pathologic Q
  waves
→ Compensated or prior congestive heart failure
→ Diabetes mellitus

MINOR

→ Advanced age
→ Abnormal electrocardiogram (left ventricular
  hypertrophy, left bundle branch block, ST-T
  abnormalities)
→ Rhythm other than sinus (e.g., atrial fibrillation)
→ Low functional capacity (e.g., inability to climb
  one flight of stairs with a bag of groceries)
→ History of stroke
→ Uncontrolled systemic hypertension

[a] The American College of Cardiology National Database Library defines recent MI as >7 days but ≤1 month.
[b] May include "stable" angina in patients who are unusually sedentary.

mellitus, restrictive or obstructive pulmonary disease, renal dysfunction, and anemia all have an increased risk of concomitant cardiac complications during the perioperative period. Optimization of management and control of noncardiac conditions may therefore reduce the risk of cardiac morbidity in the perioperative period.

Surgery-Specific Risks

Perioperative cardiac risk is related to the type of noncardiac surgery being performed. Emergency procedures are associated with a two- to fivefold increase in perioperative cardiac risk compared with elective procedures. Other types of noncardiac surgery associated with high perioperative risk include aortic and peripheral vascular surgery, and prolonged abdominal, thoracic, or head and neck procedures with large fluid shifts. The ACC/AHA Task Force Report on Perioperative Cardiac Evaluation stratifies noncardiac surgical procedures as high, intermediate, and low cardiac risk (Table 37-2).

Perioperative anesthesia technique influences the patient's cardiac physiology and may affect the perioperative cardiac risk.

TABLE 37-2

CARDIAC RISK[a] STRATIFICATION FOR NONCARDIAC SURGICAL PROCEDURES

HIGH (REPORTED CARDIAC RISK OFTEN >5%)

→ Emergent major operations, particularly in the elderly
→ Aortic and other major vascular surgery
→ Peripheral vascular surgery
→ Anticipated prolonged surgical procedures associated with large fluid shifts and/or blood loss

INTERMEDIATE (REPORTED CARDIAC RISK GENERALLY <5%)

→ Carotid endarterectomy
→ Head and neck surgery
→ Intraperitoneal and intrathoracic surgery
→ Orthopedic surgery
→ Prostate surgery

LOW (REPORTED CARDIAC RISK GENERALLY <1%)

→ Endoscopic procedures
→ Superficial procedures
→ Cataract surgery
→ Breast surgery

---

[a] Combined incidence of cardiac death and nonfatal myocardial infarction.

Although there is no one best myocardial protective anesthetic technique, differences in anesthetic techniques may favor the use of one over another for individual patients. Opioid based anesthesia generally does not affect cardiovascular function, although the commonly employed inhalational agents cause afterload reduction and decreased myocardial contractility. Hemodynamic affects are minimal when spinal anesthesia is used for infrainguinal procedures, whereas the higher dermatomal levels of spinal anesthesia required for abdominal procedures may be associated with significant hemodynamic effects, including hypotension and reflex tachycardia.

CLINICAL ASSESSMENT OF PERIOPERATIVE RISK

Patients at low risk generally require no additional testing prior to noncardiac surgery. Among patients undergoing elective noncardiac surgery in whom risk is determined to be intermediate or high, additional testing may be useful to better define risk. It is useful to employ a stepwise approach to the preoperative assessment of cardiac risk. The evaluating clinician first determines the urgency of noncardiac surgery. Then, a history of recent coronary revascularization or recent cardiac testing is taken. Clinical features including the presence of major, intermediate, or minor risk factors are noted as is an estimation of functional capacity. Finally, the nature of the planned surgical procedure is considered to determine whether additional testing may be helpful in further defining perioperative cardiac risk.

PREOPERATIVE TESTING

Resting Left Ventricular Function

Preoperative left ventricular systolic function can be assessed noninvasively using radionuclide ventriculography or echocardiography, or invasively using contrast ventriculography. Unless recently defined, preoperative assessment of left ventricular systolic function should be performed among patients with poorly controlled congestive heart failure and should be considered among patients with prior congestive heart failure and among those with dyspnea of unknown cause.

Functional Testing and Risk of Coronary Artery Disease

Because clinical factors usually serve to identify patients at low or high risk of an adverse cardiac event after noncardiac surgery, preoperative stress testing typically has the greatest utility among patients at intermediate risk. Exercise ECG study allows assessment of functional capacity as well as evaluation for evidence of coronary artery disease based on ST-segment analysis and hemodynamics. Performance of exercise echocardiographic testing or exercise nuclear perfusion imaging should be considered in the presence of significant resting ECG abnormalities that preclude diagnostic testing for coronary artery disease, such as left bundle branch block, left ventricular hypertrophy with strain, or digitalis effect. Nonexercise stress testing, such as dobutamine stress echocardiography or adenosine (or dipyridamole) thallium scintigraphy, should be considered among patients who are unable to perform adequate physical exercise.

Exercise Testing

Preoperative cardiac stress testing is useful in the objective assessment of functional capacity, to help identify patients at risk of perioperative myocardial ischemia or cardiac arrhythmias, and to aid in the assessment of long-term as well as perioperative prognosis. In a general population, the mean sensitivity and specificity of exercise ECG studies for the detection of coronary artery disease are 68 and 77 percent, respectively. In a large cohort of 4083 medically treated patients in the Coronary Artery Surgery Study, exercise testing was useful for identifying both high- and low-risk subgroups of patients. The mortality rate was 5 percent per year or more among a high-risk subset, comprising 12 percent of the total population, who were able to achieve an exercise workload of less than Bruce stage I and had an abnormal exercise ECG. In contrast, mortality was less than 1 percent per year among a low-risk subset comprising 34 percent of the total population, who were able to achieve at least Bruce stage III with a normal exercise ECG.

Nonexercise Stress Testing

Approximately 30 to 50 percent of patients undergoing noncardiac surgery are unable to achieve an adequate exercise workload for a diagnostic study. In these patients, pharmacologic stress testing for the detection of coronary artery disease can be performed using one of two general methods. Infusion of the adrenergic agonist dobutamine results in increases in heart rate, myocardial contractility, and, to a lesser degree, blood pressure, resulting in increased myocardial oxygen demand. In the setting of a limited oxygen supply, increased demand causes myocardial ischemia, which is detected as a regional wall motion abnormality on echocardiographic imaging. Alternatively, pharmacological "stress" can be achieved using the coronary vasodilators dipyridamole or adenosine. Coronary artery disease is detected as abnormal coronary vasodilator reserve, with heterogeneity of perfusion in response to maximal coronary vasodilatation as detected by nuclear imaging techniques such as thallium scintigraphy.

Although any abnormality on thallium scintigraphy is suggestive of coronary artery disease and is associated with a higher perioperative cardiac risk compared with patients who have normal scans, perioperative cardiac risk associated with a fixed perfusion defect is substantially lower than that associated with perfusion redistribution. In addition, the size of a perfusion defect is directly related to perioperative cardiac risk.

PREOPERATIVE THERAPY FOR CORONARY ARTERY DISEASE

Coronary Revascularization

There are no prospective randomized trials testing the impact of either preoperative coronary artery bypass grafting or percutaneous transluminal coronary angioplasty on perioperative cardiac morbidity and mortality rates. However, several retrospective studies suggest that patients having undergone previous successful surgical coronary revascularization have a low risk of perioperative cardiac events during noncardiac surgery, and the risk of death is comparable to that found among patients without clinical indications suggestive of coronary artery disease. The Bypass Angioplasty Revascularization Investigation (BARI) trial investigated 1049 patients undergoing noncardiac surgery. It demonstrated a low incidence of myocardial infarction or death among patients having undergone either coronary artery bypass surgery or percutaneous angioplasty. The absence of any evident difference between groups suggests that the previous percutaneous coronary angioplasty confers a protection from perioperative cardiac events that is similar to that conferred by surgical revascularization. However, based on the limited data available, indications for percutaneous coronary angioplasty among patients undergoing preoperative evaluation should be considered the same as for the general population.

The optimal timing of noncardiac surgery has not been defined for those patients requiring percutaneous revascularization. Ideally, elective surgery should be performed within 2 to 3 months of angioplasty, before restenosis can occur. However, patients who have gone more than 6 months after percutaneous coronary angioplasty with no evidence of recurrent ischemia could be considered to have undergone successful revascularization, presumably with a low perioperative risk. Furthermore, with the increasing frequency of coronary artery stenting, elective surgery within the first 28 days after the procedure is not desirable, owing to the need for intensive antiplatelet therapy after stent placement to prevent thrombosis. This may lead to unnecessary perioperative bleeding and a hypercoagulable state during the perioperative period, which may predispose to stent thrombosis.

Medical Therapy for Coronary Artery Disease

Although data are lacking to support the empiric use of nitroglycerin or calcium channel blockers, there is increasing evidence that the empiric use of perioperative beta blockers reduces the risk of an adverse cardiac event in medium- and high-risk patients. A randomized study among 112 high-risk patients undergoing vascular surgery has demonstrated a reduction in risk of perioperative myocardial infarction or death from 34 to 3 percent with the use of empiric beta-blocker therapy. Smaller retrospective studies have also supported the use of empiric perioperative beta-blocker therapy among high-risk patients undergoing intermediate or high-risk noncardiac surgery. These include, particularly, patients with established diabetes or cardiovascular disease with preoperative noninvasive tests showing myocardial ischemia during stress.

Management of Specific Conditions

Patients with a variety of medical conditions known to increase cardiovascular risk may require noncardiac surgery. Factors that contribute to increased perioperative risk include interruptions in routine medical therapy as well as physical and mental stresses associated with the surgical procedure and convalescent period. It is important to note that the period of maximum cardiac risk appears to occur in the postoperative period. Because cardiovascular risk is not limited to the intraoperative period, appropriate emphasis should be placed on the treatment of specific conditions throughout all phases of the perioperative period.

SUGGESTED READING

Bach DS, Eagle KA: Perioperative evaluation and management of patients with known or suspected cardiovascular disease who undergo noncardiac surgery. In: Fuster V, Alexander RW, O' Rourke RA, et al (eds): *Hurst's The Heart,* 10th ed. New York: McGraw-Hill; 2001:2129–2142.

Eagle KA, Brundage BH, Chaitman BR, et al: Guidelines for perioperative cardiovascular evaluation for noncardiac surgery: Report of the American College of Cardiology/American Heart Association Task Force on Practice Guidelines. *Circulation* 1996; 84:505–509.

Eagle KA, Rihal CS, Mickel MC, et al: Cardiac risk of noncardiac surgery: Influence of coronary artery disease and type of surgery in 3368 operations. CASS Investigators and University of Michigan Heart Care Program. Coronary Artery Surgery Study. *Circulation* 1997; 96:1882–1887.

Kaluza GL, Joseph J, Lee JR, Raizner AE: Catastrophic outcomes of noncardiac surgery soon after coronary stenting. *J Am Coll Cardiol* 2000; 35:1288–1294.

Poldermans D, Boersma E, Bax JJ, et al: The effect of bisoprolol on perioperative mortality and myocardial infarction in high-risk patients undergoing vascular surgery. Dutch Echocardiography Study Group. *N Engl J Med* 1999; 341:1789–1794.

38

DIABETES AND CARDIOVASCULAR DISEASE

Michael E. Farkouh
Elliot J. Rayfield
Valentin Fuster

INTRODUCTION

Diabetes mellitus, whether type 1 or type 2, is a very strong risk factor for the development of coronary artery disease (CAD) and stroke (see Table 38-1). Eighty percent of all deaths among diabetic patients are due to atherosclerosis, compared to about 30 percent among nondiabetics. A large cohort study sponsored by the National Institutes of Health (NIH) revealed that heart disease mortality in the general U.S. population is declining at a much greater rate than in diabetic subjects. However, *diabetic women* had an increase in heart disease mortality over the same time period. Of all the hospitalizations for diabetic complications, more than 75 percent are due to atherosclerosis. An increase in the prevalence of diabetes has been noted, which in part can be attributed to the aging of the U.S. population as well as an increase in the rate of obesity and the widespread sedentary lifestyle.

Diabetes accelerates the natural course of atherosclerosis in all groups of patients and involves a greater number of coronary vessels with more diffuse atherosclerotic lesions. Cardiac catheterizations in diabetic patients have shown significantly more severe proximal and distal CAD. In addition, plaque ulceration and thrombosis have been found to occur more frequently in diabetic patients. Cardiovascular complications include CAD, peripheral artery disease, nephropathy, retinopathy, cardiomyopathy, and possible neuropathy (involvement of vasa vasorum). These observations underscore the heightened risks of the diabetic patient to develop vascular disease and compel us to correct all the metabolic abnormalities. By understanding the mechanisms underlying each risk, we will be more likely to prevent them.

TABLE 38-1

CLINICAL EVALUATION OF RISK FACTORS FOR
THE DEVELOPMENT OF CARDIOVASCULAR DISEASE
IN DIABETIC PATIENTS

Cigarette Smoking
   Assess pack-years
Blood Pressure
   Duration (if known), current and previous medications,
      assess presence of orthostatic hypertension.
Serum Lipids and Lipoproteins
   Dietary habits, alcohol intake, amount of exercise and
      whether aerobic
   Family history of dyslipidemia, eruptive xanthoma,
      lipemia, retinalis, xanthelasma,
   Thyroid function tests
   LDL and HDL cholesterol, fasting triglycerides.
Spot albumin/creatinine ratio (in micro- macroalbuminuria)
   Serum creatinine
   Do not rely on dipstick protein since negative results may
      reflect lack of sensitivity of test.
Glycemic Status
   Duration of diabetes, family history of diabetes, vascular,
      renal, and retinal complications
   Laboratory—fasting plasma glucose (FPG), hemoglobin
      A1c q 3 months: Dx FPG $> 126 \times 2$: impaired fasting
      glucose 110 to 126×2. When in doubt, have patient
      undergo 2-h oral glucose tolerance test.

KEY: LDL = low-density lipoprotein; HDL = high-density lipoprotein.

CLINICAL PRESENTATIONS
OF DIABETES MELLITUS

The risk factors for the development of diabetes are well established
(Table 38-2). About 80 percent of all diabetic patients have type 2
diabetes mellitus, which characteristically occurs after the age of
40 years. The metabolic mechanisms of type 2 diabetes are the combination of insulin resistance and a genetically programmed defect
in the secretion of insulin by the pancreatic beta cells. Insulin resistance precedes the onset of type 2 diabetes by about 8 to 10 years and
is associated with other cardiovascular risk factors—dyslipidemia,

TABLE 38-2

ASSESSMENT OF PREDISPOSING RISK FACTORS
IN DIABETIC PATIENTS

Body weight and fat distribution
History
Age of onset of overweight, family history of obesity.
Physical examination
Measure body weight (kg); height (m); calculate body
mass index (BMI = kg/m^2), BMI of 25–29.9 =
overweight, >30.0 = obese; however, BMI >27 in a
diabetic should be treated as high risk; measure waist
circumference (abdominal obesity is >40 in. in men
and >36 in. in women).
Physical activity
History—job, activity in sports, walking, aerobics.
In women, child care, housework.
Physical examination—assess level of cardiovascular
fitness in cardiac rehabilitation facility.
Family history
History of heart disease, sudden death, elevated
cholesterol level, cigarette smoking; hypertension;
diabetes especially in first-degree relatives.
Laboratory
Measure fasting glucose and lipids in first-degree
relatives.

hypertension, and a procoagulant state. The combination of these risk
factors has been called syndrome X, the metabolic syndrome, and
the cardiovascular dysmetabolic syndrome. Many patients with the
metabolic syndrome exhibit either impaired fasting glucose (IFG) or
impaired glucose tolerance (IGT) for many years before they develop
overt diabetes.

There are new criteria for the diagnosis of diabetes. The fasting
plasma glucose level for the diagnosis of diabetes has been lowered
from 140 to 126 mg/dL. The upper threshold of fasting plasma glucose for normoglycemia has been lowered from 115 to 110 mg/dL.
Thus, a fasting plasma glucose of 110 to 125 mg/dl is now referred to
as an impaired fasting glucose, or IFG. These changes eliminate the
need for oral glucose tolerance testing for the diagnosis of diabetes,
and the diagnosis now depends on an elevation of the fasting plasma
glucose level.

In contrast to type 2 diabetes, type 1 diabetes (10 percent of the diabetic population) is usually induced by immunologic destruction of pancreatic beta cells. Type 1 diabetes classically has two peaks (at 4 and 13 years of age), but it can occur at any age. It typically produces microvascular disease (nephropathy, retinopathy) and also results in CAD.

Stroke

The mortality from stroke is almost three times higher among diabetics than among nondiabetics. The small paramedial penetrating arteries are the most common site of cerebrovascular disease. In addition, diabetes also increases the likelihood of severe carotid atherosclerosis. Diabetic patients are likely to suffer increased brain damage with carotid emboli that, in a nondiabetic individual, would result only in a transient ischemic attack.

Renal Disease

Nephropathy occurs in 40 percent of patients with diabetes of either type 1 or type 2. Risk factors include poor glycemic control, hypertension, and ethnicity (blacks, Mexicans, Pima Indians). Table 38-3 summarizes the key points for the assessment of renal status in a diabetic patient. The earliest clinical finding of diabetic kidney disease is microalbuminuria, which may occur at a time when renal histology is essentially normal.

There is insufficient evidence to recommend angiotensin-converting enzyme (ACE) inhibitors in normotensive diabetic patients without microalbuminuria. In predicting the progression to overt nephropathy, screening for microalbuminuria is not as useful in type 2 as in type 1 diabetes. However, once microalbuminuria develops, the rate of decline in glomerular filtration rate (GFR) in type 2 diabetes is equivalent to that in type 1. Nonetheless, for microalbuminuria, screening is still recommended on at least a yearly basis, since the risk/benefit ratio of diagnosing microalbuminuria would justify treatment with an ACE inhibitor, not only for the treatment of renal disease alone, but also to reduce the incidence of myocardial infarction (Heart Outcomes Prevention Evaluation Theory).

Patients on ACE inhibitors should be monitored for potassium, since they may develop hyperkalemia in the presence of a type 4 renal tubular acidosis. Sodium restriction will reduce hypertension and therefore is advised. Dietary protein should be adjusted to 0.8 g/kg/day to decrease intraglomerular pressure.

An optimal approach to diabetic nephropathy combines control of hypertension, preferably with an ACE inhibitor, glycemic control, sodium restriction, and adjustment of protein intake.

TABLE 38-3
EVALUATION OF RENAL STATUS

Urine albumin and protein
- Yearly screen for microalbumin in type 1 and type 2 diabetes. Microalbumin/creatinine ratio collected in a spot urine, ideally first morning urine specimen (normal <30 mg/g creatinine). Must rule out other disease that causes proteinuria.
- If urine albumin/creatinine is >300 mg/g in first morning specimen, macroalbuminuria is present and is usually not reversible with ACE inhibitors—nephrology consult.
- Nephrotic syndrome—urine protein >3 g/day— nephrology consult.
- Other reasons to consult nephrologists are diabetic patients with increasing creatinine from 1.4 to over 2.0; elevated creatinine and symptoms of uremia; micro- albuminuria which is not responding to an ACE inhibitor.

Urinalysis
- Red cells, pyuria, casts require nephrology consult.

Blood pressure evaluation
- If hypertension is present, exclude secondary causes including with advancing renal insufficiency.
- Treatment with an ACE inhibitor is preferred first choce even in African Americans (except if precluded by hyperkalemia or other complications).

Blood Urea Nitrogen, serum creatinine and glomerular fltration rate
- A yearly creatinine clearance should be obtained with a 24-h urine collection and a serum creatinine. This is the most accurate way to estimate kidney function without using a radioisotope.

DIABETES AND MECHANISMS
OF CARDIOVASCULAR RISKS

Lipoprotein Disorders

Lipid disorders constitute one of the cornerstones in the cardio- vascular management of the diabetic patient. Many factors influ- ence the lipid profile in these patients, including glycemic control, whether the diabetes is type 1 or type 2, and the presence of diabetic nephropathy.

TYPE OF DIABETES

In type 1 diabetes mellitus, the major determinant in the lipid profile is the level of glycemic control. Low-density-lipoprotein (LDL) cholesterol is moderately increased, triglycerides are markedly increased, and high-density-lipoprotein (HDL) is decreased when the level of glycemic control is impaired. For patients with type 1 diabetes, lipid abnormalities are related not only to hyperglycemia but also to the interplay of the insulin-resistant state. Patients with type 1 diabetes may have normal LDL levels but elevated levels of the very low density lipoprotein (VLDL) and triglyceride with reduced HDL levels. The expected elevation in VLDL triglycerides is usually no more than 100 percent.

MANAGEMENT OF LIPID DISORDERS

Consistent with the National Cholesterol Education Program, the American Diabetes Association has published its consensus document concerning the management of lipid disorders. For the most part, the cornerstone of therapy in diabetes comprises dietary modifications, weight loss, physical exercise, and maximized glycemic control.

Type of Diabetes   As previously mentioned, the management of lipid disorders in type 1 diabetes is closely coupled to glycemic control. For type 1 patients, the frontline strategy begins with glycemic control.

In type 1 diabetes, glycemic control can lead to marked reductions in triglyceride levels but with little or no impact on HDL levels. Pharmacotherapy is often required sooner rather than later in type 2 patients, given the modest impact of nonpharmacologic strategies.

Medical therapy for hyperlipidemia is similar in diabetic and nondiabetic patients, but diabetic patients require certain special considerations.

The hypertriglyceridemia of diabetes can be effectively treated by fibric acid derivatives without any adverse effect on glucose metabolism. Type 2 diabetics experience a reduction in the rate of cardiovascular events when they are treated with gemfibrozil. This drug causes a 5 to 15 percent drop in LDL levels in patients with normal triglyceride levels; but in patients with hypertriglyceridemia, the LDL levels go up. This elevation is probably due to the catabolism of atherogenic LDL particles, resulting in a less atherogenic LDL.

Although nicotinic acid lowers both cholesterol and triglyceride levels while raising HDL levels, it is generally not indicated in diabetes. It has an adverse effect on glycemic control due to its induction of insulin resistance.

HMG-CoA reductase inhibitors ("statins") are another group of drugs useful in lowering cholesterol levels in type 2 patients without having any adverse effect on glycemic control. In a study assessing the effectiveness of a cholesterol-lowering drug for secondary prevention of morbidity or mortality in patients with angina or prior myocardial infarction, simvastatin was found to be more efficacious in diabetic patients than in the overall group.

Bile acid–binding resins can decrease the levels of LDL in diabetic patients, but they can also cause a significant rise in triglyceride levels, especially if the VLDL level is already high or if the diabetes is poorly controlled. In patients with high levels of both LDL and VLDL, bile acid–binding resins can be used in low doses in combination with fibric acid derivatives.

Thrombosis and Diabetes

Diabetes mellitus is widely recognized as perhaps the most significant risk factor for the development of acute coronary syndromes. The relationship between diabetes and acute coronary thrombosis is multifactorial, with the interaction of plaque disruption and the interplay of local and systemic thrombogenic factors playing the primary roles.

PLAQUE DISRUPTION

The inciting role of acute plaque disruption in the development of acute coronary thrombosis is well described. Although the lipid-rich core in plaque is felt to be causative in this process, more aggressive medical management of diabetes can have a favorable effect by decreasing plaque rupture and improving clinical outcome.

It is well understood that not all disruptions of atherosclerotic plaques lead to clinical events. The complex interaction of local and systemic thrombogenic factors is an important determinant of whether clinically significant thrombus formation occurs.

CLINICAL IMPLICATIONS

Lipid Disorders

The management of diabetic patients with lipid abnormalities is a unique challenge. Important evidence from the large randomized trials of lipid-lowering therapies is based upon subgroup analyses in which diabetics represented less than 10 percent of all patients enrolled. In the Scandinavian Simvastatin Survival Study (4S), 202 diabetic patients with a prior history of CAD were enrolled. Although this number was too small, the comparison of simvastatin with placebo showed an almost 50 percent reduction in coronary events in favor of simvastatin (45 versus 23 percent, p = NS). Similar trends were observed in the Cholesterol Recurrent Event (CARE) trial, which compared pravastatin with placebo in secondary prevention. In the CARE trial, the baseline mean LDL concentration in diabetics was 136 mg/dL. LDL was reduced by 27 percent in the group receiving pravastatin, which translated into a 25 percent reduction in coronary events over 5 years when compared with the control group. These therapies are at the cornerstone of diabetes management in the current era.

In the trials of statin therapy in hyperlipidemia, the relative benefit appears similar among diabetics and nondiabetics. The concern for the clinician is that larger trials focusing on the diabetic population will have to be computed before the magnitude of the benefit of lipid-lowering therapy in reducing cardiovascular events can be determined.

Glycemic Control

The pathophysiology of type 2 diabetes is a consequence of peripheral resistance to insulin action (in muscle and fat cells), increased hepatic glucose production, and decreased secretion of insulin by the pancreatic beta cells. About 80 percent of people with type 2 diabetes are obese.

Diet and exercise remain the cornerstones of the management of type 2 diabetes. The pharmacologic agents available to treat type 2 diabetes are insulin, insulin secretagogues (sulfonylureas, repaglinide), alpha glucosidase inhibitors (acarbose, miglitol), and insulin sensitizers (biguanides, thiazolidinediones). Each of these agents targets a different mechanism responsible for hyperglycemia. Figure 38-1 shows a useful algorithm for the staged management of type 2 diabetes using these agents.

The standards of care in patients with diabetes (from the American Diabetes Association) are preprandial glucose levels of 80 to 120, bedtime glucose levels of 100 to 140, and a hemoglobin A1c (Hb-A1c) of <7 percent.

The plasma Hb-A1c reflects the average glucose level over the preceding 8 weeks and provides a uniform measure of progress as well as a gauge of the efficacy of different therapies.

Early Detection of Diabetes

Owing to the significant increase in major microvascular complications and risk of premature death among patiens with diabetes, it

Algorithm for type 2 diabetes

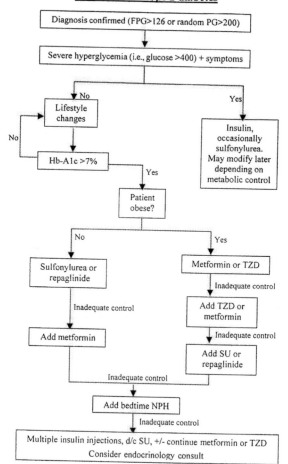

FIGURE 38-1

The algorithm shows staged management of type 2 diabetes using the agents shown. Note: Acarbose or miglitol can be added anywhere along the treatment pathway. SU = sulfonylurea; TZD = thiazolidinedione; d/c = discontinue; PG = plasma glucose; Hb-Alc = hemoglobin Alc; FPG = fasting plasma glucose.

is important that to screening for diabetes begin before age 45, the current recommendation. Within the next 10 years, the populations at highest risk for diabetes—with a view to aggressive screening strategies—will probably be selected.

Current measures of cardiovascular surveillance for CAD in asymptomatic diabetics are focused on routine stress testing in accordance with the guidelines of the American College of Cardiology/American Heart Association (ACC/AHA) (Table 38-4). Exercise testing in diabetic patients is more likely to be accurate when combined with echocardiography or radionuclide imaging. Diabetics are less likely to have an appropriate blood pressure and heart rate response to exercise; they are also less likely to experience any pain corresponding to ST-segment changes, owing in part to autonomic dysfunction. The AHA recommends that the finding of subclinical CAD should prompt clinicians to initiate more aggressive preventive measures (Table 38-4).

Hypertension and Nephropathy

To date there are no randomized trials primarily evaluating the role of hypertension treatment with nephropathy as the endpoint in type 1 diabetes without microalbuminuria. Hypertensive diabetics are primarily treated with ACE inhibitors.

As compared with nondiabetics, diabetics in the SHEP (Systolic Hypertension in the Elderly Program cooperative research group) study experienced a more pronounced benefit from treatment with clorthalidone.

The United Kingdom Prospective Diabetes Study (UKPDS) demonstrated no advantage of captopril over atenolol in reducing macrovascular complications. Clearly this illustrates the significant role that the lowering of blood pressure plays in reducing adverse events independent of the agent used. The role of further blood pressure reduction, even when high-risk patients such as diabetics are in the normal range, needs to be further delineated. The HOT (Hypertension Optimal Treatment) study showed that the risk of major cardiovascular events in diabetic patients was halved if they had a target diastolic pressure of ≤ 80 mmHg compared to those with a diastolic pressure of ≤ 90 mmHg (p for trend $= 0.005$). There was a lower but still significant decrease in the risk of silent myocardial infarction and about a 30 percent risk reduction in the rate of stroke in the ≤ 80 mmHg group compared with the ≤ 90 mmHg group.

The Captopril Prevention Projects (CAPPP) study showed a significant reduction in cardiovascular events in hypertensive patients treated with captopril instead of the standard therapy of beta blockers or diuretics. Approximately 5 percent of patients were diabetic in this trial; in these patients, similar trends in favor of captopril were

TABLE 38-4

DETECTION OF CLINICAL AND SUBCLINICAL CARDIOVASCULAR DISEASE IN THE DIABETIC PATIENT

Stress Testing for Coronary Heart Disease
  Consult AHA guidelines for exercise treadmill testing.
  Considerations for testing in diabetic patients
  - Blunting of heart rate and blood pressure responses
  - Painless ST-segment depression common in diabetic patients (autonomic neuropathy).
  - Diagnostic specificity of ST-segment depression may be reduced (previous silent myocardial infarction, etc.).
  - Exercise or pharmacologic testing perfusion scintography (with technetium 99 m or thallium-20) favorable for exercise testing in diabetic patients.
  - Ambulatory ECG monitoring may be helpful in special instances of diabetic patients to diagnose silent ischemia but not routinely.

Noninvasive Evaluation of Cardiac Function
  Echocardiography (Doppler) and radionuclide ventriculography issues in diabetic patients.
  - Diastolic function common and often precedes systolic dysfunction.
  - Left ventricular wall motion abnormalities suggest diabetic cardiomyopathy.

Evaluation of Autonomic Dysfunction
  In bedside evaluation, two or more of these tests are abnormal.
  - Resting heart rate (supine) 100.
  - Excess diastolic blood pressure response to hand-grip exercise.
  - Abnormal expiratory/inspiratory RR-interval ratio.
  - Postural hypotension.
  Significance of autonomic dysfunction in diabetic patients
  - 50% 5-year mortality.
  - Sudden death common—consider electrophysiologic study.
  - Greater complications after elective surgery.
  - Increased danger with general anesthesia.

Diagnosis of Subclinical Cardiovascular Disease
  History: symptoms of claudication, angina, dyspnea on exertion, cerebrovascular disease.
  Physical examination: routine checkup with evaluation of carotid and femoral bruits; peripheral arterial pulses; ratio of ankle-to-brachial artery systolic blood pressure (marker of subclinical peripheral vascular disease).
  Laboratory: urinary creatinine/albumin ratio (Table 38-1).
  ECG: LV hypertrophy is a strong predictor of CAD morbidity and mortality.
  Electron-beam CT: coronary calcium score correlated to some extent with total coronary atherosclerosis burden.
  Carotid ultrasound: detects subclinical carotid atherosclerosis.

KEY: AHA = American Heart Association; ECG = electrocardiogram; LV = left ventricular; CAD = covouary artery disease; CT = computed tomography.

observed. The ABCD study (Appropriate Blood pressure Control in Diabetics) also observed a benefit of ACE inhibition over conventional therapy in treatment of hypertension in diabetics.

The HOPE Study

The Heart Outcomes Prevention Evaluation (HOPE) study evaluated over 9000 high-risk patients with evidence of vascular disease or diabetes in a randomized trial comparing ramipril with placebo over a 5-year period. A total of 3578 patients were diabetic. This study demonstrated a 22 percent reduction in primary cardiovascular endpoints of death, myocardial infarction, and stroke in favor of ramipril. The beneficial effect of ramipril was observed over all predefined subgroups. This result was also observed in the CAPPP study. Ramipril lowered systolic blood pressure by a mean of 6 mmHg only. This would account for the reduction of only about 40 percent in the rate of stroke and about a 25 percent in the rate of myocardial infarction. Therefore there is some benefit of ramipril independent of the blood pressure–lowering effect, which accounts for the impressive cardiovascular protective effect. HOPE provides level-1 evidence supporting the front-line use of ACE inhibitors in the treatment of diabetic patients at risk for cardiovascular events regardless of whether they are hypertensive. In the diabetic subgroup there was an even greater relative risk reduction in primary cardiovascular events (25 percent).

Acute Coronary Syndromes

Diabetics represent a high-risk group for developing and surviving acute myocardial infarction. In particular patients with type 1 diabetes have a worse outcome than patients with type 2 disease, and diabetic women have almost twice the risk of mortality as compared with diabetic men.

Reperfusion therapy is the cornerstone of the management of acute myocardial infarction. In a meta-analysis of all major thrombolytic trials, diabetics showed a nonsignificant trend toward an increased reduction in 35 day mortality as compared with nondiabetics. The potential advantage of angioplasty over thrombolytic therapy has not been addressed in the diabetic population.

Beside the use of aspirin and beta blockers, other new treatment strategies are emerging. The utilization of insulin and glucose infusion for at least 24 h after admission for acute myocardial infarction, followed by intensive insulin long-term, was compared with usual care in the standard therapy with glucose-insulin infusion versus standard therapy (DIGAMI) trial. A total of 620 diabetic patients were randomized, and the trial demonstrated a 30 percent reduction in mortality at 12 months for the group treated with the intensive program. A new trial is under way to evaluate whether this benefit was the result of acute therapy or the intensive posthospital therapy (Smith and colleagues, unpublished).

Chronic Coronary Artery Disease

The association between CAD and diabetes is strong and has led to screening strategies in diabetics even before they are symptomatic. In addition, diabetics are often unaware of myocardial ischemic pain, so that silent myocardial infarction and ischemia are markedly increased in this population. There is a heightened concern for development of sudden cardiac death in diabetics.

Therapeutic modalities in diabetics with CAD include standard therapy with aspirin, beta blockers, calcium channel blockers, and nitrates.

Epidemiologic evidence from the Bezafibrate Infarction Prevention Study registry shows almost a 50 percent reduction in mortality for type 2 patients with chronic CAD who were treated with beta blockers as compared with controls. Other randomized trial evidence has demonstrated that diabetes is a strong predictor of earlier death and that diabetics may benefit more from beta blocker therapy than nondiabetics. In general beta blockers are extremely well tolerated; masking or prolonging of hypoglycemic symptoms appears to be highly infrequent, particularly with cardioselective beta blockers.

Coronary Revascularization

The high prevalence of CAD in diabetic patients necessitates the frequent use of revascularization procedures in these patients. Both coronary artery bypass grafting and coronary angioplasty are effective in diabetics, but the high rate of restenosis that diabetic patients experience in the first 6 months after the procedure raises concerns about the long-term benefits of angioplasty.

Prior to the use of stents and glucoprotein IIb/IIIa antagonists (see also Chap. 14), the rate of restenosis after angioplasty in diabetics has been shown to be as high as 47 to 71 percent. The mechanism of restenosis is believed to be related to neointimal hyperplasia, which is tightly linked to the interplay between platelet-thrombus deposition and various growth- factors present after injury and endothelial dysfunction.

The best evidence from randomized trials supportive of the utility of stents and abciximab comes from the Evaluation of Platelet IIb/IIIa Inhibition in Stenting (EPISTENT) trial. Of the 2399 patients randomized, 20 percent (491 patients) had diabetes. Patients were

TABLE 38-5

GUIDE TO COMPREHENSIVE RISK REDUCTION FOR PATIENTS
WITH CORONARY AND OTHER VASCULAR DISEASE
WHO HAVE DIABETES

Risk Intervention	Recommendations
Smoking Goal: complete cessation	Urge smoking cessation. Try Nicoderm patches or Xyban; bupropion enroll in smoking cessation program.
Blood Pressure control Goal: <135/ 85 mmHg	Initiate lifestyle modification: weight reduction, increased physical activity; alcohol moderation; sodium restriction in all patients with blood pressure >135/85. Add blood pressure medication if BP is not below above goal.

Lipid Management Primary goal: LDL ≤ 100 mg/dL Secondary goals: HDL > 35 mg/dL TG < 200 mg/dL	Start AHA Step II Diet in all patients: ≤30% fat, <7% saturated fat, <200 mg/dL cholesterol. Assess fasting lipid profile. Immediately start cholesterol lowering drugs when baseline LDL > 130 mg/dL.			
	LDL < 100 mg/dL No drug therapy	LDL 100–129 mg/dL Consider adding drug therapy to diet, as follows	LDL ≥ 130 mg/dL Add drug therapy as follows	HDL < 35 mg/dL Weight management, physical activity, and smoking cessation
		Suggested drug therapy		
		TG < 200 mg/dL	TG 200–400 mg/dL	TG > 400 mg/dL
		Statin Resin	Statin Fibrate	Consider combined drug therapy (statin + fibrate)
Glucose control Goal: near normal fasting glucose Goal: HbA1c ≤ 1% above normal	First-step therapy: lifestyle modifications. Second-step therapy: oral hypoglycemic agents (see Fig. 38-1). Third-step therapy: insulin therapy (see Fig. 38-1).			

(continued)

641

TABLE 38-5
(Continued)

Risk Intervention	Recommendations
Physical activity Goal: minimum 30 min 3–4 times a week	Assess risk, preferably with exercise test, to guide prescription. Encourage minimum of 30–60 min of moderate-intensity activity 3–4 times weekly (walking, jogging, cycling, etc.) supplemented by an increase in daily lifestyle activities (eg., walking breaks at work, using stairs, household work). Maximum benefit 5 to 6 h week. Advise medically supervised programs for moderate- to high-risk patients.
Weight management	Start intensive dietary therapy and appropriate physical activity, as outlined above, in patients whose BMI is ≥ 25 kg/m^2. Particularly emphasize need for weight loss in patients with hypertension, elevated triglycerides, or elevated glucose levels.
Antiplatelet agents/ anticoagulants	Start aspirin 325 mg/d day if not contraindicated. Manage warfarin to INR of 2–3.5 for post-MI patients not able to take aspirin.

ACE inhibitors in post-MI patients	Start early post-MI in stable high-risk patients [anterior MI, previous MI, Killip class II (S_3 gallop, rales, radiographic congestive heart failure)] Continue indefinitely for all with LV dysfunction (ejection fraction $\leq 40\%$) or symptoms of failure. Use as needed to manage blood pressure or symptoms in all other patients.
Beta-blockers	Start in high-risk post-MI patients (arrhythmia, LV dysfunction, inducible ischemia) at 5 to 28 days. Continue 6 months minimum. Observe usual contraindications. Appropriate use of beta-blockers not contraindicated in patients with diabetes. Use as needed to manage angina, rhythm, or blood pressure in all other patients.
Estrogen	Observational studies (but not clinical trials) suggest benefit in regard to osteoporosis but not CAD. Individualize recommendation consistent with other health risks.

Key: LDL = low-density lipoprotein; HDL = high-density lipoprotein; Hb Alc = hemoglobin Hb Alc; ACE = angiotensin-converting enzyme; MI = myocardial infarction; BP = blood pressure; AHA = American Heart Association; TG = triglycerides; BMI = body mass index; INR = International Normalized Ratio; CAD = coronary artery disease.

assigned to three treatment arms: stent implantation and placebo, stent implantation and abciximab, or angioplasty and abciximab. For diabetic patients receiving stent and abciximab versus those receiving stent treatment alone, there was a >50 percent reduction in death and nonfatal myocardial infarction at 6 months. At that point, diabetics were less likely to require repeat target-organ revascularization if they received stent and abciximab (8.1 percent) compared with those receiving either stent and placebo (16.6 percent, $p = 0.02$) or angioplasty and abciximab (18.4 percent, $p = 0.008$). It appears that the effect of abciximab is linked to stent implantation, since elastic recoil and related adverse remodeling is significantly diminished with successful stent deployment, leaving neointimal hyperplasia as the main mechanism of restenosis. With the results of the EPISTENT trial, clinicians are more comfortable recommending percutaneous intervention.

The largest randomized trial comparing angioplasty with bypass surgery in patients with multivessel CAD, the Bypass Angioplasty Revascularization Investigation (BARI) trial, was a landmark study that highlighted the marked benefit of bypass over angioplasty in diabetics as opposed to nondiabetics. In the diabetes subgroup, the 5-year mortality was reduced from 34 to 19 percent with surgical revascularization, translating into a number needed to treat to prevent one death of only 7. The most marked difference between the two groups appeared after the first year of follow-up, suggesting that mechanisms other than angioplasty-related restenosis might be playing a role.

Congestive Heart Failure

The term *diabetic cardiomyopathy* encompasses the multifactorial etiologies of diabetes-related left ventricular (LV) failure. The Framingham Heart Study showed that diabetic men with congestive heart failure (CHF) were twice as common as their nondiabetic counterparts and that diabetic females had a fivefold increase in the rate of CHF. The spectrum of heart failure ranges from asymptomatic disease to overt systolic failure. Diabetes complicated by hypertension represents a particularly high-risk group for the development of CHF. Diastolic dysfunction is exceedingly common (>50 percent prevalence in some studies) and may be linked to diabetes without the presence of concomitant hypertension.

Given the prominence of the diabetic subgroup in randomized trials of ACE inhibition in CHF, much emphasis has been placed on initiating ACE-inhibitor therapy as soon as LV dysfunction is noted, regardless of symptomatology. The results of the HOPE trial will likely translate into even earlier initiation of ACE inhibition in patients without clinical LV dysfunction.

Summary of Clinical Guidelines

Table 38-5 summarizes the AHA recommendations for risk interventions in diabetics with atherosclerotic vascular disease. It is likely that recommended levels for blood pressure and for LDL choleterol will be lowered considerably in the near future.

SUGGESTED READING

American Diabetes Association: Standard of medical care for patients with diabetes mellitus. *Diabetes Care* 2000; 23(suppl 1):S532–S542.

Farkouh ME, Rayfield EJ, Fuster V: Diabetes and cardiovascular disease. In: Fuster V, Alexander RW; O'Rourke RA, et al (eds). *Hurst's The Heart*, 10th ed. New York: McGraw-Hill; 2001: 2197–2218.

Grundy SM, Benjamin IJ, Burke GL, et al: Diabetes and cardiovascular disease: A statement for healthcare professionals from the American Heart Association. *Circulation* 1999; 100:1134–1146.

Heart Outcomes Prevention Evaluation Study Investigators: Effects of ramipril on cardiovascular and microvascular outcomes in people with diabetes mellitus: Results of the HOPE study and MICRO-HOPE sub-study. *Lancet* 2000; 355:253–259.

Lincoff AM, Califf RM, Moliterno DJ, et al for the Evaluation of Platelet IIb/IIIa Inhibition in Stenting Investigators (EPISTENT): Complementary clinical benefits of coronary artery stenting and blockade of platelet glycoprotein IIb/IIIa receptors. *N Engl J Med* 1999; 341:319–327.

Malmberg K for the DIGAMI Study Group: Prospective randomized study of intensive insulin treatment on long-term survival after acute myocardial infarction in patients with diabetes mellitus. *Br Med J* 1997; 314:1512–1515.

The Bypass Angioplasty Revascularization Investigation (BARI) Investigators: Comparison of bypass surgery with angioplasty in patients with multi-vessel disease. *N Engl J Med* 1996; 335:217–225.

The Expert Committee on the Diagnosis and Classification of Diabetes Mellitus: Report of the Expert Committee on the Diagnosis and Classification of Diabetes Mellitus. *Diabetes Care* 1997; 20:1183–1202.

39

ADVERSE CARDIOVASCULAR DRUG INTERACTIONS AND COMPLICATIONS

Lionel H. Opie
William H. Frishman

Today, knowledge of cardiovascular drug interactions is regarded as basic to our understanding of the pharmacologic properties of cardiovascular drugs. Such interactions can be either *pharmacokinetic,* whereby one agent interferes with the metabolism of another, or *pharmacodynamic,* whereby the hemodynamic properties of one agent may be additive or subtractive to those of the drugs given as cotherapy. The liver is the chief site of pharmacokinetic interactions. An example is increased danger of myopathy with statins during the coadministration of erythromycin or ketoconazole, both inhibiting the cytochrome P450 system and its CYP3A4 isoform in the liver. A second example of a pharmacokinetic interaction involves those drugs that act on the P-glycoprotein that is the digoxin transmembrane transporter, showing how basic studies can help unravel well-known but poorly understood interactions such as that between quinidine and digoxin. An example of a pharmacodynamic interaction arises when a calcium channel blocker (CCB) is added to beta-adrenergic blockade in the therapy of severe angina, sometimes with excess hypotension as a side effect.

PRINCIPLES OF CARDIAC DRUG INTERACTIONS

Hepatic Pharmacokinetic Interactions

Many cardiovascular drugs are metabolized in the liver, generally via the cytochrome oxidase system, involving one of several isoforms. Of the various isoforms, the CYP3A4 is the site of most hepatic interactions of cardiac drugs. A number of interacting drugs—such as phenytoin, barbiturates, rifampin, and the herbal remedy St John's wort—can *induce the CYP3A4 isoform.* Accordingly, such drugs accelerate the breakdown of those cardiovascular drugs that are metabolized by this isoform, such as atorvastatin, cerivastatin, cyclosporine, disopyramide, felodipine, lidocaine, lovastatin, nifedipine, nisoldipine, propafenone, and simvastatin. Thus the inducers lessen the blood concentrations of these drugs and their therapeutic efficacy. On the other hand, blood levels of these same drugs are increased by those agents that act as *inhibitors of the CYP3A4 isoform.* The prototype inhibitors are cimetidine and erythromycin, with grapefruit juice; the calcium channel blockers verapamil and diltiazem; and the antifungal agents, such as ketoconazole, all acting as inhibitors. Thus excess circulating levels may build up, with greater risk of adverse effects from statins, including greater risk of myopathy.

Cimetidine inhibits a variety of other isoforms, so that it can increase blood levels of a host of drugs, including the antiarrhythmics quinidine, lidocaine, and procainamide; the CCB verapamil; and the beta-blocker propranolol. Ranitidine inhibits fewer isoforms and is much less likely to interact in this way.

Pharmacodynamic Hepatic Interactions

These occur whenever altered hepatic blood flow changes the rate of first-pass liver metabolism. For example, when a beta blocker and lidocaine are given together, as may occur during acute myocardial infarction, the beta blocker reduces both the hepatic blood flow to the liver and the rate of hepatic metabolism of lidocaine. The consequence is an increased blood lidocaine level, with the risk of lidocaine toxicity. Conversely, by increasing hepatic blood flow, nifedipine has the opposite effect, so that the breakdown of propranolol is increased, resulting in lower blood levels of propranolol.

P-Glycoprotein

This newly discovered digoxin transporter operates whenever digoxin crosses the cell membrane—for example, during renal excretion or when being taken up through the gut wall. Inhibition of the transporter explains the major effects of quinidine and verapamil on blood digoxin levels and lays aside the previous concept that erythromycin and tetracycline increased digoxin levels by inhibiting the gut flora that break down digoxin. Rather, these agents and especially erythromycin may act at least in part by inhibiting the P-glycoprotein.

Proarrhythmic Drug Interactions

These do not fit neatly into the standard differentiation between pharmacodynamic and pharmacokinetic interactions. They must be considered separately. There are basically three possible proarrhythmic mechanisms. First, prolongation of the QT interval may occur, especially in the presence of hypokalemia and/or bradycardia. The type of arrhythmia produced by QT prolongation is highly specific—namely, torsades de pointes. Second, sympathomimetic inotropic agents that increase myocardial levels of cyclic adenosine monophosphate or cytosolic calcium cause arrhythmias through a different mechanism: the precipitation of ventricular tachycardia and/or fibrillation. Third, beta-adrenergic stimulants decrease plasma potassium levels, which, in turn, promotes automaticity.

Renal Pharmacokinetic Interactions

A number of drugs interact with each other by competing for renal clearance mechanisms by altering the rate of renal clearance of the other drug. For example, the renal clearance of digoxin is decreased by quinidine, by inhibition of the transporter P-glycoprotein, leading to an elevation of blood digoxin levels. Other antiarrhythmics that inhibit the renal excretion of digoxin include verapamil, amiodarone, and propafenone, all acting on the transporter.

Plasma Protein Binding as a Site for Drug Interactions

Sulfinpyrazone powerfully displaces warfarin, so that the dose of warfarin required may be dramatically less.

BETA-ADRENERGIC BLOCKING DRUGS

Beta-adrenergic blockers suffer from relatively few serious drug interactions (Table 39-1). Lipid-soluble beta blockers—carvedilol, labetalol, metoprolol, and propranolol—are metabolized in the liver by the cytochrome oxidase system, chiefly by CYP2D6. The latter enzyme in turn is inhibited by cimetidine, ritonavir, and quinidine, all of which would tend to increase blood levels of these beta blockers. Pharmacodynamic interactions are as expected, with added sinus and atrioventricular nodal inhibitions, by digoxin and amiodarone as well as the nondihydropyridine calcium blockers verapamil and diltiazem. Enhanced negative inotropic interactions occur in response to verapamil, diltiazem, some antiarrhythmics, and most anesthetic agents.

TABLE 39-1

INTERACTIONS OF BETA-BLOCKING DRUGS

	Interacting Drugs
HEPATIC INTERACTIONS	
Lipid-soluble drugs interact with inhibitors of CYP2D6: carvedilol, labetalol, metoprolol and propranolol (probably timolol)	Inhibitors of CYP2D6 all increase blood levels: Cimetidine, ritonavir, quinidine.
Water-soluble drugs do not interact: atenolol, nadolol, sotalol, and the major acebutolol metabolite	
PHARMACODYNAMIC INTERACTIONS	
Added nodal inhibition	Digoxin, amiodarone, verapamil, and diltiazem
Added negative inotropic effects	Verapamil and diltiazem, antiarrhythmics, most anesthetic agents

---

NITRATES

The chief drug interactions of nitrates are pharmacodynamic leading to excess hypotension (Table 39-2). For example, during triple therapy of angina pectoris (nitrates, beta blockers, calcium antagonists), the overall efficacy of the combination may be lessened, because each drug can predispose patients to excess hypotension. Even two components of triple therapy, such as diltiazem and nitrates, may interact adversely to cause moderate hypotension. Individual patients vary greatly in their susceptibility to the hypotension of triple therapy. A dangerous drug-drug interaction is that of nitrates with sildenafil, an anti-impotence drug that can intensify the hypotensive effects of nitrates. Sildenafil should not be used within 24 h of nitrate use. There is a reported beneficial interaction between nitrates and hydralazine whereby the latter drug appears to lessen nitrate tolerance.

Unexpectedly, high doses of nitroglycerin may induce heparin resistance by altering the activity of antithrombin III. Nitroglycerin can also lessen the therapeutic effects of the tissue plasminogen activator alteplase.

TABLE 39-2
NITRATES: HEMODYNAMIC INTERACTIONS

Interacting Drugs	Mechanism	Prophylaxis
CCBs	Excess vasodilation	Check BP, low initial doses
Alpha blockers	Excess vasodilation	Check BP, low initial doses
Sildenafil (Viagra)	Excess hypotension; Viagra is metabolized by 3A4 isoform, so that inhibitors, including erythromycin and ritonavir, predispose to excess Viagra levels and to nitrate interaction	Before giving nitrates for unstable angina, question on use of Viagra in preceding 24 h

CALCIUM CHANNEL BLOCKERS
(CCBs, CALCIUM ANTAGONISTS)

Hepatic interactions are important (Table 39-3). As a group, CCBs are metabolized by the CYP3A4 isoform. Therefore, blood levels will increase or decrease as the isoform is inhibited or induced during cotherapy with the agents listed in Table 39-3. Additionally, it is now increasingly recognized that verapamil and especially diltiazem (but probably not nifedipine or amlodipine) inhibit the hepatic oxidation of some drugs, the blood levels of which consequently increase. Both diltiazem and verapamil should theoretically have a similar spectrum of inhibitory effects at the level of CYP3A4. Diltiazem is already known to inhibit the breakdown of cyclosporine, some statins (lovastatin, simvastatin, and atorvastatin), and some human immunodeficiency virus (HIV) protease inhibitors. Verapamil is already known to inhibit the breakdown of the antiepileptic carbamazepine and that of prazosin, theophylline, and quinidine. A novel interaction is that verapamil inhibits the transport glycoprotein for digoxin, thereby sometimes doubling the blood digoxin levels. Concomitant grapefruit juice ingestion, by inhibiting CYP3A, can potentiate some dihydropyridine CCBs (felodipine, nifedipine). Many of the other interactions of CCBs are pharmacodynamic, such as added effects on the atrioventricular (AV) or sinus nodes (verapamil or diltiazem plus beta blockers, excess digitalis, or amiodarone) or on the systemic vascular resistance (for example, nifedipine plus beta or alpha blockers, causing excess hypotension).

ANTIARRHYTHMIC AGENTS

The three major mechanisms for the most frequent antiarrhythmic drug interactions are (1) with the digoxin transporter, causing digoxin levels to increase with quinidine, amiodarone, and verapamil (see next section); (2) at the level of the hepatic enzymes; and (3) with other drugs that prolong the QT interval (Table 39-4). Antiarrhythmics that prolong the QT interval (such as the class 1A agents quinidine, procainamide, and disopyramide) and especially the class III agents (amiodarone, sotalol, ibutilide and dofetilide) that prolong the duration of the action potential may all interact with completely different drug classes (diuretics that prolong QT interval by potassium or magnesium depletion, certain macrolide antibiotics such as erythromycin, some quinolones, some tricyclics, phenothiazines, and some antihistamines such as astemizole and terfenadine). There is also the risk of antiarrhythmic drug-drug interactions. Thus, amiodarone, when added to quinidine, enhances the risk of QT

TABLE 39-3

CALCIUM CHANNEL BLOCKER INTERACTIONS

Hepatic and Other Interactions of CCBs	Interacting Drugs
Inhibitors of CYP3A4: tend to increase blood levels of CCBs	Cimetidine, erythromycin, grapefruit juice, ketoconazole and related antifungals, amiodarone, St. John's wort (an herbal remedy)
Inducers of CYP3A4: tend to decrease blood levels of CCB, especially documented for verapamil	Barbiturates, carbamazepine, phenytoin, rifampin
CCBs as inhibitors of CYP4A4: verapamil (V) and diltiazem (D), which should have similar effects	V increases blood levels of carbamazepine, prazosin, theophylline, quinidine, cilostazol (expected) D increases blood levels of cyclosporine, some HIV protease inhibitors, some statins (lovastatin, atorvastatin, simvastatin), cilostazol
Inhibition of digoxin-transport P-glycoprotein	Digoxin blood levels are increased by verapamil and nifedipine

TABLE 39-4

INTERACTIONS (KINETIC AND DYNAMIC) OF ANTIARRHYTHMIC DRUGS[a]

Drug	Interaction with	Result
Quinidine	Digoxin	Increased digoxin level
	Other type 1 antiarrhythmics	Added negative inotropic effect and/or depressed conduction
	Beta blockers, verapamil	Enhanced hypotension, negative inotropic effect
	Amiodarone	Risk of torsades; increased quinidine levels
	Sotalol	Risk of torsades
	Diuretics	If hypokalemia, risk of torsades
	Verapamil	Increased quinidine level
	Nifedipine	Decreased quinidine level
	Warfarin	Enhanced anticoagulation
	Enzyme inhibitors	Increased blood levels
	Enzyme inducers	Decreased blood levels
Procainamide	Cimetidine	Decreases renal clearance
	Class III agents, diuretics	Torsades
	Other type 1 antiarrhythmics	Depressed conduction
Disopyramide	Amiodarone, sotalol	Torsades
	Beta-blockers, verapamil	Enhanced hypotension
	Anticholinergics	Increased anticholinergic effects

	Pyridostigmine	Decreased anticholinergic effect
	Enzyme inducers	Decreased blood levels
	Enzyme inhibitors	Increased blood levels
Lidocaine	Beta blockers, cimetidine, halothane	Reduced liver blood flow (increased blood levels)
	Enzyme inducers	Decreased blood levels
	Enzyme inhibitors	Increased blood levels
Flecainide	Major kinetic interaction with amiodarone; also cimetidine, quinidine, and ritonavir	Increased blood flecainide levels; with amiodarone, use half-dose
	Beta blockers, quinidine, disopyramide	Added negative inotropic effects
	Quinidine, procainamide	Conduction block
	Digoxin, verapamil, diltiazem, beta blockers	Added AV nodal block
Moricizine	Enzyme inhibitors	Moricizine levels increased
	Beta blockers, quinidine, disopyramide	Enhanced nodal and myocardial depression
Propafenone	Digoxin	Digoxin level increased
	Warfarin	Anticoagulant effect enhanced

(continued)

TABLE 39-4
(Continued)

Drug	Interaction with	Result
Sotalol	Diuretics, class IA agents, amiodarone, tricyclics, phenothiazines, others	Risk of torsades; avoid hypokalemia; check QT interval
Amiodarone (NB very long half life, with long-lasting interactions)	As for sotalol	Risk of torsades, check QT and potassium
	Digoxin	Increased digoxin levels
	Quinidine	Increase quinidine levels, torsades risk
	Phenytoin	Increased phenytoin levels
	Flecainide	Increased flecainide levels
	Warfarin	Increased warfarin effect
Ibutilide Dofetilide	As for sotalol (all agents prolonging QT)	As for sotalol
Verapamil Diltiazem	Beta blockers, excess digoxin, myocardial depressants, quinidine	Increased myocardial or nodal depression

[a] Enzyme inducers = hepatic enzyme inducers (i.e., barbiturates, phenytoin, rifampin, St. John's wort); enzyme inhibitors = cimetidine, erythromycin, verapamil, diltiazem, ketoconazole, grapefruit juice, ritonavir.

SOURCE: Compiled by L. H. Opie and adapted from Opie LH, Gersh B (eds): *Drugs for the Heart*, 5th ed. Philadelphia: Saunders; 2001, with permission.

prolongation while quinidine levels increase, so that quinidine toxicity is also more likely. Although the combination of two arrhythmic drugs, amiodarone and beta blockers, can occasionally lead to life-threatening bradycardia, this combination may be lifesaving in postinfarct patients with severe ventricular arrhythmias. Of all the antiarrhythmics, quinidine is associated with the most interactions. Although there is no evidence that it prolongs life and there is a bold death warning in the package insert, quinidine inexplicably continues to be used.

Among the antiarrhythmic drugs that prolong life are beta blockers, already discussed, and amiodarone. Besides QT prolongation, note that amiodarone, with its very long half-life, potentiates warfarin and increases the International Normalized Ratio (INR) (prothrombin time) for months, so that the combination must be avoided. The mechanism is not fully known, but may be by an interaction of the hepatic CYP2C9 isoform.

Regarding hepatic interactions, these are now known to be much more complex than previously thought (cimetidine decreases hepatic metabolism of quinidine; phenytoin and barbiturates have an opposite effect). When hepatic CYP3A isoenzymes are induced by drugs such as phenytoin, phenobarbital, rifampin, and theophylline as well as by the herbal remedy St. John's wort, the hepatic metabolism of quinidine may markedly increase with decreased steady-state concentrations of quinidine. Conversely, cimetidine, verapamil, diltiazem, ketoconazole, amiodarone, grapefruit juice, and ritonavir can inhibit these isoenzymes to decrease the metabolism of quinidine and increase quinidine levels. Similar principles apply to propafenone, disopyramide, and lidocaine, which are also broken down by hepatic CYP3A. Flecainide, broken down by CYP2D6, has levels increased by amiodarone, cimetidine, quinidine, and ritonavir.

Adenosine interacts markedly with aminophylline or theophylline, which compete with adenosine for the receptor sites, thereby inhibiting the therapeutic nodal effects of adenosine. Dipyridamole, on the other hand, inhibits the breakdown of adenosine and/or its uptake into the tissues, so that the amount of adenosine available for the antiarrhythmic effect is enhanced. Effective doses of adenosine in patients receiving sustained dipyridamole therapy may only be one-quarter to one-eighth of the normal doses.

POSITIVE INOTROPIC AGENTS

Digoxin

The digoxin transmembrane transporter, P-glycoprotein, which transports digoxin across renal epithelial cell membranes, is markedly inhibited by quinidine, verapamil, and amiodarone, with a large rise in blood digoxin levels. The previous dose of digoxin should be halved and the plasma digoxin rechecked. *Diuretics* may indirectly precipitate digitalis toxicity by causing hypokalemia, which, when really severe (plasma potassium below 2 to 3 meq/L), may stop the tubular secretion of digoxin. Potassium-sparing diuretics (amiloride, triamterene, and spironolactone) as well as captopril decrease digoxin clearance by about 20 to 30 percent and may also elevate serum potassium levels. Cancer chemotherapeutic agents may damage intestinal mucosa to depress digoxin absorption. Nonsteroidal anti-inflammatory drugs (NSAIDs) decrease the renal clearance of digoxin, thereby increasing plasma digoxin levels. Rifampin and phenobarbital, through hepatic enzyme induction, can reduce plasma digoxin levels. (See Table 39-5.)

Dopamine and Dobutamine

Monoamine-oxidase inhibitors decrease dopamine breakdown; the dose of dopamine should be one-tenth of the usual. Dobutamine decreases plasma potassium and should be given with care together with diuretics, especially when QT-prolonging drugs are used.

DIURETICS

Loop Diuretics

Hypokalemia, as may occur when loop diuretics are given acutely and intravenously, may precipitate digitalis toxicity. Complex interactions between furosemide and captopril have emerged. Captopril decreases the renal excretion of furosemide, which is required for the diuretic effect of the latter. When captopril is given in a standard dose of 25 mg, furosemide has little or no diuretic effect. On the other hand, only minute doses of captopril, such as 1 mg, enhance the diuretic effect of furosemide. In patients with low serum sodium, which is an indirect indicator of a high-renin state, it is the high aldosterone level that retains sodium and stimulates vasopressin secretion, the latter causing the hyponatremia. Therapy of such patients by furosemide alone is ineffective; the addition of captopril in a standard dose may achieve improvement.

Thiazide Diuretics

Steroids, estrogens, and indomethacin and other NSAIDs lessen the antihypertensive effect of thiazide diuretics and may worsen congestive heart failure. Angiotensin converting enzyme (ACE) inhibitors

TABLE 39-5

DRUG INTERACTIONS OF DIGOXIN (D)

Interacting Drug	Mechanism	Result
Amiodarone	Reduced renal clearance of D; P-glycoprotein inhibition	D level may double
Atorvastatin	Not known	D level may rise 20%
Captopril	Reduced D clearance	Blood D increases
Diltiazem	Variable decrease of D clearance; inhibits P-glycoprotein	Variable blood D increases
Diuretics: potassium-sparing amiloride or triamterene; spironolactone (S)	Reduced extrarenal D clearance;	D levels vary, may rise by 20%
	S reduces D clearance, inhibits P-glycoprotein	D levels increase
Erythromycin	Inhibits P-glycoprotein	Decreased D loss into bowel; increased D levels
Nifedipine	Variable effect on D clearance	Variable blood D rises
Prazosin (PZ)	PZ displaces D from binding sites	Blood D rises
Propafenone	Inhibits P-glycoprotein	D level increases
Quinidine, quinine	Inhibits P-glycoprotein	Blood D doubles
Verapamil	Inhibits P-glycoprotein	Blood D doubles or more

and angiotensin II receptor blockers are potassium-retaining and may cause hyperkalemia if combined with other potassium retainers, especially if there is renal impairment.

ANGIOTENSIN-CONVERTING ENZYME INHIBITORS AND ANGIOTENSIN II TYPE 1–RECEPTOR BLOCKERS (ARBs)

In general, these agents have few drug interactions apart from risk of first-dose hypotension with high diuretic doses. There is potential hyperkalemia with potassium-sparing diuretics; yet in heart failure, spironolactone in low doses can improve outcome provided that the plasma potassium is carefully monitored and renal failure excluded. Aspirin may annul some of the vasodilating effects of ACE inhibitors, so that it may be best to select low-dose aspirin.

ANTITHROMBOTIC AND THROMBOLYTIC AGENTS

Aspirin

Blood levels of uric acid may be increased by both aspirin and thiazide diuretics, so that special care is required in patients with a history of gout. Conversely, aspirin may decrease the uricosuric effects of sulfinpyrazone and probenecid. Aspirin can have some effects similar to those of the other NSAIDs, inhibiting the effects of vasodilatory prostaglandins. Aspirin-induced gastrointestinal bleeding may be a greater hazard in patients receiving other NSAIDs or corticosteroid therapy. Inducers of the hepatic cytochrome oxidase system (barbiturates, phenytoin, rifampin) increase aspirin breakdown. Aspirin tends to cause hypoglycemia in patients receiving oral hypoglycemics or insulin. Aspirin, especially in high doses, may exaggerate a bleeding tendency and anticoagulant-induced bleeding. All these drug interactions should be less intense if the aspirin doses are kept low, as is the current trend. (See Table 39-6.)

Ticlopidine and Clopidogrel

These antiplatelet drugs do not appear to interfere with the vasodilating activity of ACE inhibitors.

Warfarin (Coumadin)

NUMEROUS DRUG AND DIET-DRUG INTERACTIONS

Warfarin may be subject to many (up to 80) drug interactions. Furthermore, there is a *diet-drug interaction*. Warfarin has its effects lessened by a diet rich in the prothrombin precursor vitamin K, found in dark green vegetables, and certain plant oils, including those used in margarines and salad dressings. Dose adjustments may be required when potentially interfering drugs including herbal agents are added.

MECHANISMS

The major known sites of interaction are, first, the plasma proteins, where warfarin is bound while circulating, and second, the hepatic cytochrome P450 system, where warfarin is broken down by the CYP2C9 isoform. For example, with amiodarone, a given dose of warfarin has a greater inhibition of prothrombin with increased risk of bleeding, resulting from the inhibition by amiodarone of the CYP2C9 isoform. Any drug impairing platelet function, such as aspirin, ticlopidine, or clopidogrel, may indirectly promote bleeding due to warfarin. Very high doses of aspirin (six to eight tablets per day) may act differently by impairing synthesis of clotting factors. Heparin also potentiates the risk of bleeding with large individual variations.

Interfering drugs include those that reduce absorption of vitamin K, warfarin (cholestyramine), or sulfinpyrazone (which displaces warfarin from the plasma protein binding sites) and those that induce hepatic enzymes (barbiturates, phenytoin, rifampin). The latter drugs, and also the herbal agent St. John's wort, increase the rate of warfarin degradation in the liver.

Potentiating drugs decrease warfarin degradation by inhibiting the CYP2C9 isoform. These include a variety of antibiotics such as metronidazole (Flagyl) and cotrimoxazole (Bactrim). Other antifungals such as fluconazole and vaginal suppository miconazole also potentiate warfarin. Cimetidine inhibits hepatic degradation; ranitidine does not. Other potentiating drugs include the cardiovascular agents allopurinol, propafenone, quinidine, and amiodarone. Amiodarone is especially dangerous because of its excessively long half-life, so that this interaction can occur even after withdrawal of amiodarone. Grapefruit juice does not act on the CYP2C9 so that there is no interaction with warfarin. Potentiation also results from displacement of warfarin from blood proteins by sulfinpyrazone and the fibrates (fenofibrate, gemfibrozil). Sulfinpyrazone does this so powerfully that the dose of warfarin may have to be reduced to only 1 mg in some patients.

TABLE 39-6

DRUG INTERACTIONS OF ANTITHROMBOTIC AGENTS

Cardiac Drug	Interacting Drugs	Mechanism	Consequence
Aspirin (A)	ACE inhibitors	Vasodilation ↓	Less antifailure effect
	Hepatic enzyme inducers (barbiturates, phenytoin, rifampin)	Increased A metabolism	Decreased A effect
	Sulfinpyrazone (S), probenecid (P)	A decreases urate excretion	Decreased uricosuric effect of S or P
	Thiazide diuretics	A decreases urate excretion	Hyperuricemia
	Warfarin (W)	A is antithrombotic	Excess bleeding
Sulfinpyrazone (S)	Warfarin	S displaces W from plasma proteins	Excess bleeding

Warfarin (W)		
Potentiating drugs		
Allopurinol	Mechanism unknown	Excess bleeding
Amiodarone	Mechanism unknown	Sensitizes to W for months
Aspirin	Added bleeding tendency	Excess bleeding
Cimetidine	Decreased W degradation	Excess bleeding
Quinidine	Hepatic interaction	Excess bleeding
Statins	Hepatic interaction?	Excess bleeding
Sulfinpyrazone	Displaces W from plasma proteins	Excess bleeding
Fibrates	As above	Excess bleeding
Inhibitory drugs		
Cholestyramine, colestipol	Decrease absorption of W	Decreased W effect
Nitrates	Decreased tPA effect	
Alteplase, t-PA		Less thrombolytic benefit

663

LIPID-LOWERING DRUGS

Fibrates may markedly potentiate warfarin (see above), while the statins in general have little or no effect. The latter is not too surprising, because most of them (exceptions: pravastatin and fluvastatin) are metabolized by the CYP3A4 isoform that does not metabolize warfarin. In the case of fluvastatin, the absence of interaction noted in the package insert is surprising because this statin, unlike the others, inhibits the hepatic CYP2C9, according to the Georgetown University website data. Nonetheless, caution is advised with all statins. On first principles, the simplest statin to combine with warfarin would be pravastatin, because it is metabolized quite differently from the cytochrome P450 system.

Whenever potentially interfering drugs or over the counter agents are added more frequent measurements of the prothrombin time (International Normalized Ratio, or INR) and possible dose adjustments are required.

LIPID-LOWERING AGENTS

There are not many serious interactions (Table 39-7). A number of lipid-lowering agents may interact with warfarin, either by decreased absorption (cholestyramine) or by hepatic interference (bezafibrate, fenofibrate, gemfibrozil). The exact mechanism is not clear. The fibrates (fenofibrate, gemfibrozil) and many of the statins increase the effects of warfarin.

Simvastatin, lovastatin, atorvastatin, and cerivastatin are metabolized by the hepatic CYP3A4 isoform. The risk of myopathy with these statins is increased substantially by concomitant use of the few drugs that substantially inhibit P450 CYP3A4, including ketoconazole, erythromycin, and verapamil. Cyclosporine, diltiazem, and grapefruit juice are weaker inhibitors. Pravastatin is not metabolized by P450, so it is free of these interactions. There is a positive interaction of pravastatin with cyclosporine, with increased immunosuppression (Table 39-7). Fluvastatin is metabolized by the CYP2C9 isoform, so that its clearance is decreased by cimetidine and probably ranitidine but increased by rifampin. Statins should ideally not be combined with the fibrates or niacin because of the higher risk of myositis with rhabdomyolysis and possible renal failure. Yet in clinical practice, the advantages of better lipid control with combined therapy seem to outweigh these risks. Likewise, concurrent therapy with niacin or ketoconazole or erythromycin may also carry a small risk of rhabdomyolysis. Serum creatine kinase levels should be checked periodically, especially after increasing doses or after starting combination therapy.

TABLE 39-7
DRUG INTERACTIONS OF LIPID-LOWERING AGENTS

Lipid Drug	Interacting Drugs	Mechanisms	Consequence
Fibrates (gemfibrozil, bezafibrate, fenofibrate)	Warfarin	Hepatic interference and/or displacement of warfarin from plasma proteins	Risk of bleeding
Bile acid sequestrants (cholestyramine, colestipol)	Warfarin (W)	Decreased absorption	Decreased W effect
	Many other drugs	Decreased absorption	Decreased drug effect
Statins Lovastatin Simvastatin Atorvastatin Cerivastatin	Fibrates	Added damage to muscle with myositis	Rhabdomyolysis and risk of renal failure; increased cyclosporine levels
	Inhibitors of CYP3A4 (erythromycin, antifungal azoles, others)		
	Nicotinic acid		
	Cyclosporine		
Fluvastatin	CYP2C9 metabolizers	Cimetidine, ranitidine	Levels increase, toxic risk
		Enzyme inducers	Levels decrease
Pravastatin	Cyclosporine	Hepatic interaction; cyclosporine hepatotoxicity	Rhabdomyolysis and risk or renal failure; increased cyclosporine levels
All statins	Warfarin	Hepatic interaction	Increased risk of bleeding

HERBAL MEDICINE

Herbal supplements are commonly used by patients in the hope of benefiting cardiac conditions. Many of these herbs cause cardiac toxicity or can interact unfavorably with known cardiac drugs. Chamomile has antispasmodic and warfarin-like effects. Feverfew, garlic, and ginger have antiplatelet actions and can pose safety problems in patients taking warfarin. Gingko and ginseng should be avoided in patients receiving warfarin and heparin. Herbal acquaretics can inhibit diuretics or other antihypertensive therapy. Gossypol and licorice may cause renal loss of potassium and should not be used with thiazide and loop diuretics or digoxin. Plantain and hawthorn berries can mimic or potentiate digoxin toxicity. Kelp can interfere with the antiarrhythmic effects of amiodarone. St. Johns's wort can lower serum digoxin levels by reducing digoxin absorption. It stimulates hepatic CYP3A to lower serum warfarin and should be added to the list of hepatic enzyme inducers.

SUGGESTED READING

Abernethy DR, Flockhart DA: Molecular basis of cardiovascular drug metabolism. Implications for predicting clinically important drug interactions. *Circulation* 2000; 101:1749–1753.

Frishman WH, Cheng-Lai A, Chen J (eds): Antiarrhythmic agents. In: *Current-Cardiovascular Drugs,* 3d ed. Philadelphia: Current Medicine; 2000:54–84.

Fromm MF, Kim RB, Stein M, et al: Inhibition of P-glycoprotein–mediated drug transport. A unifying mechanism to explain the interaction between digoxin and quinidine. *Circulation* 1999; 99:552–557.

Opie LH: Adverse cardiovascular drug interactions. *Curr Probl Cardiol* 2000; 25:621–676.

Opie LH, Frishman WH: Adverse cardiovascular drug interactions and complications. In: Fuster V, Alexander RW, O'Rourke RA, et al (eds): *Hurst's The Heart,* 10th ed. New York: McGraw-Hill; 2001:2251–2269.

Opie LH, Gersh BJ: *Drugs for the Heart,* 5th ed. Philadelphia: Saunders; 2001.

40

HEART DISEASE AND PREGNANCY

John H. McAnulty
James Metcalfe
Kent Ueland

An understanding of the cardiovascular changes of a normal pregnancy is important for optimal care. This is even more important if a woman has heart disease. With successful treatment of heart disease during childhood, usually with surgery, the number of women with heart disease is increasing. They now can survive to the age of childbearing and are able to conceive.

HEART ISSUES UNIQUE TO PREGNANCY

Some basic issues must be considered when treating any woman with heart disease during pregnancy.

Health Priorities

Mother and child—the health of one importantly influences the other. The well-being of the fetus should be considered, but the safety of the mother is always the highest priority. Ideally, treatment of the mother with drugs, diagnostic studies, or surgery should be avoided, but if required for maternal safety, each should be used.

Maternal Fragility

Despite advances in the management of heart disease, pregnancy puts the mother at risk. The risk is so great with some cardiovascular abnormalities that a recommendation of avoidance or interruption of pregnancy is supportable (Table 40-1).

TABLE 40-1

CARDIOVASCULAR ABNORMALITIES PLACING A MOTHER
AND INFANT AT EXTREMELY HIGH RISK

Advise *avoidance or interruption of pregnancy*
  Pulmonary hypertension
  Dilated cardiomyopathy with congestive failure
  Marfan's syndrome with dilated aortic root
  Cyanotic congenital heart disease
Pregnancy counseling and close clinical follow-up
    required
  Prosthetic valve
  Coarctation of the aorta
  Marfan's syndrome
  Dilated cardiomyopathy in asymptomatic women
  Obstructive lesions

Fetal and Newborn Vulnerability

The fetus depends completely on its mother for a continuous supply
of oxygen and nutrients. Although the maternal commitment to the
fetus is exceptional, if the mother's safety is threatened, blood is preferentially diverted away from the uterus. In the woman with heart
disease, where uterine blood flow may already be compromised, the
chance of inadequate uterine perfusion increases. In addition, diagnostic studies, drugs, or surgery required to protect the mother may
increase fetal loss, result in teratogenicity, or alter fetal growth. A
newborn infant is also fragile, possibly due to previous marginal
uterine blood flow during pregnancy or to lingering effects of medications used to treat the mother. Early infant nourishment may be
jeopardized if maternal heart disease is severe enough to interfere
with breast feeding. If the mother is on medications, breast feeding
could further threaten the infant. Finally, the infant is at risk of losing
a parent, since life expectancy with many forms of heart disease is
significantly less than normal.

Maternal Heart Disease
Is Not "Corrected"

Many women with heart disease who become pregnant will have
had previous mechanical therapy— usually surgery, but increasingly
with a catheter. It is best not to consider a previous lesion "corrected,"
because there is always some residual disease. In some cases, this

disease—a shunt, ventricular dysfunction, an arrhythmia, or persistent obstruction—may adversely affect the mother and, in turn, the fetus.

CARDIOVASCULAR ADJUSTMENTS DURING A NORMAL PREGNANCY

Maternal adaptation to pregnancy includes remarkable cardiovascular changes. This may result in symptoms and physical signs even in a normal pregnancy that are difficult to distinguish from those occurring with heart disease and explains why some abnormalities are not well tolerated during pregnancy (Table 40-1).

Hemodynamic Changes

Resting cardiac output increases by over 40 percent during pregnancy. The increase begins early, with cardiac output reaching its highest levels by the 20th week. Body position influences cardiac output, particularly in the second half of pregnancy, as the enlarged uterus reduces venous return from the lower extremities. When compared with measurements made with the woman in the left lateral position, cardiac output falls by 0.6 L/min when she is supine and by 1.2 L/min when she assumes the upright position. In general, this results in few or no symptoms; in some, however, maintenance of the supine position may result in symptomatic hypotension—the "supine hypotensive syndrome of pregnancy." This can be corrected by having the woman turn onto her side. Cardiac output increases still further at the time of labor and delivery. With each uterine contraction, its value rises by over 30 percent, resulting in a cardiac output that can be as great as 9 L/min. The cardiac output falls rapidly to near normal nonpregnant values within days to weeks after delivery, although there is a slight elevation that can persist as long as lactation occurs.

Associated with and influencing these changes of cardiac output are changes in other hemodynamic parameters. The stroke volume increases dramatically and early in pregnancy and then levels off or falls slightly as venous return is inhibited during the second half of pregnancy. Ventricular end-diastolic volume increases; the ejection fraction does not change. The heart rate increases steadily throughout pregnancy but rarely reaches a value greater than 100 beats per minute in the normal resting woman. Blood pressure falls slightly early in pregnancy, then returns to normal values for the rest of gestation. There is an early fall in systemic vascular resistance associated with the early rise in cardiac output, with a gradual return of vascular resistance to near normal levels by term. Oxygen consumption increases steadily during pregnancy, reaching a value that is 30 percent above nonpregnant levels by the time of delivery.

Distribution of Blood Flow

Where does it go? This is not fully understood, but the distribution is affected by changes in local vascular resistance. During pragnancy, renal blood flow increases by approximately 30 percent. Blood flow to the skin increases by 40 to 50 percent—a mechanism for heat dissipation. Not surprisingly, mammary flood flow increases; usually this is approximately 1 percent of the cardiac output, and it increases to 2 percent by term. In the nonpregnant woman, uterine blood flow is approximately 100 mL/min (2 percent of the cardiac output). This doubles by the 28th week of pregnancy and increases to approximately 1200 mL/min at term. During pregnancy, uterine blood vessels are maximally dilated; flow can increase, but it must result from increased maternal arterial pressure and flow. As mentioned earlier, the mother makes a remarkable commitment to a fetus, but if redistribution of total flow is required by the mother or if there is a fall in maternal blood pressure and cardiac output, uterine blood flow falls preferentially. Vasoconstriction caused by endogenous catecholamines, vasoconstrictive drugs, mechanical ventilation, and some anesthetics—also that associated with preeclampsia and eclampsia—can decrease perfusion of the uterus. Uterine blood flow can potentially be compromised even in a healthy woman. In the mother with heart disease, whose blood flow may already be compromised, the concern about diversion of flow from the uterus is greatest.

The mechanisms for the hemodynamic changes are also not fully understood. They may in part be due to volume changes. Total body water increases steadily throughout pregnancy by 6 to 8 L (most is extracellular). As early as 6 weeks after conception, plasma volume increases and approaches its maximum of 1 1/2 times normal by the second trimester, where it stays throughout the pregnancy. Red blood cell mass also increases, but not to the same degree; thus, the hematocrit falls during pregnancy, though rarely to a value less than 30 percent. Vascular changes are importantly related to the hemodynamic changes of pregnancy. Arterial compliance increases and there is an increase in venous vascular capacitance. These changes are advantageous in maintaining the hemodynamics of a normal pregnancy. There may be disadvantages as well. The arterial changes are associated with increased fragility and, when vascular accidents occur in women, they frequently do so in pregnancy. The increased level of circulating steroid hormones may be the major explanation for the vascular and myocardial changes.

DIAGNOSIS OF HEART DISEASE

Recognition and definition of heart disease may be difficult at any time. This is particularly true during pregnancy. Symptoms suggesting heart disease—fatigue, dyspnea, orthopnea, pedal edema, and chest discomfort—occur commonly in pregnant women with normal hearts. Still, they should at least alert the caregiver to the possibility of heart disease. The concern should increase if the dyspnea or orthopnea is progressive and limiting or if a woman develops hemoptysis, syncope with exertion, or chest pain clearly related to effort. Likewise, the examination can be confusing. Pedal edema, basilar pulmonary rales, a third heart sound, a systolic murmur, and visible neck vein pulsations are also part of a normal pregnancy. Cyanosis, clubbing, a loud systolic murmur ($>3/6$), cardiomegaly, a "fixed split" second heart sound, or evidence for pulmonary hypertension (a left parasternal lift and loud P_2) do not occur as part of a normal pregnancy and deserve attention (see Chap. 1). A diastolle murmur is unusual enough that its presence is an indication of heart disease, although the murmurs can be confused with a venous hum or internal mammary flow sounds (souffle), which are normal findings during pregnancy.

Diagnostic Studies

It is preferable to evaluate the cardiovascular status with history and physical alone, but if the safety of the mother requires it, diagnostic studies should be performed. The electrocardiogram is safe and useful. Echocardiography with evaluation of flow by Doppler is so safe and diagnostically useful that overuse is the only significant concern. Expense and potential misinterpretations are reasons to consuler its use only when required to answer a specific question. Transesophageal echocardiography has been used safely during pregnancy with no apparent increased risk.

All x-ray procedures should generally be avoided, particularly early in pregnancy, as they increase the risk of fetal organogenesis or of a subsequent malignancy in the child, particularly leukemia. If required, a study should be delayed to as late in pregnancy as possible, and shielding of the fetus should be optimal. Every woman of childbearing age should be questioned about the possibility of pregnancy before any x-ray procedure. Chest x-rays are performed on occasion when pregnancy is not recognized (or intentionally when it is). The exposure to a fetus is small (estimated between 10 to 1400 μGY) and has not been associated with recognizable increase in problems. Information can be given to worried parents if a chest x-ray was performed. Magnetic resonance imaging has been used for other purposes during pregnancy and without recognized adverse effects. Radionuclide studies are preferably avoided. Most radionuclide should attach to albumin and thus not reach the fetus, but separation can occur and fetal exposure is possible.

CARDIOVASCULAR DRUGS AND PREGNANCY

Nearly all cardiac drugs cross the placenta and are secreted in breast milk. Information about them all is incomplete, and it is best, when possible, to avoid their use. Again, if required for maternal safety, they should not be withheld.

Diuretics

These can and should be used for treatment of congestive heart failure uncontrolled by sodium restriction, and they are effective therapy for hypertension. Experience is greatest with the thiazide diuretics and with furosemide. Diuretics should not be used for prophylaxis against toxemia or for the treatment of pedal edema.

Inotropic Agents

Digoxin and digitoxin cross the placenta; fetal serum levels are approximately those of the mother's. Maternal serum levels during pregnancy are often lower than in nonpregnancy, given the same digoxin dose. Measuring levels may be helpful, but the assay used should not be one that is affected by an immunoreactive substance found in pregnancy. Digitalis may shorten the duration of gestation and labor due to an effect on the myometrium, which is similar to that on the myocardium. Intravenous inotropic and vasopressor agents (dopamine, dobutamine, and norepinephrine) should be used if necessary to protect the mother, but the fetus is jeopardized because of a reduction in uterine blood flow and the tendency to stimulate uterine contractions. Ephedrine is an appropriate initial vasopressor drug as—at least in animal models—it does not adversely affect uterine blood flow. There is no available information about the use of phosphodiesterase inhibitors during pregnancy.

Adrenergic Receptor Blocking Agents

There have been concerns about the use of beta-blocking drugs during pregnancy, but their safe use in large numbers of pregnant women without adverse effects justifies their use for usual clinical indications. All available beta blockers cross the placenta and are present in human breast milk. If beta blockers are used, beta$_1$-selective agents are preferable; recent concerns of low birth weight with atenolol make metropolol the preferred drug. The newborn infant's heart rate, blood sugar, and respiratory status should be assessed immediately after delivery. Experience with the alpha-blocking agents is sparse. Clonidine, prazosin, and labetalol have been used for hypertension without clear detrimental effects.

Calcium Channel Blocking Drugs

Nifedipine, verapamil, diltiazem, nicardipine, isradipine, and amlodipine have been used to treat hypertension and arrhythmias without adverse effects on the fetus or newborn infant. The drugs may cause relaxation of the uterus; nifedipine has been used specifically for this purpose.

Antiarrhythmic Agents

Atrioventricular (AV) node blockade is occasionally required during pregnancy. This can be achieved with digoxin, beta blockers, and calcium channel blockers; early reports suggest that adenosine can be safely used as well.

When essential for recurrent arrhythmias or maternal safety, the standard antiarrhythmic agents should be used, but there is insufficient accumulated information to know whether or not they increase the risk to the fetus or child. If oral antiarrhythmic therapy is required, it may still be appropriate to begin with quinidine, since, given its long-term availability, it has most frequently been used without clear adverse fetal effects. There is some information about procainamide, disopyramide, mexiletine, flecainide, and atenolol, but it is insufficient to recommend their use unless the drug is essential for the mother. The early available information concering amiodarone would suggest an increased likelihood of fetal loss and deformity.

If intravenous drug therapy is required, lidocaine is reasonable first-line therapy, keeping maternal levels below 4 μg/L. There is no information about the effects of intravenous procainamide, amiodarone, ibutilide, or bretylium during pregnancy.

Vasodilator Agents

When needed for emergency treatment of a hypertensive crisis or pulmonary edema, nitroprusside is the vasodilator drug of choice. This controversial recommendation is made despite a paucity of information about its use during pregnancy because the drug is so effective, works instantly, is easily titrated, and its effects dissipate immediately when the drug is stopped. A concern about the use of this drug is that its metabolite, cyanide, can be detected in the fetus, but this has not been demonstrated to be a significant problem in humans. It is a reason to limit the duration of the use of this drug whenever possible. Intravenous hydralazine, nitroglycerin, and labetalol are options for parenteral therapy.

Chronic afterload therapy to treat hypertension, aortic or mitral regurgitation, or ventricular dysfunction during pregnancy has been achieved with the calcium blocking drugs, hydralazine, and methyldopa. The angiotension-converting enzyme (ACE) inhibitors are contraindicated in pregnancy because they increase the risk of fetal renal development abnormalities. There are no data available on the angiotension II blocking agents losartin and valsartin.

Antithrombotic Agents.

Warfarin crosses the placenta, and fetal exposure during the first 3 months is associated with a 15 to 25 percent incidence of malformations that make up the "warfarin embryopathy syndrome" (facial abnormalities, optic atrophy, digital abnormalities, epithelial changes, and mental impairment). This appears to be particularly true in women exposed to the drug during the seventh to twelfth weeks of gestation. Warfarin use at any time during pregnancy increases the risk of fetal bleeding and maternal uterine hemorrhage. In women who require anticoagulation during pregnancy, heparin is preferable. The drug does not cross the placenta. Self-administered subcutaneous high-dose heparin (16,000 to 24,000 U/day) has proved feasible and efficacious; accumulating data suggests that low-molecular-weight heparin may be equally effective (used once or twice daily without the need for serial blood tests), and it is as safe as standard heparin therapy. When anticoagulation is required, some have advocated using heparin for the first trimester, warfarin for the next 5 months, and a return to heparin prior to labor and delivery. Successful pregnancy has been achieved with this approach, but avoidance of warfarin during pregnancy is preferable.

Antiplatelet agents increase the chance of maternal bleeding, and they, too, cross the placenta. There are theoretical and demonstrated reasons to have concern about aspirin, but it has been used so frequently without problems and, in fact, has been recommended as prophylaxis against preeclampsia by some. Like any drug, aspirin is probably best avoided during pregnancy, but it can be used if necessary with reasonable safety. There are no data on the effects of ticlopidine or clopidigril during pregnancy or on the effects of the glycoprotein IIb/IIIa receptor site blockers.

MANAGEMENT OF CARDIOVASCULAR SYNDROMES

Cardiovascular complications can occur with any form of heart disease. Management must be individualized, but some recommendations are applicable in most cases.

Low Cardiac Output Syndrome

A low cardiac output syndrome is ominous in any patient; this is particularly true in pregnancy. It results in signs of poor perfusion (mental obtundation, peripheral vascular constriction, low urine output, and often a low blood pressure). Potentially reversible causes such as tamponade or severe valvular stenosis should be considered, but in pregnancy it is most often due to intravascular volume depletion. While it is a concern in any pregnant woman, volume depletion is particularly dangerous in those with lesions that limit blood flow, such as pulmonary hypertension, aortic or pulmonic valve stenosis, hypertrophic cardiomyopathy, or mitral stenosis. The measures outlined in Table 40-2 are exceptionally important; they are necessary to prevent or treat a fall in central blood volume during pregnancy.

TABLE 40-2

MEASURES TO PROTECT AGAINST A FALL IN CENTRAL BLOOD VOLUME

Position
    45–60° left lateral
    10° Trendelenburg
Full-leg stocking
Volume preloading for surgery and delivery
    1500 mL of glucose-free normal saline
Drugs
    Avoid vasodilator drugs
    Ephedrine for hypotension unresponsive to fluid
        replacement
    Anesthetics (if required)
    Regional: serial small boluses
    General: emphasis on benzodiazepines and
        narcotics, low-dose inhalation agents

Congestive Heart Failure

Management of congesitve heart failure during pregnancy should not differ greatly from that at other times. Standard therapy can and should be used, remembering that ACE inhibitors are contraindicated. Congestive heart failure is one situation where maintaining a woman in the supine position may be beneficial by causing preload reduction with reduction of return of inferior vena cava blood to the heart (see Chap. 3).

Thromboembolic Complications

The risk of venous thromboemboli increases fivefold during and immediately after pregnancy, and there is arguably an increase in arterial emboli as well. Both may be the result of a woman's hypercoagulable state during pregnancy, and venous thrombosis is enhanced by increased venous stasis. Prevention is optimal; prophylactic full-dose or low-molecular-weight heparin is indicated in those at particularly high-risk—for example, those with a hypercoagulable state. If a thrombus or embolus is identified, 5 to 10 days of intravenous therapy followed by full-dose subcutaneous heparin is recommended. If a thromboembolus is life-threatening (for example, a massive pulmonary embolism or a thrombosed prosthetic valve), thrombolytic therapy can be used.

Hypertension

Hypertension can be present before pregnancy (in 1 to 5 percent) and may persist throughout pregnancy, or it can develop with pregnancy. When normotensive women become pregnant, 5 to 7 percent will develop hypertension. Because of the early fall in systemic vascular resistance, this often does not occur until the second half of pregnancy. It has been called *pregnancy-induced* or *gestational hypertension* or *toxemia.* When associated with proteinuria, pedal edema, central nervous system (CNS) irritability, elevation of liver enzymes, and coagulation disturbances, the hypertension syndrome is called *preeclampsia.* If convulsions occur, the diagnosis is *eclampsia.* It is not clear that hypertension alone puts the mother or fetus at risk during pregnancy, but preeclampsia increases maternal risk (a 1 to 2 percent chance of CNS bleed, convulsions, or severe systemic illness) and may cause fetal growth retardation (10 to 15 percent). This increases further with eclampsia.

Treatment guidelines are evolving. Until more is known, an argument can be made for keeping the systolic pressure at least below 160 mmHg and the diastolic pressure below 100 mmHg. Nonpharmacologic therapy is preferable and possible, although it is not clearly defined. Strict bed rest is not generally recommended, although limitation of activity and reduction of stress is commonly advised. Unless the patient has previously demonstrated salt-sensitive hypertension, sodium restriction is generally inadvisable, since pregnant women have lower plasma volumes than normotensive women. If drug treatment is required, experience is greatest with methyldopa. This otherwise infrequenlty used antihypertensive agent has been demonstrated to promote fetal survival and to result in children with normal mental and physical development. It may be that other drugs will achieve the same goal. Initial therapy can also include a beta$_1$-selective beta blocker or diuretic. As mentioned earlier, ACE inhibitors should not be used.

Pulmonary Hypertension

No matter what its cause, pulmonary hypertension is associated with a maternal mortality rate ranging from 30 to 70 percent and a fetal loss exceeding 40 percent. Maternal death can occur at any time during pregnancy, but the mother is most vulnerable during the time of labor and delivery and in the first postpartum week. If pulmonary hypertension is recognized early in pregnancy, interruption is advised. If this is declined or if pulmonary hypertension is recognized late in pregnancy, close follow-up is required. Intravascular volume depletion puts these patients at greatest risk, emphasizing again the need to follow the measures outlined in Table 40-2. When pulmonary hypertension is due to increased pulmonary vascular resistance and associated with right-to-left shunting (Eisenmenger's syndrome), meticulous attention to avoidance of air emboli or thromboemboli from intravenous catheters is essential to avoid systemic emboli in these patients. At the time of labor and delivery, a central venous line allows adequate fluid administration, and a radial artery catheter makes determinations of blood pressure and oxygen saturation easier. These lines should be used for 48 to 72 h postdelivery.

Arrhythmias

The rules for the treatment of arrhythmias should be the same as in the nonpregnant patient, with the possible exception that a rhythm causing hemodynamic instability should be treated somewhat more rapidly because of the concern about a diversion of blood flow away from the uterus. As always, if a potentially reversible cause can be identified, it should be corrected. If treatment is required, it should never be instituted without electrocardiographic documentation of the rhythm.

Tachyarrhythmias are as frequent during pregnancy as at other times. Atrial and ventricular premature beats, or sinus tachycardia, are reasons to look for and correct the cause but not to initiate specific treatment.

Paroxysmal supraventricular tachycardia is the most common sustained abnormal rhythm of pregnancy. Initial treatment with vagal maneuvers is as appropriate as at other times. If medical treatment is required to convert the rhythm, intravenous adenosine and verapamil are effective. Cardioversion can be used, remembering that the rule "never cardiovert an awake patient" is just as applicable during pregnancy as at any other time. If recurrent episodes require day-to-day therapy, beta blockers or verapamil are optimal choices. Management of atrial fibrillation and flutter should be as in the nonpregnant women. If they occur in a women with mitral stenosis, severe left ventricular dysfunction, or a previous thromboembolic event, antithrombotic therapy with heparin is indicated.

Ventricular tachycardias should be treated as in a nonpregnant woman. Recurrent, sustained monomorphic ventricular tachycardia that has the appearance of originating in the right ventricle (i.e., a left bundle brach morphology) may be effectively treated with beta-blocker therapy.

Bradyarrhythmias may also occur during pregnancy. They, too, are a reason to look for a reversible cause. Treatment is generally not required unless the patient has clear hemodynamic compromise. Complete heart block, usually congenital in origin in this population, is consistent with a successful pregnancy; however, if necessary, a permanent pacemaker can be inserted.

Loss-of-Consciousness Spells

The supine hypotensive syndrome can result in loss of consciousness; treatment, again, is to avoid the supine position. If a seizure cannot be excluded in the pregnant women with loss of consciousness, appropriate evaluation with electroencephalography is indicated. If a seizure is unlikely, the syncope should include a consideration of the usual causes.

Endocarditis

The clinical presentation of endocarditis is the same during pregnancy as at other times. *Streptococcus* is the most common cause. Intravenous drug abusers are more likely to have staphylococcal infections, and women with genitourinary tract infections are more likely to have gram-negative infections, most commonly *Escherichia coli* (see also Chap. 36).

Optimal management includes prevention. The use of antibiotics as prophylaxis against endocarditis in women with structural heart disease is as appropriate during pregnancy as at other times. Most physicians caring for women with heart disease recommend antibiotic prophylaxis at the time of labor and delivery. If endocarditis does occur, it should be treated aggressively with medical therapy, and the usual indications for surgery are appropriate during pregnancy.

Surgery

While heart disease is not exactly a complication of pregnancy, pregnant women with such disease have the same 0.5 to 2 percent chance of requiring surgery during pregnancy as those with a normal heart. If surgery is required, it is important to maintain venous return. Again, the rules in Table 40-2 apply. If possible, anesthesia is optimally achieved locally.

SPECIFIC FORMS OF HEART DISEASE

RHEUMATIC HEART DISEASE

Worldwide, rheumatic fever is common and virulent; it is probably the most common cause of heart disease during pregnancy. In the United States, clinically recognized rheumatic fever is uncommon. In a women presenting with myocarditis, rheumatic fever as a cause should be considered, particularly if it is associated with fever, joint discomfort, subcutaneous nodules, erythema marginatum, or chorea and if there is evidence of a group A streptococcal infection.

Rheumatic fever is the cause of almost all mitral stenosis; some isolated mitral, aortic, or tricuspid regurgitation; and of some double- and triple-valve disease. Echocardogrpahy will help define valve morphology and thus the etiology. Recognition of rheumatic fever as the cause of heart disease is important because it identifies those who need antibiotic prophylaxis to prevent recurrence of the disease. Twice-daily penicillin is the treatment regimen of choice, and this should be continued throughout pregnancy.

Valve Disease

MITRAL STENOSIS

Due almost exclusively to rheumatic fever, the lesion is more common in women than in men (see Chap. 23). The increased tachycardia and fluid retention of pregnancy may double the resting pressure gradient across a stenotic mitral valve. Symptoms associated with pulmonary vascular congestion occur in 25 percent of patients with mitral stenosis during pregnancy. This usually becomes apparent by about the 20th week and may be aggravated at the time of labor and delivery. While potentially at risk from the elevated left atrial pressure, the patient with mitral stenosis also depends on an adequate pressure to fill left ventricle and maintain cardiac output. Preservation of an adequate intravascular volume is essential to prevent a dramatic fall in cardiac output (Table 40-2).

A woman with symptomatic mitral valve stenosis who is contemplating pregnancy should be treated with balloon dilation or valve surgery before conception. If mitral stenosis is first recognized during pregnancy and symptoms develop, standard medical therapy is appropriate. Balloon valvuloplasty can be performed (with appropriate radiation shielding of the fetus). Mitral valve surgery can also be performed. Atrial fibrillation is of particular concern during pregnancy—a reason to use daily digoxin on a prophylactic basis (recognizing some inadequacy of rate control with this drug).

MITRAL REGURGITATION

In a young woman, mitral regurgitation may also be due to rheumatic fever. Myxomatous changes in the valve, with prolapse, is the other common cause. Regurgitation is generally well tolerated during pregnancy. Recognized congestive heart failure should be treated as described earlier. Afterload reduction is an important component of this therapy, but the ACE inhibitors should not be used. While the examination findings of mitral valve prolapse may change during pregnancy, the possibly associated arrhythmias, endocarditis, cerebral emboli, and hemodynamically significant regurgitation are rare complications and no more likely to occur in pregnancy than at other times. The physical examination is sufficient for diagnosis.

AORTIC STENOSIS

Almost always congenital in etiology, aortic stenosis is more common in males but does occur in women of childbearing age (see also Chap. 22). Recent information suggests that pregnancy can succeed with little or no maternal mortality and with no clear increase in fetal loss. If severe stenosis is recognized before pregnancy, balloon valvotomy or surgical commissurotomy is recommended. If pregnancy does occur in the presence of severe aortic stenosis, measures to avoid hypovolemia are important (see Table 40-2). If severe symptoms persist, a balloon valvuloplasty or aortic valve surgery can be performed during pregnancy.

AORTIC REGURGITATION

This lesion is generally well tolerated during pregnancy, but it is important to define the cause. Etiologies include rheumatic fever, endocarditis, dilation of the aortic root, or, more ominously, aortic dissection. An associated dilated root or dissection should raise the consideration of Marfan's syndrome as a cause. If congestive heart failure occurs, standard treatment is appropriate—once again, with a warning to avoid ACE inhibitors. If endocarditis occurs and the infection cannot be controlled, surgical therapy is indiacted.

PULMONIC VALVE DISEASE

Much pulmonary valve disease will have been altered by previous surgery. The residual stenosis and the invariable regurgitation are potential concerns but in general do not adversely affect the outcome of pregnancy. In the rare patient presenting with pulmonic stenosis during pregnancy, it is again important to avoid intravascular volume depletion. If severe symptoms occur (recurrent syncope, uncontrolled dyspnea, and chest pain), balloon valvuloplastly can be peformed.

TRICUSPID VALVE DISEASE

Tricuspid regurgitation (most often the result of previous intravenous drug use) usually requires no specific therapy during pregnancy. Tricuspid stenosis is of course rare. If it is encountered, avoiding intravascular volume depletion would seem to be important.

PROSTHETIC VALVE DISEASE

While many have benefited from a prosthetic valve, all are left with "prosthetic heart valve disease," consisting of one or more of the major complications of thromboemboli, bleeding (from anticoagulation), endocarditis, valve dysfunction, reoperation, or death (see Chap. 26). This affects patients at a rate of 5 percent per year throughout their lives. Pregnancy increases the risk of each of these complications, and the prosthetic valve and its treatment can adversely affect the fetus as well. All these are reasons that a prosthetic valve is a relative contraindication to pregnancy. In women with mechanical valves, anticoagulation is required. Full-dose subcutaneous heparin (maintaining the partial thromboplastin time between 1.5 and 2.5 times normal) is the therapy of choice. Low-molecular-weight heparin is increasingly appearing to be a preferable alternative. A heterograft or homograft is an alternative to a mechanical prosthesis. The opportunity to avoid anticoagulation is a logical argument for using these prostheses in young women. However, these valves do not completely eliminate the concern about thromboemboli, and the rate of heterograft degeneration is high in young women, resulting in the need for early valve replacement. The choice between insertion of a mechanical or a tissue valve in a woman of childbearing age is difficult. A young woman capable of safely using warfarin when not pregnant and heparin during pregnancy is best treated with a mechanical valve. If a woman's social situation or attention to her health are questionable in regard to the safety of anticoagulation therapy, a biological valve is more appropriate.

Congenital Heart Disease

Congenital heart disease is now the most common heart disease encountered in women of childbearing age in the United States (see Chap. 29). It has often been altered by surgery. Each abnormality is unique, but there are some issues that should be considered with all. First, some abnormalities significantly increase maternal morbidity and mortality (see Table 40-1). Second, there is an increased risk of fetal death, which increases with the severity of the maternal lesions. Third, the presence of a congenital cardiac lesion in either a parent or a sibling increases the risk of cardiac and congenital abnormalities in the fetus. Congenital heart disease is recognized in 0.8 percent of all live births in the United States. Its presence in a parent increases this risk to 2 to 15 percent—actually in up to 50 percent if the abnormality is transmitted as an autosomal dominant trait—for example, Marfan's syndrome, the congenital long-QT syndrome, or the hypertrophic obstructive cardiomyopathy. Fourth, as a general rule, when maternal congenital heart disease is recognized, it should be corrected prior to pregnancy. Fifth, residual or inoperable lesions require careful understanding before pregnancy is undertaken. Finally, as with valve disease, antibiotic prophylaxis against endocarditis is as appropriate during pregnancy as at other times in patients with lesions that render them susceptible to this complication.

LEFT-TO-RIGHT SHUNTS

Although left-to-right shunting increases the chance of pulmonary hypertension, right ventricular failure, arrhythmias, and emboli, it is not clear that these are made more likely by pregnancy. The degree of shunting is affected by the relative resistances of the systemic and pulmonary vascular circuits—both fall to a similar degree during pregnancy and, in general, there is no significant alteration in the degree of shunting. In the United States, most patients with left-to-right shunts will have undergone surgical correction prior to pregnancy. There is no clear increase in mortality in these patients with pregnancy when they are compared to women with normal hearts. Correction does not influence the incidence of congenital heart disease in the offspring.

Atrial Septal Defect   Since the symptoms and signs of an atrial septal defect can be subtle, this abnormality is occasionally encountered uncorrected during pregnancy. In women with an ostium secundum defect, pregnancy is generally well tolerated. Ostium primum defects are equally well tolerated unless they are associated with other congenital abnormalities. Surgical correction prior to pregnancy does not lower the 5 to 10 percent chance that offspring will have congenital heart disease.

Ventricular Septal Defect   Over half of ventricular septal defects (VSDs) close in childhood, and most of the remainder will have heen corrected prior to the age of pregnancy. In women with a VSD, however, pregnancy is generally well tolerated. Congestive heart failure or arrhythmias can be managed as previously discussed. The child has a 5 to 8 percent chance of being born with a cardiac defect. Again, this incidence is not altered by previous surgical correction.

Patent Ductus Arteriosus   This left-to-right shunt is also well tolerated during pregnancy. The occasional congestive heart failure can be treated in the standard fashion.

RIGHT-TO-LEFT SHUNT ("CYANOTIC" HEART DISEASE)

Right-to-left shunting can occur through an atrial or VSD or a patent ductus arteriosus. This occurs when pulmonary vascular resistance exceeds systemic vascular resistance (Eisenmenger's syndrome) or when there is obstruction to right ventricular outflow with normal pulmonary vascular resistance. All are forms of "cyanotic" heart disease, and the presence of cyanosis, especially when sufficient to result in elevated hemoglobin levels, is associated with high maternal mortality, fetal loss, prematurity, and reduced infant birth weights. Eisenmenger's syndrome was discussed earlier with pulmonary hypertension—it is worth repeating that with this problem it is advisable to avoid or interrupt pregnancy. When the cyanosis is not due to an elevated pulmonary vascular resistance but rather to right ventricular outflow obstruction, maternal mortality is less, but cardiovascular complications are still increased.

Tetralogy of Fallot   This is the most common form of right-to-left shunting, resulting from obstruction to pulmonary flow with normal pulmonary vascular resistance. Successful pregnancy can be achieved if the lesion is uncorrected, but maternal mortality is high. After surgical correction, maternal mortality does not clearly exceed that of women without heart disease. The offspring have a 5 to 10 percent chance of having congenital heart disease.

OBSTRUCTIVE LESIONS

Two treatment recommendations apply in women with obstructive cardiac lesions. First, volume depletion should be avoided (Table 40-2), since it can result in a significant fall in cardiac output. Second, surgical or catheter treatment for obstructive lesion is recommended prior to pregnancy, not only to increase maternal safety but also because of the observation that it reduces the chance of congenital heart disease in the offspring.

The two most common forms of obstruction to the right ventricle have already been mentioned—pulmonic valve stenosis and tetralogy of Fallot. Obstructions to the left side of the heart include the previously described aortic valve stenosis. Experience with isolated supravalvular or subvalvular bands is sparse; the approach recommended for aortic valve stenosis would seem applicable.

Coarctation of the Aorta   Certainly a form of left ventricular obstruction, this condition is more common in men but may occur in women and may be associated with a bicuspid aortic valve. Maternal mortality can range from 3 to 8 percent. Surgical correction or balloon dilation reduces the risk or aortic dissection or rupture, and thus death, to less than 1 percent; its effects on the rate of rupture of associated intracranial aneurysms is not known. If pregnancy occurs in a woman with a coarctation, blood pressure control, as previously described, is recommended.

Hypertrophic Obstructive Cardiomyopathy   Increasingly recognized as a left ventricular outflow tract obstructive lesion during pregnancy, this abnormality is inherited as an autosomal dominant trait with variable penetrance. It has been shown to result in increased symptoms of dyspnea and chest discomfort and palpitations during pregnancy. Hypertrophic obstructive cardiomyopathy is associated with an approximately 1 to 3 percent chance per year of sudden death. It is not clear whether pregnancy increases this, although a death has been reported with this syndrome during pregnancy. This is still one more obstructive lesion where it is important to avoid hypovolemia (Table 40-2). Beta-blocker therapy is recommended at the time of labor and delivery.

COMPLEX CONGENITAL LESIONS

The predictability of outcome of pregnancy is more difficult as complexity increases, but in general, maternal and fetal morbidity and mortality are high, particularly when the abnormality results in maternal cyanosis.

Transposition of the Great Vessels   While pregnancy has been reported in women with this syndrome, maternal and fetal outcome are poor. Partial or complete correction of the lesion prior to pregnancy improves the outcome for the mother and the fetus. If "corrected" transposition is not complicated by cyanosis, ventricular dysfunction, or heart block, pregnancy should be well tolerated.

Ebsteins's Anomaly of the Tricuspid Valve   This condition may be mild and may go unrecognized during pregnancy. Maternal risk increases in a woman with associated right ventricular dysfunction, right ventricular outflow tract obstruction, and right-to-left shunting with cyanosis. This latter—the right-to-left shunting—is a reason to avoid pregnancy.

Marfan's Syndrome   It may be difficult to diagnose Marfan's syndrome, but it is important to do so because pregnancy is particularly dangerous for affected women. First, the risk of death from aortic rupture or dissection, particulary if the aortic root is enlarged (greater than 40 mm by echocardiography has been used as one criterion), is high. Second the woman's life span is reduced, implying that her years of motherhood will be limited. Third, half of the offspring will be affected. These are reasons that women with Marfan's syndrome should be advised to avoid pregnancy. In the woman with a dilated aortic root, the risks are sufficient to recommend interruption if pregnancy has occurred. Should the parents elect to continue the pregnancy, activity should be restricted and hypertension prevented. The prophylactic use of beta blockers, while unproven, seems reasonable. This is the one cardiovascular syndrome where cesarean section is recommended because of the hemodynamic stresses of labor.

Myocardial Disease

HYPERTROPHIC CARDIOMYOPATHY

The asymmetrical form of hypertrophic cardiomyopathy has been discussed as an obstructive lesion. A concentric hypertrophic cardiomyopathy may be the result of aortic stenosis or hypertension. When *not* due to either of these, the cause, prognosis, and management are often unclear, even unrelated to pregnancy. Again, hypovolemia should be avoided, and if congestive heart failure occurs, standard therapy is appropriate (see Chap. 34).

DILATED CARDIOMYOPATHY

This is a reason to recommend that pregnancy should be avoided. This recommendation is not supported by the data from prospective trials but is given because myocardial dysfunction is the feature associated with increased maternal and fetal mortality in many forms of heart disease (see Chapt. 30). On occasion, the cardiomyopathy may be caused by pregnancy—a *peripartum cardiomyopathy.* This occurs almost exclusively in the third trimester or in the first 6 weeks postpartum, suggesting that it is a unique entity. Myocarditis has been implicated as being an initial part of the syndrome, but data are limited. In the woman with a dilated cardiomyopathy during pregnancy, standard treatment for heart failure, thromboemboli, or arrhythmias is appropriate.

A subsequent pregnancy should be discouraged, even when function returns to normal, because the maternal mortality can approach 10 percent.

CORONARY ARTERY DISEASE

Chest discomfort is common during pregnancy but is due most often to gastroesophageal reflux or abdominal distention. Coronary artery disease, however, can cause angina and myocardial infarctions during pregnancy. The disease is rarely due to atherosclerosis. Other explanations have included dissection of the coronary artery, spasm, emboli, or vasculitis. Kawasaki's or Takayasu's disease has been implicated in some cases. When suspected or demonstrated, coronary artery disease should be treated with standard medical therapy. If symptoms are not relieved, angioplasty or surgery can be performed.

Pregnancy following Cardiac Transplantation

Many cardiac transplant recipients are women of childbearing age. Successful pregnancies have been reported after transplantation. The potential hazards to the mother and fetus—which include maternal heart failure, immunosuppressive therapy, maternal infections, and serial diagnostic studies as well as a potential for a shortened maternal life-span—are reasons that a patient, at very best, should be counseled about the advisability of proceeding with pregnancy.

SUGGESTED READING

Haemostasis and Thrombosis Task Force: Guidelines on the prevention, investigation and management of thrombosis associated with pregnancy. Maternal and neonatal haemostasis working papers of the haemostasis and thrombosis task force. *J Clin Pathol* 1993; 46:489–496.

McAnulty JH, Metcalfe J, Ueland K: Heart disease and pregnancy. In: Fuster V, Alexander RW, O'Rourke RA (eds): *Hurst's The Heart,* 10th ed. New York, McGraw-Hill; 2001:2271–2288.

National High Blood Pressure Education Program: Working Group report on high blood pressure in pregnancy. *Am J Obstet Gynecol* 1990; 163:1691–1712.

Presbytero P, Sommerville J, Stone S, et al: Pregnancy and cyanotic congenital heart disease, outcome of mother and fetus. *Circulation* 1994; 89:2673–2676.

Robson SC, Hunter S, Boys RJ, Dunlop W: Serial study of factors influencing changes in cardiac output during human pregnancy. *Am J Physiol* 1989; 256:H1060—H1065.

Whittemore R, Hobbins JCC, Engle MA: Pregnancy and its outcome on women with and without surgical treatment of congenital heart disease. *Am J Cardiol* 1982; 50:641–651.

41

WOMEN AND CORONARY ARTERY DISEASE

Pamela Charney

INTRODUCTION

Only recently has coronary artery disease (CAD) been perceived by both patients and physicians as a major contributor of morbidity and mortality in women. The increasing focus on women and CAD reflects both greater attention to older populations and enthusiasm for improving women's health. Initial CAD research focused on middle-aged populations, among whom men have a dramatically higher rate of coronary artery disease than women. As research has expanded to include elderly subjects, less dramatic differences in mortality rates between women and men have been documented (Fig. 41-1).

In this chapter, the prevention, diagnosis, and management of CAD in women is addressed. More detailed discussions can be found in *Hurst's The Heart* or in *Coronary Artery Disease in Women: Prevention, Diagnosis and Management* (see "Suggested Reading" at the end of this chapter).

PREVENTION OF CAD IN WOMEN

Tobacco exposure is the most important CAD risk factor, followed by diabetes and hypertension. Other important risk factors with clinically important gender differences are reviewed in Table 41-1. Risk factors are additive, and women without traditional cardiovascular risk factors (tobacco, hypertension, high cholesterol, diabetes, physical inactivity, family history, and old age) are at relatively low risk for coronary events. The largest treatment benefit is derived from aggressive preventive measures in women with multiple risk factors or prior coronary events.

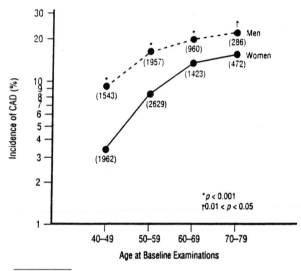

FIGURE 41-1

Framingham data: 10-year incidence of coronary artery disease (angina, myocardial infarction, coronary insufficiency, or death) among women and men by age. (From Eaker ED, Castelli WP: Coronary heart disease and its risk factors among women in the Framingham study. In: Eaker ED, Packard B, Wenger NK, et al., (eds): *Coronary Heart Disease in Women: Proceedings of an NIH Workshop.* New York: Haymark Doyma; 1987:122–130, and Future directions. In: Charney P, ed. *Coronary Artery Disease in Women.* Philadelphia: American College of Physicians; 1999:576, with permission.)

Tobacco

Exposure to tobacco is the single most important CAD risk factor for both women and men. Cigarette smoking has been associated with an increased risk of myocardial infarction and an earlier age of first myocardial infarction. Tobacco use also lowers the age of reported menopause. Over the last several decades, tobacco use among American women has not decreased as dramatically as it has among men. The prevalence of cigarette use among women reflects both higher initiation and lower successful tobacco cessation.

As noted in the 1996 Smoking Cessation: Clinical Practice Guidelines: "Simple advice by one's physician to stop smoking is more effective than no advice at all, and as the physician-delivered smoking intervention becomes more intensive, the effects are greater." Women

TABLE 41-1

ADDITIONAL CAD RISK FACTORS WITH SIGNIFICANT
GENDER DIFFERENCES

Risk Factor	Clinically Important Issues for Women
Lipids	—Total cholesterol peaks in women from age 55 to 64 (in men at about age 50). LDL is higher with greater age.
	—HDL in women is greater than in men, remaining similar with aging.
	—HDL may be most predictive for women, especially low HDL.
	—Triglyceride levels may be important in women.
	—Because women usually develop clinical coronary artery disease (CAD) 10 years later than men, many primary prevention trials have inadequate power to assess treatment for women.
	—There has been adequate power to show that secondary prevention decreases CAD events in women.
	—However, these agents are underprescribed after myocardial infarction in women and target treatment levels are often not reached.
	—Women at high risk, such as women with diabetes, should be aggressively treated for lipid abnormalities.
	—There is controversy about aggressive treatment in the woman at low risk for vascular disease while results of further primary prevention clinical trials are pending.
Obesity	—The prevalence of obesity increasing, with >30% of white women and 50% black or Mexican-American women being obese. Racial differences in body-mass index as well as glycosylated hemoglobin start in childhood.

(continued)

TABLE 41-1
(Continued)

Risk Factor	Clinically Important Issues for Women
Physical activity & exercise	—Obesity is linked to multiple cardiac risk factors. —Behavioral interventions to decrease weight have been most successful when there is an exercise component. —Generally, women have smaller hearts, and cardiac output is increased by raising heart rate. —In national surveys, sedentary lifestyles are reported by as many as 70% of adult women, with higher rates among black and Hispanic women and those with less education or lower income. —Most studies focus on leisure activities and do not include housework or walking. —Especially for women, increased activity during daily routines is more helpful than an exercise program. —Women more likely to exercise regularly with prior successful weight loss and exercise and are encouraged by their school-age children.
Menopause	—Importance is not fully defined. Historically, women with early surgical menopause have been considered at higher risk for CAD and osteoporosis. However, the Nurse's Health Study found that only women smokers with a younger age of menopause have a greater risk of CAD.

(continued)

TABLE 41-1
(Continued)

Risk Factor	Clinically Important Issues for Women
Hormone replacement therapy	—While both retrospective and prospective epidemiologic evidence suggests that users of hormonal therapy have substantially lower rates of CAD, results from clinical trials have not been confirmatory to date. —The Heart & Estrogen/Progestin Replacement Study (HERS), the only completed secondary prevention clinical trial of hormonal therapy, revealed no overall reduction in CAD events but substantially more venous thrombotic events and gallbladder disease with hormonal therapy. —An increased risk of breast cancer with long-term use (greater than 5 years) is based on a worldwide review of the epidemiologic literature.
Race and coronary artery disease	—Young black women (age <55) had more than twice the rate of CAD mortality (sudden and nonsudden) than young white women. —Importantly, family income, educational level, and occupational status accounted for more of this observed difference than traditional coronary risk factors.

(continued)

TABLE 41-1

(Continued)

Risk Factor	Clinically Important Issues for Women
Psychosocial factors	—Depression, an independent risk factor for CAD, is diagnosed twice as often in women than men. —Depression after myocardial infarction also predicts greater morbidity as well as higher subsequent mortality in women more than men. —Coronary disease morbidity and mortality is greater among those with lower socioeconomic status (SES)— described as years of formal education, owning a car, income defined by absolute or relative amount, and parental status. More recently, SES has also been defined independent of race. —Lower SES has also been related to higher rates of tobacco use and higher inpatient mortality after myocardial infarction. — Differences in event rates were greater for women than men with different SES.

KEY: LDL = low-density lipoprotein; HDL = high-density lipoprotein.

have more difficulty quitting cigarette use, both initially and in the long term, although successful tobacco cessation for women, as for men, dramatically decreases the risk of further coronary events. For women, the frequent 7- to 10-lb weight gain with tobacco cessation is often a substantial barrier to trying to stop smoking cigarettes. While fewer than 10 percent of those who stop smoking gain more than 20 lb, women smokers report that they are unwilling to experience any or minimal weight increase as they stop smoking. To avoid weight gain with tobacco cessation, it is helpful to develop realistic expectations, encourage exercise and careful choice of snacks, and provide appropriate pharmacotherapy. Social pressure from others is an important stimulus for women to stop smoking.

Diabetes

Once a woman is diagnosed with diabetes, her "female advantage" in relation to the risk of coronary artery disease is lost. After myocardial infarction, diabetic women have been observed to have a higher risk of death and congestive heart failure (CHF) than diabetic men. The mechanisms for these observations are suspected to be at least partially related to lipid abnormalities as well as insulin resistance.

While treatment trials to prevent CAD and its complications in diabetic patients are in progress, aggressive management of lipoprotein abnormalities and hypertension, if present, are beneficial. There is some evidence that glucose control decreases vascular disease. Regular exercise can also improve glucose control and insulin resistance. For women at risk of developing diabetes, regular physical activity and weight control may decrease the risk of subsequently developing diabetes.

Hypertension

Both systolic and diastolic blood pressures have been found in population and cohort studies to predict coronary events in women and men. Generally, women are more likely to have controlled blood pressure (BP) than men. While treatment trials have also documented that lower blood pressure decreases the incidence of a first myocardial infarction and sudden death, this effect has been less dramatic than the decrease in stroke occurrence with BP control. As Kannel states, "coronary disease is the most common and lethal sequela of hypertension, equaling in incidence all the other cardiovascular outcomes combined."

In epidemiologic studies, use of thiazide diuretics has been associated with a lower incidence of hip fracture. Angiotensin-converting enzyme (ACE) inhibitors should be cautiously utilized in women of reproductive age because they are potentially teratogenic. Cough, a common side effect of first-generation ACE inhibitors, occurs substantially more frequently in women than in men.

DIAGNOSIS OF CORONARY ARTERY DISEASE

CAD is often diagnosed clinically by a careful history. Women generally visit physicians more often than men and report more symptoms, including chest pain. Too often, older women ascribe their decreased ability to complete housework or to walk to "getting old." Therefore regular exploration of a patient's exercise tolerance while considering CAD in the differential diagnosis is essential. The physician's preconceived biases can affect the diagnosis of CAD. In one study, where an actress portrayed a woman twice, with the same script but different clothes and affect, physicians who reviewed the scene in which the actress described her chest pain with "exaggerated emotional presentation style" predicted less CAD than when the same scene was presented with a "businesslike affect."

Exercise stress testing is a commonly used, noninvasive modality to assess CAD risk. If a completed exercise stress test reveals ST-segment changes and depression greater than 1 mm, especially in younger women (when the prevalence of ST-segment depression is less), this may indicate significant CAD, since smaller ST-segment changes are often seen in women. In comparison, a negative exercise stress test with adequate exertion is often helpful because it decreases the need to consider cardiac catheterization.

Generally, stress imaging techniques are favored in assessing a woman for possible CAD or staging the severity of disease. Local expertise is an important consideration in deciding whether to use nuclear medicine or echocardiography techniques. Nuclear stress perfusion testing with the use of thallium in women can be potentially hindered by soft tissue attenuation from breast tissue, so technetium may be preferred. Stress echocardiography is highly dependent on operator expertise and may be technically difficult in obese patients. Many authors prefer stress imaging tests with lower false-positive rates than an exercise stress test for women.

MANAGEMENT OF CLINICAL CORONARY ARTERY DISEASE IN WOMEN

Chronic Angina

In the Framingham study, the commonest presenting coronary artery symptom in women is angina. Women with angina, compared with men, more frequently report anginal symptoms with emotional or mental stress. Managing angina in women is complicated by the observation that anginal symptoms in women are less predictive of abnormal coronary anatomy than in men. Women may more often demonstrate vasospastic responses.

Acute Coronary Ischemia Including Acute Myocardial Infarction

There are significant gender differences in acute ischemia at the time of presentation and during short-term follow-up. Women tend to delay arrival for medical care longer after symptoms begin; have less

ST-segment elevation on the initial electrocardiogram; receive less thrombolytic treatment, aspirin, or beta blockers as well as less invasive interventions [catheterization, percutaneous transluminal coronary angioplasty (PTCA), and coronary artery bypass grafting (CABG)]. Women more often developed acute pulmonary edema or cardiogenic shock. Data analyzed from the National Registry of Myocardial Infarction-II for a possible interaction of gender and age found that the 30-day mortality after myocardial infarction was about twice as high for women aged 30 to 50 than in men of the same age and that it decreased progressively with increasing age until it reached unity at age 75.

Myocardial infarctions can also present as sudden death or without painful symptoms (silent myocardial infarction) with a high percentage of lethal first myocardial infarctions in women. In Framingham, silent myocardial infarctions are more common in women than in men (35 versus 28 percent).

In long-term follow-up after myocardial infarction, women have more symptoms than men, although long-term mortality is better or similar. Women tend to have more angina and congestive heart failure despite better systolic left ventricular function. Therapies that are efficacious in women as well as in men are, in observational studies, often not prescribed for women (i.e., aspirin and agents to lower cholesterol). Furthermore, even when such drugs are prescribed, treatment goals have often not been met (such as achieving improved cholesterol levels). Rehabilitation is also less often recommended for women, although it is equally effective. To improve the prognosis of women after myocardial infarction, it is essential to encourage less tobacco exposure (secondary as well as primary exposure) and to use medications in adequate doses documented to decrease mortality and morbidity (beta blockers and aspirin) and to address other risk factors. Ischemic heart disease is the commonest etiology of CHF in women as well as in men.

Interventions for Coronary Artery Disease: Angioplasty and Coronary Artery Bypass Grafting

Both of these procedures are utilized less in women than men, and there has been controversy as to whether women are undertreated or men overtreated. With the development of smaller coronary artery catheters, angioplasty outcomes and complications are similar for women and men. Conduit selection in CABG is less often the internal mammary artery in women than in men, although this graft is associated with the best short- and long-term results. Reasons the internal mammary artery is avoided might include higher rates of diabetes in women undergoing CABG and the presence of osteoporosis. Since women compared with men undergoing CABG tend to be older and to have more comorbid conditions, a higher postoperative complication rate—including slower postoperative recovery and higher rates of depression—is not unexpected. With follow-up after several years, gender differences are less apparent.

Arrhythmias

Palpitations are reported more commonly by women than men. It is generally known that torsades de pointes occurs more commonly in women. Small preliminary studies have considered heart rate variability and QT duration as potential contributors to the development of torsades de pointes.

SUGGESTED READING

Charney P: Women and coronary artery disease. In: Fuster V, Alexander RW, O'Rourke, et al (eds): *Hurst's The Heart,* 10th ed. New York: McGraw-Hill; 2001:2357–2371.

Charney P (ed): *Coronary Artery Disease in Women: Prevention, Diagnosis, and Management.* ACP/ASIM Women's Health Book Series. Philadelphia: American College of Physicians; 1999.

Fiore M, Bailey W, Cohen S, et al: *Smoking Cessation: Clinical Practice Guidelines No. 18.* Publication 96-0692. Rockville, MD: USDHHS, PHS, AHCPR; 1996.

Hochman JS, Tamis J, Thompson TD, et al: Sex, clinical presentation, and outcome in patients with acute coronary syndromes. *N Engl J Med* 1999; 341:226–232.

Hu FB, Grodstein F, Hennekens CH, et al: Age at natural menopause and risk of cardiovascular disease. *Arch Intern Med* 1999; 159:1061–1066.

Hulley S, Grady D, Bush T, et al: Randomized trial of estrogen plus progestin for secondary prevention of coronary heart disease in postmenopausal women. *JAMA* 1998; 280(7):605–613.

Kannel WB: Blood pressure as a cardiovascular risk factor: Prevention and treatment. *JAMA* 1996; 275:1571–1576.

Lerner DS, Kannel W: Patterns of heart disease morbidity and mortality in the sexes: A 26-year follow-up of the Framingham population. *Am Heart J* 1986; 111:383–390.

Vaccarino V, Parsons L, Every NR, et al: Sex-based differences in early mortality after myocardial infarction. *N Engl J Med* 1999; 341:217–225.

Winkleby MA, Robinson TN, Sundquist J, Kraemer HC: Ethnic variations in cardiovascular disease risk factors among children and young adults: Findings from the third national health and nutrition examination survey, 1988–1994. *JAMA* 1999; 281:1006–1013.

42

DIAGNOSIS AND TREATMENT OF DISEASES OF THE AORTA

Joseph Lindsay, Jr.

DEFINITION

The aorta is affected by a diversity of disease processes, but its uncomplicated structure and function limit the number of clinical syndromes that result. Weakening of the aortic wall by congenital or acquired disease may lead to aneurysm, rupture, or dissection. When the process affects the proximal aorta, aortic valvular incompetence may result from dilatation of the aortic ring or from involvement of the valve leaflets themselves. Disease may also narrow the aorta or, more often, the origin of one of its branches.

ETIOLOGY

Atherosclerosis of the aorta accompanies aging in most individuals in the western world but varies in severity from subject to subject. It is accelerated by diabetes, hypercholesterolemia, hypertension, and smoking. Aortic atherosclerosis is clinically manifest most frequently by embolization of plaque material from its luminal surface to more distal arterial segments. Because of its predilection for the infrarenal segment, atherosclerosis may produce obstruction of that segment. Infrarenal abdominal aneurysms have, in the past, been attributed to atherosclerosis, but recent evidence provides reason to doubt that atherosclerosis is the sole cause.

Medial degeneration also accompanies aging. As a consequence, the aorta becomes elongated, tortuous, and inelastic in older individuals. Severe and premature medial degeneration is the cardiovascular hallmark of Marfan's syndrome. A genetic mutation(s) resulting in the production of abnormal fibrillin, a matrix protein of the aorta and other connective tissue, has been identified. Aneurysmal dilatation of the proximal aorta, including the sinuses of Valsalva, is

701

characteristic of this heritable disease. The resulting bulb-shaped aortic root has been described as reflecting *annuloaortic ectasia*. While characteristic of Marfan's syndrome, annuloaortic ectasia is encountered clinically with even greater frequency in subjects with no other manifestations of that genetic disorder. Medial degeneration may be severe enough to produce clinical disease in individuals with coarctation of the aorta, bicuspid aortic valve, polycystic kidneys, and Turner's syndrome. Its association with these congenital/heritable diseases adds credence to the idea that additional genetically determined medial defects await identification.

Light microscopic changes in the aortic media, termed *cystic medial necrosis* by Erdheim, were long thought to be diagnostic of medial degeneration. Its features include fragmentation of elastic fibers, loss of nuclei of smooth muscle cells, increase in collagen, and replacement of the degenerated tissue by basophilic-staining ground substance. More recent studies suggest that this is a nonspecific finding reflecting the effects of prolonged stress on the aortic wall.

Infectious aortitis may result from extension of aortic valve endocarditis to the adjacent wall and, less often, from direct spread of infection from periaortic soft tissue. Finally, although the intact aortic intima is resistant to blood-borne infection, areas damaged by atherosclerosis or other disease may be invaded by pathogens from the bloodstream. The late effects of syphilitic aortitis (coronary artery ostial obstruction, aneurysm, and aortic regurgitation) are still encountered.

Nonspecific aortitis, often associated with evidence of an "autoimmune" process, has been termed *Takayasu's aortitis.* Moreover, aortitis of the proximal aorta often accompanies giant-cell arteritis as well as ankylosing spondylitis and Reiter's syndrome, the HLA-B27 arthropathies.

Common congenital anomalies encountered after early childhood include aortic coarctation and aneurysm of the sinuses of Valsalva.

Trauma that is not immediately fatal may result in false aneurysm formation at the site of injury.

CLINICAL MANIFESTATIONS

Aneurysms

Most aortic aneurysms are asymptomatic and are first detected in the course of a routine physical examination or an imaging study directed at another organ. The onset of symptoms attributable to an aneurysm signal expansion or threatened rupture, since pain results from impingement on or erosion into an adjacent structure. Aneurysms of the aortic arch are special cases. They may produce hoarseness or dysphagia as a result of pressure on an adjacent mediastinal structure.

Rupture of an aneurysm is life-threatening and demands immediate operative treatment. The sudden onset of abdominal discomfort in a patient with an abdominal aneurysm or of chest pain in one with aneurysm of the thoracic aorta heralds such events. Evidence of blood loss often accompanies the pain and alerts the examiner to the vascular nature of the illness.

Aortic Regurgitation

Aortic valvular incompetence is a common manifestation of proximal aortic disease. Currently, severe incompetence most often results from annuloaortic ectasia, with its characteristic dilatation of the aortic sinuses, ascending aorta, and aortic valve ring. When a regurgitant valve is the initial manifestation of aortic root disease, as is often the case, the underlying nature of the disease may not be suspected until echocardiography is performed.

Aortic Dissection

Characterized by longitudinal splitting of the medial fibers, aortic dissection produces a dramatic clinical syndrome almost always including the abrupt onset of severe midline chest, back, or abdominal pain or, less commonly, by sudden syncope. The aortic valve is often rendered incompetent when the ascending aorta is involved. Moreover, a major branch vessel off the aorta may be obstructed, producing absent arterial pulses and evidence of obstruction to flow to the brain, spinal cord, kidneys, viscera, or limbs.

About 65 percent of all dissections originate in the ascending aorta and extend distally, often to the iliac bifurcation. These were classified as type I by DeBakey and as type A by the Stanford surgical group. One-quarter originate just beyond the left subclavian artery and, like proximal dissections, extend distally. These comprise type III of DeBakey and Stanford type B. The remainder do not fall readily into these typical patterns. They are often limited in their extent, but one relatively common pattern originates distal to the left subclavian artery and extends retrogradely into the ascending aorta as well as distally along the descending aorta.

Because of their proximity to the aortic valve, proximal dissections frequently result in aortic regurgitation. They also, more often than those originating beyond the arch, produce obstruction to an aortic branch. This may be particularly destructive if the blood supply to the brain is affected.

Obstruction

Narrowing of one or more of the ostia of branches of the aorta, as a consequence of aortitis or atherosclerosis, may produce ischemic symptoms of the heart, the central nervous system, or an upper extremity. Atherosclerotic obstruction of the infrarenal aorta may produce the Leriche syndrome—effort-produced discomfort of the low back, buttocks, or thighs. Abrupt occlusion of the aortic bifurcation by a saddle embolus, aortic dissection, or in situ thrombosis results in limb-threatening lower extremity ischemia accompanied by weakness or frank paralysis.

Embolization from the Aorta

Atherosclerotic aortic segments or aortic aneurysms may be the source of emboli to the central nervous system, to the viscera, or to the extremities. Such events are the most frequent clinical consequences of aortic atherosclerosis. *Cholesterol embolization* is a special clinical syndrome produced by a shower of small atherosclerotic fragments from "raw" aortic surfaces to distal organs and limbs. The hallmark physical finding, blue toes, is accompanied by other evidence of lower extremity ischemia and by injury to the kidneys and other viscera. Most often a complication of cardiac catheterization, it may be spontaneous.

PHYSICAL EXAMINATION

Detection of the murmur of aortic regurgitation, of a supraclavicular or abdominal bruit, or of diminution of one or more of the carotid, radial, or femoral pulses may direct the examiner's attention to aortic disease or may support a suspicion of that possibility aroused from other information (see also Chap.1). Moreover, every abdominal examination should include a search for the expansile mass of an abdominal aneurysm. The presence of a tracheal tug or of a lift of either sternoclavicular joint may reflect aneurysm or dissection of the aortic arch.

   One should be particularly alert for evidence of aortic disease in patients whose body habitus suggests either Marfan's or Turner's syndrome.

X-RAY STUDIES

The aortic silhouette on the plain chest film is usually distorted in the presence of disease of the thoracic aorta. An important exception to this generalization are processes limited to the aortic root (aortitis and annuloaortic ectasia). In that case, any aortic deformity may lie entirely within the cardiac shadow. Notching of the underside of the ribs is virtually pathognomonic of aortic coarctation.

Abdominal x-rays, particularly when proper techniques are employed, frequently disclose the calcified outline of an infrarenal aneurysm. A "cross-table lateral" may be rewarding.

DIFFERENTIAL DIAGNOSIS

The possibility of aortic disease should be considered in a variety of clinical situations. It may be responsible for newly discovered aortic insufficiency. It may manifest as pain, suggesting myocardial infarction or an acute abdominal illness. At times an infectious or autoimmune process may be suggested. Moreover, the mass of an aneurysm may lead to an initial suspicion of a neoplasm.

SPECIAL DIAGNOSTIC EVALUATION

The aorta may be imaged in exquisite detail by several techniques. Computed tomography is perhaps the most widely available modality for confirming the presence of aneurysm or dissection. Properly performed, it has a high level of sensitivity and specificity. Abdominal ultrasound, long a valuable tool for examining the abdominal aorta, has been joined by transesophageal echocardiography, which provides diagnostic images of the thoracic aorta. The latter may be the diagnostic method of choice in acutely ill patients suspected of dissection in whom its ability to provide diagnostic information "on-line" is particularly valuable. Magnetic resonance imaging and angiography now produce images with astounding detail and may be the final arbiters in difficult cases of aortic disease. Once the "gold standard," contrast aortography can now be reserved for special needs.

NATURAL HISTORY AND PROGNOSIS

Rupture of an aneurysm or the occurrence of an aortic dissection are acute, life-threatening emergencies. Survival for more than a few days is rare unless surgical repair can be effected. An exception to this generalization is dissection located distal to the aortic arch. Such patients may survive with effective medical management.

Aortic aneurysms tend to enlarge gradually. The greater their size, the more likely they are to rupture. An abdominal aneurysm of 5 cm

TABLE 42-1

ANTIHYPERTENSIVE AGENTS FOR
ACUTE AORTIC DISSECTION

Labetalol	BP control: 20 mg over 2 min IV, additional 40–80 mg at 5-min intervals[a]
	Maintenance: 1–2 mg/min infusion
Nitroprusside	0.5–10.0 μg/kg/min IV if labetalol is ineffective or in a patient with a contraindication to beta blockade
Esmolol	As an alternative to labetalol: 0.5 mg/kg over 1 min, 0.05–0.3 mg/kg/min[b]

[a] Until effect or a total of 300 mg.
[b] Dilute to $\leq$ 10 mg/mL before administration.

is considered a sufficient threat to the patient to justify operation. In the thorax, 6 cm is the critical dimension usually cited, although some now advise operative treatment of 5-cm aneurysms in patients with Marfan's syndrome. Smaller aneurysms also rupture, but less often. One should bear in mind that for some patients, advanced age or associated illness may be a greater threat to life or well-being than the aneurysm.

Aortic regurgitation and aortic branch obstruction also tend to be progressive.

TREATMENT

Surgical repair of aortic lesions is now usually possible in suitable patients, and is the only definitive approach in most cases. For rupture of an aneurysm or for dissection of the proximal aorta, surgical treatment is the lifesaving option.

Recently, considerable enthusiasm has been generated for catheter-based exclusion of aneurysms or dissections from the lumen of the aorta as an alternative to operative treatment. Endovascular stent-grafts of various designs have been employed, mostly for abdominal aneurysm, with at least satisfactory initial success and with less morbidity than operative repair.

Medical treatment of dissection or unruptured aneurysm generally is supportive or is aimed at preventing progression of a demonstrated lesion. For example, the patient with medial degeneration and annuloaortic ectasia may be given beta-blocking agents and other antihypertensive medications to reduce wall stress and the severity of aortic regurgitation.

Aggressive reduction of blood pressure has a special role in many cases of acute aortic dissection. Systolic arterial pressure should be lowered promptly to 100 to 120 mmHg using a drug regimen such as those suggested in Table 42-1. This antihypertensive program should be maintained through the preoperative period. In selected patients whose dissection begins beyond the aortic arch, chronic antihypertensive therapy may be preferable to surgery. The table outlines the drug regimen currently favored by intensivists at the author's institution.

SUGGESTED READING

Ernst CB: Abdominal aortic aneurysm. *N Engl J Med* 1993; 328: 1167–1172.

Goldstein SA, Mintz GS, Lindsay J Jr: Aorta: Comprehensive evaluation by transesophageal echocardiography. *J Am Soc Echocardiogr* 1993; 6:634–659.

Lindsay J Jr: Diagnosis and treatment of diseases of the aorta. *Curr Probl Cardiol* 1997; 22:490–542.

Lindsay J Jr: Diagnosis and treatment of diseases of the aorta. In: Fuster V, Alexander RW, O'Rourke RA, et al (eds): *Hurst's The Heart,* 10th ed. New York: McGraw-Hill; 2001: 2375–2395.

Lindsay J Jr: *Diseases of the Aorta.* Philadelphia: Lea & Febiger; 1994.

CHAPTER

43

CEREBROVASCULAR DISEASE AND NEUROLOGIC MANIFESTATIONS OF HEART DISEASE

Louis R. Caplan

CARDIOGENIC BRAIN EMBOLISM

Diagnostic criteria for cardiogenic embolism were formerly very restrictive. Embolism was diagnosed when sudden focal neurologic signs, maximal at onset, developed in patients with peripheral systemic embolism and recent myocardial infarction or rheumatic mitral stenosis. Using these criteria, cardiogenic embolism was diagnosed in only 3 to 8 percent of stroke patients. None of these criteria is secure. About 20 percent of patients do not have maximal symptoms at onset. Many other cardiac lesions are now well-accepted sources of emboli. Only about 2 percent of patients with cardiogenic brain embolism have clinically recognized peripheral emboli. Symptoms of peripheral embolism are often so minor and nonspecific (transient abdominal discomfort, leg cramp, etc.) that they are seldom diagnosed correctly.

Cardiac sources can be divided into three groups: (1) *cardiac wall and chamber abnormalities*—e.g., cardiomyopathies, hypokinetic and akinetic ventricular regions after myocardial infarction, atrial septal aneurysms, ventricular aneurysms, atrial myxomas, papillary fibroelastomas and other tumors, septal defects, and patent foramen ovale; (2) *valve disorders*—e.g., rheumatic mitral and aortic disease, prosthetic valves, bacterial endocarditis, fibrous and fibrinous endocardial lesions, mitral valve prolapse, and mitral annulus calcification; and (3) *arrhythmias,* especially atrial fibrillation and "sick-sinus" syndrome. Some cardiac sources have much higher rates of initial and recurrent embolism. The Stroke Data Bank divided potential sources into *high-risk sources* and *medium-risk sources* (Table 43-1).

TABLE 43-1

STROKE DATA BANK CATEGORIZATION OF CARDIAC RISK

High-risk categories
    Valve surgery
    Atrial fibrillation or flutter, sick sinus node with or
        without valve disease
    Left ventricular aneurysm
    Left ventricular mural thrombus
    Cardiomyopathy or left ventricular hypokinesis
    Akinetic region of left ventricle
Medium-risk categories
    Myocardial infarct within 6 months
    Valve disease without atrial fibrillation/flutter or sick
        sinus node
    Congestive heart failure
    Decreased left ventricular function
    Hypokinetic left ventricular segment
    Mitral valve prolapse (by history or echocardiogram)
    Mitral annulus calcification

Mitral Valve Prolapse

Several clinical series indicate that mitral valve prolapse (MVP) is associated with stroke. Morphologic lesions, such as thrombi and fibrous lesions, clearly suggest embolism; fibrin-platelet depositions on the surfaces of the mitral leaflets and thrombi in the angle between the posterior mitral valve leaflet and the left atrial wall have been noted. Patients with MVP also often have atrial fibrillation, syncope, and migraine. The rate of recurrence of stroke in patients with MVP as the only known cause is very low. Given the very high incidence of MVP, the frequency of MVP-related stroke is extremely low. Warfarin anticoagulants are ordinarily not indicated in prophylaxis of patients with MVP (see also Chap. 24), even after an initial stroke. Aspirin prophylaxis (80 to 325 mg/day) is, however, advisable. Demonstration by echocardiography of an intracardiac thrombus related to MVP would change that recommendation to warfarin.

Mitral Annulus Calcification

Mitral annulus calcification is an important, often unrecognized cause of embolism. Ulceration and extrusion of calcium through overlapping cusps have been seen at necropsy, thrombi have been found on valves attached to the ulcerative process, and calcific emboli have been seen in surgical embolectomies. Bacterial endocarditis can also develop on the calcified mitral annulus.

Some disorders are associated with fibrous and fibrinous lesions of the heart valves and endocardium. Similar valve lesions occur in patients with systemic lupus erythematosus (Libman-Sacks endocarditis), the antiphospholipid antibody syndrome, and cancer and other debilitating diseases (nonbacterial thrombotic endocarditis). Mobile fibrous strands are also often found during echocardiography. Fibrin-platelet aggregates attach to these fibrous and fibrinous lesions. Warfarin anticoagulants are not effective in the prevention of embolism in these conditions.

Embolic complications are common in patients who have infective endocarditis. (see also Chap. 36). Mycotic aneurysms can cause fatal subarachnoid bleeding. Embolization usually stops when infection is controlled. Warfarin does not prevent embolization and is probably contraindicated unless there are other important lesions, such as prosthetic valves or life-threatening pulmonary embolism. In children and young adults with congenital heart defects, especially those with right-to-left shunts and polycythemia, brain abscess is an important complication.

Emboli often arise from sources other than the heart, such as the aorta, proximal arteries, leg veins (paradoxical emboli), fat in the liver or bones, and materials introduced by the patient or physician (drug particles or air). The types of embolic material also vary (Table 43-2).

Atheromatous plaques in the aortic arch and ascending aorta are a very important and previously neglected source of embolism to the brain. Transesophageal echocardiography (TEE) often shows these atheromas. The aorta can also be insonated by B-mode ultrasound probes placed in the supraclavicular fossae on each side. *Large (>4 mm), protruding mobile aortic atheromas are especially likely to cause embolic strokes and are associated with a high rate of recurrent strokes.*

Onset, Clinical Course, and Diagnostic Approaches

Most embolic events occur during activities of daily living, but some embolic strokes have their onset during rest or sleep. Sudden coughing, sneezing, or arising at night to urinate can precipitate embolism. Although the deficit is most often maximal at outset, 11 percent of embolic stroke patients in the Harvard Stroke Registry had a stuttering or stepwise course, whereas 10 percent had fluctuations or progressive deficits. Later progression, if it occurs, is usually within the first 48 h. Progression is usually due to distal passage of emboli. "Nonsudden embolism" is explained by an embolus moving from its initial location, as demonstrated by angiography, to a more distal branch. Early angiography in embolic stroke patients demonstrates

TABLE 43-2

TYPES OF EMBOLIC MATERIALS

Cardiac	Arterial
Red erythrocyte–fibrin thrombi	Red erythrocyte–fibrin thrombi
White platelet–fibrin thrombi	White platelet–fibrin thrombi
Bacterial endocarditis	Cholesterol crystals
Fibrin strands and bland vegetations	Atheromatous plaque debris
Calcium (valves and mitral annulus calcification)	Calcium
Myxoma and other tumor particles	Tumor particles
	Air
	Fat
	Talc and microcrystalline cellulose (drug injection)

intracranial emboli with high frequency, but angiography after 48 h is associated with a much lower rate of arterial blockage, presumably because of spontaneous lysis of thrombus.

Transcranial Doppler (TCD) sonography shows a high incidence of middle cerebral artery blockage acutely in patients with sudden-onset hemispheric strokes. Brain edema and swelling may develop during the 24 to 72 h after stroke, with headache, decreased alertness, and worsening of neurologic signs. The edema is often cytotoxic (inside cells) and usually does not respond to corticosteroid treatment.

Emboli usually cause occlusion of distal branches and produce surface infarcts that are roughly triangular, with the apex of the triangle pointing inward. Computed tomography (CT) and magnetic resonance imaging (MRI) findings can suggest the presence of embolism by the location and shape of the lesion, the presence of superficial wedge-shaped infarcts in multiple different vascular territories, hemorrhagic infarction, and visualization of thrombi within arteries. MRI is more sensitive for detection of brain infarcts than CT and is also superior in detecting hemorrhagic infarction by imaging hemosiderin. Hemorrhagic infarction has long been considered characteristic of embolism, especially when the artery leading to the infarct is patent. The mechanism of hemorrhagic infarction is reperfusion of ischemic zones, which occurs with spontaneous passage of emboli, after iatrogenic opening of an occluded artery (e.g., end-arterectomy, fibrinolytic treatment), or after restoration of the circulation after a period of systemic hypoperfusion. At times, it is also possible to image the acute embolus on CT. Aortic plaques, atrial or septal aneurysms, and atrial septal defects, potential sources of emboli, are best seen with TEE, but echocardiography has limitations. Particles the size of 2 mm can block major brain arteries but are beyond the imaging resolution of current technology. Thromboembolism is a dynamic process. When a clot forms in the heart and embolizes, there may be no residual evidence until a clot re-forms. Cardiac thrombi are imaged differently on sequential echocardiograms; even large thrombi seen on one echocardiogram can appear to disappear later. Embolic signals are now detected by monitoring with TCD. Embolic particles passing under TCD probes produce transient, short-duration, high-intensity signals. TCD monitoring of patients with atrial fibrillation, cardiac surgery, prosthetic valves, left ventricular assist devices, carotid artery disease, and carotid endarterectomy have shown a relatively high frequency of embolic signals.

Prevention and Treatment

Early studies showed that warfarin was effective in preventing brain embolism in patients with rheumatic mitral stenosis and atrial fibrillation (AF). Previously, the intensity of anticoagulation was higher than that currently used, and brain hemorrhages and other bleeding complications were common. Trials now show that low-dose warfarin [International Normalized Ratio (INR) 2.0 to 3.0] is effective in preventing brain emboli in patients with nonrheumatic AF. Warfarin is about 50 percent more effective than aspirin in preventing stroke in patients with atrial fibrillation who do not have valvular disease. Warfarin may not be effective in preventing calcific, myxomatous, bacterial, and fibrin-platelet emboli, and warfarin has been posited to worsen cholesterol crystal embolization. Embolic brain infarcts often become hemorrhagic, and serious brain hemorrhage has occurred after anticoagulation. Large infarcts, hypertension, large bolus doses of heparin, and excessive anticoagulation are associated with hemorrhage. In most patients with brain hemorrhagic infarction, the cause is embolic. Hemorrhagic infarction occurs equally with and without anticoagulation, and development of hemorrhagic infarction is rarely accompanied by clinical worsening. Patients with hemorrhagic transformation continued on anticoagulants usually do not worsen. The risk of reembolism must be balanced against the small but definite risk of important bleeding. In patients with large brain infarcts, heparin should be delayed and bolus heparin infusions avoided. If the risk for reembolism is high, immediate heparinization is advisable, but if the risk seems low, it is prudent to delay anticoagulants for at least 48 h. Patients with atrial fibrillation with embolic strokes who are treated with well-controlled heparin anticoagulation soon after stroke onset fare better than patients treated later.

Paradoxical Embolism

Emboli entering the systemic circulation through right-to-left shunting of blood are now, with the advent of newer diagnostic technologies, often recognized. By far the most common potential intracardiac shunt is a patent foramen ovale (PFO). The high frequency of PFOs in the normal adult population make it difficult to be certain in an individual stroke patient with a PFO whether paradoxical embolism through the PFO was the cause of their stroke or whether the PFO was an incidental finding. About 30 percent of adults have a probe PFO at necropsy. The frequency of PFOs declines with age: 34.3 percent during the first three decades of life, 25.4 percent during the fourth through eighth decades, and 20.2 percent during the ninth and tenth decades. The average diameter of a PFO is 4.9 mm, and the size tends to increase with age. There is a high degree of certainty of paradoxical embolism when four or more of five criteria are met: (1) a situation that promotes thrombosis of leg or pelvic veins (e.g., long sitting in one position, recent surgery, etc.); (2) increased coagulability (e.g., the use of oral contraceptives, presence of Leiden factor with resistance to activated protein C, dehydration); (3) sudden onset of stroke during sexual intercourse, straining at stool, or other activity that includes a Valsalva maneuver or that promotes right-to-left shunting of blood; (4) pulmonary embolism shortly before or after the neurologic ischemic event; and (5) the absence of other putative causes of stroke after thorough evaluation.

Brain Hypoperfusion Due to Cardiac Pump Failure (Cardiac Arrest)

Very severe damage after cardiac arrest leads to mortal injury to the cortex and brainstem, irreversible coma, and brain death. When first examined, such patients have no brainstem reflexes (pupillary, corneal, or oculovestibular and oculocephalic reflexes) and no response to stimuli except perhaps a decerebration response. These findings do not improve, and respiratory control is absent or lost. When cerebrocortical damage is very severe but brainstem ischemic changes are reversible, brainstem reflexes are preserved but there is no meaningful response to the environment. Automatic facial movements such as blinking, tongue protrusion, and yawning usually persist. The eyes may rest slightly up and move from side to side. When this state does not improve, it is referred to as the *persistent vegetative state* or "wakefulness without awareness." Laminar cortical necrosis causes seizures. These are often multifocal myoclonic twitches or jerks of the facial and limb muscles, which are difficult to control with anticonvulsants. With severe border-zone injury, there is weakness of the arms and proximal lower extremities with preservation of face, leg, and foot movement (the "man in a barrel" syndrome). With less severe ischemia, the symptoms and signs are predominantly visual. Patients describe difficulty seeing and cannot integrate the features of large objects or scenes despite retained ability to see small objects in some parts of their visual fields. Reading is impossible. Apathy and inertia are also common and are due to damage to the frontal lobe. Amnesia is also very common. Patients cannot record new memories and have patchy, retrograde amnesia for events during and before hospitalization.

Shortly after arrest, patients with less severe brain injury show reactivity to the environment. Eye opening and restless limb movements develop. The eyes fixate on objects. Noise, a flashlight, or a pinch arouses patients to avoid or react to stimuli. Soon patients awaken and begin to speak. Cognitive and behavioral abnormalities detected after awakening depend on the degree of injury. The initial neurologic findings and course are helpful in predicting outcome. Among patients with meaningful responses to pain at 1 h, almost all survivors have preserved intellectual function. Patients who do not respond to pain by 24 h either die or remain in a vegetative state. Coma predicts a poor prognosis. *The presence or absence of coma and the response to pain predict neurologic outcome very early.*

Neurologic imaging and other tests are relatively unhelpful. CT is used to exclude other causes of coma such as brain hemorrhage. Electroencephalography (EEG) is helpful in studying cortical activity in unresponsive patients and in assessing brain death.

Neurologic Effects of Cardiac Drugs and Cardiac Encephalopathy

Digitalis can cause visual hallucinations, yellow vision, and general confusion. Quinidine can cause confusion with delirium, seizures and coma, vertigo, tinnitus, and visual blurring. Chronic cognitive and behavioral changes and "quinidine dementia" sometimes occur. Similar toxicity has been seen with lithium. Patients may become acutely comatose while being treated with intravenous lidocaine. This effect has been associated with the accidental administration of very large doses; more common CNS effects include sedation, irritability, and twitching. Amiodarone often causes ataxia, weakness, tremors, paresthesias, visual symptoms, a parkinsonian-like syndrome, and occasionally delirium.

Patients with congestive heart failure often have encephalopathy characterized by decreased alertness, sleepiness, decrease in all intellectual functions, asterixis, and variability of alertness and cognitive functions from minute to minute and hour to hour. These patients may not have pulmonary, liver, or renal failure or electrolyte abnormalities. This cardiac encephalopathy is probably multifactorial: decreased brain perfusion due to low cardiac output and high central venous pressure; intracranial fluid effusion similar in etiology to pericardial and pleural effusions and ascites; and side effects of cardiac and other drugs.

NEUROLOGIC AND CEREBROVASCULAR COMPLICATIONS OF CARDIAC SURGERY

The frequency of abnormalities of intellectual function and behavior after cardiac surgery is quite high. Fortunately, most changes are reversible with time. Prospectively, transient complications are noted in 61 percent of patients. A major concern has been that the hemodynamic and circulatory stress of heart surgery will lead to underperfusion of areas supplied by already stenosed or occluded arteries, leading to brain infarcts. This concern underlies neck auscultation for bruits, ultrasound carotid artery testing, and often cerebral angiography prior to coronary artery bypass graft surgery (CABGS). However, hemodynamically induced infarction related to preexisting atherosclerotic occlusive cervicocranial arterial disease is rare. Embolism arising from cardiac and aortic sources is much more common and a much greater concern. *Patients with carotid bruits have a very low rate of stroke after elective surgery. In a retrospective study of CABGS patients with known carotid disease, ipsilateral strokes occurred in 1.1 percent of arteries with 50 to 90 percent stenosis, in 6.2 percent of arteries with >90 percent stenosis, and in only 2 percent of vessels with carotid occlusion.* Thromboembolic infarction often occurs in the days following surgery, when cessation of anticoagulation and the activation of coagulation factors promotes hypercoagulability.

Strokes occur most often *after* recovery from the anesthetic. If the mechanism of stroke was hemodynamic, the major circulatory stress would be intraoperative and patients would awaken with the deficit. Emboli may arise from preexisting cardiac abnormalities, such as hypofunctioning ventricles, dilated atria, and from aortic atheromas or postoperative arrhythmias. *Mounting evidence links operative and postoperative embolism to aortic ulcerative atherosclerotic lesions. Cross-clamping of the ascending aorta and aortotomy liberate cholesterol or calcific plaque debris.* About one-third of embolic signals are detected as the aortic cross clamps are removed and another 24 percent as aortic partial occlusion clamps are removed. The number of microemboli detected correlates with abnormalities of cognitive function studied after surgery. Necropsy examination of patients dying after cardiac surgery have shown severe bilateral, predominantly border-zone infarcts. The small arteries of the brain and other viscera (heart, kidney, spleen, pancreas) may be packed with birefringent cholesterol crystal emboli. *Atherosclerosis of the ascending aorta is a very important risk factor for post-CABGS stroke. Patients who are to undergo elective cardiac surgery and have evidence of extensive peripheral vascular disease should be considered for preoperative noninvasive assessment of the extent of disease in the carotids and thoracic aorta.* In some patients, hypercoagulability related to surgery can precipitate occlusive thrombosis in atherostenotic arteries, and the newly formed thrombus can lead to intraarterial embolism. Cardiac, aortic, and intraarterial embolism accounts for the vast majority of cardiac surgery–related focal neurologic deficits.

Drugs are a very common cause of encephalopathy in the postoperative period. Particularly important are haloperidol, narcotics, and sedatives. Morphine is sometimes used heavily intraoperatively, and opiate withdrawal with restlessness and hyperactivity can result. Agitation and restlessness are often early signs of organic encephalopathy and may lead to the administration of haloperidol, barbiturates, phenothiazines, or benzodiazepines for calming and sedation. When these drugs wear off and patients begins to awaken, agitation may occur and more sedatives may be given. Haloperidol causes rigidity, restlessness, agitation, hallucinations, and confusion. In experimental animals, haloperidol delays recovery from strokes by months and its use clinically in this setting is not advised. Phenothiazines and sedatives are also problematic; *in general, use of sedatives and narcotics should be minimized and they should be tapered as soon as possible.*

CARDIAC EFFECTS OF BRAIN LESIONS

Cardiac Lesions

The most common lesions found in the hearts of patients dying with acute CNS lesions are patchy regions of myocardial necrosis and subendocardial hemorrhage. The abnormalities range from eosinophilic muscle cell staining with preserved striations to transformation of myocardial cells into dense eosinophilic contraction bands. These changes are referred to as *myocytolysis.* Subendocardial petechiae and hemorrhages are also noted. Stress-related release of catecholamines and corticosteroids may be responsible for these cardiac lesions.

In stroke patients, especially those with subarachnoid hemorrhage, ECGs may show a prolonged QT interval; giant, wide, roller-coaster inverted T waves; and U waves. Patients with stroke who have continuous ECG monitoring have a high incidence of T-wave and ST-segment changes, various arrhythmias, and cardiac enzyme abnormalities. ECG changes also may include a prolonged QT interval, depressed ST segments, flat or inverted T waves, and U waves. Less often, tall, peaked T waves and elevated ST segments are noted. Cardiac and skeletal muscle enzymes, including the MB isoenzyme of creatine kinase (MB-CK), are often abnormal in stroke patients. During the 4 to 7 days after stroke, MB-CK levels show a slow rise and later fall in serum, a pattern different from that found in acute myocardial infarction. The temporal pattern of cardiac isoenzyme release is compatible with smoldering low-grade necrosis, such as focal myocytolysis. The ST-segment and T-wave abnormalities and cardiac arrhythmias correlate with raised levels of MB-CK.

Various cardiac arrhythmias have been found in stroke patients, most often sinus bradycardia, tachycardia, and premature ventricular contractions. Some arrhythmias are due to primary cardiac problems, but others are undoubtedly secondary to the brain lesions. Ventricular bigeminy, atrioventricular dissociation and block, ventricular tachycardia, atrial fibrillation, and bundle branch blocks are found less often. Arrhythmias are more common in patients who have brainstem lesions or brainstem compression. Acute pulmonary edema may complicate strokes, especially *subarachnoid hemorrhage* and posterior circulation ischemia and hemorrhage.

Sudden death associated with stressful situations, including "voodoo death," must involve CNS mechanisms. Ventricular fibrillation can be reliably elicited by stimulation of cardiac sympathetic nerves in both normal and the ischemic hearts. Ischemia reduces the threshold for ventricular fibrillation. Stress causes CNS stimulation that triggers autonomic activation. Sudden vagotonic stimulation can cause bradycardia and cardiac standstill. Patients with lateral medullary and lateral pontine infarcts affecting structures of the reticular formation die unexpectedly; these patients have a high incidence of various types of autonomic dysregulation, such as labile blood pressure, syncope, tachycardia, flushing, and failure of automatic respiration.

SUGGESTED READING

Barbut D, Caplan LR: Brain complications of cardiac surgery. *Curr Probl Cardiol* 1997; 22:455–476.

Barbut D, Hinton RB, Szatrowski TP, et al: Cerebral emboli detected during bypass surgery are associated with clamp removal. *Stroke* 1994; 25:2398–2402.

Caplan LR: *Caplan's Stroke: A Clinical Approach,* 3d ed. Boston: Butterworth-Heinemann; 2000.

Caplan LR: Cerebrovascular disease and neurologic manifestations of heart disease. In: Fuster V, Alexander RW, O'Rourke RA, et al (eds): *Hurst's The Heart,* 10th ed. New York: McGraw-Hill; 2001:2397–2420.

Caplan LR, Hurst JW, Chimowitz MI: *Clinical Neurocardiology.* New York: Marcel Dekker; 1999:186–225.

Chamorro A, Vila N, Ascaso C, Blanc R: Heparin in acute stroke with atrial fibrillation. Clinical relevance of very early treatment. *Arch Neurol* 1999; 56:1098–1102.

Cohen A, Chauvel C: Transesophageal echocardiography in the management of transient ischemic attack and ischemic stroke. *Cerebrovasc Dis* 1996; 6(suppl 1):15–25.

Kanter MC, Hart RG: Neurologic complications of infective endocarditis. *Neurology* 1991; 41:1015–1020.

Pessin MS, Estol CJ, Lafranchise F, Caplan LR: Safety of anticoagulation after hemorrhagic infarction. *Neurology* 1993; 43:1298–1303.

The French Study of Aortic Plaques in Stroke Group: Atherosclerotic disease of the aortic arch as a risk factor for recurrent ischemic stroke. *N Engl J Med* 1996; 334:1216–1221.

DIAGNOSIS AND MANAGEMENT OF DISEASES OF THE PERIPHERAL ARTERIES AND VEINS

Paul W. Wennberg
Thom W. Rooke

PERIPHERAL ARTERIAL DISEASE

History and Physical Examination

Claudication is reproducible, predictable distress brought on by sustained exercise and relieved by rest. It occurs in single or multiple muscle groups and is independent of position. If a specific position is required for relief, *pseudoclaudication* should be considered (Table 44-1). Severe peripheral arterial disease (PAD) may cause rest pain (typically worse at night) that is relieved with dependency. The femoral, iliac, aortic, carotid, and subclavian arteries should be routinely palpated and auscultated for bruits. Pulses are graded on a scale of 0 to 5 : 0 absent, 4 normal, and 5 aneurysmal. When a pulse is not palpable, a Doppler examination may be performed. Skin temperature, color, and integrity should be compared to those of the proximal limb and the contralateral limb.

Laboratory Assessment

Continuous-wave Doppler examination should be performed in evaluating PAD. The normal triphasic signal becomes biphasic, then monophasic, and eventually absent as severity of stenosis increases. *Ankle brachial indices* (ABIs) are determined by dividing the systolic pressure at the ankle by the brachial artery systolic pressure. Severity

TABLE 44-1

DIFFERENTIAL DIAGNOSIS OF CLAUDICATION

Atherosclerosis obliterans	Popliteal entrapment
Arteritis (Takayasu's, giant-cell, etc.)	Venous claudication/ varicosities
Embolic disease/acute arterial occlusion	Baker's cyst
Degenerative joint disease (hip, back, knee)	Deconditioning
Spinal stenosis	Aortic dissection
Myopathy	Aortic coarctation
Thromboangiitis obliterans	Retroperitoneal fibrosis

of disease is guided by the ABI (Table 44-2). *Exercise studies* can further classify severity of disease as well as document a baseline walking distance. Poorly compressible or noncompressible vessels due to arterial calcification (especially in diabetes) limit universal applicability of the ABI. The *transcutaneous partial pressure of oxygen* ($TcpO_2$) is useful in a number of situations, especially with noncompressible vessels. $TcpO_2$ predicts whether cutaneous perfusion is adequate for healing an ulcer or in planning an amputation site. *Angiography* is the "gold standard" in the evaluation of arterial disease and is usually necessary in planning revascularization. *Ultrasound* is useful in locating and estimating stenosis. The use of *magnetic resonance angiography* (MRA) is increasing; in diabetic patients or others at risk of contrast nephropathy, it should be considered as an alternative to contrast angiography.

CLINICAL SYNDROMES

Peripheral Arterial Disease

Arteriosclerosis obliterans (ASO) is the most common cause of lower extremity ischemic syndromes in western societies. The presentation varies depending upon rate of progression, presence and extent of collateral vessels, comorbidities, and activity of the patient. Risk factors for ASO are similar to those for coronary artery disease. The prevalence of PAD increases with age. Diabetes increases the risk of PAD threefold. The risk of death, usually due to a cardiovascular event, increases dramatically as the ABI decreases, independent of age. Amputation rates are low, around 1 percent per year. However, diabetes and continued smoking substantially increase the rate of amputation.

TABLE 44-2

THE ANKLE/BRACHIAL INDEX[a]

	Preexercise	Postexercise	Claudication	Walking Time
Normal	>0.95	>0.95	None	5 min
Minimal	>0.95	<0.95	None	5 min
Mild	>0.80	>0.50	Present late	5 min
Moderate	<0.80	<0.50	Present, limiting	<5 min
Severe	<0.50	<0.15	Early, limiting	<3 min

[a]The anke/brachial index (ABI) is the systolic blood pressure at the ankle divided by the systolic blood pressure of the arm measured in the supine position. Postexercise values are taken after walking 5 min on a 10 percent grade at 2 mph. (Speed and distance will vary as tolerated by each patient.)

TREATMENT

Risk-factor modification and a walking program are the cornerstones of therapy. Smoking cessation is necessary. Control of lipids, hypertension, and diabetes should be optimized. A *walking program* should be initiated in all patients, with a goal of 20 to 30 min 4 to 5 days per week. Diligent foot care and protective footwear must be emphasized, particularly in diabetics. *Pentoxifylline* has proven effective in some patients with ASO. *Cilostazol* has recently been approved for use for patients with claudication and may effectively increase walking distance. Beta blockade should be given as needed to patients with coronary artery disease and should not be withheld from patients with concurrent PAD. Revascularization should be considered in the patients with rest pain, impending tissue loss, or significant lifestyle limitation. Surgical revascularization is well established and durable. Percutaneous balloon angioplasty, with or without stent placement, is beneficial for proximal lesions, such as iliac or renal arteries. In arteries that are more distal, it has been less beneficial; however, for patients deemed poor surgical candidates, it is reasonable to attempt distal angioplasty for limb salvage.

Acute Arterial Occlusion

Acute arterial occlusion presents with one or more of the following clinical pentad: pain, pallor, paresthesia, paralysis, and pulselessness. The limb may also be cold (polar). Restoration of flow should occur quickly. Etiology may be due to trauma (including dissection), thrombosis in situ, or embolism. Distal changes caused by microembolization may be present. A search for an embolic source should be undertaken, especially in patients with atrial fibrillation. Immediate treatment measures include heparinization, limb protection, and pain control. Angiography is often required to plan intervention. If cardiac disease increases surgical risk, the heart should be stabilized over a few hours before intervention. Thrombolysis in acute occlusion can be effective when performed early.

Other Causes

Claudication and ischemia may result from numerous disorders (see Table 44-1). *Ergot* compounds can induce Raynaud's phenomenon, claudication, acute ischemia, or tissue infarction. The incidence of ergot toxicity is decreasing as alternatives for migraine treatment become available, but it should be considered in patients with ischemia and few or no risk factors. Intravenous nitroprusside infusion may help acute ischemia. *Fibromuscular dysplasia* most commonly affects women in the fourth decade. Renal artery disease is most common, but any artery may be affected. It is frequently treatable by angioplasty. *Microembolism* usually originates from an ulcerative plaque or aneurysm and only rarely from the heart. Diffuse microembolization often requires biopsy to differentiate it from vasculitis or other entities. Events may be spontaneous or precipitated by surgery, instrumentation, or anticoagulant therapy. Livedo reticularis or overt ischemia ("blue-toe syndrome") may be present. Solitary plaques are potentially treated surgically. When lesions are diffuse or at several levels, surgical repair is more difficult. Antiplatelet agents or systemic anticoagulation may prevent recurrences; however, the efficacy of these drugs is less well documented.

Upper Extremity Arterial Disease

Arterial disease in the upper extremity is less common and more varied in etiology than it is in the lower extremity. Associated vasospasm is more common. Arm claudication is less frequent, since arm use is more intermittent and less severe because of generally better collateral circulation. *Thoracic outlet syndrome* usually results from the clavicle and the first rib and/or a cervical rib impinging on the subclavian artery like a scissors. This predisposes to subclavian artery aneurysm, thrombus formation, distal embolization, and Raynaud's phenomenon. Venous and neurogenic complaints may also be present. Imaging for the presence of a functional stenosis with duplex ultrasound or arteriography can be used to document the presence of a functional hemodynamic obstruction. Clinical correlation is required for the diagnosis. Resection of a cervical rib or first rib is frequently required. Improvement of symptoms is variable, particularly for neurogenic complaints. *Hammer hand syndrome* is the result of trauma to the hypothenar area by using the hand as a hammer or by repetitive force on levers or other devices. These activities may produce aneurysm formation of the ulnar artery, usually at the level of the hammate bone. Ischemia of one or more digits can result from emboli.

Takayasu's arteritis and *giant-cell (temporal) arteritis* (GCA) are similar in pathologic process and typically but not exclusively affect arteries above the diaphragm. In general, Takaysu's occurs in the younger patient and GCA in the older. The process is usually bilateral although not symmetrical and progresses briskly (months). Both conditions are associated with characteristic clinical and laboratory findings, including an elevated sedimentation rate and typical arteriographic features. These diseases are unique among arteriopathies in that the stenotic lesions improve with steroid therapy. Adjunctive cytotoxic drugs are often useful.

TABLE 44-3

RAYNAUD'S PHENONMENON: SECONDARY CAUSES

Collagen vascular disease	Pulmonary hypertension
Scleroderma	Neurogenic
Mixed connective tissue disease	Thoracic outlet irritation
Rheumatoid arthritis	Carpal tunnel syndrome
Myositis	Neuropathy
Sjögren's syndrome	Medications
Necrotizing vasculitis	Beta blockers
Hematologic disorders	Ergotamine
Myxedema	Methysergide
Acromegaly	

Raynaud's Phenomenon

In Raynaud's phenomenon, cold or emotional stimuli induce digital color changes from blue to white to red. Many patients describe only the white phase. Fingers are involved more often than toes. *Primary Raynaud's*, as defined by Allen and Brown, is bilateral and shows no evidence of ischemia or other disease for 2 consecutive years. Patients without laboratory evidence of digital occlusive, thrombophilic, or serologic abnormalities have a benign course. *Secondary Raynaud's phenomenon* has many etiologies (Table 44-3). Patients with primary Raynaud's phenomenon require no therapy and quickly learn to keep not only hands but also the whole body warm. Treatment of secondary forms is directed at the underlying cause when feasible. Calcium channel and alpha-adrenergic blockade, alone or in combination, may suppress or reduce the episodes.

VENOUS DISEASE

Varicose Veins

Primary varicosities are often familial and may be exacerbated by obesity or pregnancy. Symptoms—such as pain, bursting, or burning—are aggravated by prolonged dependency. Edema and skin changes due to venous stasis are rarely present in primary varicosities; when they are present, a secondary process should be sought. *Secondary varicosities* are due to a shift in venous return from the deep to the superficial veins. Common causes of secondary varicosities are extrinsic venous compression, prior deep venous thrombosis (DVT), congenital lesions, arteriovenous fistulas, and right heart pressures. Varicosity enlargement and superficial thrombophlebitis may occur over time. Both symptoms and progression can be ameliorated by appropriately fit graduated compression hose of 20 to 30 mmHg or more. Ablation of varicose veins should be considered if complications arise or discomfort is present. Sclerotherapy is effective for most small varicosities and cutaneous "spider veins." Surgical removal is indicated for long proximal varicosities, especially if incompetence of the perforator vein or saphenofemoral junction is present.

Deep Venous Thrombosis

The morbidity and mortality of DVT remain high. Risk factors for DVT and pulmonary embolism have been well defined (Table 44-4). Objective testing to confirm and define the extent of DVT should be obtained whenever DVT is suspected. Treatment with heparin (acutely) and warfarin (chronically) is highly effective in preventing clot propagation and pulmonary embolism. Recent literature suggests treatment for a minimum of 6 to 12 months for patients with spontaneous DVT and indefinitely if a primary coagulopathy is present. Low-molecular-weight heparin has been approved for the initial treatment of uncomplicated DVT.

Thrombus isolated to the calf is less dangerous than in the thigh. However, with time, 20 percent will extend proximally and 10 percent will embolize. Laboratory surveillance is required if anticoagulants are not used primarily. Inferior vena cava filters should be considered when anticoagulation is contraindicated or has failed. Early thrombolytic therapy accelerates recovery and may reduce the incidence and severity of postphlebitic syndrome. Well-defined indications

TABLE 44-4

RISK FACTORS FOR DEEP VENOUS THROMBOSIS

Age	Residency in a health care facility
Immobility	
Recent surgery	Prior superficial venous thrombosis
Progesterone therapy	
Prior deep venous thrombosis	Hospitalization
Underlying coagulopathy	Malignancy
	Trauma

for thrombolysis in DVT have not yet been established, but extensive thrombus in the ileofemoral system with severe symptoms is a reasonable indication. Indefinite use of compression stockings (30 mmHg or greater) reduces the incidence of postphlebitic syndrome, venous stasis changes, and venous ulceration. *Phlegmasia cerulea dolens* is a rare complication of DVT. It is characterized by rapid, massive edema, severe pain, and cyanosis in the setting of extensive iliofemoral thrombosis. One-third of patients die due to pulmonary embolism, and half develop distal gangrene. It is seen most commonly with advanced malignancy or severe infections but can follow surgery, fractures, and other common precipitants of thrombosis. Urgent treatment including placement of a caval filter, heparinization, thrombectomy, or thrombolysis is often required to minimize loss of life or limb.

LABORATORY ASSESSMENT

Venography is considered the gold standard for imaging deep venous thrombosis. Venous duplex ultrasound is the most commonly used method, although it is less sensitive than venography above the groin and below the knee. Duplex has the potential advantage of differentiating acute from chronic thrombus based on the presence or absence of distention (acute) and increased echogenicity (chronic). Continuous-wave Doppler (CWD) provides information about the presence of reflux or obstruction. Impedance plethysmography (IPG) is the best-studied plethysmographic technique and the most widely employed. The ease of performance, low cost, and reasonable overall accuracy of IPG continue to make it a useful screening tool.

Chronic Venous Insufficiency

Chronic deep venous incompetence with or without obstruction (postphlebitic syndrome) is characterized by leg edema, venous dilation, and intradermal deposition of proteins and hemosiderin. Symptoms include heavy, congested limbs; venous claudication; pruritus; and painless ulceration. Cutaneous changes include fibrosis, lichenification, cellulitis, and ulceration. Edema of the foot (with sparing of the toes) differentiates edema of chronic venous insufficiency from lymphedema. Once ulceration has occurred, reduction of the edema must be accomplished first, ulcer healing will then follow. Indefinite use of 30- to 40-mmHg compression hose is indicated.

LYMPHEDEMA

Primary lymphedema may be present at birth as an isolated occurrence or as part of a congenital familial syndrome. Onset of lymphedema in the teens or early twenties is called *lymphedema praecox* and is seen more often in females (usually around menarche). *Lymphedema tarda* is primary lymphedema with onset in later years. This is a diagnosis of exclusion, since a secondary cause is more likely in this age group. *Secondary lymphedema* is more common than primary. Etiologies include trauma, recurrent infection, mass obstruction, infiltrative processes, or direct damage to the lymphatics (e.g., radiation.)

Recurrent cellulitis is common in patients with lymphedema. Repeated infection damages and eventually obliterates the vessel. Unlike edema and lipedema, lymphedema involves the toes. The skin is thickened and rough, giving it the characteristic orange-peel *(peau d' orange)* appearance. Lymphangiography and lymphoscintigraphy are the currently available imaging techniques. Lymphoscintigraphy is easier to perform than lymphangiography and poses a lower risk of lymphangitis. While this procedure has good ability to differentiate lymphedema from other causes of edema, it cannot as reliably distinguish primary from secondary lymphedema.

The mainstay of treatment for lymphedema is compression. The leg must be reduced in size by elevation and mechanical pumping or manual massage. Wrapping of the distal-to-proximal portion of the affected limb(s) is required whenever the patient is upright. Once the leg volume has been decreased, a fit-to-measure compression garment at 40 to 50 mmHg should be worn. Early and aggressive treatment of cellulitis and of fungal infection, including tinea pedis, is beneficial.

VASCULAR ULCERS

Ulceration due to a vascular etiology is common and can be classified into four categories: arterial, small-vessel, venous, and neurotrophic (Table 44-5). Multifactorial ulcerations are common, particularly in diabetes and with immunosuppression. Nonvascular etiologies—such as dermatologic, oncologic, hematologic, infectious, and factitious causes—are also common and must be kept in mind when a properly treated ulcer is not responding to therapy.

Treatment is guided by etiology. In general, protection, treatment of infection, and establishment of an ulcer base conducive to the formation of granulation tissue are needed. The wound base should guide selection of a dressing. In general, one should choose an absorbent dressing for wet wounds, a moistening agent for dry wounds, and an antibiotic agent for infected wounds. Moisture-neutral dressings are also available. Nonstick products to prevent irritation are often required. Manual debridement or mechanical debridement using wet-to-dry gauze dressing changes may be necessary.

TABLE 44-5

ULCERS OF VASCULAR ETIOLOGY

Type	Venous	Arterial	Neurotrophic	Small-Vessel
Location	Above medial and lateral malleoli	Shins, toes, sites of injury	Plantar surface, pressure points	Shin, calf
Pain	No, unless infected	Yes	No	Exquisite
Skin	Stasis pigmentation Thickening with lipodermatosclerosis	Shiny, pale decreased hair, may see livedo	Callous, normal to changes of ischemia	Normal or "satellite" ulcers in various stages
Edges	Clean	Smooth	Trophic, callused	Serpiginous
Base	Wet, weeping, healthy granulation	Dry, pale with eschar	Healthy to pale depending on ASO	Dry, punched-out, pale, thin eschar
Cellulitis	Common	Often	Common	No
Treatment	Compression	Revascularize	Relieve pressure +/− revascularize	Treat underlying disease and pain

SUGGESTED READING

Ballard JL, Bergan JJ (eds): *Chronic Venous Insufficiency.* London: Springer-Verlag; 1999.

Dormandy JA, Heeck L, Vig S: Peripheral arterial occlusive disease: Clinical data for decision making. *Semin Vasc Surg* 1999; 12(2):93–162.

Rutherford RB (ed): *Vascular Surgery,* 5th ed. Philadelphia: Saunders; 2000.

Wennberg PW, Rooke TW: Diagnosis and management of diseases of the peripheral arteries and veins. In: Fuster V, Alexander RW, O'Rourke RA, et al (eds): *Hurst's The Heart,* 10th ed. New York: McGraw-Hill; 2001: 2421–2441.

Young JR, Olin JW, Bartholomew JR (eds): *Peripheral Vascular Diseases,* 2d ed. St. Louis: Mosby Year Book; 1996.

Paul Poirier
Robert H. Eckel

INTRODUCTION

Populations of industrialized countries are becoming more overweight as a result of changes in lifestyle. Both overweight and obesity must be regarded as serious medical problems in our time, since obesity is associated with reduced life expectancy. Obesity represents an independent predictor of cardiovascular disease, and this association is more pronounced in individuals younger than 50 years. Thus the American Heart Association has stated that obesity is a major modifiable risk factor for heart disease. Obesity is a complex multifactorial chronic disorder that develops from an interaction of genotype and the environment. Because weight reduction is difficult to achieve and maintain, obesity is a self-perpetuating condition, wherein homeostatic mechanisms attempt to restrain further weight loss.

There are several definitions for overweight and obesity. Although body weight that exceeds ideal standards as determined by age, sex, and height may be accounted for by a greater muscle mass or bone mass, most individuals who weigh over their calculated ideal body weight have excessive adipose tissue mass. Because body-mass index (BMI) is an assessment of total fat content that avoids frame size and gender, it has replaced relative weight as an index of body composition. Overweight is defined as a BMI (weight in kilograms divided by the square of height in meters) of 25 to 29.9 kg/m^2 and obesity as a BMI $\geq$ 30 kg/m^2 (Table 45-1). At present, all overweight and obese adults (aged >18 years with a BMI $\geq$ 25 kg/m^2) are considered to be at risk for developing comorbidities (Table 45-2). Importantly, adipose tissue is not to be regarded as merely a passive storehouse for fat but rather as a diffuse, vascular organ in

TABLE 45-1

CLASSIFICATION OF OVERWEIGHT AND OBESITY BY PERCENTAGE OF BODY FAT, BODY-MASS INDEX, WAIST CIRCUMFERENCE, AND ASSOCIATED DISEASE RISK

	BMI[b] (kg/m²)	DISEASE RISK[a] RELATIVE TO NORMAL WEIGHT AND WAIST CIRCUMFERENCE	
		Men, ≤102 cm Women, ≤88 cm	Men, >102 cm Women, >88 cm
Underweight	<18.5		
Normal	18.5–24.9	—	—
Overweight	25.0–29.9	Increased	High
Obesity, class			
I	30.0–34.9	High	Very high
II	35.0–39.9	Very high	Very high
III (extreme obesity)	≥40	Extremely high	Extremely high

[a] Disease risk for type 2 diabetes, hypertension, and cardiovascular disease.
[b] Body-mass index.
SOURCE: Bouchard et al., with permission.

TABLE 45-2

DISEASES ASSOCIATED WITH OBESITY

Heart disease
Stroke
Hypertension
Dyslipidemia
Type 2 diabetes mellitus
Gallbladder disease
Osteoarthritis
Sleep apnea and respiratory problems
Endometrial, breast, prostate, and colon cancers

which synthesis of a variety of molecules important to cardiovascular medicine is carried out (Table 45-3).

ADAPTATION OF THE CARDIOVASCULAR SYSTEM IN OBESITY

Cardiac Output

Any increase in body mass requires a higher cardiac output and expanded intravascular volume to meet the higher metabolic demands. Because of the need to move excess body weight, the cardiac workload is greater for obese subjects than for nonobese individuals at any given level of activity. Thus, obese subjects are known to have higher cardiac outputs and lower total peripheral resistance. The high cardiac output is mostly attributable to increased stroke volume. The increase in blood volume and cardiac output in obesity is in proportion to the amount of excess body weight and duration of obesity.

TABLE 45-3

PARTICLES PRODUCED BY ADIPOCYTES

Interleukin-6 (IL-6)
Tumor necrosis factor alpha (TNF-α)
Plasminogen activator inhibitor-1 (PAI-1)

TABLE 45-4

HEART ADAPTATIONS TO WEIGHT LOSS

↓ Resting oxygen consumption
↓ Cardiac output
↓ Stroke volume (↓ blood volume and heart volume)
↓ Systemic arterial pressure
↓ Filling pressures of the right and the left side of the heart
No change in systemic arterial resistance

Also, in obesity, left ventricular filling pressure and volume increase, shifting left ventricular function to the left on the Frank-Starling curve and inducing chamber dilatation (Table 45-4). The volume of the dilated chamber increases inappropriately to the stress on the left ventricular wall. The myocardium adapts by increasing contractile elements and myocardial mass. The end product is left ventricular hypertrophy, often of the eccentric type. If this hemodynamic burden is sustained, premature impairment of left ventricular contractile function may result. Left atrial enlargement is also frequent in normotensive obese individuals and is associated with increased left ventricular mass. Provided that arterial pressure does not change, the increase in cardiac output is associated with a decrease in vascular resistance. When obesity and hypertension are present, obesity increases preload and hypertension postload. The heart of the obese hypertensive individual is now confronted with a double burden, which may result in early left ventricular dysfunction and premature heart failure. Obesity is also associated with persistence of elevated cardiac filling pressures. A decrease in blood volume accompanies weight reduction, and relief of edema and dyspnea, when present, accompanies this improvement.

FREQUENTLY PERFORMED PROCEDURES IN CARDIOLOGY AND OBESITY

Physical Examination

Fat mass is distributed differently in men and women. The android, or male, pattern is characterized by fat distributed predominantly in the upper body above the waist; whereas the gynecoid, or female, pattern demonstrates fat predominantly in the lower body, that is, the lower abdomen, buttocks, hips, and thighs. Although obesity is often

TABLE 45-5
ENDOCRINE DISEASES ASSOCIATED WITH OBESITY

Hypothalamic disease (inflammation, trauma, tumor)
Pituitary (Cushing's disease)
Thyroid (hypothyroidism)
Adrenal (Cushing's syndrome)
Ovarian (polycystic ovarian syndrome)

held to be an endocrine disease, less than 1 percent of obese patients have any significant endocrine dysfunction (Table 45-5).

The presence of obesity may limit the accuracy of the physical exam. Jugular venous pulse is often not seen, and heart sounds are usually distant. A common finding in massive obesity is pedal edema, which can occur in part as a consequence of elevated ventricular filling pressure, despite elevation in cardiac output. Obese individuals can also have increases in demand for ventilation and breathing workload, especially in the supine position. Accurate blood pressure measurement is crucial, since many obese patients are hypertensive. A small cuff size can cause considerable increases in blood pressure. This could incorrectly classify up to 35 percent of normotensive obese individuals as hypertensive. One should always evaluate the presence of *cor pulmonale* when examining an obese individual. In obese patients, the split S_2, when either inaudible or very poorly defined in the second interspace, is often best heard at the first left interspace. Therefore an increase in the intensity of P_2, suggestive of pulmonary hypertension, may be missed at the bedside.

Surface Electrocardiogram

Obesity has the potential to affect the electrocardiogram (ECG) in several ways: (1) displacement of the heart by elevating the diaphragm in the supine position, (2) increasing the cardiac workload, and (3) increasing the distance between the heart and the recording electrodes. The voltage of the QRS complexes is attenuated by its passage through a fat-laden chest wall and is related to several factors, including the anatomy of the thorax, degree of fatty infiltration of the heart, degree of associated chronic lung disease, increase in left ventricular muscle mass and—most importantly—the selection of the ECG leads for measuring voltage. Overall, the effect of weight loss in obese patients on the QRS voltage is a source of controversy in the literature; studies report a decrease, no change, or an increase in the QRS amplitude after weight reduction. In some instances, low QRS voltage after drastic weight loss could be secondary to loss of lean mass and myocardial atrophy. It is important to keep in mind that weight loss with modifications in the anatomy of the thorax (decrease in the amount of fat mass) may counterbalance a real decrease in left ventricular mass. These factors, acting in opposite directions, may affect the resultant QRS amplitudes differently. Heart rate, PR interval, QRS interval, QRS voltage, and QTc interval all showed an increase with increasing obesity. An increased incidence of false-positive criteria for inferior myocardial infarction was reported in both obese individuals and in women in the final trimester of pregnancy, presumably because of diaphragmatic elevation.

Left ventricular hypertrophy (LVH) is strongly associated with cardiac morbidity and mortality. As left ventricular mass increases, electrical forces usually become more posteriorly oriented and the S wave in lead V_3 may be the most representative voltage for evaluating posterior forces. In obesity, it was proposed that for men at all ages, LVH is present by QRS voltage alone when the amplitude of the R wave in lead aV_L and the S wave in lead V_3 are >35 mm. For women at all ages, the same criteria were set at >25 mm. When slightly different ECG voltage criteria in the same leads were compared with left ventricular mass estimated by echocardiography, a sensitivity of 49 percent, specificity of 93 percent, and overall accuracy of 76 percent were revealed. These percentages are higher than most widely used criteria (Table 45-6).

TABLE 45-6

DETECTION OF LEFT VENTRICULAR HYPERTROPHY BY QRS VOLTAGE IN OBESITY

	Sensitivity in Obesity	Specificity in Obesity	Accuracy in Obesity
Sokolow-Lyon[a]	20%	93%	65%
Romhilt-Estes point score ≥4[b]	31%	83%	63%
Cornell[c]	49%	93%	76%

[a] Sokolow-Lyon voltage criteria: R in V_5 or V_6 + S in V_1 > 35 mm.
[b] Romhilt-Estes point score: *Am Heart J* 1968; 75:752–758.
[c] Cornell voltage criteria: R in aV_L + S in V_3 > 28 mm in men, >20 mm in women.
SOURCE: Adapted from Casale et al: *J Am Coll Cardiol* 1985, 6:572–580.

Radiology

In obesity, the chest x-ray generally shows an elevated diaphragm with a widened heart in a horizontal direction, with the apex displaced outward to the left. The heart appears enlarged and the left ventricle hypertrophied, based on the criteria of a total transverse diameter of the heart more than half the maximum internal thoracic diameter. This is often discordant with the findings on the surface ECG (see above). The apex or the lower portion of the left border of the heart could be hazy in outline, owing to the presence of apical pericardial fat. Moreover, portable bedside radiographs are usually of a very poor quality in obese patients, limiting the value of this important diagnostic tool in an emergency situation. Also, many computed tomography (CT) tables have weight restrictions (about 160 kg) that often prohibit imaging of severely obese patients.

Echocardiography

Transthoracic echocardiography can be technically difficult in obese patients, and obtaining a good echocardiographic window is often difficult. This is of importance in evaluating the presence of left ventricular diastolic dysfunction. Pulmonary venous Doppler evaluation may be used; but if this is not technically accessible, transmitral Doppler image with the use of the Valsalva maneuver may properly evaluate the presence of left ventricular diastolic dysfunction. Another feature of the echocardiographic assessment in obese patients is the differentiation between subepicardial adipose tissue and pericardial effusion, which can sometimes be difficult. Epicardial adipose tissue is known to be a common cause of pseudopericardial effusion, and this adipose tissue depot may cause an underestimation of the amount of pericardial fluid. Another issue is the presence of fat within the heart. Fat can accumulate in a variety of places, but the site of predilection tends to be the interatrial septum. Lipomatous hypertrophy of the interatrial septum should be suspected in the presence of a dumbbell-shaped appearance of the septum with thick echogenic tissue surrounding a thin echo at the level of the fossa ovalis. Also, accumulation of fat may simulate a mass.

Nuclear Medicine

Cardiac function can adequately be assessed in severely obese subjects using nuclear cardiology imaging techniques. Due to obvious limitations, a dipyridamole thallium-201 or technetium-99m perfusion scan may be used instead of exercise testing in very obese patients for the evaluation of the presence of ischemic heart disease. In spite of the attenuation factor caused by obesity, prolonged transmission scanning with thallium-201 is not required in the obese. Triple-head simultaneous emission transmission tomography using technetium-99m is also accurate in obesity.

Cardiac Catheterization

Obese individuals may have several limitations in the catheterization laboratory. The catheterization laboratory table usually does not accommodate subjects weighing more than 160 kg. Moreover, vascular access to the femoral vein and artery may be difficult. The percutaneous radial approach has advantages in the very obese patient, in whom the percutaneous femoral technique may be technically difficult and bleeding hard to control after catheter removal. Indeed, the frequency of complications using the percutaneous radial technique is very low, and this should be contemplated when the evaluation of extremely obese individuals is necessary in the catheterization laboratory.

OBESITY AND CARDIOVASCULAR DISEASE

Visceral Obesity

Accumulation of intraabdominal (visceral) fat is associated with type 2 diabetes mellitus, hypertension, and coronary artery disease. There is ample evidence to suggest that increased cardiovascular risk is at least partly accounted for by the metabolic abnormalities associated with excessive abdominal fat distribution. Indeed, disturbances in lipoprotein metabolism, plasma insulin-glucose homeostasis, elevations of blood pressure, and hemostatic factors—which are risk factors for cardiac disease (Table 45-7)—have all been reported in subjects with visceral adiposity. There is a beneficial impact of weight loss on plasma plasminogen activator inhibitor-1 (PAI-1) activity and other hemostatic factors in overweight individuals. Waist circumference is positively correlated with abdominal fat content; it is the most practical anthropometric measurement for assessing a patient's abdominal fat content. In patients with a BMI $\geq$ 35 kg/m^2, the waist circumference cutoffs lose their incremental predictive power. When obese subjects are matched for their levels of total body fat; subjects with high levels of visceral fat have dyslipidemia (see Table 45-7).

Blood Glucose and Hyperinsulinemia

The increased risk of diabetes mellitus as weight increases has been shown by prospective studies in numerous countries. The relative

TABLE 45-7

METABOLIC AND HEMOSTATIC ABNORMALITIES
ASSOCIATED WITH OBESITY

↑ Triglycerides
↓ HDL cholesterol
↑ Apolipoprotein B levels
↑ Proportion of small, dense LDL
↑ Fibrinogen
↑ Factor VII activity
↑ Factor VIIIc activity
↑ TPA antigen
↑ PAI-1 antigen and activity

KEY: HDL = high-density lipoprotein; LDL = low-density lipoprotein; TPA =
tissue plasminogen activator; PAI-1 = plasminogen activator inhibitor.

risk of diabetes increases by approximately 25 percent for each additional unit of BMI over 22 kg/m^2. Of importance is that it was recently reported in three European cohorts (> 17,000 men) followed for over 20 years that nondiabetic men with higher blood glucose had a significantly higher risk of death from cardiovascular and coronary heart disease. Thus, asymptomatic glucose intolerance is not a benign metabolic condition, and features associated with the insulin resistance syndrome should be taken seriously. This is further reinforced by the Quebec Cardiovascular Study, which showed that hyperinsulinemia might be an independent risk factor for coronary artery disease. Furthermore, in a 5-year follow-up after coronary artery bypass, it was shown that patients with the components of the insulin resistance syndrome showed angiographic progression of atherosclerosis in nongrafted coronary arteries (see also Chap. 38).

Dyslipidemia

The relationship between obesity and altered plasma lipid profile is well established. Generally, increased fasting plasma triglycerides and reduced plasma HDL-C levels characterize obesity. A BMI change of 1 unit is associated with an HDL-C change of 1.1 mg/dL for young adult men and an HDL-cholesterol change of 0.69 mg/dL for young adult women. Plasma cholesterol and LDL-C levels may be marginally elevated, but the number of apoprotein B–carrying lipoproteins is usually increased. However, a remarkable metabolic heterogeneity is observed among obese subjects, and the presence of visceral obesity worsens the lipid profile. There is evidence that weight loss produced by lifestyle modifications in overweight individuals is accompanied by reductions in serum triglycerides and by increases in HDL-C. Weight loss occasionally produces some reductions in serum total cholesterol and LDL-C levels (see also Chap. 12).

Coronary Artery Disease

Obesity may be an independent risk factor for ischemic heart disease. The association between obesity and ischemic heart disease seems evident only after two decades of follow-up. A high BMI was significantly associated with development of myocardial infarction, coronary insufficiency, and sudden death; among those adverse events, the association was strongest with sudden death. Although obesity per se is considered a major modifiable risk factor for ischemic heart disease, it is important to remember that overweight individuals present a cluster of other traditional and nontraditional risk factors—i.e., dyslipidemia, hypertension, type 2 diabetes mellitus, prothrombotic state, hyperinsulinemia, hypertriglyceridemia, and elevated apolipoprotein B—that are all potentially deleterious. In the ECAT angina pectoris study, there was a strong relationship between obesity and impairment in the fibrinolytic system even after adjusting for total triglycerides, cholesterol, age, and sex.

Hypertension

The majority of patients with high blood pressure are overweight, and hypertension is about six times more frequent in obese than in lean subjects. Not only is hypertension more frequent in obese subjects but weight gain in young people is an important risk factor for subsequent development of hypertension. A 10-kg increase in body weight is associated with a 3.0-mmHg higher systolic and 2.3-mmHg higher diastolic blood pressure. These increases translate into an estimated 12 percent increased risk for coronary heart disease (CHD) and 24 percent increased risk for stroke. The Framingham Heart Study reported that obesity was significantly correlated with increased left ventricular mass and that a 10 percent reduction in the weight of obese hypertensive patients not only reduced blood pressure but also decreased left ventricular wall thickness and left ventricular mass. The effect on left ventricular mass was seen in both hypertensive and nonhypertensive patients. There is strong and consistent evidence from lifestyle trials in overweight patients—hypertensive and nonhypertensive—that weight loss produced by lifestyle modifications reduces blood pressure levels. Weight reduction is one of the rare antihypertensive strategies that decreases blood pressure in normotensive as well as hypertensive persons.

Left Ventricular Hypertrophy and Left Ventricular Diastolic Dysfunction

A longer duration of obesity is associated with higher left ventricular mass, poorer left ventricular systolic function, and greater impairment of left ventricular diastolic function. It has been shown by echocardiography that the eccentric left ventricular hypertrophy in obese subjects causes an abnormal left ventricular diastolic filling pattern similar to the concentric left ventricular hypertrophy of hypertension. In the normotensive obese, the increase in left ventricular mass is not always accompanied by myocardial fibrosis, and normal diastolic function is commonly found. In addition, it was reported that only obese subjects with increased left ventricular mass appeared to have impaired left ventricular diastolic dysfunction and that group of subjects had improvements in left ventricular function after weight loss. Importantly, substantial weight loss may improve the abnormal pattern of ventricular filling and increased left ventricular dimension in diastole. Furthermore, in hypertensive obese subjects, weight loss was associated with a greater decrease in ventricular and posterior wall thickness and left ventricular mass than in subjects treated with metoprolol, suggesting that changes in weight independent of changes in blood pressure were directly associated with changes in left ventricular mass (see also Chap.18). Pathologically, there is a proportionality between heart weight and body weight, and echocardiographic studies have shown that LV end-diastolic dimension as well as septal and posterior wall dimensions are greater in obese subjects. Of note, during weight loss, between 14 to 25 percent of the reduction in left ventricular mass could be explained by the change in body weight. Premature ventricular complexes increase with body weight and are 30 times more frequent in obese patients with eccentric left ventricular hypertrophy compared with lean subjects.

Obstructive Sleep Apnea, Hypoventilation, Pulmonary Hypertension, Right Ventricular Failure

There are numerous respiratory complications of obesity, including an increased breathing workload, respiratory muscle inefficiency, decreased functional reserve capacity and expiratory reserve volume, and closure of peripheral lung units. These often result in a ventilation/perfusion mismatch, especially in the supine position. Obesity is a classic cause of alveolar hypoventilation. The prevalence of sleep-disordered breathing and sleep disturbances rises dramatically in obese subjects, and obesity is by far the most important modifiable

TABLE 45-8

CARDIAC COMPLICATIONS ASSOCIATED
WITH SLEEP APNEA

Diurnal hypertension
Nocturnal dysrhythmias
Pulmonary hypertension
Right and left ventricular failure
Myocardial infarction
Stroke
Increased mortality

risk factor for sleep-disordered breathing. It is estimated that 40 million Americans suffer from sleep disorders and that the vast majority of these patients remain undiagnosed. Despite careful screening by history and physical examination, sleep apnea is revealed only by polysomnography in most patients. Although there are some clinical features that could be useful in screening for sleep apnea, their diagnostic accuracy is inadequate. The prevalence of pulmonary hypertension in subjects with obstructive sleep apnea is 15 to 20 percent; however, pulmonary hypertension is rarely observed in the absence of daytime hypoxemia. The extent of pulmonary hypertension in patients with obstructive sleep apnea is generally mild to moderate (pulmonary artery pressures ranging between 20 and 35 mmHg) and does not necessitate specific treatment. The physician who evaluates an obese patient referred for hypertension should address related symptoms such as habitual snoring, nocturnal gasping or choking, witnessed episodes of apnea, and daytime sleepiness. Also, there are several cardiac complications associated with sleep apnea (Table 45-8). Weight loss should always be advocated in obese patients.

Arrhythmia, Sudden Death, and QT$_c$ Interval

Obese subjects of both sexes, even without dieting, have an increased risk of arrhythmias and sudden death in the absence of cardiac dysfunction. Hence, the annual sudden cardiac mortality rate in obese men and women is estimated at 65 per 100,000 patients, about 40 times higher than the rate of unexplained cardiac arrest in a matched nonobese population. In severely obese men between the ages of 25 and 34 years, a 12-fold excess mortality rate was seen, whereas in men between the ages of 35 and 44 years, a substantial risk with a sixfold excess mortality rate was demonstrated. There is a correlation between BMI and QT_c, with longer intervals observed in obese subjects. Weight loss through starvation, liquid protein diets, very low calorie diets, or even obesity surgery can be associated with prolongation of the QT_c interval. To some extent, this phenomenon is unrelated to the biological value of the constituent protein or the addition of mineral and trace supplements. In addition, it has been shown that liquid protein diets are frequently associated with potentially life-threatening arrhythmias, a relationship documented by 24-h Holter recording but not in a study using routine ECG. Ventricular tachycardia (torsades de pointes) and fibrillation have often been documented in subjects who died under observation. Treatment with different drug regimens or techniques is usually ineffective. ECG changes in the course of weight loss in obese patients appear to be common. However, because extremely obese patients often have a dilated cardiomyopathy, fatal arrhythmias may be the most frequent cause of death.

Cardiac Surgery

Health care professionals often cite obesity as a risk factor for perioperative morbidity and mortality. The presence of hypertension, coronary artery disease, dyslipidemia, and type 2 diabetes mellitus as well as the technical difficulties inherent in the surgical and postsurgical care of the obese patients likely contribute to this perception. Sternal wound infection is increased in obese patients, and obesity has also been identified as a risk factor for infection of the saphenous vein harvest site and atrial dysrhythmias. These complications increase with increasing BMI. On the other side, obesity was not associated with an increased risk of operative mortality, stroke, renal failure, acquired respiratory distress syndrome, prolonged mechanical ventilation, pneumonia, sepsis, pulmonary embolism, or ventricular arrhythmias. Strangely, despite well-documented alterations in respiratory physiology in obese patients, pulmonary complications were comparable to those seen in nonobese patients. Obese patients have been shown to have a higher incidence of postoperative thromboembolic disease in noncardiac surgery. Nevertheless, the high risk of thromboembolic disease in obese patients may warrant an aggressive approach to prophylaxis for deep venous thrombosis.

CARDIOMYOPATHY OF OBESITY (ADIPOSITAS CORDIS)

Excess epicardial fat and fatty infiltration of the myocardium in the hearts of obese subjects, which may have interfered with cardiac function, is well documented. Characteristically, the thickness of the atrial septum is increased (lipomatous hypertrophy). Of interest,

myocardial fatty infiltration has also been described without any relationship to obesity. Myocardial fat infiltration is an uncommon
autopsy finding, with an incidence of approximately 3 percent. This
condition is more prevalent in women. The presence of excess adipose tissue on the surface of the right ventricle represents an exaggeration of the normal architecture. Thus, at least at first, the fatty heart is
probably not an infiltrative process but most likely a metaplastic phenomenon. With time, fat can infiltrate between muscle fibers and/or
result in myocyte degeneration. With progressive disease, fatty heart
can result in cardiac conduction defects. Fatty heart can also result in
a restrictive cardiomyopathy. In general, the right ventricle is more
likely to be involved than the left ventricle and the anterior wall is
involved to a greater extent than the posterior. Most of the time, cardiac hypertrophy is a direct reflection of BMI and the hypertrophy
is from myocyte change and not from excessive fat infiltration or
fibrosis.

TREATMENT

The general goals of weight loss and management are, at a minimum,
to prevent further weight gain, reduce body weight, and maintain a
lower body weight indefinitely. Patients should have their BMI and
levels of abdominal fat measured, with goals of weight reduction
established to favorably affect outcomes, including cardiovascular
health. Obesity treatment includes counseling, diet, exercise, drugs,
and/or surgery.

Lifestyle Modifications (Behavioral, Diet, Exercise)

Behavioral strategies to reinforce changes in diet and physical activity in obese adults can produce weight loss in the range of 10 percent
over a period of 6 months. Weight-loss programs that result in a
slow but steady weight reduction—e.g., 1 to 2 lb per week, may be
more effective than those that result in rapid weight loss. Long-term
follow-up results of patients undergoing behavioral therapy show a
return to baseline weight for the majority of subjects in the absence
of continued behavioral intervention. In obese patients who smoke,
smoking cessation is mandatory. However, a major obstacle to cessation has been the attendant weight gain observed in about 80 percent
of quitters.

DIET

Diets for weight reduction should be restricted not only in total calories but also in fat and sugar. Approximately 1 lb per week can be lost

with no change in physical activity if 500 Kcal/day are eliminated. Such diets would continue to include foods that are low in saturated fat and cholesterol but enriched in nutrients that are associated with a reduced risk for cardiovascular disease—e.g., fruits, vegetables, legumes, and whole-grain products.

EXERCISE

Aerobic exercise alone produces only a modest weight reduction, generally 2 to 3 percent; however, it is extremely important in sustaining the weight-reduced state. Fat loss through dieting and/or exercise produces comparable and favorable changes in HDL-C and its subfractions HDL_2 and HDL_3 as well as triglycerides and can normalize the metabolic profile of obese subjects even if the subjects remain very obese at the end of the program. Of interest, even if weight loss is minimal, physically fit obese individuals are less vulnerable to mortality from cardiovascular disease then lean subjects who are not physically fit. Initially, moderate levels of physical activity for 30 to 45 min 3 to 5 days a week should be encouraged. Thereafter, all adults should set a long-term goal to accumulate at least 30 min or more of moderate-intensity physical activity on most and preferably all days of the week.

DRUGS

Weight-loss drugs can be useful adjuncts to dietary therapy and physical activity for some patients—i.e., with a BMI $\geq$ 30 kg/m^2 with or without concomitant comorbidities and for patients with a BMI $\geq$ 27 kg/m^2 with concomitant risk factors or diseases. The comorbidities considered of sufficient importance to warrant pharmacotherapy at a BMI of 27 to 29.9 kg/m^2 are hypertension ($\geq$140/90 mmHg), dyslipidemia (LDL $\geq$160 mg/dL, HDL <35 mg/dL), coronary artery disease, type 2 diabetes, and obstructive sleep apnea. The two main categories of obesity drugs are anorectics, which act centrally in the brain on adrenergic or serotonergic pathways, and nutrient absorption inhibitors, which decrease macronutrient absorption from the gastrointestinal tract.

SURGERY

Weight-loss surgery, including gastric plication and gastric bypass with a Roux-en-Y anastomosis, represents an option in a limited number of patients with extreme obesity—i.e., BMI $\geq$ 40 kg/m^2 or BMI $\geq$ 35 kg/m^2—with comorbid conditions. Weight-loss surgery should be reserved for extremely obese patients in whom efforts at medical therapy have failed. An acceptable operative risk must also be present. Furthermore, lifelong medical surveillance after surgery is necessary.

CONCLUSIONS

Obesity is a chronic metabolic disorder associated with cardio-vascular disease and increased morbidity and mortality. When the BMI is ≥ 30 kg/m^2, mortality rates from all causes, and especially cardiovascular disease, are increased by 50 to 100 percent. There is strong evidence that weight loss in overweight and obese individuals reduces risk factors for diabetes and cardiovascular disease. Additional evidence indicates that weight loss reduces blood pressure in both overweight hypertensive and nonhypertensive individuals, reduces serum triglyceride levels and increases high-density-lipoprotein cholesterol (HDL-C) levels, and may produce some reduction in low-density-lipoprotein cholesterol (LDL-C) levels. Weight loss also reduces blood glucose levels and hemoglobin A$_{1c}$ levels in patients with type 2 diabetes, signs and symptoms of left ventricular failure, and obstructive sleep apnea. Although there have been no prospective trials to convincingly show changes in mortality with weight loss in obese patients, reductions in risk factors would at least predict a reduced incidence of cardiovascular disease and perhaps cardiovascular disease–related mortality.

SUGGESTED READING

Alpert MA, Lambert CR, Panayiotou H, et al: Relation of duration of morbid obesity to left ventricular mass, systolic function, and diastolic filling, and effect of weight loss. *Am J Cardiol* 1995; 76:1194–1197.

Birkmeyer NJ, Charlesworth DC, Hernandez F, et al: Obesity and risk of adverse outcomes associated with coronary artery bypass surgery. Northern New England Cardiovascular Disease Study Group. *Circulation* 1998; 97:1689–1694.

Bouchard C, Després JP, Mauriège P: Genetic and nongenetic determinants of regional fat distribution. *Endocr Rev* 1993; 14:72–93.

Clinical Guidelines on the Identification, Evaluation, and Treatment of Overweight and Obesity in Adults—The Evidence Report. National Institutes of Health. *Obes Res Suppl* 1998; 2:51S–209S.

Eckel RH, Krauss RM: American Heart Association call to action: Obesity as a major risk factor for coronary heart disease. AHA Nutrition Committee. *Circulation* 1998; 97:2099–2100.

Executive summary of the clinical guidelines on the identification, evaluation, and treatment of overweight and obesity in adults. *Arch Intern Med* 1998; 158:1855–1867.

Krauss RM, Deckelbaum RJ, Ernst N, et al: AHA dietary guidelines for healthy American adults. *Circulation* 1996; 94:1795–1800.

Lee CD, Blair SN, Jackson AS: Cardiorespiratory fitness, body composition, and all-cause and cardiovascular disease mortality in men. *Am J Clin Nutr* 1999; 69:373–380.

Lemieux S, Després JP: Metabolic complications of visceral obesity: Contribution to the aetiology of type 2 diabetes and implications for prevention and treatment. *Diabetes Metab* 1994; 20:375–393.

Marik P, Varon J: The obese patient in the ICU. *Chest* 1998; 113:492–498.

Poirier P, Eckel RH: The heart and obesity. In: Fuster V, Alexander RW, O'Rourke RA, et al (eds): *Hurst's the Heart,* 10th ed. New York: McGraw-Hill; 2001:2289–2303.

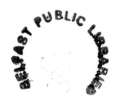

INDEX

Note: Page numbers followed by *f* indicate figures; those followed by *t* indicate tables.

A

AAI pacing, 143
ABIs (ankle brachial indices), in peripheral arterial disease, 721–722, 723*t*
Accelerated ventricular rhythm, 77
Acebutolol, dosage and kinetics of, 66*t*
Acid maltase deficiency, restrictive cardiomyopathy in, 555
ACI inhibitors. *See* Angiotensin-converting enzyme (ACE) inhibitors
Acromegaly, cardiomyopathy and, 571
Acute myocardial infarction (AMI), 277–324
 angioplasty for, 321, 339–341
  rescue, 347–348
  thrombolytic therapy versus, 339–340
 circadian variation in occurrence of, 279
 in diabetes mellitus, 638–639
 diagnosis of, 282–287
  diagnostic markers in plasma and, 283–287, 284*f*, 292–293

 differential diagnosis, 282
 electrocardiographic, 282–283
 discharge from coronary care unit and, 317–321
  coronary angioplasty and percutaneous transluminal coronary angioplasty and, 321
  noninvasive risk stratification and, 318–321
 electrocardiogram in, 27, 28*f*, 29*f*
 emergency department management of, 288–308
  initial approach, detection, and assessment or risk and, 289, 290*f*, 291*t*, 291–295
  with ischemic-type chest pain and without ST-segment elevation, 305–308
  with ST-segment elevation, 295–305, 296*f*
  after triage into electrocardiographic subgroups, 295–308

Acute myocardial infarction
(AMI) (*Cont.*):
imaging in, 285, 287
inpatient management of,
308–318
activity and, 308
education in, 308
of high-risk patient,
310–317
of low-risk patients,
309–310
pharmacologic, 308, 309
intra-aortic balloon pumping
for, 345–347
misdiagnosis of, 288–289
physical findings in,
280–281
platelet inhibitors for, 345,
346t
precipitating events for,
278–279
predisposing characteristics
and circumstances for,
278
prehospital care for, 287–288
secondary prevention and
cardiac rehabilitation
and, 321–324
lifestyle modification and
cardiac rehabilitation
and, 323–324
pharmacotherapy in,
322–323
risk-factor reduction and,
321–322
stents for, 341, 344t,
344–345
symptoms of, 279–280
in women, 696–697
Acylated plasminogen-
streptokinase activated
complex (APSAC), for
acute myocardial
infarction, 298, 300
Adenoidectomy, for cor
pulmonale, 411

Adenosine (Adenocard)
actions of, 94t
dosage of, 67t, 110–111
interactions and
complications of, 657
kinetics of, 67t
plasma concentration range
for, 110–111
for pulmonary hypertension,
381
for supraventricular
tachycardia, 65, 65t, 67t
Adipositas cordis, 745–746
Adriamycin (doxorubicin),
cardiac effects of,
575–576, 576
AF (atrial flutter), 71–72, 72t
after acute myocardial
infarction, 316
pacing for, 145
Age
as risk factor for
atherosclerosis, 233
sudden cardiac death and,
166, 167
Aging, 39–47
aortic stenosis and, 47
atrial fibrillation and, 47
congestive heart failure and,
46
exercise cardiovascular
function and, 41, 43,
43t
hypertension and, 46
ischemic heart disease and,
44, 45t
resting cardiovascular
function and, 41, 42t
structural changes associated
with, 39, 40t, 41
Airway obstruction, 212
Alcoholic cardiomyopathy,
572
Alcohol intake, sudden cardiac
death and, 168, 185
Aldactone, for heart failure, 57

Aldosterone receptor antagonists, for heart failure, 57

Aldosteronism, primary, evaluation for, 358–359

Alpha-adrenergic blockers, for hypertension, 361

Alteplase, interactions and complications of, 663t

Alveolar hypoventilation, pulmonary hypertension and, 380

Ambulatory blood pressure monitoring, 354

Ambulatory electrocardiogram, 62
  in aortic regurgitation, 424
  in hypertrophic cardiomyopathy, 543

American trypanosomiasis cardiomyopathy and, 538, 566
  sudden cardiac death and, 180

AMI. *See* Acute myocardial infarction (AMI)

Amiloride, interactions and complications of, 659t

Amiodarone (Cordarone)
  actions of, 94t
  for atrial fibrillation, 74
  during cardiopulmonary resuscitation, 211
  dosage of, 67t, 99t, 107–109
  interactions and complications of, 656t, 659t, 715–716
  kinetics of, 67t
  pharmacokinetics of, 96t
  plasma concentration range for, 99t, 107–109
  for sudden cardiac death prevention, 196t, 198t, 199–201
  for ventricular arrhythmias, 84, 84t, 214, 305

Amoxicillin, for infective endocarditis prophylaxis, 613t

Ampicillin
  for infective endocarditis prophylaxis, 613t
  for infective endocarditis treatment, 604t, 607t, 609t

Amsacrine, cardiac effects of, 575

Amyloidosis
  cardiomyopathy and, 552–553, 568–569
  sudden cardiac death and, 180

Anabolic steroids, cardiac effects of, 578

Anacrotic limb, 5

Analgesia, in acute myocardial infarction, 293–294, 308

Aneurysms, aortic, 702–703

Angina pectoris, 237–255
  with aortic stenosis, 415
  classification of, 3, 4t, 238, 238t
  diagnosis of, 239–243
    history and physical examination in, 239t, 239–241
    tests in, 241–243
  differential diagnosis of, 243, 245t
  etiology of, 237–238
  myocardial revascularization for, 252, 253t–254t, 255
  pathophysiology of, 245–426
  prognosis and risk stratification in, 263, 264t–265t, 266
  risk stratification of patients with, 246–247, 248t, 249t
  stable, treatment of, 247, 249–252

Angina pectoris (*Cont.*):
stress testing and coronary angiography in, 266–267
treatment of, 267–275, 268*f*
unstable, 257–275
classification of, 257–259, 258*t*, 259*t*
definition of, 257
diagnosis and risk stratification in, 259–263
variant (Prinzmetal's), 259
in women, 696

Angiography
antithrombotic therapy and, 489
coronary. *See* Coronary angiography
left ventricular
in aortic regurgitation, 424
in mitral regurgitation, 445–446
magnetic resonance, in peripheral arterial disease, 722
in peripheral arterial disease, 722
radionuclide, in mitral regurgitation, 446
stress, 243, 244*t*

Angioplasty. *See also* Percutaneous coronary interventions (PCI); Percutaneous transluminal coronary angioplasty (PTCA)
in acute myocardial infarction, 339–341
thrombolytic therapy versus, 339–340
coronary
for acute myocardial infarction, 301, 302
for unstable angina pectoris, 274

laser, 334*t*, 335
rescue, for acute myocardial infarction, 347–348

Angiotensin-converting enzyme (ACE) inhibitors. *See also* *specific drugs*
for acute myocardial infarction, 309, 323
for coronary heart disease prevention, 235
in diabetic patients, 630
for heart failure, 51, 52*t*, 54, 54*t*
for hypertension, 361
interactions and complications of, 660
for sudden cardiac death prevention, 194

Angiotensin II receptor blockers, interactions and complications of, 660

Ankle brachial indices (ABIs), in peripheral arterial disease, 721–722, 723*t*

Annuloaortic ectasia, 702

Anthracyclines, cardiac effects of, 575–576
cardiomyopathy and, 537, 573

Antiarrhythmic agents, 93–111. *See also specific agents*
classification of, 93, 94*f*, 95, 96*t*, 98*t*–99*t*
interactions and complications of, 652, 654*t*–656*t*, 657
during pregnancy, 673
for premature ventricular contractions, 81–82
sudden cardiac death and, 184–185
for sudden cardiac death prevention, 194–195, 196*t*–198*t*, 199–201

torsades de pointes due to, 86, 97

Antibiotics. *See also specific drugs*
for infective endocarditis prophylaxis, 612, 613t–614t, 615
in aortic regurgitation, 425
in aortic stenosis, 418
in mitral regurgitation, 447
in mitral stenosis, 437, 438t
in mitral valve prolapse, 458, 459t
with prosthetic valves, 477
for infective endocarditis treatment, 601–602, 604t, 606t–610t

Anticoagulant therapy. *See also specific drugs*
after acute myocardial infarction, 323
with atrial fibrillation, 75, 76t
complications of, 396
for coronary heart disease prevention, 234
for hypertrophic cardiomyopathy, 547
for mitral stenosis, 438
novel agents for, 396
for pulmonary hypertension, 381–382

Antidepressants, cardiac effects of, 576–577

Antihypertensive therapy. *See also specific drugs and drug types*
adverse reactions and side effects of, 369–370
cost of, 370–371
matching goal blood pressure to cardiovascular risk and, 362
tailoring for specific clinical situations, 363–369

Antithrombotic therapy. *See also specific drugs*
for angina pectoris, 247
for coronary heart disease prevention, 234
interactions and complications of, 660, 662t–663t
for non-Q-wave myocardial infarction, 306
with percutaneous coronary interventions, 335
during pregnancy, 674
with prosthetic valves, 480–481
in valvular heart disease, 483–492, 484t
with altered native valves, 487, 487t
angiography and, 489
cardiac catheterization and, 489
dental care and, 488–489
infective endocarditis and, 492
native valve disease, 484t, 484–486, 485f
during pregnancy, 487–488
prosthetic valve disease, 486–487, 487t
surgery and, 488–489
at time of active thromboembolic event, 489–490
at time of bleed, 490, 492

Anxiolytics, for acute myocardial infarction, 308

Aorta, coarctation of, 519–520
during pregnancy, 684

Aortic disorders, 701–707
clinical manifestations of, 702–704
of aneurysms, 702–703
of aortic dissection, 703

Aortic disorders (*Cont.*):
  of aortic regurgitation, 703
  of embolization from the
    aorta, 704
  of obstruction, 704
  differential diagnosis of, 705
  etiology of, 701–702
  natural history and prognosis
    of, 705–706
  physical examination in, 704
  treatment of, 706*t*, 706–707
  x-ray studies in, 704–705
Aortic dissection, 703
  acute myocardial infarction
    and, 291
  antihypertensive agents for,
    706*t*, 707
Aortic regurgitation (AR),
    419–428
  clinical features of, 422–424,
    703
  definition of, 419
  etiology and pathology of,
    420–421
  natural history and prognosis
    of, 424–425
  pathophysiology of, 421–422
  during pregnancy, 680–681
  treatment of
    medical, 425
    surgical, 425, 426*t*–427*t*,
      427–428
Aortic stenosis (AS), 413–419
  clinical features of, 415–417
  definition of, 413
  in elderly people, 47
  etiology and pathology of,
    413–414
  hypertension in, treatment of,
    365
  laboratory studies in,
    417–418
  murmurs in, 15
  natural history and prognosis
    of, 418
  pathophysiology of, 414–415

  during pregnancy, 680
  rheumatic, 414
  rheumatoid, 414
  sudden cardiac death and,
    181
  supravalvular, 510–511
  treatment of
    medical, 418
    surgical, 419, 420*t*
Aortic valve replacement
  for aortic regurgitation, 425,
    426*t*–427*t*, 427–428
  for aortic stenosis, 419, 420*t*
Aortitis
  infectious, 702
  nonspecific, 702
APSAC (acylated plasminogen-
    streptokinase activated
    complex), for acute
    myocardial infarction,
    298, 300
AR. *See* Aortic regurgitation
    (AR)
Arrhythmias. *See also*
    Antiarrhythmic agents
  after acute myocardial
    infarction, 316
  in acute myocardial
    infarction, 303–305
  in congenital heart disease,
    523
  drug-induced, 649
  heritable, 505, 506*t*–507*t*
  obesity and, 744–745
  during pregnancy, 677–678
  following stroke, 718
  syncope related to, 158–159
  in women, 698
Arrhythmogenic right
    ventricular dysplasia
    (ARVD)
  familial, dilated
    cardiomyopathy in,
    497–498
  sudden cardiac death and,
    178

Arterial blood gases, in pulmonary hypertension, 378
Arterial pressure pulse, 5f, 5–6
Arteriosclerosis obliterans (ASO), 722, 724
Arteriovenous malformations, gastrointestinal, with aortic stenosis, 415
Arteritis, 725
ARVD (arrhythmogenic right ventricular dysplasia)
  familial, dilated cardiomyopathy in, 497–498
  sudden cardiac death and, 178
AS. See Aortic stenosis (AS)
Aschoff's nodule, 431
ASD (atrial septal defect), 515–516
  familial, 509
  during pregnancy, 682
ASO (arteriosclerosis obliterans), 722, 724
Aspirin
  after acute myocardial infarction, 323
  for acute myocardial infarction, 295
  with atrial fibrillation, 75, 76t
  for coronary heart disease prevention, 234
  interactions and complications of, 660, 662t
  for non-Q-wave myocardial infarction, 307
  with percutaneous coronary interventions, 335
  for pericarditis, 310
  with prosthetic valves, 480–481, 486, 487t
  for unstable angina pectoris, 270
  for valve thrombosis, 491t

Asystole, 215–216
  in acute myocardial infarction, 303
  differential diagnosis of, 215–216
Atherectomy, 335
  directional, 334t
  extraction, transluminal, 334t
  rheolytic, 334t
Atherogenic diet, 226
Atherosclerosis
  of aorta, 701
  noncoronary forms of, coronary heart disease risk and, 223
  plaque disruption in, thrombosis and, 633
  sudden cardiac death and, 173, 175
Athletes, sudden cardiac death in, 170
Atorvastatin, interactions and complications of, 659t, 664t, 665
Atrial fibrillation, 72–75
  after acute myocardial infarction, 316
  chronic, 75
  in elderly people, 47
  familial, 506t, 507t, 509
  first episode of, 73
  in hypertrophic cardiomyopathy, 545
  pacing for, 145
  paroxysmal, 73–74, 145
  persistent, 74–75
  stroke risk with, 484–485
Atrial flutter (AF), 71–72, 72t
  after acute myocardial infarction, 316
  pacing for, 145
Atrial premature beats, after acute myocardial infarction, 316

Atrial septal defect (ASD), 515–516
  familial, 509
  during pregnancy, 682
Atrial septostomy, for pulmonary hypertension, 382
Atrial standstill, familial, 507t
Atrial tachycardia
  ectopic, 70
  multifocal, 70–71
Atrioventricular block
  in acute myocardial infarction, 303
  complete, 89–90, 146
  congenital, 90, 137
  familial, 507t, 509
  first-degree, 88–89
  intermittent, 146
  pacing for, 136–137, 138t–139t, 146
  second-degree, 89
  sudden cardiac death and, 189
Atrioventricular dissociation, 90
Atrioventricular junctional rhythms, 75–77
Atrioventricular junctional tachycardia, 78
Atrioventricular nodal reentry, supraventricular arrhythmias due to, 64–65, 65t–67t, 68–69
Atrioventricular septal defect (AVSD), 517
Atropine
  for accelerated junctional and ventricular rhythms, 77
  actions of, 94t
  for asystole, 215
  for bradycardia, in acute myocardial infarction, 303
  during cardiopulmonary resuscitation, 211

Auscultation, 10
  dynamic, in mitral valve prolapse, 454
Austin-Flint murmur, 18
Autograft valves, 476
Automatic external defibrillators, after prehospital arrest, 210, 212
Automatic mode switch, 145
Autonomic nervous system, arrhythmias and, 172–173
AVSD (atrioventricular septal defect), 517
a waves, 6–8, 7f

B
Balloon angioplasty. See Percutaneous transluminal coronary angioplasty (PTCA)
Ball valves, 475
Baroreflex sensitivity, sudden cardiac death and, 192
Barth syndrome, dilated cardiomyopathy in, 497
Benazepril, for heart failure, 54t
Benzafibrate, interactions and complications of, 664t
Bepridil, actions of, 94t
Beta-adrenergic agonists, cardiac effects of, 577
Beta-adrenergic blockers. See also specific drugs
  after acute myocardial infarction, 322–323
  for acute myocardial infarction, 297
  for angina pectoris, 251
  during cardiopulmonary resuscitation, 211
  for coronary heart disease prevention, 234–235

dosage and kinetics of, 68
for heart failure, 53, 55t, 56
for hypertrophic
cardiomyopathy, 545,
546t
interactions and
complications of, 649,
650t
for non-Q-wave myocardial
infarction, 307
during pregnancy, 672–673
for sudden cardiac death
prevention, 193–194
for unstable angina pectoris,
269
Betapace. *See* Sotalol
(Betapace)
Bile acid sequestrants,
interactions and
complications of, 664t
Bileaflet valves, 476
Biochemical markers
in acute myocardial
infarction, 283–285,
284f, 292–293
in unstable angina, 263
Biological valves,
antithrombotic therapy
for, 486–487
Bisferiens pulse, 5f, 6
Bisoprolol, for heart failure,
55t
Bivalirudin, for venous
thromboembolism
treatment, 396
Bjork-Shiley tilting-disk valve,
475–476
Bleeding, in cyanotic heart
disease, 522t
Blood flow
distribution of, during
pregnancy, 670
mechanisms of, 208–209,
209t
Blood glucose, obesity and,
740–741

Blood pressure. *See also*
Antihypertensive
therapy; Hypertension;
Hypotension
measurement of, 353–354
"Blue-toe syndrome," 725
Blunt trauma, tricuspid valve
disease following, 465
Bounding pulse, 5–6
Bovine pericardial heterograft
valves, 476–477
Bradyarrhythmias, 87–91
bradycardia, in acute
myocardial infarction,
303–304
during pregnancy, 678
in sudden cardiac death, 171
Bradycardia-tachycardia
syndrome, 158
Brain, hypoperfusion of,
cardiac arrest and,
714–715
Brain embolism, 709–714, 710t
cardiac arrest and, 714–715
cardiac drugs and cardiac
encephalopathy and,
715–716
with mitral annulus
calcification, 710–711,
712t
with mitral valve prolapse,
710
onset, clinical course, and
diagnostic approaches
for, 711–713
paradoxical embolism and,
714
prevention and treatment of,
713–714
Brain lesions, cardiac effects
of, 717–718
Bretylium (Bretylol)
actions of, 94t
dosage of, 67t, 99t, 106
kinetics of, 67t
pharmacokinetics of, 96t

Bretylium (Bretylol) (*Cont.*):
  plasma concentration range
    for, 99*t*, 106
  for ventricular arrhythmias,
    305
  for ventricular tachycardia,
    84*t*
Brugada syndrome, 506*t*,
  508–509
Bundle branch block, familial,
  507*t*

C
CABG. *See* Coronary artery
  bypass grafting
  (CABG)
CAD. *See* Coronary artery
  disease (CAD)
Calcium-channel blockers. *See
  also specific drugs*
  for angina pectoris, 251–252
  for hypertension, 361
  for hypertrophic
    cardiomyopathy,
    545–546, 546*t*
  interactions and
    complications of, 652,
    653*t*
  for non-Q-wave myocardial
    infarction, 307
  overdose of, 215
  during pregnancy, 673
  for unstable angina pectoris,
    269–270
Calcium chloride
  for calcium-channel blocker
    overdose, 215
  during cardiopulmonary
    resuscitation, 211,
    218
Calcium excess, sudden cardiac
  death and, 186
Calcium gluconate, during
  cardiopulmonary
  resuscitation, 211

Candesartan, for heart failure,
  52*t*
Captopril
  for heart failure, 52*t*, 54*t*
  interactions and
    complications of,
    659*t*
Carbomedics valve, 476
Carbon monoxide, cardiac
  effects of, 581
Carcinoids
  cardiomyopathy and, 570
  restrictive cardiomyopathy
    and, 555
  tricuspid valve disease
    following, 464–465
Cardiac arrest. *See also* Sudden
  cardiac death (SCD)
  brain hypoperfusion due to,
    714–715
  diagnosis of, 209
  identification of, 209
  implantable cardioverter-
    defibrillator therapy for,
    122
  out-of-hospital, clinical
    presentation and
    management of,
    186–187
  pathology of, 187–188
  preliminary patient
    evaluation and triage in,
    210, 211*t*
  primary versus secondary,
    188, 188*t*
  prognosis after, 187
  risk stratification for sudden
    cardiac death and, 189,
    190*t*–191*t*, 192–193
  survival after, 187
Cardiac auscultation, 10
Cardiac catheterization
  antithrombotic therapy and,
    489
  in aortic regurgitation, 424
  in aortic stenosis, 417

in constrictive pericarditis, 590
in infective endocarditis, 601
in mitral regurgitation, 445
in mitral stenosis, 436
in mitral valve prolapse, 456
in obesity, 740
in pulmonic valve disease, 469
in restrictive cardiomyopathy, 550
right-sided, in cor pulmonale, 409–410
in tricuspid valve disease, 469
Cardiac evaluation, in hypertension, 355–356
Cardiac examination, in acute myocardial infarction, 281–282
Cardiac memory, 24–25
Cardiac output
in obesity, 735–736, 736*t*
syncope related to obstruction of, 157–158
Cardiac rehabilitation, after acute myocardial infarction, 323–324
Cardiac surgery. *See also specific procedures*
neurologic and cerebrovascular complications of, 716–717
obesity and, 745
Cardiac tamponade, 588–589
Cardiac transplantation, pregnancy following, 686
Cardiogenic shock, after acute myocardial infarction, 314–315
Cardiomyopathy. *See also Myocarditis; Restrictive cardiomyopathy*
alcoholic, 572

carnitine deficiency causing, 501–502
classification of, 527–529, 528*t*
diabetic, 644
idiopathic, 573–574
mitochondrial, 502–503
of obesity, 745–746
specific, 529
Cardiopulmonary resuscitation (CPR), 207–220
asystole and, 215–216
automatic external defibrillators and, 210, 212
chain of survival and, 207–208
diagnosis and identification of cardiac arrest and, 209
drugs used during, 217–218
electromechanical dissociation and, 216
intravenous route establishment and, 216–217
mechanisms of blood movement and, 208–209, 209*t*
postarrest care and, 219–220
preliminary patient evaluation and triage and, 210, 211*t*
respiratory arrest and, 212
termination of, 218–219
ventilation during, 212–213
ventricular tachycardia or fibrillation and, 213–215
Cardiovascular disorders. *See also specific disorders*
in cyanotic heart disease, 522*t*

Cardiovascular drugs. *See also specific drugs and drug types*
interactions and complications of, 647–666
  of angiotensin-converting enzyme inhibitors and angiotensin II receptor blockers, 660
  of antiarrhythmic agents, 652, 654t–656t, 657
  of antihypertensive agents, 369
  of antithrombotic and thrombolytic agents, 660–661, 662t–663t, 665
  of beta-adrenergic blocking drugs, 649, 650t
  of calcium-channel blockers, 652, 653t
  of diuretics, 658, 660
  of herbal supplements, 666
  of lipid-lowering agents, 664t, 665
  of nitrates, 650, 651t
  P-glycoprotein and, 648
  pharmacodynamic hepatic interactions and, 648
  pharmacokinetic hepatic interactions and, 647–648
  pharmacokinetic renal interactions and, 649
  plasma binding and, 649
  of positive inotropic agents, 657–658
  proarrhythmic interactions and, 649
neurologic effects of, 715–716
during pregnancy, 672–674
Cardiovascular system adaptation in obesity, 735–736

age-related structural changes in, 39, 40t, 41
Cardioversion
  for atrial fibrillation, 73
  for atrial flutter, 71, 72t
  in mitral stenosis, 437–438
  for ventricular tachycardia, 84
Carditis, rheumatic, mitral stenosis due to, 431
Carey-Coombs murmur, 18
Carnitine, deficiency of, cardiomyopathy due to, 501–502
Carotid sinus hypersensitivity, 155
Carotid sinus massage, 71
Carotid sinus syndrome, pacing for, 137, 141t, 142, 146
Carvedilol, for heart failure, 55t, 56
Catheter balloon commissurotomy (CBC), for mitral stenosis, 439, 440t, 442t
Catheter balloon valvuloplasty, for aortic stenosis, 419
CCA (congenital contractual arachnodactyly), 504
Cefazolin, for infective endocarditis prophylaxis, 614t
Ceftriaxone, for infective endocarditis, 606t, 609t, 610t
Cellulitis, recurrent, 729
Cerebrovascular syncope, 153, 155
Cerivastatin, interactions and complications of, 664t, 665
Cerubidine (daunorubicin), cardiac effects of, 575
Chagas' disease cardiomyopathy and, 538, 566

sudden cardiac death and, 180

Chain of survival concept, 207–208

Chamomile, interactions and complications of, 666

CHD. *See* Coronary heart disease (CHD)

Chemotherapeutic agents, cardiac effects of, 573, 575–576

Chest pain. *See also* Angina pectoris
    differential diagnosis of, 1, 2*t*, 3
    in mitral valve prolapse, 453

Chest radiography
    in acute myocardial infarction, 285
    in angina pectoris, 241
    in aortic disorders, 704–705
    in aortic regurgitation, 422
    in aortic stenosis, 416
    in cor pulmonale, 409
    in hypertrophic cardiomyopathy, 543
    in mitral regurgitation, 444
    in mitral stenosis, 435
    in mitral valve prolapse, 455
    in pulmonary embolism, 389
    in pulmonary hypertension, 375
    in pulmonic valve disease, 468
    in tricuspid valve disease, 468

CHF. *See* Congestive heart failure (CHF)

Chloroquine, cardiac effects of, 578

Cholestyramine, interactions and complications of, 664*t*

Chronic obstructive pulmonary disease (COPD)
    cor pulmonale due to, 403–405

pulmonary hypertension and, 378

Cigarette smoking
    cessation of, 229, 230*t*, 322
        for reduction of coronary artery disease risk, 690, 694
    sudden cardiac death and, 168, 170

Cilostazol, for arteriosclerosis obliterans, 724

Circadian rhythm
    acute myocardial infarction and, 279
    of coronary ischemia, 246

CK-MB, in acute myocardial infarction, 284–285, 286*t*, 292–293

Claudication, 721

Clindamycin, for infective endocarditis prophylaxis, 613*t*

Clopidogrel
    interactions and complications of, 660
    with percutaneous coronary interventions, 335
    for unstable angina pectoris, 270–271

Coarctation of the aorta, 519–520
    during pregnancy, 684

Cocaine
    cardiac effects of, 578–579
    cardiomyopathy and, 572–573
    sudden cardiac death and, 185

Colestipol, interactions and complications of, 664*t*

Compensatory mechanisms, progression of myocardial failure and, 529–532, 530*f*, 531*f*

Computed tomography (CT), in pulmonary embolism, 390

Conduction disorders
  in congenital heart disease, 523
  heritable, 505, 507t, 508–509
  intraventricular, electrocardiogram in, 29, 31–34

Congenital contractual arachnodactyly (CCA), 504

Congenital heart disease, 515–524
  during pregnancy, 682–685
  pulmonary hypertension and, 376–377
  sudden cardiac death and, 180–181

Congestive heart failure (CHF)
  in acute myocardial infarction, 311–315
  in diabetes mellitus, 644
  in elderly people, 46
  encephalopathy with, 716
  in infective endocarditis, 602, 605
  neurocardiogenic, 142
  during pregnancy, 676

Connective tissue disorders
  heritable, 503–505
  pulmonary hypertension and, 379–380

Consciousness, loss of, during pregnancy, 678

Continuous electrocardiogram monitoring, 62

Contraception, in congenital heart disease, 523

Contrast venography, for deep vein thrombosis detection, 391

COPD (chronic obstructive pulmonary disease)
  cor pulmonale due to, 403–405

pulmonary hypertension and, 378

Cordarone. See Amiodarone (Cordarone)

Coronary angiography
  in acute myocardial infarction, 321
  in aortic stenosis, 417–418
  in mitral stenosis, 436
  in non-Q-wave myocardial infarction, 307–308
  stress, 243, 244t
  in unstable angina, 266–267

Coronary angioplasty. See Percutaneous transluminal coronary angioplasty (PTCA)

Coronary artery bypass grafting (CABG)
  for acute myocardial infarction, 302
  for angina pectoris, 252, 253t, 254t, 255
  in elderly people, 44
  before noncardiac surgery, 623–624
  percutaneous transluminal coronary angioplasty versus, 328, 329t
  stents versus, in multivessel disease, 330–331
  for sudden cardiac death prevention, 203–204
  for unstable angina pectoris, 274
  in women, 697–698

Coronary artery disease (CAD)
  in diabetes mellitus, 639
  hypertension in, treatment of, 367
  obesity and, 742
  during pregnancy, 686
  preoperative functional testing and, 621–622
  preoperative therapy for, 623–624

sudden cardiac death and, 173, 175–176
in women, 689–698, 690f
  diabetes and, 695
  diagnosis of, 695–696
  hypertension and, 695
  management of, 696–698
  prevention of, 689–690, 691t–694t, 694–695
  surgical interventions for, 697–698
  tobacco use and, 690, 694
Coronary care unit, discharge from, after acute myocardial infarction, 317–321
Coronary heart disease (CHD)
  absolute risk for, 222, 222t
  risk factors for, 221–235
    assessment of, 221–225
    pharmacologic therapy and, 234–235
    unmodifiable, 233–234
    for which interventions are likely to lower risk, 230–233
    for which interventions are proven to lower risk, 226–230
Coronary syndromes, evolution of, electrocardiogram and, 27–28
Cor pulmonale, 374, 379
  chronic, 403–412
    clinical manifestations of, 408–410
    etiologies of, 403–406, 404t
    pathophysiology of, 406–408, 407t
    treatment of, 410–412
    workup for, 410
  obesity and, 737
Corvert. See Ibutilide (Corvert)
Cost, of antihypertensive therapy, 370–371

Cough syncope, 156
Coumadin. See Warfarin (Coumadin)
CPR. See Cardiopulmonary resuscitation (CPR)
Creatine kinase
  in acute myocardial infarction, 284–285, 286t, 292–293
  in unstable angina, 263
CREST syndrome, pulmonary hypertension and, 379–380
CT (computed tomography), in pulmonary embolism, 390
Cyanotic heart disease, 521, 522t
  during pregnancy, 683
Cyclophosphamide, cardiac effects of, 573, 575
Cystic fibrosis, pulmonary hypertension and, 378
Cystic medial necrosis, of aorta, 702

D
Daunorubicin (Cerubidine), cardiac effects of, 575
DCM. See Dilated cardiomyopathy (DCM)
DDD pacing, 144f, 144–145
DDI pacing, 145
Deep vein thrombosis (DVT), 727t, 727–728
  diagnosis of, 387–392
    history and physical examination in, 388
    imaging studies in, 389–392
    laboratory testing in, 388–389
  pathogenesis of, 385–386
  risk factors for, 385, 386t
Defecation syncope, 156

Defibrillation. *See also* Automatic external defibrillators; Implantable cardioverter-defibrillator (ICD)
   public-access, 212
   for ventricular fibrillation, 87, 213–214
   for ventricular tachycardia, 213–214
Defibrillation threshold (DFT), 129, 129*f*, 130*t*
Dental care, antithrombotic therapy and, 488–489
Depression, 233
Dexamethasone sodium phosphate, following cardiac arrest, 219
Dexfenfluramine, cardiac effects of, 578
Dexrazoxane, cardiac effects of, 576
DFT (defibrillation threshold), 129, 129*f*, 130*t*
Diabetes mellitus, 627–645
   acute coronary syndromes and, 638–639
   cardiomyopathy and, 572
   chronic coronary artery disease in, 639
   clinical presentation of, 628–631, 629*t*
   congestive heart failure and, 644
   coronary artery disease and, in women, 695
   coronary revascularization and, 639, 644
   early detection of, 634, 636, 637*t*
   glycemic control in, 634
   HOPE study, 638
   hypertension and nephropathy in, 636, 638
   hypertension in, treatment of, 363–364
   lipid abnormalities in, 631–634
   mechanisms of cardiovascular risk and, 631–633
   risk factors for cardiovascular disease in, 627, 628*t*
   risk reduction guidelines for, 640*t*–643*t*
   type 2, coronary heart disease risk and, 223
Diastolic rumble, in mitral stenosis, 434
Diastolic thrill, in mitral stenosis, 433
Diazepam, for acute myocardial infarction, 294
Dicrotic pulse, 5*f*, 6
Diet
   atherogenic, 226
   interaction with drugs, 661
   for weight reduction, 746–747
DiGeorge anomaly, 512
Digitalis, interactions and complications of, 715
Digitalis glycosides. *See also specific drugs*
   for heart failure, 57
Digitoxin, during pregnancy, 672
Digoxin
   actions of, 94*t*
   for acute myocardial infarction, 313
   for atrial fibrillation, 73
   dosage and kinetics of, 67*t*, 68
   interactions and complications of, 657–658, 659*t*
   during pregnancy, 672

for supraventricular
tachycardia, 65t
Dihydropyridine, for
hypertension, 361
Dilated cardiomyopathy
(DCM), 527–538
anthracycline, 537
Chagas', 538
compensatory mechanisms
and, 529–532, 530f,
531f
in familial arrhythmogenic
right ventricular
dysplasia, 497–498
HIV infection and, 565–566
hypertensive, 535
idiopathic, 496–497,
536–537
ischemic, 532, 534
in mucopolysaccharidoses,
498–499
myocarditis due to, 561t
neurocardiogenic, 142
postpartum, 537
during pregnancy, 685–686
premature ventricular
contractions following,
81
scope of, 532, 533t–534t
sudden cardiac death and,
176–177
valvular, 535
in X-linked cardioskeletal
myopathy, 497
Diltiazem
actions of, 94t
for atrial fibrillation, 73–74
dosage and kinetics of, 67t,
68
interactions and
complications of, 656t,
659t
for pulmonary hypertension,
381
for supraventricular
tachycardia, 65t

D-Dimer, pulmonary embolism
and, 389
Directional atherectomy, 334t
Disk valves, 475–476
Disopyramide (Norpace)
actions of, 94t
for atrial fibrillation, 74
dosage of, 66t, 98t, 103
for hypertrophic
cardiomyopathy, 546,
546t
interactions and
complications of,
654t–655t
kinetics of, 66t
pharmacokinetics of, 96t
plasma concentration range
for, 98t, 103
for premature ventricular
contractions, 81
Diuretics
for acute myocardial
infarction, 313
for heart failure, 56–57
interactions and
complications of, 658,
659t, 660
during pregnancy, 672
sudden cardiac death and,
185
DM (myotonic dystrophy),
dilated cardiomyopathy
in, 500–501
DMD (Duchenne muscular
dystrophy), dilated
cardiomyopathy in,
499–500
Dobutamine
for acute myocardial
infarction, 313–314
interactions and
complications of, 658
Dofetilide (Tikosyn)
dosage of, 99t, 109–110
interactions and
complications of, 656t

Dofetilide (Tikosyn) (*Cont.*):
  pharmacokinetics of, 96*t*
  plasma concentration range
    for, 99*t*, 109–110
  for sudden cardiac death
    prevention, 198*t*, 200
Dopamine
  for acute myocardial
    infarction, 314
  during cardiopulmonary
    resuscitation, 217–218
  interactions and
    complications of, 658
  for pulmonary embolism,
    398
Doppler ultrasonography
  in aortic regurgitation, 423
  in aortic stenosis, 417
  for deep vein thrombosis
    detection, 391
  in mitral regurgitation,
    445
  in mitral stenosis, 436
  in peripheral arterial disease,
    721
  with prosthetic valves,
    479–480
Down's syndrome, 511
Doxorubicin (Adriamycin),
    cardiac effects of,
    575–576
Drug interactions. *See*
    Cardiovascular drugs,
    interactions and
    complications of
Duchenne muscular dystrophy
    (DMD), dilated
    cardiomyopathy in,
    499–500
DVT. *See* Deep vein
    thrombosis (DVT)
Dynamic auscultation, in mitral
    valve prolapse, 454
Dyslipidemia, 226–229
  after acute myocardial
    infarction, 322

low-density lipoprotein
    lowering and, 226–228,
    227*t*
  obesity and, 741–742
Dyspnea
  with aortic stenosis, 415
  in hypertrophic
    cardiomyopathy, 542

E
EA (electrical axis), 23–24
Ebstein's anomaly, 521
  during pregnancy, 684–685
  sudden cardiac death and,
    181
ECG. *See* Electrocardiogram
    (ECG)
Echocardiography
  in acute myocardial
    infarction, 285, 287,
    293
  in aortic regurgitation, 423
  in aortic stenosis, 417
  in hypertrophic
    cardiomyopathy, 543
  in infective endocarditis,
    600*f*, 600–601
  in mitral regurgitation, 445
  in mitral stenosis, 436
  in mitral valve prolapse,
    455–456, 457*t*
  obesity and, 739
  with prosthetic valves,
    479–480
  in pulmonary embolism,
    390–391
  in pulmonary hypertension,
    375
  in pulmonic valve disease,
    468–469
  rest, in angina pectoris, 242
  stress, in angina pectoris, 243
  in tricuspid valve disease,
    468–469
  in unstable angina, 263

ECT (electroconvulsive therapy), cardiac effects of, 580

EDMD (Emery-Dreyfuss muscular dystrophy), dilated cardiomyopathy in, 500

Ejection sound, 13

Elderly people
hypertension in, treatment of, 368
syncope in, 160

Electrical axis (EA), 23–24

Electrical injuries, cardiac effects of, 579–580

Electrocardiogram (ECG), 21–38
abnormal Q waves on, 26
abnormal segment changes on, 25
acute coronary syndrome evolution and, 27–28
in acute myocardial infarction, 27, 28*f*, 29*f*, 282–283, 292
ambulatory, 62
in angina pectoris, 241
in aortic regurgitation, 423
in aortic stenosis, 416–417
in cor pulmonale, 409–410
electrical axis and, 23–24
heart rhythm and, 61–62
in hypertrophic cardiomyopathy, 542–543
in infective endocarditis, 599
intraventricular conduction defects and, 29, 31–34
ischemic T-wave changes on, 26
leads for, 22–23
left ventricular hypertrophy and, 34
in mitral regurgitation, 444

in mitral stenosis, 435
in mitral valve prolapse, 454–455
nonspecific ST-T-wave changes on, 27
pericarditis and, 29
in pulmonary embolism, 389
in pulmonary hypertension, 375
in pulmonic valve disease, 468
Q-wave myocardial infarction location and, 28, 30*t*
right ventricular hypertrophy and enlargement and, 34–36
secondary S-T-T-wave changes on, 26
spatial vectorcardiography and, 36–38
ST-segment elevation in right precordial leads on, 25–26
surface, obesity, 737–738, 738*t*
in tricuspid valve disease, 468
in unstable angina, 262
ventricular depolarization and repolarization and, 21–22, 23
ventricular gradient and, 24–25

Electroconvulsive therapy (ECT), cardiac effects of, 580

Electrolyte abnormalities, sudden cardiac death and, 185–186

Electromagnetic interference (EMI), with pacemaker function, 147

Electromechanical dissociation (EMD), 216

Electrophysiologic studies (EPSs)
  intracardiac, 62
  ventricular arrhythmias and, 193
Electrovectorcardiography, spatial vectorcardiography versus, 37–38
Embolism. *See also* Thromboembolic disease
  of brain. *See* Brain embolism
  peripheral arterial disease due to, 725
Embolization, from aorta, 704
EMD (electromechanical dissociation), 216
Emery-Dreyfuss muscular dystrophy (EDMD), dilated cardiomyopathy in, 500
EMF (endomyocardial fibrosis), 555, 556t
EMI (electromagnetic interference), with pacemaker function, 147
Enalapril, for heart failure, 54t
Encainide
  actions of, 94t
  dosage and kinetics of, 66t
  for sudden cardiac death prevention, 196t
Encephalopathy
  cardiac, 716
  following cardiac surgery, 717
Endocarditis. *See* Infective endocarditis
Endocrine disorders, cardiomyopathy due to, 571–572
Endomyocardial biopsy, diseases diagnosed by, 564t

Endomyocardial fibrosis (EMF), 555, 556t
Endotracheal intubation, during cardiopulmonary resuscitation, 213
Enoxaparin, for venous thromboembolism treatment, 395t
Eosinophilic heart disease, cardiomyopathy and, 562t, 570–571
Epinephrine
  for asystole, 215
  during cardiopulmonary resuscitation, 211, 216, 217
  with defibrillation, 214
  for ventricular arrhythmias, 305
Epoprostenol (Flolan; PGI$_2$; prostacyclin), for pulmonary hypertension, 381
EPSs (electrophysiologic studies)
  intracardiac, 62
  ventricular arrhythmias and, 193
Ergotamine, cardiac effects of, 577
Ergot compounds, peripheral arterial disease due to, 724
ERT (estrogen replacement therapy), 232
Erythrocytosis, in cyanotic heart disease, 522t
Erythromycin
  interactions and complications of, 659t
  for mitral stenosis, 438t
Esmolol
  for aortic dissection, 706t
  dosage and kinetics of, 66t, 68

for supraventricular tachycardia, 65*t*

Esophageal disorders, acute myocardial infarction and, 292

Estrogen replacement therapy (ERT), 232
coronary artery disease and, 693*t*

Exercise. *See also* Physical activity
in congenital heart disease, 523
gender differences in, 692*t*
for weight reduction, 747

Exercise cardiovascular function, aging and, 41, 43, 43*t*

Exercise stress testing, 62
in angina pectoris, 241–242
before noncardiac surgery, 622
in peripheral arterial disease, 722

Expressivity, 493

Extremity leads, for electrocardiogram, 22

F

Fabry's disease, restrictive cardiomyopathy in, 554

Factor V Leiden mutation, deep vein thrombosis and, 385–386

Familial arrhythmogenic right ventricular dysplasia, dilated cardiomyopathy in, 497–498

Familial hypertrophic cardiomyopathy, 494–496, 495*t*

Family history, as risk factor for atherosclerosis, 234

Fascicular block, electrocardiogram in, 31

Fat embolism, 399–400

Fenfluramine, cardiac effects of, 578

Fenofibrate, interactions and complications of, 664*t*

Fetus. *See also* Pregnancy
vulnerability of, 668

Feverfew, interactions and complications of, 666

Fibrates, interactions and complications of, 664*t*

Fibromuscular dysplasia, peripheral arterial disease due to, 724–725

Flecainide (Tambocor)
actions of, 94*t*
dosage of, 66*t*, 98*t*, 105–106
interactions and complications of, 655*t*
kinetics of, 66*t*
pharmacokinetics of, 96*t*
plasma concentration range for, 98*t*, 105–106
for sudden cardiac death prevention, 196*t*

Flolan (epoprostenol; PGI$_2$; prostacyclin), for pulmonary hypertension, 381

5-Fluorouracil, cardiac effects of, 575

Fluvastatin, interactions and complications of, 664*t*

Fosinopril, for heart failure, 54*t*

Friction rub, pericardial, 19

Fusion beat, 83

G

Garlic, interactions and complications of, 666

Gas exchange, abnormalities of, pulmonary embolism and, 387

Gastrointestinal system, arteriovenous malformations of, with aortic stenosis, 415

Gated blood pool radionuclide scans, in aortic regurgitation, 424

Gaucher's disease, restrictive cardiomyopathy in, 554

Gemfibrozil, interactions and complications of, 664t

Gender. See also Coronary artery disease (CAD), in women; Pregnancy as risk factor for atherosclerosis, 233
    risk of coronary artery disease related to, 689, 691t–694t
    sudden cardiac death and, 166

Genetic abnormalities, 493–512. See also Congenital heart disease
    cardiovascular disease due to single-gene mutations, 494–512. See also specific disorders
    genotype and phenotype and, 493

Genome, 493

Genotype, 493

Gentamicin
    for infective endocarditis, 604t, 606t–609t
    for infective endocarditis prophylaxis, 613t

Gestational hypertension, 676

Giant-cell arteritis, 725

Giant-cell myocarditis, 563t, 567–568

Ginger, interactions and complications of, 666

Ginkgo, interactions and complications of, 666

Ginseng, interactions and complications of, 666

Glycemic control, in diabetes mellitus, 634, 635f

Glycolipid accumulation, restrictive cardiomyopathy and, 554

P-Glycoprotein, 648

Gossypol, interactions and complications of, 666

Granulomas, cardiomyopathy and, 553–554, 569–570

H
HACEK infections, endocarditis due to, 596t, 597

Halogenated hydrocarbons, cardiac effects of, 581

Hammer hand syndrome, 725

Hawthorn, interactions and complications of, 666

HCM. See Hypertrophic cardiomyopathy (HCM)

Heart block, after acute myocardial infarction, 316–317

Heart failure, 49–58
    after acute myocardial infarction, 314–315
    in acute myocardial infarction, 311, 312t
    cardiomyopathy and. See Cardiomyopathy; Dilated cardiomyopathy (DCM); Hypertrophic cardiomyopathy (HCM)
    congestive. See Congestive heart failure (CHF)
    diagnosis of, 50–51

hypertension in, treatment of, 364–365

pathophysiology of, 49–50

with symptoms, treatment of, 56–57

without symptoms, treatment of, 51

treatment of, 51–58

Heart-lung transplantation, for cor pulmonale, 411–412

Heart murmurs. *See* Murmurs

Heart rate, variability of, sudden cardiac death and, 192

Heart rhythm
analysis of, 61–63
disturbances of. *See* Arrhythmias; *specific arrhythmias*

Heart sounds, 10–13, 11*f*
in mitral stenosis, 433–434

Heart transplantation, pregnancy following, 686

Heart valves. *See* Prosthetic heart valves; Valvular heart disease

Heimlich maneuver, 212

Hemochromatosis
cardiomyopathy and, 570
restrictive cardiomyopathy in, 554
sudden cardiac death and, 180

Hemodynamic management, for pulmonary embolism, 398–399

Hemodynamics
in hypertrophic cardiomyopathy, 544
during pregnancy, 669–670
pulmonary embolism and, 387
pulmonary hypertension and, 374

Heparin. *See also* Low molecular weight heparin (LMWH)
for acute myocardial infarction, 301–302
with atrial fibrillation, 75
for brain embolism prevention, 713–714
for mitral stenosis, 438
during pregnancy, 488
with prosthetic valves, 481
for unstable angina pectoris, 272–273
for valve thrombosis, 490
for venous thromboembolism treatment, 393–394, 394*t*

Herbal therapies
cardiac effects of, 580
interactions and complications of, 666

Herceptin, cardiac effects of, 575, 576

Heterograft valves, 476–477

Heteroplasmy, 503

Hirudin, for venous thromboembolism treatment, 396

History taking, 1, 2*t*, 3, 4*t*

HIV, dilated cardiomyopathy due to, 565–566

HMG-CoA (hydroxymethylglutaryl-coenzyme A) reductase inhibitors, for hypertriglyceridemia of diabetes, 633

Holosystolic murmurs, 15, 16*f*

Holter monitoring, 62
in hypertrophic cardiomyopathy, 543

Holt-Oram syndrome, 509–510

Homocysteine, 233
deep vein thrombosis and, 385–386

Homocystinuria, cardiomyopathy due to, 502

Homograft valves, 476

Hormone replacement therapy (HRT), 232
coronary artery disease and, 693t

Human immunodeficiency virus (HIV), dilated cardiomyopathy due to, 565–566

Hunter syndrome, dilated cardiomyopathy in, 498

Hurler-Scheie syndrome, dilated cardiomyopathy in, 498

Hurler syndrome, dilated cardiomyopathy in, 498

Hydrocarbons, halogenated, cardiac effects of, 581

Hydroxymethylglutaryl-coenzyme A (HMG-CoA) reductase inhibitors, for hypertriglyceridemia of diabetes, 633

Hypercalcemia, sudden cardiac death and, 186

Hypercoagulable conditions, antithrombotic therapy in, 486

Hypereosinophilic syndrome, 555, 556t

Hyperinsulinemia, obesity and, 740–741

Hyperkalemia, treatment of, 214

Hyperkinetic pulse, 5f, 5–6

Hypersensitivity myocarditis, 562t, 567

Hypertension, 229–230, 351–371. See also Antihypertensive therapy; Pulmonary hypertension
cardiomyopathy and, 535, 571
sudden cardiac death and, 178
coronary artery disease and, in women, 695
definition of, 351, 352t
in diabetes mellitus, nephropathy and, 636, 638
diagnosis of, 352–354
in elderly people, 46
evaluation of, 354–359
cardiac evaluation in, 355–356
renal evaluation in, 356
routine, 355
for secondary of hypertension, 356, 357t, 358–359
of vasculature, 356
obesity and, 742
during pregnancy, 676–677
renovascular, evaluation for, 356, 358
treatment of, 359–371
lifestyle modifications in, 360
pharmacologic. See Antihypertensive therapy
"white-coat," 354

Hypertensive urgencies and emergencies, 368–369

Hypertriglyceridemia, of diabetes, 632–633

Hypertrophic cardiomyopathy (HCM), 541–547
clinical manifestations of, 542
definition of, 541
diagnostic tests for, 542–544
differential diagnosis of, 545
etiology of, 541
familial, 494–496, 495t
murmurs in, 15

natural history of, 544–545
neurocardiogenic, 142
obstructive, during
    pregnancy, 684
pathology of, 541–542
during pregnancy, 685
premature ventricular
    contractions following,
    81
sudden cardiac death and,
    177–178
treatment of, 545–547, 546t
Hyperventilation, 156
with defibrillation, 214
Hypokalemia, sudden cardiac
    death and, 185
Hypokinetic pulse, 5f
Hypomagnesemia, sudden
    cardiac death and,
    185–186
Hypotension
    after acute myocardial
        infarction, 314–315
    orthostatic, 153, 154t, 155t
Hypoventilation
    alveolar, pulmonary
        hypertension and, 380
    cor pulmonale due to, 405
    obesity and, 743
Hypoxemia, pulmonary
    embolism and, 389

I
IABP (intra-aortic balloon
        pumping)
    for acute myocardial
        infarction, 345–347
    for congestive heart failure,
        in acute myocardial
        infarction, 312–313
    for unstable angina pectoris,
        273
Ibutilide (Corvert)
    actions of, 94t
    dosage of, 67t, 99t, 109

interactions and
    complications of, 656t
kinetics of, 67t
pharmacokinetics of, 96t
plasma concentration range
    for, 99t, 109
ICD. See Implantable
    cardioverter-
    defibrillator
    (ICD)
Idiopathic cardiomyopathy,
    496–497, 536–537,
    573–574
Iloprost, for pulmonary
    hypertension, 381
Impedance plethysmography
    (IPG), for deep vein
    thrombosis detection,
    391–392
Implantable cardioverter-
    defibrillator (ICD),
    113–132
    in asymptomatic high-risk
        patients, 124
    in cardiac arrest survivors,
        122
    complications of, 130, 131t,
        132, 133t
    dual-chamber devices, 128
    evidence base for therapy
        using, 113–119
    future directions for, 132
    implantation of, 128–129
    long-term follow-up of, 130
    in severe left ventricular
        dysfunction, 123
    for sudden cardiac death
        prevention, 197t,
        201–202, 202f
    primary, 116t–117t,
        118–119, 119f
    secondary, 114t, 115, 115f,
        118
    in sustained monomorphic
        ventricular tachycardia,
        122–123

Implantable (*Cont.*):
  in syncope of undetermined
    origin, 123
  tachyarrhythmia detection
    by, 124, 125*f*, 126, 127*t*
  testing, 129, 129*f*, 130*t*
  for ventricular fibrillation,
    126
  for ventricular tachycardia,
    85, 128
Infections. *See also* Infective
    endocarditis
  myocarditis due to, 559,
    560*t*–561*t*, 564–567
  with pacemakers, 146
Infectious aortitis, 702
Infective endocarditis, 593–615
  antibiotic prophylaxis of. *See*
    Antibiotics,
    prophylactic
  clinical features of, 597,
    598*t*, 599
  complications of, 602, 605,
    611*t*, 612, 612*t*
  in congenital heart disease,
    523
  diagnostic criteria for, 601,
    602*t*, 603*t*
  echocardiography in, 600*f*,
    600–601
  epidemiology of, 593–594
  etiology of, 595, 596*t*, 597
  laboratory findings in, 599
  native valve, microbiologic
    cure rates for, 611*t*
  pathogenesis of, 594*f*,
    594–595
  during pregnancy, 678–679
  prevention of, 612,
    613*t*–614*t*, 615
  prosthetic valve,
    microbiologic cure rates
    for, 611*t*
  treatment of, 601–602, 604*t*,
    606*t*–610*t*
  tricuspid valve disease in, 465

Inferior vena cava (IVC) filters,
    for pulmonary
    embolism, 396
Inotropic agents
  interactions and
    complications of,
    657–658
  during pregnancy, 672
Insulin resistance syndrome,
    230–231
Interferon alpha, cardiac effects
    of, 575
Interleukin-2, cardiac effects
    of, 575
Interstitial lung disease
  diffuse, cor pulmonale due
    to, 405
  fibrotic, pulmonary
    hypertension and, 378
Intra-aortic balloon pumping
    (IABP)
  for acute myocardial
    infarction, 345–347
  for congestive heart failure,
    in acute myocardial
    infarction, 312–313
  for unstable angina pectoris,
    273
Intravenous route,
    establishment of, during
    cardiopulmonary
    resuscitation, 216–217
Intraventricular conduction
    defects
  electrocardiogram in, 29,
    31–34
  sudden cardiac death and,
    189
IPG (impedance
    plethysmography), for
    deep vein thrombosis
    detection, 391–392
Iron deficiency, in cyanotic
    heart disease, 522*t*
Iron deposition
  cardiomyopathy and, 570

restrictive cardiomyopathy and, 554

Ischemia
assessment of, 319
in elderly people, 44, 45*t*
electrocardiogram in, 26
electrophysiologic effects of, 171–172
recurrent, after acute myocardial infarction, 310
in women, 696–697

Ischemic dilated cardiomyopathy, 532, 534

Isosorbide dinitrate (ISDN), for angina pectoris, 250

Isosorbide mononitrate (ISMO), for angina pectoris, 250

IVC (inferior vena cava) filters, for pulmonary embolism, 396

J

Jervell and Lange-Nielsen long-QT-syndrome, 506*t*, 508

Jugular venous pressure, in mitral stenosis, 433

Jugular venous pulse, 6–8, 7*f*

K

Kelp, interactions and complications of, 666

Kussmaul's sign, 8

L

Labetalol, for aortic dissection, 706*t*

Laser angioplasty, 334*t*, 335

LBBB (left bundle branch block), complete, electrocardiogram in, 32

Leads
for electrocardiogram, 22–23
of pacemakers, breakage of, 146

Left bundle branch block (LBBB), complete, electrocardiogram in, 32

Left-to-right shunts, during pregnancy, 682–683

Left ventricular angiography
in aortic regurgitation, 424
in mitral regurgitation, 445–446

Left ventricular dysfunction
antithrombotic therapy in, 485
cor pulmonale and, 408
implantable cardioverter-defibrillator therapy for, 118–119, 123
mitral valve prolapse and, 458
sudden cardiac death and, 189, 190*t*–191*t*

Left ventricular ejection fraction, assessment of, 319

Left ventricular failure, pulmonary hypertension and, 376

Left ventricular function
assessment of, 319
in hypertrophic cardiomyopathy, 544
preoperative testing of, 621

Left ventricular hypertrophy (LVH)
electrocardiogram in, 34
hypertension in, treatment of, 364
obesity and, 738, 738*t*, 743

Left ventricular outflow tract obstruction, 518–519

Lev-Lengre syndrome, 507t
Licorice, interactions and
    complications of, 666
Lidocaine (Xylocaine), 97,
        100–101
    actions of, 94t
    dosage of, 66t, 98t
    interactions and
        complications of, 655t,
        715
    kinetics of, 66t
    pharmacokinetics of, 96t
    plasma concentration range
        for, 98t
    for ventricular arrhythmia
        prevention, 305
    for ventricular arrhythmia
        treatment, 305
    for ventricular tachycardia,
        84, 84t
Lifestyle modification
    after acute myocardial
        infarction, 323–324
    for hypertension, 360
Lightning injuries, cardiac
        effects of, 579–580
Lipid(s), gender differences in,
        691t
Lipid disorders, in diabetes
        mellitus, 631–634
Lipid-lowering agents
    for angina pectoris, 249–250
    interactions and
        complications of, 664t,
        665
Lipoprotein(a), 229
Lisinopril, for heart failure, 54t
Lithium
    cardiac effects of, 577
    interactions and
        complications of, 715
Livedo reticularis, 725
LMWH. See Low molecular
        weight heparin
        (LMWH)
Loeffler's syndrome, 555, 556t

Long-QT syndrome (LQTS)
    sudden cardiac death and,
        181
    torsades de pointes due to,
        86–87
Loop diuretics
    for heart failure, 56–57
    interactions and
        complications of, 658
Losartan, for heart failure,
        52t
Loss of consciousness, during
        pregnancy, 678
Lovastatin, interactions and
        complications of, 664t,
        665
Low cardiac output syndrome,
        during pregnancy, 675,
        675t
Low molecular weight heparin
        (LMWH)
    for acute myocardial
        infarction, 301–302
    for deep vein thrombosis
        prophylaxis, 392–393
    for non-Q-wave myocardial
        infarction, 306–307
    during pregnancy, 488
    for unstable angina pectoris,
        273
    for venous thromboembolism
        treatment, 393–394,
        395t
LQTS (long-QT syndrome)
    sudden cardiac death and,
        181
    torsades de pointes due to,
        86–87
Lungs
    biopsy of, in pulmonary
        hypertension, 375–376
    examination of, in acute
        myocardial infarction,
        281
Lung scans, in pulmonary
        hypertension, 375

Lung transplantation
   for cor pulmonale, 411–412
   for pulmonary hypertension, 382
LVH (left ventricular hypertrophy)
   electrocardiogram in, 34
   hypertension in, treatment of, 364
   obesity and, 738, 738t, 743
Lyme carditis, 566
Lymphangiography, 729
Lymphedema, 728–729
Lymphoscintigraphy, 729

M

Magnesium deficiency, sudden cardiac death and, 185–186
Magnetic resonance angiography (MRA), in peripheral arterial disease, 722
Magnetic resonance imaging (MRI)
   for deep vein thrombosis detection, 392
   in pulmonary embolism, 391
Magnet mode, with pacemakers, 143
MAOIs (monoamine oxidase inhibitors), cardiac effects of, 576–577
Marfan syndrome, 503–505, 521–522, 524
   during pregnancy, 685
Marine toxins, cardiac effects of, 581
Maroteaux-Lamy syndrome, dilated cardiomyopathy in, 498–499
MB-CK, in acute myocardial infarction, 284–285, 286t, 292–293

Mechanical valves, antithrombotic therapy for, 486
Mechanoelectrical feedback, sudden cardiac death and, 172
Medial degeneration, of aorta, 701–702
Memory, cardiac, 24–25
Menopause, 232–233
   coronary artery disease and, 692t
Metabolism, defects of, causing cardiomyopathy, 501–502
Methylprednisolone, following cardiac arrest, 219
Methylxanthines, cardiac effects of, 577
Methysergide, cardiac effects of, 577
Metoprolol, for heart failure, 55t, 56
Mexiletine (Mexitil)
   actions of, 94t
   dosage of, 66t, 98t, 101
   kinetics of, 66t
   pharmacokinetics of, 96t
   plasma concentration range for, 98t, 101
   for premature ventricular contractions, 81–82
   for sudden cardiac death prevention, 196t
MI. *See* Acute myocardial infarction (AMI); Myocardial infarction (MI)
Microalbuminuria, hypertension in, treatment of, 366
Microembolism, peripheral arterial disease due to, 725
Micturition syncope, 156
Midsystolic clicks, 13

Midsystolic murmurs, 15, 16f
Mitochondrial cardiomyopathy, 502–503
Mitral annulus calcification, brain embolism and, 710–711, 712t
Mitral regurgitation (MR), 439–449
  clinical manifestations of, 443–444
  definition of, 439
  etiology and pathology of, 440–441
  laboratory tests in, 445–446
  murmurs in, 15–16
  natural history and prognosis of, 446
  pathophysiology of, 441, 443
  during pregnancy, 680
  treatment of, 447–449
    medical, 447
    surgical, 447, 448t, 449
Mitral stenosis (MS), 431–439
  clinical manifestations of, 432–436
  definition of, 431
  etiology and pathology of, 431–432
  laboratory tests in, 436–437
  natural history and prognosis of, 437
  during pregnancy, 679–680
  treatment of
    interventional, 439, 440t–442t
    medical, 437–438, 438t
Mitral valve disease
  hypertension and, treatment of, 365
  pulmonary hypertension and, 376
Mitral valve prolapse (MVP), 451–460
  brain embolism and, 710
  clinical manifestations of, 453–454, 455t

complications of, 458, 459t
diagnostic studies in, 454–458
natural history and prognosis of, 458
pathophysiology of, 453
primary, 451–452, 452t
secondary, 452, 452t
sudden cardiac death and, 179
treatment of, 459–460
Mitral valve repair
  for mitral regurgitation, 447, 448t, 449
  for mitral valve prolapse, 460
Mitral valve replacement, for mitral stenosis, 439, 441t
Mobitz type II block, 89
Monoamine oxidase inhibitors (MAOIs), cardiac effects of, 576–577
Moricizine
  actions of, 94t
  dosage and kinetics of, 66t
  interactions and complications of, 655t
Morphine sulfate, for acute myocardial infarction, 294
Morquio syndrome, dilated cardiomyopathy in, 498
Morrow procedure, for hypertrophic cardiomyopathy, 546t, 546–547
MPSs (mucopolysaccharidoses), dilated cardiomyopathy in, 498–499
MR. See Mitral regurgitation (MR)
MRA (magnetic resonance angiography), in peripheral arterial disease, 722

MRI (magnetic resonance imaging)
for deep vein thrombosis detection, 392
in pulmonary embolism, 391
MS. *See* Mitral stenosis (MS)
Mucopolysaccharidoses (MPSs), dilated cardiomyopathy in, 498–499
Murmurs, 13–14, 14*f*
in aortic regurgitation, 422
continuous, 18–19
diastolic, 17*f*, 17–18
in mitral stenosis, 434
systolic, 15–17, 16*f*
Muscular dystrophy
Duchenne, dilated cardiomyopathy in, 499–500
Emery-Dreyfuss, dilated cardiomyopathy in, 500
MVP. *See* Mitral valve prolapse (MVP)
Myocardial failure
progression of, compensatory mechanisms and, 529–532, 530*f*, 531*f*
pulmonary hypertension and, 376
Myocardial infarction (MI). *See also* Acute myocardial infarction (AMI)
ischemic cardiomyopathy and, 532, 534
location of, Q waves and, 28, 30*t*
pacing after, 139*t*
premature ventricular contractions following, 80–81
subacute phase of, sudden cardiac death during, 172
tricuspid valve disease following, 465

Myocardial perfusion imaging, in angina pectoris, 242
Myocarditis, 559–567
causes of, 560*t*–563*t*
giant cell, 563*t*, 567–568
infectious, 559, 560*t*–561*t*, 564–567
peripartum, 563*t*, 568
sudden cardiac death and, 180
Myocytolysis, brain lesions and, 717–718
Myoglobin
in acute myocardial infarction, 284–285, 286*t*
in unstable angina, 263
Myotonic dystrophy (DM), dilated cardiomyopathy in, 500–501

N
Nafcillin, for infective endocarditis, 604*t*, 608*t*, 609*t*
Native valve infective endocarditis, microbiologic cure rates for, 611*t*
Nephropathy
in diabetes mellitus, hypertension and, 636, 638
diabetes mellitus and, 630, 631*t*
Neurocardiogenic syncope, 151–153
Newborns, vulnerability of, 668
New York Heart Association functional classification, 3, 4*t*
Nifedipine
interactions and complications of, 659*t*
for pulmonary hypertension, 381

Nitrates. *See also specific drugs*
for angina pectoris, 250–251
interactions and
complications of, 650,
651*t*
tolerance of, 250–251
Nitric oxide, for pulmonary
hypertension, 381
Nitroglycerin
for acute myocardial
infarction, 294–295,
313
for angina pectoris
stable, 250–251
unstable, 268–269
Nitroprusside, for aortic
dissection, 706*t*
Noncardiac drugs. *See also
specific drugs and drug
types*
cardiac effects of, 575–579
Noncardiac surgery, 617–624
clinical assessment of
perioperative risk and,
621
clinical determinants of
perioperative
cardiovascular risk and,
617–618, 619*t*, 620–621
comorbid diseases and,
618, 620
history and, 618
physical examination and,
618
surgery-specific risks and,
620*t*, 620–621
during pregnancy, 679
preoperative testing for,
621–623
preoperative therapy for
coronary artery disease
and, 623–624
Nonejection clicks, 13
Nonexercise stress testing,
before noncardiac
surgery, 622–623

Non-Q-wave myocardial
infarction, patient
approach for, 305–308
Norepinephrine
during cardiopulmonary
resuscitation, 217
for pulmonary embolism,
398
Norpace. *See* Disopyramide
(Norpace)
Nuclear medicine. *See also*
Radionuclide *entries*
in obesity, 739–740

O
Obesity, 232, 733–748, 734*t*,
735*t*
arrhythmias and, 744–745
blood glucose and
hyperinsulinemia and,
740–741
cardiac catheterization in,
740
cardiac surgery and, 745
cardiomyopathy of, 745–746
cardiovascular system
adaptation in, 735–736
coronary artery disease and,
742
dyslipidemia and, 741–742
echocardiography in, 739
gender differences in,
691*t*–692*t*
hypertension and, 742
hypoventilation and, 743
left ventricular hypertrophy
and, 743
nuclear medicine in,
739–740
obstructive sleep apnea and,
743–744, 744*t*
physical examination in,
736–737, 737*t*
pulmonary hypertension and,
744

radiology in, 739
surface electrocardiogram in, 737–738, 738t
treatment of, 746–747
ventricular diastolic dysfunction and, 743
visceral, 740, 741t
Obliterative myocardial disease, 570–571
Obstructive cardiac lesions, during pregnancy, 683–684
Obstructive sleep apnea, obesity and, 743–744, 744t
Opening snap (OS), 12
in mitral stenosis, 434
Oral contraceptives, cardiac effects of, 578
Orthostatic syncope, 153, 154t, 155t
OS (opening snap), 12 in mitral stenosis, 434
Oxidative stress, 233
Oxygen therapy
for acute myocardial infarction, 293
for cor pulmonale, 411

P
Pacemakers, 135–150
AAI pacing with, 143
abnormal pacing rates and, 147, 148f
after acute myocardial infarction, 303–304, 317
for asystole, 215
for atrioventricular block, 136–137, 138t–139t
for carotid sinus syndrome, 137, 142, 146
complications of, 146–147
for congestive heart failure, 142

DDD pacing with, 144f, 144–145
DDI pacing with, 145
for dilated cardiomyopathy, 142
hardware for, 142–143
for hypersensitive carotid sinus, 141t
for hypertrophic cardiomyopathy, 142
indications for, 90–91
loss of capture and, 149
modes for, 143
after myocardial infarction, 139t
for neurocardiac syncope, 141t, 142
oversensing by, 149
in paroxysmal atrial fibrillation, flutter, and other tachyarrhythmias, 145
permanent, indications for, 136–137, 138t–141t, 142
for sinus node dysfunction, 137, 140t
for sudden cardiac death prevention, 203
temporary, 136
in third-degree atrioventricular block, 146
undersensing by, 149–150
for vasovagal syncope, 146
Pacemaker syndrome, 146–147
Paclitaxel, cardiac effects of, 575, 576
PACs (premature atrial contractions), 63–64
PAD. See Peripheral arterial disease (PAD)
Pain
in chest. See also Angina pectoris

Pain (*Cont.*):
  differential diagnosis of, 1,
    2*t*, 3
  in mitral valve prolapse,
    453
  quality of, 3
Pansystolic murmurs, 15,
    16*f*
Papillary muscle dysfunction,
    after acute myocardial
    infarction, 315
Paroxysmal supraventricular
    tachycardia (PSVT)
  after acute myocardial
    infarction, 316
  during pregnancy, 678
Patent ductus arteriosus, during
    pregnancy, 683
Patent foramen ovale (PFO),
    brain embolism with,
    714
PCIs. *See* Percutaneous
    coronary interventions
    (PCIs)
Peau d'orange, 729
Penetrance, 493
Penicillin G
  for infective endocarditis,
    606*t*, 607*t*, 610*t*
  for mitral stenosis, 438*t*
Penicillin V, for mitral stenosis,
    438*t*
Pentoxifylline, for
    arteriosclerosis
    obliterans, 724
Percutaneous coronary
    interventions (PCIs),
    327–337. *See also*
    Percutaneous
    transluminal coronary
    angioplasty (PTCA)
  for acute myocardial
    infarction, 300
  for angina pectoris, 252,
    253*t*, 254*t*, 255
  complications of, 336
  in elderly people, 44
  future directions for, 337
  indications for, 331–335
    lesion selection and,
      332–335
    patient selection and,
      331–332
  performance of, 335–336
  results with, 336
  stents for, 329–331
    coronary artery bypass
      grafting versus, in
      multivessel disease,
      330–331
Percutaneous transluminal
    coronary angioplasty
    (PTCA)
  for acute myocardial
    infarction, 301, 302,
    321
  coronary artery bypass
    grafting versus, 328,
    329*t*
  development of, 327
  before noncardiac surgery,
    623–624
  randomized trials of,
    327–328
  for unstable angina pectoris,
    274
  in women, 697
Perfusion imaging, in unstable
    angina, 263
Pericardial disease, restrictive
    cardiomyopathy and,
    557
Pericardial effusion, 586–587
Pericardial friction rub, 19
Pericardiectomy, for
    constrictive pericarditis,
    590
Pericarditis
  acute, 583–584, 586, 586*f*,
    587*t*
    acute myocardial
      infarction and, 292

after acute myocardial infarction, 292, 310–311
constrictive, 589–590
restrictive cardiomyopathy versus, 549–550, 551*t*
electrocardiogram in, 29
Pericardium
diseases of, 583, 585*t*. *See also specific diseases*
congenital, 591
functions of, 583, 584*t*
Perindopril, for heart failure, 54*t*
Peripartum cardiomyopathy, 685
Peripartum myocarditis, 563*t*, 568
Peripheral arterial disease (PAD), 721–726
causes of, 724–725
clinical manifestations of, 722
laboratory assessment of, 721–722, 723*t*
Raynaud's phenomenon and, 726, 726*t*
treatment of, 724
of upper extremities, 725
PFO (patent foramen ovale), brain embolism with, 714
PGI₂ (epoprostenol; Flolan; prostacyclin), for pulmonary hypertension, 381
P-glycoprotein, 648
Pharmacotherapy. *See also specific drugs and drug types*
for weight reduction, 747
Phenotype, 493
Phentermine, cardiac effects of, 578
Pheochromocytoma, evaluation for, 358

Phlebotomy, in cyanotic heart disease, 522*t*
Phlegmasia cerulea dolens, 728
Physical activity. *See also Exercise*
in acute myocardial infarction, 308
gender differences in, 692*t*
lack of, 231
after acute myocardial infarction, 322
sudden cardiac death and, 170
Physical examination, 3, 5
Plant(s), poisonous, 580
Plantain, interactions and complications of, 666
Platelet glycoprotein IIb/IIIa receptor inhibitors
as adjunct to coronary intervention, 331
with percutaneous coronary interventions, 335–336
for unstable angina pectoris, 271–272, 272*t*
Platelet inhibitors, for acute myocardial infarction, 345, 346*t*
Polysomnography, in cor pulmonale, 410
Pompe's disease, restrictive cardiomyopathy in, 555
Porcine heterograft valves, 476
Postpartum dilated cardiomyopathy, 537
Postphlebitic syndrome, 728
Postprandial syncope, 156
Potassium
deficiency of, sudden cardiac death and, 185
excess of, treatment of, 214
PPH (primary pulmonary hypertension), 380–382
definition of, 380–381
treatment of, 381–382

Pravastatin, interactions and complications of, 664t
Prazosin, interactions and complications of, 659t
Precordial leads, for electrocardiogram, 22–23
Precordial palpation, 8, 9f, 10
Precordium, in mitral stenosis, 433
Prednisone, for pericarditis, 586
Preeclampsia, 676
Preexcitation syndromes, wide QRS complexes in, 32–33
Pregnancy, 667–686
  antithrombotic therapy during, 487–488
  arrhythmias during, 677–678
  blood flow distribution during, 670
  cardiovascular drugs during, 672–674
  in congenital heart disease, 523, 682–685
  congestive heart failure during, 676
  diagnosis of heart disease during, 671–672
  endocarditis during, 678–679
  fetal and newborn vulnerability and, 668
  health priorities during, 667
  following heart transplantation, 686
  hemodynamic changes during, 669–670
  hypertension during, 676–677
  loss-of-consciousness spells during, 678
  low cardiac output syndrome during, 675, 675t
  maternal fragility during, 667, 668t

  myocardial disease during, 685–686
  normal, cardiovascular adjustments during, 669–670
  pulmonary hypertension during, 677
  rheumatic heart disease during, 679
  surgery during, 679
  thromboembolic complications in, 676
  uncorrected maternal heart disease and, 668–669
  valvular heart disease during, 679–681
Pregnancy-induced hypertension, 676
Premature atrial contractions (PACs), 63–64
Premature ventricular contractions (PVCs), 78–82
  in absence of significant structural disease, 79
  in acute settings, 79–80
  in chronic cardiac cases, 80–82
Preventive cardiology, barriers to implementing, 235
Primary pulmonary hypertension (PPH), 380–382
  definition of, 380–381
  treatment of, 381–382
Prinzmetal's angina, 259
Procainamide (Procan-SR; Pronestyl)
  actions of, 94t
  for atrial fibrillation, 74
  dosage of, 66t, 98t, 101–103
  interactions and complications of, 654t
  kinetics of, 66t
  pharmacokinetics of, 96t

plasma concentration range for, 98*t*, 101–103
for supraventricular tachycardia, 65*t*
for ventricular tachycardia, 84, 84*t*

Propafenone (Rhythmol)
actions of, 94*t*
dosage of, 66*t*, 99*t*, 105
interactions and complications of, 655*t*, 659*t*
kinetics of, 66*t*
pharmacokinetics of, 96*t*
plasma concentration range for, 99*t*, 105

Propranolol
actions of, 94*t*
dosage and kinetics of, 66*t*, 68
for supraventricular tachycardia, 65*t*

Prostacyclin (epoprostenol; Flolan; PGI$_2$), for pulmonary hypertension, 381

Prosthetic heart valves, 475–481
antithrombotic therapy for, 486–487, 487*t*
biological, 476–477
clinical reporting guidelines for, 477
disease of, during pregnancy, 681
infective endocarditis and, microbiologic cure rates for, 611*t*
management of, 477–481, 480*t*
antithrombotic therapy in, 480–481
mechanical, 475–476
selection criteria for, 477, 478*t*, 479*t*

Pseudoclaudication, 721

PSVT (paroxysmal supraventricular tachycardia) after acute myocardial infarction, 316
during pregnancy, 678

Psychosocial factors, coronary artery disease and, 694*t*

Psychotropic agents, cardiac effects of, 576–577

PTCA. *See* Percutaneous transluminal coronary angioplasty (PTCA)

Public-access defibrillation, 212

Pufferfish, cardiac effects of, 581

Pulmonary arteriography, in pulmonary embolism, 390

Pulmonary edema, cor pulmonale and, 408

Pulmonary embolectomy, for cor pulmonale, 411

Pulmonary embolism, 385–400
acute, 387
acute myocardial infarction and, 291
chronic, 399
cor pulmonale and. *See* Cor pulmonale
deep vein thrombosis and, 385–386, 386*t*
diagnosis of, 387–392
history and physical examination in, 388
imaging studies in, 389–392
laboratory testing in, 388–389
fat embolism, 399–400
management of, 392–399
anticoagulation therapy in, 393–394, 394*t*, 395*t*, 396
hemodynamic, 398–399

Pulmonary embolism (*Cont.*):
  prophylaxis of deep vein
    thrombosis and,
    392–393
  thrombolytic therapy in,
    397*t*, 397–398
  vena cava filters in, 396
  miscellaneous causes of,
    400
  pathophysiology of, 387
Pulmonary hypertension,
    373–382
  clinical manifestations of,
    374
  definition of, 373–374
  diagnostic studies in,
    375–376
  heart sounds in, 11–12
  hemodynamics and, 374
  mitral stenosis and, 432
  obesity and, 744
  during pregnancy, 677
  primary, 380–382
    definition of, 380–381
    treatment of, 381–382
  right ventricular response to,
    407
  secondary, 376–380
    with connective tissue
      diseases, 379–380
    with respiratory disorders,
      378–379
Pulmonary stenosis, isolated,
    518
Pulmonary valve disease
  clinical manifestations of,
    466–467, 468, 469
  definition of, 465
  etiology and pathology of,
    465, 466*t*
  natural history and prognosis
    of, 470
  during pregnancy, 681
  treatment of
    medical, 470–471
    surgical, 473

Pulmonary vascular disease,
    cor pulmonale due to,
    405–406
Pulse
  arterial pressure, 5*f*, 5–6
  hypokinetic, 5*f*
  jugular venous, 6–8, 7*f*
Pulsus alternans, 5*f*, 6
Pulsus paradoxus, 6
Pulsus parvus, 5, 5*f*
Pulsus tardus, 5, 5*f*
PVCs (premature ventricular
    contractions), 78–82
  in absence of significant
    structural disease, 79
  in acute settings, 79–80
  in chronic cardiac cases,
    80–82

Q
QRS complexes, wide
  in preexcitation syndromes,
    32–33
  ventricular pacing and,
    33–34
QT interval
  long-QT syndrome and
    sudden cardiac death and,
    181
  torsades de pointes due to,
    86–87
  normal, prolonged, and
    dispersed, 35–36
Quinapril, for heart failure, 54*t*
Quinidine
  actions of, 94*t*
  for atrial fibrillation, 74
  dosage of, 66*t*, 98*t*, 103–105
  interactions and
    complications of, 654*t*,
    659*t*, 715
  kinetics of, 66*t*
  pharmacokinetics of, 96*t*
  plasma concentration range
    for, 98*t*, 103–105

for premature ventricular contractions, 81
for sudden cardiac death prevention, 196*t*
Quinine, interactions and complications of, 659*t*
Q waves
abnormal, 26
myocardial infarction location and, 28, 30*t*

R
Race
coronary artery disease and, 693*t*
hypertension and, treatment of, 368
sudden cardiac death and, 166
Radiation
cardiac effects of, 581
myocarditis due to, 563*t*
during pregnancy, 671–672
Radionuclide imaging
in hypertrophic cardiomyopathy, 544
in mitral regurgitation, 446
Ramipril, for heart failure, 54*t*
Raynaud's phenomenon, 726, 726*t*
RBBB (right bundle branch block)
complete, electrocardiogram in, 31
incomplete, electrocardiogram in, 32
ST-segment elevation in, 25–26
Remodeling
in cardiomyopathy, 531–532
in heart failure, 49
Renal dysfunction
diabetes mellitus and, 630, 631*t*

hypertension in, treatment of, 366–367
Renal evaluation, in hypertension, 356
Renovascular hypertension, evaluation for, 356, 358
Respiratory arrest, 212
Respiratory disorders. *See also specific disorders*
pulmonary hypertension and, 378–379
Restenosis
in-stent, 332–333
predictors of, 332
Resting cardiovascular function, aging and, 41, 42*t*
Restrictive cardiomyopathy, 549, 550*t*
constrictive pericarditis versus, 549–550, 551*t*
infiltrative, 552–554
in amyloidosis, 552–553
in Gaucher's disease, 554
myocarditis due to, 561*t*
in sarcoidosis, 553–554
noninfiltrative, 552
nonobliterative endomyocardial diseases and, 555, 557
obliterative, 555, 556*t*
in storage diseases, 554–555
Reteplase, for acute myocardial infarction, 298–299
Revascularization. *See also* Coronary artery bypass grafting (CABG); Percutaneous transluminal coronary angioplasty (PTCA)
for angina pectoris, 252, 253*t*–254*t*, 255
in diabetes mellitus, 639, 644
before noncardiac surgery, 623–624

Revascularization (*Cont.*):
  for unstable angina pectoris,
    274–275
Rheolytic atherectomy, 334*t*
Rheumatic carditis, 567
  mitral stenosis due to, 431
Rheumatic fever
  heart disease due to, during
    pregnancy, 679
  tricuspid valve disease
    following, 463–464
Rhythmol. *See* Propafenone
  (Rhythmol)
Rifampin, for infective
  endocarditis, 609*t*
Right bundle branch block
  (RBBB)
  complete, electrocardiogram
    in, 31
  incomplete,
    electrocardiogram in, 32
  ST-segment elevation in,
    25–26
Right-to-left shunts, during
  pregnancy, 683
Right ventricular dysplasia,
  arrhythmogenic,
  familial, dilated
  cardiomyopathy in,
  497–498
Right ventricular hypertrophy
  (RVH)
  electrocardiogram in, 34–36
  pulmonary hypertension and,
    407
Right ventricular infarction,
  311, 312*t*
Romano-Ward long-QT
  syndrome, 505, 506*t*,
  508

S
SAECG (signal-averaging
  electrocardiography),
  192–193

St. John's wort, interactions and
  complications of, 666
St. Jude bileaflet valve, 476
Sanfilippo syndrome, dilated
  cardiomyopathy in, 498
Sarcoidosis
  cardiomyopathy and,
    569–570
  restrictive cardiomyopathy
    in, 553–554
  sudden cardiac death and,
    180
SCD. *See* Sudden cardiac death
  (SCD)
Scheie syndrome, dilated
  cardiomyopathy in,
  498
Scorpion fish venom, cardiac
  effects of, 581
Scorpion venom, cardiac
  effects of, 580
Selective serotonin reuptake
  inhibitors (SSRIs),
  cardiac effects of, 576
Septal blocks,
  electrocardiogram in, 31
Septal myotomy-myectomy, for
  hypertrophic
  cardiomyopathy, 546*t*,
  546–547
Serum cardiac markers
  in acute myocardial
    infarction, 283–285,
    284*f*, 292–293
  in unstable angina, 263
Sex. *See also* Coronary artery
  disease (CAD), in
  women; Pregnancy
  as risk factor for
    atherosclerosis, 233
  risk of coronary artery
    disease related to, 689,
    691*t*–694*t*
  sudden cardiac death and,
    166
Sick sinus syndrome, 88, 158

SIDS (sudden infant death syndrome), 508

Signal-averaging electrocardiography (SAECG), 192–193

Simvastatin, interactions and complications of, 664t, 665

Sinus arrhythmias, 63

Sinus bradycardia, 88

Sinus nodal dysfunction, pacing for, 137, 140t

Sinus rhythm, 63
  familial absence of, 507t

Sinus tachycardia, 63
  after acute myocardial infarction, 316
  acute myocardial infarction and, 281

Situational syncope, 156

Skeletal abnormalities, thoracic, in mitral valve prolapse, 454, 455t

Sleep apnea, obesity and, 743–744, 744t

Sly syndrome, dilated cardiomyopathy in, 498

Smoking
  cessation of, 229, 230t, 322
    for reduction of coronary artery disease risk, 690, 694
  sudden cardiac death and, 168, 170

Snake venoms, cardiac effects of, 580

Socioeconomic status, sudden cardiac death and, 170

Sodium bicarbonate, during cardiopulmonary resuscitation, 211, 218

Solid-angle, 22

Sotalol (Betapace)
  actions of, 94t
  for atrial fibrillation, 74
  dosage of, 67t, 99t, 106–107
  interactions and complications of, 656t
  kinetics of, 67t
  pharmacokinetics of, 96t
  plasma concentration range for, 99t, 106–107
  for sudden cardiac death prevention, 195, 197t, 198t, 199

Spatial vectorcardiography, 36–38
  electrovectorcardiography versus, 37–38

Spironolactone, interactions and complications of, 659t

SSRIs (selective serotonin reuptake inhibitors), cardiac effects of, 576

Standard leads, for electrocardiogram, 22

Staphylococcal infections, endocarditis due to, 596t, 597

Starr-Edwards valve, 475

Statins
  for hypertriglyceridemia of diabetes, 633
  interactions and complications of, 664t

Steinert's disease, dilated cardiomyopathy in, 500–501

Stents, 329–331, 334t
  for acute myocardial infarction, 341, 344t, 344–345
  coronary artery bypass grafting versus, in multivessel disease, 330–331
  as primary treatment, 333

Steroids. See also specific steroids
  anabolic, cardiac effects of, 578

Stingray venom, cardiac effects of, 581

Storage diseases, restrictive cardiomyopathy and, 554–555

Streptococcal infections, endocarditis due to, 595, 596t

Streptokinase
for acute myocardial infarction, 298, 300
for pulmonary embolism, 397t
for valve thrombosis, 489

Stress, sudden cardiac death and, 170

Stress angiography, 243, 244t

Stress testing
exercise, 62
in angina pectoris, 241–242
before noncardiac surgery, 622
in peripheral arterial disease, 722
nonexercise, before noncardiac surgery, 622–623
in unstable angina, 266–267

Stroke
antithrombotic therapy to prevent. See Antithrombotic therapy, in valvular heart disease
cardiac effects of, 718
following cardiac surgery, 716–717
diabetes mellitus and, 630
hypertension following, treatment of, 367–368

ST segment
elevation of, acute myocardial infarction and, 295–305, 296f
non-ischemic elevation in right precordial leads, 25–26

ST waves
nonspecific changes in, 27
secondary changes in, 26

Subarachnoid hemorrhage, cardiac effects of, 718

Sudden cardiac death (SCD), 165–204, 506t. See also Cardiac arrest
age and, 166, 167
with aortic stenosis, 415
assessment of risk of, 319–321
cardiomyopathy and, 176–178
congenital heart disease and, 180–181
definition of, 165
electrical abnormalities and, 181–184
gender and, 166
incidence of, 165–166
ischemic heart disease and, 173, 175–176
mechanism of, 171–173
mitral valve prolapse and, 458
myocardial disease and, 180
prevention of
implantable cardioverter-defibrillator therapy for. See Implantable cardioverter-defibrillator (ICD)
pacemaker for, 203
pharmacologic therapy for, 193–201
surgical therapy for, 203–204
race and, 166
risk factors for, 167–170, 168t, 169f
risk stratification for, 189, 190t–191t, 192–193
stress and, 718
syncope and, 160
toxic agents and, 184–186

valvular heart disease and, 178–179

in young people, 167

Sudden infant death syndrome (SIDS), 508

Sulfadiazine, for mitral stenosis, 438t

Sulfinpyrazone, interactions and complications of, 662t

Sumatriptan, cardiac effects of, 577

Supraventricular arrhythmias, 63–75

  atrial fibrillation, 72–75

  atrial flutter, 71–72, 72t

  due to atrioventricular nodal reentry, 64–65, 65t–67t, 68–69

  due to Wolff-Parkinson-White syndrome, 69–70

  ectopic atrial tachycardias, 70

  familial, 507t

  multifocal atrial tachycardia, 70–71

  premature atrial contractions, 63–64

  sinus rhythm and sinus tachycardia, 63

  tachycardia, 63, 64

    after acute myocardial infarction, 316

    antidromic, 69

    intraoperative mapping of, 62

    paroxysmal, 316, 678

    during pregnancy, 678

Surgery. See also Noncardiac surgery; specific procedures

  antithrombotic therapy and, 488–489

  for weight reduction, 747

Swallowing syncope, 156

Syncope, 151–163

  with aortic stenosis, 415

  cardiac, 157t, 157–159

    cardiac arrhythmias and, 158–159

    obstruction of cardiac output and, 157–158

  diagnostic evaluation of, 161, 162f, 163

  in elderly persons, 160

  implantable cardioverter-defibrillator therapy for, 123

  multifactorial, 160, 161f

  neurocardiogenic, 142

  noncardiac, 151–156, 152t

    carotid sinus hypersensitivity, 155

    cerebrovascular, 153, 155

    neurocardiogenic, 151–153

    orthostatic, 153, 154t, 155t

    situational, 156

  pacing for, 142

  recurrent, 161

  sudden death and, 160

  of undetermined cause, 159–160

Systolic murmurs, 15–17, 16f

  ejection, 15, 16f

  in mitral stenosis, 434

T

Tachyarrhythmias

  implantable cardioverter-defibrillator detection of, 124, 125f, 126, 127t

  pacing for, 145

  during pregnancy, 678

  in sudden cardiac death, 171

Takayasu's aortitis, 702

Takayasu's arteritis, 725

Tambocor. See Flecainide (Tambocor)

TEE (transesophageal echocardiography), in mitral stenosis, 436

Tetralogy of Fallot, 517–518
  during pregnancy, 683
  sudden cardiac death and,
      180
TGA (transposition of the great
      arteries), 520
  congenitally corrected,
      520–521
  during pregnancy, 684
  sudden cardiac death and,
      180
Thiazide diuretics, interactions
      and complications of,
      658, 660
Thoracic outlet syndrome, 725
Thromboembolic disease. See
      also Brain embolism;
      Deep vein thrombosis
      (DVT); Pulmonary
      embolism
  antithrombotic therapy
      for. See Antithrombotic
      therapy, in valvular
      heart disease
  during pregnancy, 676
  pulmonary hypertension and,
      377–378
  screening for patients at high
      risk for, 486
Thrombolytic therapy
  for acute myocardial
      infarction, 297–301,
      299t, 300t
  in elderly people, 44
  for pulmonary embolism,
      397t, 397–398
  for unstable angina pectoris,
      271–274
Thrombosis. See also Deep
      vein thrombosis (DVT);
      Thromboembolic
      disease
  diabetes mellitus and, 633
Thyroid disease,
      cardiomyopathy and,
      571

Ticlopidine
  interactions and
      complications of, 660
  for unstable angina pectoris,
      270–271
Tikosyn. See Dofetilide
      (Tikosyn)
Tinzaparin, for venous
      thromboembolism
      treatment, 395t
Tissue-type plasminogen
      activator (t-PA)
  for acute myocardial
      infarction, 298, 300
  interactions and
      complications of,
      663t
  for pulmonary embolism,
      397t
Tissue valves. See Biological
      valves
Tocainide
  actions of, 94t
  dosage of, 66t, 98t
  kinetics of, 66t
  pharmacokinetics of, 96t
  plasma concentration range
      for, 98t
  for premature ventricular
      contractions, 81–82
Torsades de pointes, 81, 86–87,
      97
  drugs causing, 577
Toxins, 580–581
  cardiomyopathy and, 563t,
      572–573
t-PA (tissue-type
      plasminogen activator)
  for acute myocardial
      infarction, 298, 300
  interactions and
      complications of, 663t
  for pulmonary embolism,
      397t
Trandolapril, for heart failure,
      54t

Transcutaneous partial pressure of oxygen, in peripheral arterial disease, 722

Transesophageal echocardiography (TEE), in mitral stenosis, 436

Transluminal extraction atherectomy, 334*t*

Transposition of the great arteries (TGA), 520
congenitally corrected, 520–521
during pregnancy, 684
sudden cardiac death and, 180

Transthoracic echocardiography (TTE), in infective endocarditis, 600*f*, 600–601

Trauma, aortic, 702

Treadmill exercise test, in aortic regurgitation, 424

Triamterene, interactions and complications of, 659*t*

Tricuspid valve disease
clinical manifestations of, 465–469
definition of, 463
Ebstein's anomaly, 521
during pregnancy, 684–685
sudden cardiac death and, 181
etiology and pathology of, 463–465, 464*f*
natural history and prognosis of, 469–470
during pregnancy, 681
treatment of
medical, 470
surgical, 471–473, 472*t*

Tricyclic antidepressants, cardiac effects of, 576

Trisomy 21, 511

Troponins
in acute myocardial infarction, 284
in unstable angina, 263

Trypanosomiasis, American cardiomyopathy and, 538, 566
sudden cardiac death and, 180

TTE (transthoracic echocardiography), in infective endocarditis, 600*f*, 600–601

Tumors, infiltrating, of heart, restrictive cardiomyopathy and, 555–556

Turner's syndrome, 511–512

T wave(s)
ischemic changes in, 26
nonspecific changes in, 27
secondary changes in, 26

T-wave alternans, sudden cardiac death and, 192

U

Ulcers, vascular, 729, 730*t*

Ultrasonography. *See also* Doppler ultrasonography
in peripheral arterial disease, 722

Urokinase, for valve thrombosis, 489

Uvulopalatopharyngoplasty, for cor pulmonale, 411

V

Valsartan, for heart failure, 52*t*

Valves, prosthetic. *See* Prosthetic heart valves

Valvular heart disease. *See also specific disorders*

Valvular heart disease (*Cont.*):
  antithrombotic therapy in.
    See Antithrombotic
    therapy, in valvular
    heart disease
  dilated cardiomyopathy, 535
  hypertension in, treatment of,
    365
  during pregnancy, 679–681
  sudden cardiac death and,
    178–179
Vancomycin
  for infective endocarditis
    prophylaxis, 613*t*, 614*t*
  for infective endocarditis
    treatment, 604*t*,
    606*t*–609*t*
Variant angina, 259
Varicose veins, 726–727
Vascular ulcers, 729, 730*t*
Vasculature, evaluation of, in
    hypertension, 356
Vasodilators
  during pregnancy, 673–674
  for pulmonary hypertension,
    378
Vasopressin, during
    cardiopulmonary
    resuscitation, 211, 217
Vasovagal syndrome, pacing
    for, 146
Vectorcardiography (VCG),
    spatial, 36–38
  electrovectorcardiography
    versus, 37–38
Vena cava filters, for pulmonary
    embolism, 396
Venography, contrast, for deep
    vein thrombosis
    detection, 391
Venous disease, 726–728
Venous insufficiency, chronic,
    728
Ventilation, during
    cardiopulmonary
    resuscitation, 212–213

Ventilation/perfusion scan, in
    pulmonary embolism,
    390
Ventricular arrhythmias, 78–87
  fibrillation, 87
    after acute myocardial
      infarction, 316
    in acute myocardial
      infarction, 304–305
    cardiopulmonary
      resuscitation and,
      213–215
    familial, 508–509
    implantable cardioverter-
      defibrillator for,
      126
    sudden cardiac death and,
      183–184
  premature ventricular
    contractions, 78–82
  sudden cardiac death and,
    189, 192
  tachycardia
    after acute myocardial
      infarction, 316
    in acute myocardial
      infarction, 304–305
    cardiopulmonary
      resuscitation and,
      213–215
    familial, 506*t*
    implantable cardioverter-
      defibrillator for,
      128
    implantable cardioverter-
      defibrillator therapy for,
      118, 122–123
    intraoperative mapping of,
      62
    nonsustained, 82
    polymorphic, 86–87
    during pregnancy,
      678
    sudden cardiac death and,
      182–183
    sustained, 83*t*, 83–86

Ventricular depolarization, electrocardiogram and, 21–22, 23
Ventricular diastolic dysfunction, obesity and, 743
Ventricular ectopy
after acute myocardial infarction, 316
in acute myocardial infarction, 304–305
Ventricular function, in congenital heart disease, 523
Ventricular gradient, 24–25
Ventricular pacing, wide QRS complexes produced by, 33–34
Ventricular repolarization, electrocardiogram and, 21–22
Ventricular septal defect (VSD), 516–517
murmurs in, 15
during pregnancy, 683
Ventricular septal rupture, after acute myocardial infarction, 315
Verapamil
actions of, 94t
for atrial fibrillation, 73–74
dosage and kinetics of, 67t, 68
for hypertrophic cardiomyopathy, 545, 546t
interactions and complications of, 656t, 659t
for supraventricular tachycardia, 65t
Visceral obesity, 740, 741t
"Voodoo death," 718

VSD (ventricular septal defect), 516–517
murmurs in, 15
during pregnancy, 683
VVI mode, with pacemakers, 143

W
Warfarin (Coumadin)
with atrial fibrillation, 75, 76t
for brain embolism prevention, 713
interactions and complications of, 661, 663t, 665
for mitral stenosis, 438
for mitral valve prolapse, 458
during pregnancy, 674
with prosthetic valves, 480, 481, 487t
sulfinpyrazone interaction with, 649
surgical procedures and, 488–489
for valve thrombosis, 489, 490, 491t
Weight-loss medications, cardiac effects of, 578
Wenckebach phenomenon, 89
Williams syndrome, 510, 511
Wolff-Parkinson-White (WPW) syndrome, 507t
concealed, 69–70
sudden cardiac death and, 181, 182
supraventricular arrhythmias due to, 69–70
wide QRS complexes in, 32–33
Women. See Coronary artery disease (CAD), in women; Pregnancy

X
X descent, 7
X-linked cardioskeletal
    myopathy, dilated
    cardiomyopathy in, 497
X-rays. *See also specific
    imaging modalities*
  during pregnancy, 671–672

Xylocaine. *See* Lidocaine
    (Xylocaine)

Y
y descent, 7
Young people, sudden cardiac
    death in, 167